Handbook of Gynecology

Donna Shoupe
Editor

Handbook of Gynecology

Volume 2

With 213 Figures and 169 Tables

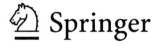 Springer

Editor
Donna Shoupe
Department of Obstetrics and Gynecology
Keck School of Medicine, University of Southern California
Los Angeles, CA, USA

ISBN 978-3-319-17797-7   ISBN 978-3-319-17798-4 (eBook)
ISBN 978-3-319-17799-1 (print and electronic bundle)
DOI 10.1007/978-3-319-17798-4

Library of Congress Control Number: 2017943810

Printed on acid-free paper

This Springer imprint is published by Springer Nature
The registered company is Springer International Publishing AG
The registered company address is: Gewerbestrasse 11, 6330 Cham, Switzerland

This book is dedicated to the many physicians, health care providers, scientists, researchers, and publishers who have provided valuable care or advanced the field of women's health for women and girls of all ages. We thank you.

Preface

The *Handbook of Gynecology* is a comprehensive textbook that is designed to guide management and understanding of the many complex issues surrounding women's health. The book addresses issues in adolescents such as congenital adrenal hyperplasia, amenorrhea, genital tract anomalies, or other common problems in adolescents. The book has separate chapters on the multiple issues of reproductive-aged women, including management of bleeding issues, sexually transmitted diseases, vaginitis and chronic recurrent vulvovaginitis, sexual issues, premenstrual syndrome, obesity, abnormal Pap smears, recurrent pregnancy loss, infertility, preconception management, and androgen excess. For the perimenopausal and menopausal women, chapters include assessment of risk factors for osteoporosis and cardiovascular disease, perimenopausal/menopausal symptoms, guidelines for hormone replacement therapy, management of pelvic pain, benign breast disease, vulvar disease, and abnormal bleeding and also on common office procedures such as endometrial, vulvar, or cervical biopsy. There are multiple chapters on surgical techniques such as operative hysteroscopy, robotic surgery, laparoscopic hysterectomy, minimal invasive procedures, stress incontinence procedures, avoiding surgical complications, and management of postoperative complications. There are also detailed chapters addressing vulvar, vaginal, cervical, uterine, and ovarian premalignant and malignant lesions as well as chapters on their management. Most importantly, the book includes chapters addressing fertility and ovarian sparing operative procedures for these premalignant and malignant lesions.

The authors, section editors, and editor hope that this book will be highly educational and very valuable for its readers.

June 2017   Donna Shoupe

Acknowledgments

There were many hardworking and outstanding contributors to this book. The contributors, who are leaders in their field around the world, share their own clinical experience as well as the current studies, common practices, and national and international society recommendations. I would especially like to thank my section editors Drs. Marc Gualtieri, Jennifer Israel, Begüm Özel, Paulette Mhawech-Fauceglia, and Koji Matsuo for their many hours of work, their expertise, their outstanding judgment on selecting the best authors, and for sticking with the writing and editing process all the way to the completion of this book.

Thanks also to Springer and their representatives including Sylvia Blago and Rebecca Urban who tirelessly worked with me and my section editors. Thanks to my family for support and Juni Joy during the completion of this book. Thanks to all.

Contents

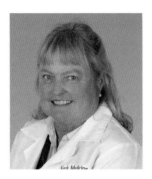

Donna Shoupe, M.D., M.B.A., is a professor in the Department of Obstetrics and Gynecology and the Keck School of Medicine, University of Southern California. She graduated from Massachusetts Institute of Technology in 1974 and the Ohio State College of Medicine. She also graduated from the Marshall School of Business at the University of Southern California in 2002. She did her residency in Obstetrics and Gynecology and her Reproductive Endocrinology and Infertility Fellowship at Los Angeles County University of Southern California School of Medicine and was appointed to the faculty in 1984. She has received many awards and served in many leadership positions. She has published more than 90 peer review papers, more than 60 book chapters, and has edited 8 books. She is also an editor of the journal *Contraception and Reproductive Medicine*. She is a member of several national organizations and reviewer for multiple journals.

Her main interests include menopause, ovarian conservation, contraception, osteoporosis, polycystic ovarian syndrome, insulin resistance, hormone therapy, uterine anomalies, androgen excess, osteoporosis, and cardiovascular disease in women.

Section Editors

Part I: General Office Gynecology
Part III: Gynecologic Care During the Early Reproductive Years

Marc Gualtieri Division of Reproductive Endocrinology and Infertility, Department of Obstetrics and Gynecology, University of Southern California, Los Angeles, CA, USA
marcgualtieri@gmail.com

Part VII: Gynecologic Office and Minimally Invasive Procedures

Jennifer Israel Department of Obstetrics and Gynecology, Keck School of Medicine, University of Southern California, Los Angeles, CA, USA
Jennifer.Israel@med.usc.edu

Part IX: Management of Gynecologic Neoplasms and Cancers

Koji Matsuo Division of Gynecologic Oncology, Department of Obstetrics and Gynecology, University of Southern California, Los Angeles, CA, USA
Koji.Matsuo@med.usc.edu

Part X: Pathology of the Female Gynecologic System

Paulette Mhawech-Fauceglia Division of Gynecologic Oncologic Pathology, Department of Pathology, Keck School of Medicine, University of Southern California, Los Angeles, CA, USA
pfauceglia@hotmail.com

Part IV: Gynecologic Care During the Early and Late Reproductive Years
Part VIII: Gynecologic Operative Procedures

Begüm Özel Division of Female Pelvic Medicine and Reconstructive Surgery, Department of Obstetrics and Gynecology, Keck School of Medicine, University of Southern California, Los Angeles, CA, USA
ozel@usc.edu

Part V: Work-Up and Management: Reproductive Endocrinology and Infertility
Part VI: Gynecologic Care During the Perimenopausal and Menopausal Years

Alexander M. Quaas Section of Reproductive Endocrinology and Infertility, Department of Obstetrics/Gynecology, Oklahoma University Health Science Center, Oklahoma City, OK, USA
alexander-quaas@ouhsc.edu

Part II: Gynecologic Care of the Adolescent

Donna Shoupe Department of Obstetrics and Gynecology, Keck School of Medicine, University of Southern California, Los Angeles, CA, USA
donna.shoupe@med.usc.edu

Contributors

Yalda Afshar Division of Maternal Fetal Medicine, Department of Obstetrics and Gynecology, University of California, Los Angeles, CA, USA

Fausto F. Andrade Department of Obstetrics and Gynecology, University of Miami/Jackson Memorial Hospital, Miami, FL, USA

Kate C. Arnold Department of OBGYN, University of Oklahoma Health and Science Center, Oklahoma City, OK, USA

Benjamin J. Barenberg The University of Oklahoma Health Sciences Center, Oklahoma City, OK, USA

Amanda Barnes University of Miami Miller School of Medicine, Miami, FL, USA

Tania Basu Department of Obstetrics and Gynecology, Cedars-Sinai Medical Center, Los Angeles, CA, USA

Erin A. Blake Department of Obstetrics and Gynecology, University of Colorado, Aurora, CO, USA

Claudia Borzutzky Department of Pediatrics, Division of Adolescent and Young Adult Medicine, Keck School of Medicine of USC/Children's Hospital Los Angeles, Los Angeles, CA, USA

Janet Bruno-Gaston Department of Obstetrics and Gynecology, Keck School of Medicine, University of Southern California, Los Angeles, CA, USA

Lindsey Buckingham Department of Obstetrics and Gynecology, Pennsylvania Hospital, Philadelphia, PA, USA

Sigita S. Cahoon Department of Obstetrics and Gynecology, University of Southern California, Los Angeles, CA, USA

Amy R. Carroll WellStar Gynecologic Oncology, Austell, GA, USA

Antonio V. Castaneda Department of Obstetrics and Gynecology, University of Southern California, Los Angeles, CA, USA

Judy Hall Chen Department of Health Services, Los Angeles County, Keck School of Medicine, Los Angeles, CA, USA

Alexander Chiang Department of Obstetrics and Gynecology, David Geffen School of Medicine at UCLA, Los Angeles, CA, USA

T. Justin Clark Birmingham Women's NHS Foundation Trust, Edgbaston, UK

Elizabeth Stephens Constance Department of Obstetrics and Gynecology, University of Michigan Health System, Ann Arbor, MI, USA

Christina Dancz University of Southern California, Los Angeles, CA, USA

Mohamed Mokhtar Desouki Department of Pathology, Microbiology and Immunology, Vanderbilt University Medical Center, Nashville, TN, USA

Dalal Eldick Department of Obstetrics and Gynecology, University of Miami/Jackson Memorial Hospital, Miami, Fl, USA

M. Blake Evans Oklahoma State University Department of Obstetrics and Gynecology, Tulsa, OK, USA

Oluwole Fadare Department of Pathology, University of California San Diego, San Diego, CA, USA

Caroline J. Flint Department of OBGYN, University of Oklahoma Health and Science Center, Oklahoma City, OK, USA

Christina Fotopoulou Department of Gynaecological Oncology, West London Gynecological Cancer Centre, Imperial College NHS Trust, Queen Charlottes and Hammersmith Hospital, London, UK

Morgan Elizabeth Fullerton Department of Obstetrics and Gynecology, University of Southern California, Los Angeles, CA, USA

Jocelyn Garcia-Sayre Division of Gynecologic Oncology, Department of Obstetrics and Gynecology, University of Southern California, Los Angeles, CA, USA

Mitchell E. Geffner Center for Endocrinology, Diabetes and Metabolism, Children's Hospital Los Angeles, University of Southern California, Los Angeles, CA, USA

Bree Anna Gibson University of Oklahoma Health Science Center, Oklahoma City, OK, USA

Elizabeth S. Ginsburg Division of Reproductive Endocrinology, Brigham and Women's Hospital, Boston, MA, USA

Martha Goetsch Center for Women's Health, Oregon Health and Science University, Portland, OR, USA

Saketh Guntupalli Division of Gynecologic Oncology, Department of Obstetrics and Gynecology, University of Colorado, Aurora, CO, USA

Ardeshir Hakam Department of Pathology, University of South Florida/ H. Lee Moffitt Cancer Center, Tampa, FL, USA

Kristina Haley Division of Pediatric Hematology/Oncology, Department of Pediatrics, Oregon Health and Science University, Portland, OR, USA

Christina S. Han Division of Maternal Fetal Medicine, Department of Obstetrics and Gynecology, University of California, Los Angeles, CA, USA
Center for Fetal Medicine and Women's Ultrasound, Los Angeles, CA, USA

Micah Hill Reproductive Endocrinology and Infertility/Obstetrics and Gynecology, USU, National Institutes of Health and Walter Reed Natl. Military Medical Center, Bethesda, MD, USA

Jacqueline R. Ho Department of Obstetrics and Gynecology, Keck School of Medicine, University of Southern California, Los Angeles, CA, USA

Pardis Hosseinzadeh Baylor College of Medicine, Houston, TX, USA

Helena Hwang University of Texas Southwestern Medical Center, Dallas, TX, USA

Jennifer Israel Department of Obstetrics and Gynecology, Keck School of Medicine, University of Southern California, Los Angeles, CA, USA

Julie Jaffray Children's Hospital Los Angeles, Keck School of Medicine, University of Southern California, Los Angeles, CA, USA

Pouya Javadian Division of Female Pelvic Medicine and Reconstructive Surgery, Department of Obstetrics and Gynecology, University of Oklahoma Health Sciences Center, Oklahoma City, OK, USA

Mamoru Kakuda Department of Obstetrics and Gynecology, Osaka University Graduate School of Medicine, Suita, Osaka, Japan

Mahiru Kawano Department of Obstetrics and Gynecology, Osaka University Graduate School of Medicine, Suita, Osaka, Japan

Angela S. Kelley Department of Obstetrics and Gynecology, University of Michigan Health System, Ann Arbor, MI, USA

Courtney Ketch University of Oklahoma Health Science Center, Oklahoma City, OK, USA

Anam Khaja University of Miami Miller School of Medicine, Miami, FL, USA

Sana N. Khan Wayne State University, Detroit, MI, USA

Grace N. Kim Department of Pathology, University of Texas MD Anderson Cancer Center, Houston, TX, USA

Mimi S. Kim Center for Endocrinology, Diabetes and Metabolism, Children's Hospital Los Angeles, University of Southern California, Los Angeles, CA, USA

Tadashi Kimura Department of Obstetrics and Gynecology, Osaka University Graduate School of Medicine, Suita, Osaka, Japan

Abigail Kingston Great Western Hospitals NHS Foundation Trust, Swindon, UK

Emily Ko Division of Gynecologic Oncology, University of Pennsylvania Health System, Philadelphia, PA, USA

Eiji Kobayashi Department of Obstetrics and Gynecology, Osaka University Graduate School of Medicine, Suita, Osaka, Japan

Christina M. Koppin Center for Endocrinology, Diabetes and Metabolism, Children's Hospital Los Angeles, University of Southern California, Los Angeles, CA, USA

Katsumi Kozasa Department of Obstetrics and Gynecology, Osaka University Graduate School of Medicine, Suita, Osaka, Japan

Kavitha Krishnamoorthy Department of Obstetrics and Gynecology, University of Miami, Miller School of Medicine/Jackson Health System, Miami, FL, USA

Hiromasa Kuroda Department of Obstetrics and Gynecology, Osaka University Graduate School of Medicine, Suita, Osaka, Japan

Trevin C. Lau Massachusetts General Hospital, Boston, MA, USA

Jacob Lauer Department of Obstetrics and Gynecology, The University of Wisconsin, School of Medicine and Public Health, Madison, WI, USA

John P. Lenihan Jr. Department of Obstetrics and Gynecology, University of Washington School of Medicine, Medical Director of Robotics and Minimally Invasive Surgery, MultiCare Health System, Tacoma, WA, USA

Seiji Mabuchi Department of Obstetrics and Gynecology, Osaka University Graduate School of Medicine, Suita, Osaka, Japan

Heather R. Macdonald Keck School of Medicine, University of Southern California, Los Angeles, CA, USA

Hiroko Machida Division of Gynecologic Oncology, Department of Obstetrics and Gynecology, University of Southern California, Los Angeles, CA, USA

Gillian Mackay University of Oklahoma Health Sciences Center, Oklahoma City, OK, USA

Yuri Matsumoto Department of Obstetrics and Gynecology, Osaka University Graduate School of Medicine, Suita, Osaka, Japan

Koji Matsuo Division of Gynecologic Oncology, Department of Obstetrics and Gynecology, University of Southern California, Los Angeles, CA, USA

E. Clair McClung Department of Gynecologic Oncology, University of South Florida/H. Lee Moffitt Cancer Center, Tampa, FL, USA

Alexander Melamed Department of Obstetrics, Gynecology and Reproductive Biology, Harvard Medical School, Boston, MA, USA

Paulette Mhawech-Fauceglia Division of Gynecologic Oncologic Pathology, Department of Pathology, Keck School of Medicine, University of Southern California, Los Angeles, CA, USA

Devin T. Miller The Department of Obstetrics and Gynecology and Women's Health, Albert Einstein College of Medicine, Bronx, NY, USA

Aida Moeini Division of Gynecologic Oncology, Department of Obstetrics and Gynecology, University of Southern California, Los Angeles, CA, USA

Molly B. Moravek Department of Obstetrics and Gynecology, University of Michigan Health System, Ann Arbor, MI, USA

Youssef Mouhayar Department of Obstetrics and Gynecology, Jackson Memorial Hospital, Jackson Health System, Miami, FL, USA

Anita L. Nelson David Geffen School of Medicine at UCLA, Los Angeles, CA, USA

Laurice Bou Nemer Obstetrics and Gynecology, University of Texas Southwestern Medical Center, Dallas, TX, USA

Mikio A. Nihira Division of Female Pelvic Medicine and Reconstructive Surgery, Department of Obstetrics and Gynecology, University of Oklahoma Health Sciences Center, Oklahoma City, OK, USA

Katherine Nixon Department of Gynecology, Imperial College NHS Trust, Queen Charlottes and Hammersmith Hospital, London, UK

Begüm Özel Division of Female Pelvic Medicine and Reconstructive Surgery, Department of Obstetrics and Gynecology, Keck School of Medicine, University of Southern California, Los Angeles, CA, USA

William H. Parker Department of Obstetrics and Gynecology, David Geffen School of Medicine at UCLA, Los Angeles, CA, USA

Stephanie D. Pickett The University of Oklahoma Health Sciences Center, Oklahoma City, OK, USA

Alexander M. Quaas Section of Reproductive Endocrinology and Infertility, Department of Obstetrics/Gynecology, Oklahoma University Health Science Center, Oklahoma City, OK, USA

Alexandra Regens University of Oklahoma Health Sciences Center, Oklahoma City, OK, USA

Jessica Reid Keck School of Medicine, University of Southern California, Los Angeles, CA, USA

Caryl S. Reinsch Kaiser Permanente Southern California, San Diego, CA, USA

Valentina M. Rodriguez-Triana University of California Los Angeles, Los Angeles, CA, USA

Cassandra M. Roeca Division of Reproductive Endocrinology, Brigham and Women's Hospital, Boston, MA, USA

Renee Rolston Division of Female Pelvic Medicine and Reconstructive Surgery, Department of Obstetrics and Gynecology, Keck School of Medicine, University of Southern California, Los Angeles, CA, USA

Lynda D. Roman Division of Gynecologic Oncology, Department of Obstetrics and Gynecology, University of Southern California, Los Angeles, CA, USA

Brianne D. Romeroso Department of Obstetrics and Gynecology, David Geffen School of Medicine at UCLA, Los Angeles, CA, USA

Michael Saad-Naguib Department of Obstetrics and Gynecology, Jackson Health System, Jackson Memorial Hospital/ University of Miami Miller School of Medicine, Miami, FL, USA

Alejandra Salazar Department of Obstetrics and Gynecology, University of Miami/Jackson Memorial Hospital, Miami, FL, USA

Parisa Samimi Department of Obstetrics and Gynecology – Resident Physician, Cedars-Sinai Medical Center, Los Angeles, CA, USA

Daman Samrao University of Southern California, Los Angeles, CA, USA

Laboratory Medicine Consultants, Las Vegas, NV, USA

Tomoyuki Sasano Department of Obstetrics and Gynecology, Osaka University Graduate School of Medicine, Suita, Osaka, Japan

Anastasiya Shabalova University of Southern California, Los Angeles, CA, USA

Mian M. K. Shahzad Department of Gynecologic Oncology, University of South Florida/H. Lee Moffitt Cancer Center, Tampa, FL, USA

Mariko Shindo Department of Obstetrics and Gynecology, Osaka University Graduate School of Medicine, Suita, Osaka, Japan

Donna Shoupe Department of Obstetrics and Gynecology, Keck School of Medicine, University of Southern California, Los Angeles, CA, USA

Paul P. Smith Birmingham Women's NHS Foundation Trust, Edgbaston, UK

Lisa B. Spiryda Obstetrics and Gynecology, University of Florida, College of Medicine, Gainesville, FL, USA

Ryoko Takahashi Department of Obstetrics and Gynecology, Osaka University Graduate School of Medicine, Suita, Osaka, Japan

Yoko Takashima Department of Obstetrics and Gynecology, Keck School of Medicine, University of Southern California, Los Angeles, CA, USA

Katherine E. Tierney Division of Gynecologic Oncology, Department of Obstetrics and Gynecology, Kaiser Permanente Orange County, California, Irvine, CA, USA

Emma Torbé Great Western Hospitals NHS Foundation Trust, Swindon, UK

Teresa Tseng Center for Endocrinology, Diabetes and Metabolism, Children's Hospital Los Angeles, University of Southern California, Los Angeles, CA, USA

Yutaka Ueda Department of Obstetrics and Gynecology, Osaka University Graduate School of Medicine, Suita, Osaka, Japan

Katrina Wade Department of Obstetrics and Gynecology, Section of Gynecologic Oncology, Ochsner Medical Center, New Orleans, LA, USA

Saloni Walia Department of Pathology and Laboratory Medicine, Los Angeles County and University of Southern California Medical Center, Los Angeles, CA, USA

Alexandra Walker Obstetrics and Gynecology, University of Florida College of Medicine, Jacksonville, FL, USA

Yan Wang Department of Pathology, Kaiser Roseville Medical Center, Roseville, CA, USA

Kristy Ward Division of Gynecologic Oncology, Department of Obstetrics and Gynecology, University of Florida College of Medicine Jacksonville, Jacksonville, FL, USA

Elizabeth Weedin University of Oklahoma Health Science Center, Oklahoma City, OK, USA

Jamie Wilkerson Department of Obstetrics and Gynecology, University of Oklahoma, Oklahoma City, OK, USA

Kristina Williams Department of Obstetrics and Gynecology, Pennsylvania Hospital, Philadelphia, PA, USA

Irene Woo Division of Reproductive Endocrinology and Infertility, Department of Obstetrics and Gynecology, University of Southern California, Keck School of Medicine, LAC+USC Hospital, Los Angeles, CA, USA

Terri L. Woodard The University of Texas MD Anderson Cancer Center, Houston, TX, USA

Baylor College of Medicine, Houston, TX, USA

Terez A. Yonan Division of Adolescent and Young Adult Medicine, Children's Hospital Los Angeles, Los Angeles, CA, USA

Kiyoshi Yoshino Department of Obstetrics and Gynecology, Osaka University Graduate School of Medicine, Suita, Osaka, Japan

Steve Yu Department of Obstetrics and Gynecology, David Geffen School of Medicine at UCLA, Los Angeles, CA, USA

Austin Zanelotti University of Miami/Jackson Memorial Hospital, Miami, FL, USA

Mya Rose Zapata UCLA Medical Center, University of California, Los Angeles, CA, USA

Part VII

Gynecologic Office and Minimally Invasive Procedures (Jennifer Israel)

Office Procedures: Endometrial, Cervical, and Vulvar Biopsy

Donna Shoupe

Abstract

Bleeding abnormalities along with disorders of the uterus, cervix, and vulva are common causes for outpatient visits to the gynecologist. Most of these disorders are benign in nature, but it is the job of the examining physician to establish the severity of the disorder by distinguishing benign versus more serious lesions. A biopsy in many cases will establish a specific diagnosis and direct treatment options.

Keywords

Endometrial biopsy • Cervical biopsy • Vulvar biopsy • Cervical lesion • Abnormal uterine bleeding • Vulvar lesion • HPV

Contents

1 Introduction

In-office gynecologic procedures are now a mainstay of women's healthcare. Biopsies of the endometrium, cervix, and vulva can be safely done in the office, and they usually allow the woman to quickly resume her normal activities. The biopsy is primarily done to exclude the diagnosis of cancer and potentially establish the diagnosis and treatment options.

2 Endometrial Biopsy

2.1 Evaluation

It is estimated that one-third of outpatient gynecologic visits yearly in the USA are for abnormal uterine bleeding (Awwad et al. 1993; Cooper 2000). Differential diagnosis of abnormal uterine bleeding includes anovulation, leiomyoma, polyps, endometrial hyperplasia, cancer, medications, and coagulation disorders (Table 1). Women with

D. Shoupe (✉)
Department of Obstetrics and Gynecology, Keck School of Medicine, University of Southern California, Los Angeles, CA, USA
e-mail: donna.shoupe@med.usc.edu; shoupe@usc.edu

© Springer International Publishing AG 2017
D. Shoupe (ed.), *Handbook of Gynecology*,
DOI 10.1007/978-3-319-17798-4_89

Table 1 Causes of abnormal uterine bleeding

Uterine etiology	Medications
Leiomyoma, adenomyosis	Contraceptives, hormone replacement
Polyp	Psychotropic drugs, MAO inhibitors
Endometrial hyperplasia, cancer	Anticoagulants
Infection: endometritis	SERMs
Congenital anomalies	Corticosteroids
Vascular lesions, hemangioma	Chemotherapeutic agents
Atrophic endometrium	Dilantin, digoxin
Systemic etiology	Other
Liver disease	Anovulation, PCO
Thyroid disorders	Perimenopausal transition, perimenarchal DUB
Adrenal disorders, late-onset CAH	Pregnancy, accidents of pregnancy
Leukemia, thrombocytopenia	Lactation, hyperprolactinemia
Thrombophilias [von Willebrand's disease]	Foreign body, trauma
Ovarian tumors	

abnormal bleeding are at risk for anemia and disability from heavy bleeding, and they may suffer occupational, sexual, social, or psychological impact. In most cases, management of abnormal bleeding can be handled on an age-specific basis in an outpatient setting, often starting with an endometrial biopsy. Abnormal genital bleeding can also originate from the vulva, vagina, and cervix.

Evaluation of the patient presenting with abnormal uterine bleeding starts with a detailed history of the patient's normal bleeding pattern, time when abnormal bleeding began, and pattern and quantity of bleeding. Additional details should include associated symptoms, current and past medical problems, and medication history. Gynecologic history should include last Pap test, any prior endometrial biopsy or dilation and curettage, known fibroids, and prior ultrasound results. Vital signs, height and weight, and general physical exam are important. Evaluation of the skin for bruising or petechiae, conjunctiva, thyromegaly, galactorrhea, and evidence of androgen excess can suggest etiology of abnormal bleeding. An abdominal exam should evaluate for signs of infection, trauma, distention,

guarding, abdominal mass, or ascites. A pelvic exam should check for vulvar, vaginal, or cervical lesions; determine size and shape of the uterus; quantify bleeding; identify masses and tenderness; and establish that bleeding is coming from the cervical os or vaginal trauma. In reproductive-age women at risk for pregnancy, a pregnancy test should be done (Table 2).

An endometrial biopsy is often an important first test for women over 35 with irregular bleeding [metrorrhagia] or heavy bleeding [menorrhagia], women under 35 with long-standing abnormal bleeding > 6–12 months, and women with postmenopausal bleeding. In addition to identifying neoplasia or malignancy, an endometrial biopsy can provide useful information regarding ovulatory status when secretory endometrium is identified or in diagnosing chronic endometritis. For persistent bleeding, adjunctive testing may be indicated (Table 3). Ordering of adjunctive testing depends on the age of patient, length of time and heaviness of abnormal bleeding, gynecologic history, prior imaging results, medical conditions, contraceptive or hormonal use, other medications, size of the uterus, the presence of androgen, or steroid excess. Acute heavy bleeding may need acute surgical intervention or transfusion.

2.2 Contraindications

The presence of a viable and desired pregnancy is the only absolute contraindication to endometrial biopsy. Caution should be used when considering a biopsy in women with bleeding abnormalities, severe liver disease, use of anticoagulation medications, acute cervical or pelvic infection, obstructing lesion, or cervical cancer. A low-suction pipelle device can generally be used safely in the presence of an intrauterine device.

2.3 Sampling Technique

An in-office endometrial biopsy is a relatively easy procedure, especially in young, parous women. An endometrial biopsy can be done with a variety of instruments including disposable low-pressure

Table 2 Etiology of abnormal uterine bleeding by age groups

Childhood < 10 years
Newborn withdrawal from placental hormones
Foreign objects
Vaginitis
Trauma
Sexual abuse
Ovarian tumor [with secondary sexual characteristics
Contraceptive pill/HRT/hormonal ingestion
Precocious puberty
Adolescents 10–18 years
Physiological anovulation [2–3 years after menarche
Coagulation defect, thrombophilia [von Willebrand's disease]
Thrombocytopenic purpura
Leukemia, aplastic anemia, hypersplenism
Platelet dysfunction from medications
Premature ovarian failure, gonadal dysgenesis
Congenital reproductive tract anomalies
Medications: hormones, anticoagulants, chemo
Systemic disease: thyroid, liver, adrenal
Reproductive 19–39 years
Pregnancy-related complications
Anovulation, PCO
Fibroids [particularly submucous], polyp
Medications: hormones, anticoagulants, chemo, psychoactive
Systemic disease: thyroid, liver, adrenal
Endometrial hyperplasia [rare cancer]
Late reproductive 40–49 years
Perimenopausal transition, anovulation
Leiomyoma [particularly submucous], adenomyosis
Endometrial polyp
Medications: hormones, anticoagulants, chemo, psychoactive
Systemic disease: thyroid, liver, adrenal
Endometrial hyperplasia, infrequent cancer
Menopausal 50 and above
Early menopausal transitional bleeding
Hormone therapy
Systemic disease: thyroid, liver, adrenal
Medications: anticoagulants, chemo, psychoactive
Endometrial hyperplasia, endometrial cancer
Polyps, submucous leiomyomas

Cervical etiologies discussed in cervical biopsy sections

Table 3 Adjunctive testing: evaluation of abnormal bleeding [when indicated]

Transvaginal and transabdominal pelvic ultrasound [MRI, CT], hydrosonogram
Pap smear, gonorrhea, and *Chlamydia* screening
Hormone labs: **pregnancy test,** androgens, 17-hydroxyprogesterone, prolactin, progesterone, FSH, LH, estradiol
Other labs: CBC, liver function tests, thyroid function tests, renal function tests, ferritin glucose tolerance test, HgA1c, 24-hour urinary free cortisol, coagulation testing
Office or hospital hysteroscopy

devices [pipelle catheter], or high-pressure devices [vacuum aspirating biopsy retrieval apparatus (VABRA), Karman cannula], or reusable low-pressure devices [metal pipette, Randall curette, Novak curette]. These methods collect strips or sections of the endometrium by suction and/or scraping of the endometrial surface. The pipelle is one of the most popular methods used. The outer diameter of the sheath is about 3 mm with a 2.1–2.4 mm opening at the distal end for collection of the sample. The sheath is made of flexible polypropylene, and it contains a firm plastic internal plunger that slides up and down. The pipelle samples only a small section of the endometrial surface, 4.5–15% (Eddowes 1990; Rodriguez et al. 1993; Guido et al. 1995). However, the pipelle is relatively easy to use, causes less pain, and is less expensive than the other methods that collect a larger proportion of the endometrial surface (Stovall et al. 1991; Silver et al. 1991). Importantly, the combined technique of using endometrial scraping or curettage, with a corkscrew twisting motion, is reported to result in a 95% success rate for obtaining adequate tissue for diagnosis (Sierecki et al. 2008). The recommendation is that even if an adequate sample was obtained, if bleeding persists, further evaluation is needed (Meniru and Hopkins 2006). Further evaluation may be necessary such as repeat pipelle sampling, ultrasound evaluation, VABRA, hysteroscopy, or dilation and curettage depending on clinical presentation and risk factors.

There is a 4–10% risk that cervical stenosis may interfere with getting the catheter through the cervical canal (Guido et al. 1995). In these cases, the use of either a disposable Os Finder or non-disposable dilators, 1–5 mm diameter, can be used to dilate the cervix in office. Pretreatment with vaginal or buccal misoprostol and/or NSAIDS may be helpful in patients with stenosis. The steps for an endometrial biopsy using a pipette are listed in Table 4. Rare complications include 0.1–0.2% perforation (Kaunitz et al. 1998; McElin et al. 1974; Leclair 2002), bleeding, vasovagal reaction, severe cramping during or after procedure, and infection. Desired pregnancy is a contraindication to endometrial biopsy. Relative contraindications include coagulation disorder, use of anticoagulation medication, and coagulopathy from other causes such as liver failure and endometritis. The use of prophylaxis antibiotics to prevent bacterial endocarditis is not required (Dajani et al. 1997).

There is also a disposable endometrial brush that is available. It is similar to the brush used for endocervical sampling. The use of the brush in addition to the endometrial low-pressure suction device was reported to result in a 100% specificity and diagnosis rate for hyperplasia or cancer (Del Priore et al. 2001). Serial endometrial biopsies can be considered in high risk patients, those with recurrent bleeding or refractory to treatment.

2.4   Treatment Options

For younger women with anovulatory bleeding, treatment with the levonorgestrel-releasing IUD, combination of birth control pills or ring, or progestins can regulate and generally decrease menstrual flow. Younger women with hyperplasia without atypia can be appropriately treated with cyclic or continuous progestins. Pre- or postmenopausal women with hyperplasia with atypia should be referred to a gynecologist or gynecologic oncologist. Younger women with ovulatory bleeding should first be treated by addressing any clear structural or medical causes. After these problems are addressed, management may also include the levonorgestrel-releasing IUD; combination of oral contraceptive pills, ring, or patch; tranexamic acid; or nonsteroidal anti-inflammatory drugs (Sweet et al. 2012). Treatment for postmenopausal bleeding is also directed at the underlying cause, including removal of polyps or full evaluation of endometrial lesions by hysteroscopy, dilatation and curettage, or hysterectomy. Treatment

options also include vaginal estrogen for vaginal atrophy, correction of systemic illness, or adjustment of hormone replacement therapy.

2.5   Complications and Side Effects

Cramping generally resolves within a few minutes of the procedure. The high-suction devices are associated with more cramping than the low-suction devices. After the procedure, patients should be encouraged to stay supine for a few minutes in order to avoid a vasovagal reaction. Rare complications include perforation, excessive bleeding, and infection. Unless prolonged dilation is needed, a paracervical block is generally not needed. A paracervical block interrupts the sensory fibers of the cervix, upper vagina, and lower uterus. Intravascular injection or absorption of the anesthetic agent may cause headache, syncope, excessive sedation, or generalized convulsions.

3   Cervical Biopsy

3.1   Evaluation

Evaluation of the cervix is an integral part of the standard pelvic exam, and it includes both a visual and manual inspection as well as timely cervical cytology. Visual inspection of the cervix includes clear visualization of the cervical os, noting color changes, signs of infection, raised lesions, the presence of endocervical polyp or mass, trauma, foreign body, and discharge. The nonpregnant cervix is generally 2.5–3 cm in diameter and 3–5 cm in length. It is usually angled slightly backward and downward. The external cervical os in nonparous women is usually small and round, while in parous women there is often a transverse slit. The canal is approximately 8 mm wide and has longitudinal ridges. A cervical biopsy can either be a visually directed biopsy on the surface of the cervix using a cervical biopsy instrument or a blind scraping of the endocervical canal using an EndoCurette [endocervical curettage].

Table 4 Steps for performing an endometrial biopsy

Consent signed and questions answered [consider vaginal or buccal Cytotec to soften the cervix the night before and morning of and/or 1 hour prior to procedure oral NSAID]
Bimanual exam to establish size and position of the uterus
Evaluation of the vulva and vagina and cervix for lesion; Betadine solution to clean the cervix
Evaluate the cervical os and take note of possible stenosis, parous versus nonparous, amount of bleeding, and the absence of infection
If there is stenosis of the cervix that prevents introduction of the biopsy catheter, dilation of the cervix may be necessary. The use of a tenaculum or paracervical block may facilitate this procedure
There are multiple disposable as well as non-disposable dilators. A popular disposable dilator is the Os Finder. Having several dilation options available is helpful as the amount of beveling, diameter, and degree of flexibility of the dilator may play an important role in determining whether or not the dilation is possible. A very stenotic os requires a firm, tapered dilator to initiate the dilation, while canals that are very tortuous may need the more flexible and less pointed dilators

When dilation is necessary or high-suction device is used, consider:

1.	Paracervical block (prepackaged kits that include a needle guide and plastic needle spacer that control the depth of needle penetration
2.	Or 21–22 gauge [15 cm] extended length spinal needle
	10 ml syringe with a large 18–20 gauge needle to draw up 10–20 ml lidocaine, with or without epinephrine 1% or with vasopressin 3–5 units to 4:00 and 8:00 sites on the cervix; prior to injection, reverse pressure on the plunger to insure no backflow of blood, to avoid direct injection into the vessel
	Up to six sites on ectocervix, depth 3–7 mm
	Topical anesthetic cervical gels or creams can be used

Consider: Single-toothed tenaculum applied to upper cervix to stabilize the cervix and in some cases straighten out the cervix for easier insertion. After removal, insure hemostasis at sites of cervical perforation. Cotton tip swab can be pressed against any bleeding area with or without Monsel's solution. The use of a tenaculum and sound is standard when using a VABRA or high-suction device
Insertion of uterine sound is not always necessary but can be used to establish a tract and measure the length of the uterus [generally 6–8 cm] and always used when using high-suction device
Endometrial sampler is gently introduced into the uterine cavity; several passes are usually performed unless the patient is too uncomfortable to continue. The combined technique of endometrial curetting with a corkscrew twisting motion while using suction is recommended
The sample is placed into specimen container and sent to pathology lab
The presence of hemostasis insured
Procedure note and orders entered into the chart
Patient allowed to rest supine on the exam table for about 1–10 min after the procedure generally until moderate to severe cramping resolves. The patient should be then allowed to sit on the exam table, making sure she has no lightheadedness for 1–2 min before she stands up
She should be counseled that although unlikely to happen, she should to return to clinic and seek medical help if she has fever, chills, continued cramping past 24–48 h, or abnormally heavy bleeding. The use of nonsteroidal anti-inflammatory drugs can be used during the day and before bedtime for moderate to severe cramping

There are other types of cervical biopsies that are not covered in this chapter as they are often done in the operating room as an outpatient surgery. The loop electrosurgical excision procedure [LEEP] and various forms of cone biopsy procedures remove large, cone-shaped pieces of tissue from the cervix.

3.2 Differential Diagnosis

While most cervical biopsies are done as part of colposcopy for abnormal Pap smear or HPV testing, visual inspection of the cervix may reveal abnormal lesions that may warrant biopsy. The following are clinically significant cervical findings:

- Cervical or endocervical polyps are generally red, smooth, fingerlike growths often arising from within the cervical canal. The etiology of cervical polyps is not well understood, but they are likely due to estrogen stimulation of endocervical cells. Other possible etiologies include chronic infection or congestion of blood vessels. Cervical polyps are often asymptomatic but may cause bleeding or vaginal discharge. They can be very small, pea-sized, or large, several centimeters. While they are usually single, multiple cervical polyps can form. Removal of most cervical polyps is relatively simple and can be done in office using a ring forceps. Polyps with a thick diameter that originate deep within the cervical canal can be difficult to remove in office. Endometrial polyps can also extrude from the cervical os and are not easily distinguished from cervical polyps. There are a variety of histologic patterns that can occur: (1) typical endocervical polyp [mucosal], (2) granulation tissue, and (3) vascular, fibrous, pseudodecidual, endometrial or mixed endometrial and endocervical, and malignant area on part of polyp. The removal technique is described in Table 5.
- Microglandular hyperplasia is a polypoid growth measuring 1–2 cm occurring most often in women on oral contraceptives or depot medroxyprogesterone acetate. It can also occur in pregnant or postpartum women. It is thought to be due to progesterone activity. Removal is the same as a typical cervical polyp (Table 5) (Nichols and Fidler 1971).
- Nabothian cysts are mucus-filled, firm cysts that appear on the surface of the cervix. They are thought to be caused when stratified squamous epithelium of the ectocervix grow over and cover the columnar epithelium of the endocervix. The result is that cervical crypts (usually 2–10 mm in diameter) are formed by trapped cervical mucus inside the crypts. Nabothian cysts, clearly seen as cysts filled with mucus, are benign and do not need to be biopsied.
- Currently, there are more than 40 HPV serotypes that can infect mucosal surfaces.

Table 5 Steps in removing a cervical/endocervical polyp

Removal can usually be done by grasping the polyp with a ring forceps
The ring forceps are then twisted. The thicker the stalk, the slower the twisting to allow hemostasis at the base of the polyp. Polyps with a very thick stalk may require surgical removal
After removal of the polyp, the cervical os or base of polyp if visible should be checked for bleeding
If there is bleeding after the removal, a small Q-tip dipped in Monsel's solution can be placed into the cervical canal to the level of the base of the polyp. Good hemostasis should be insured
Specimen sent to pathology. Procedure note and orders entered into the chart
Although many of these removals are associated with minimal pain, patients with moderate to severe pain should be encouraged to stay in a supine position for a few minutes to avoid a vasovagal reaction

Exophytic warts, from HPV 6 or 11, can occur on the vulva, vagina, and cervix, while flat warts on the cervix, from 16, 18, 31, 33, and 35, are associated with CIN. Pap testing now includes identification of the serotype of HPV present on the cervix. HPV is therefore associated with both flat and warty-like lesions on the cervix. The flat lesions are better visualized when treated with 3–5% acetic acid, which causes cellular dehydration and increased nuclear density and acetowhite appearance in dysplastic lesions. Lesions suggestive of HPV should be biopsied under colposcopic guidance for confirmation.

- Cancer generally will often appear as a friable ulcer or cauliflower-like growth. Biopsy of any raised or suspicious lesion on the cervix should be carefully considered. The technique for cervical biopsy is shown in Table 6.
- Squamous papilloma is a benign, small, solid, cervical lesion that commonly arises from inflammation or trauma. They are generally 2–5 mm in diameter. Treatment is removal (Table 6).
- Leiomyomas [smooth muscle tumors] may originate in the cervix accounting for about 8% of all uterine myomas. They are similar to lesions in the fundus but usually are small

Table 6 Techniques for cervical biopsy

Consents signed, questions answered
Area cleaned with Betadine or equivalent
Consider use of a tenaculum for stabilization of the cervix
Consider use of a local anesthetic injection [not typically done for in-office procedures]
Paracervical block [see above for technique]
Local injection under lesion
Cervical biopsy forceps used to remove lesion [under direct visual or using colposcopy]. Specimen placed in formalin and sent to pathology
Insure hemostasis following procedure using a long [Q-tip] cotton-tipped applicator [8 inches long], pressure for 30 sec–2 min or more
Addition of Monsel's solution applied to cotton-tipped applicator and placed directly with pressure at site of biopsy when necessary
Removal of tenaculum [if used] and careful to insure hemostasis at site of tenaculum puncture sites. Use of cotton-tipped applicators with or without Monsel's solution when necessary
Post-procedure patient counseling to avoid sex or anything in the vagina for at least 3 days. Report to clinic if heavy persistent bleeding, fever, and pain

5–10 mm in diameter. Removal can be performed with ring forceps if pedunculated (Table 5).

- Mesonephric duct remnants are usually located at the 3 or 9 o'clock position deep within the cervical stoma. These are remnants of the mesonephric or Wolffian ducts. They are usually only a few millimeters in diameter and usually incidental findings on 15–20% of sectioned cervices (Ferry and Scully 1990).
- Endometriosis is usually an incidental finding but may appear as a mass or cause abnormal or typically postcoital bleeding. It often appears as a bluish-black or bluish-red lesion 1–3 mm in diameter. Diagnosis is made by biopsy, often colposcopically directed biopsy (Phadins et al. 2005).
- Papillary adenofibroma is an uncommon neoplasm that appears as a polypoid structure. Similar growths may appear in the fallopian tubes or endometrium.
- Hemangiomas are also rare and similar to those found in the rest of the body. They can cause

vaginal bleeding or pain. The differential diagnosis included cervical cancer and treatment if surgical removal ((Gupta et al. 2006)–(Gusdon 1965)).

3.3 Contraindications and Complications

There are a very limited number of relative contraindications for cervical biopsy, and they are mainly various etiologies of active cervicitis. Although control of post-procedure bleeding with ferric subsulfate, Monsel's solution, silver nitrate, or pressure is very effective for most patients, a careful risk-benefit analysis is important in evaluating patients with known bleeding disorders, liver failure, or other coagulopathies. Generally, if colposcopy is done in a pregnant patient, biopsies, particularly endocervical curettage, are avoided.

Bleeding at the site of biopsy is the most common complication. Other complications include failure to biopsy the correct site or, rarely, post-procedure infection.

3.4 Follow-Up Care

Patients should avoid coitus, use of tampons, or any another intravaginal item for at least 3–14 days after the biopsy to allow healing. The patient should be instructed to return to the clinic or seek medical care if she experiences heavy prolonged bleeding, moderate to severe [worsening] pain over the next few days, or persistent fever.

4 Vulvar Biopsy

4.1 Evaluation

Symptoms related to vulvar lesions are common, often chronic, and can have a significant effect on a woman's sexual function, self-esteem, and quality of life. Inquiring about specific complaints as well as onset, duration, location, prior treatments, and any possible aggravating or precipitating factors is important in determining the etiology. Important past history includes childbirth, over-the-counter-treatments, cryotherapy, prior treatment for condyloma, vulvar laser, or prior vulvar biopsy or surgery.

The examination should begin with a thorough examination with good lighting. Adding colposcopic examination can often be helpful. Color changes, vaginal discharge, swelling, edema, visible lesions, tenderness, changes in architecture, fissures, and vascular lesions should be noted. These findings as well as size, nature of the border, contour, raised areas, and the presence of ulcerated areas should be accurately recorded. Biopsy of lesions showing hyperpigmentation, raised exophytic areas, changes in vascular patterns, or those that remain unresolved after treatment should be performed to rule out carcinoma and aid in diagnosis. White or hypopigmented lesions or those with pebbling, skin thickening, or thinning may represent skin conditions where biopsy is particularly useful for diagnosis and directing treatment.

- *Dermatitis*is a common finding, reportedly occurring in half of patients complaining of chronic vulvar complaints of an "itchy rash." It is often called contact dermatitis as it is often due to vulvar irritants including chronic vaginal discharge, semen, spermicides, soaps, propylene glycol found in many medicines, and allergic reactions. A comprehensive interview regarding hygiene practices, the presence of chronic vaginal discharge, and vulvar product use is very important. The skin lesions are sometimes poorly demarcated, erythematous, scaly, cracked and lichenified, thin "cigarette-paper" skin often with gray or white color. **Chronic cases may benefit from a biopsy**. Avoiding chronic "wetness" in the vulva and discontinuing any contributing irritants are important counseling point. The use of protective emollient, topical antibiotics [A&D ointment], and topical steroids is a treatment option (Schlosser 2010).

- Acute or chronic vulvovaginitis candidiasis is associated with vulvar burning and itching, erythema and edema of the vulva including the labia and vestibule, patches of thrush, and thick curd-like vaginal discharge.
  - Chronic conditions may show lichenification of the vulva and may be associated with pain and dyspareunia (Krapf 2016). Treatment with local or systemic antifungal products plus local drying hygiene techniques is indicated. Additional treatment for concomitant bacterial infection may need to be added if clinically indicated.
- Atrophic vaginitis often plays a role in this condition and it may positively respond to local or systemic estrogen therapy. Normal vaginal epithelial and cervical discharge is an alkaline transudate with a pH ranging from 3.8 to 4.5. *Lactobacillus* produces acetic acid and helps to maintain a low vaginal pH. Lack of estrogen results in a higher vaginal pH and resultant change in vaginal flora.
- *Lichen sclerosus* is a chronic skin condition whose definite cause is not currently known. Lichen sclerosus is strongly associated with low endogenous estrogen levels, autoimmune diseases, and genetic factors (Higgins and Cruickshank 2012). Estimates are that between 1 in 70 and 1 in 1000 women have vulvar lichen sclerosus, a rate that is tenfold higher than men. On examination, typical lesions are shiny, flat, blanched white plaques with "crinkled tissue paper" affecting the vulva. There can be associated narrowing of the introitus, thinning, fusion of labia, phimosis of the clitoral hood, and fissures surrounded by purple or red borders (Eva 2012). A biopsy is recommended to confirm the diagnosis and rule out cancer. First-line treatment is high-dose topical steroid, clobetasol propionate, nightly for 4 weeks, then every other night for 4 weeks, and then twice weekly for maintenance (Chi et al. 2012; Thorstensen and Birenbaum 2012). Fissures, ecchymoses, hyperkeratosis, and erosions are expected to

heal, but pigmentation changes may remain (Thorstensen and Birenbaum 2012). Avoiding chronic vulvar moisture is an important counseling point. The use of protective emollients, topical antibiotics, A&D ointment, and other topical hormones or steroids is optional treatment. Follow-up is critically important.

- *Vulvar HPV lesions and VIN.* There are at least 35 HPV subtypes that infect the anogenital tract. HPV infections in the vulva often appear as bumps or growths. They can be asymptomatic or cause itching, burning, bleeding, or pain. They can range in appearance from flat-topped papules, keratotic warts, or dome-shaped, flesh-colored papules to the true condylomata acuminate, cauliflower-like appearance (Boardman and Cooper 2007). Differentiating genital warts from a vulvar neoplasia from appearance alone can be difficult. **Generally, indurated, fixed, hyperpigmented, or ulcerative lesions or lesions that do not respond to treatment should be biopsied**. VIN can be white, red, dark, eroded, or raised. If the biopsy returns VIN, the patient should receive colposcopy and/or referral to gynecologic oncology (Boardman and Cooper 2007).

- *Paget's disease of the vulva* is a rare type of skin disease that is most often found in postmenopausal women. The most common complaint is itching or pruritus. It is very slow in spreading, but in some cases an invasive cancer of the vulva is found below the affected area (Shaco-Levy et al. 2010). The appearance of Paget's disease is sharply demarcated patches of red and white scaly skin, similar to the appearance of eczema. Biopsy confirms the diagnosis and rule out the underlying risk of cancer. Referral to gynecologic oncology is recommended as wide resection and further evaluations are the mainstay of treatment (Edey et al. 2013).

- *Squamous cell carcinomas* are the most common vulvar malignancy, but other pathologies include basal cell, melanoma, Bartholin's gland cancer, and non-squamous cell malignancy. These lesions present as a nodule or exophytic mass, asymptomatic lump, or flat or raised lesion with ulceration or excoriation. Melanomas are usually brown to bluish black, but they may be nonpigmented. Lesions with these findings or any lesion that the patient reports have changed in size and shape should be biopsied.

- *An acrochordon* or skin tag may first present as a tiny soft bump on the skin. With time it may grow into a flesh-colored or darker lesion that is attached to the skin below often on a small stalk. A skin tag is generally painless but it can become irritated if rubbed or moved often. Biopsy is not necessary unless there are suspicious features or symptoms.

4.2 Biopsy Techniques

The Threshold for Performing a Vulvar Biopsy Should Be Low Chronic, recently changing, or exophytic lesions require a biopsy. Other indications are listed below. Techniques for three types of vulvar biopsies are detailed in Table 7.

Indications
Indications for performing a vulvar biopsy include the following:

- Possible malignancy
- Chronic, changing, or exophytic lesion
- Visible lesion and no definitive diagnosis
- Visible lesion, particularly white lesion not responding to usual therapy
- Lesions with atypical vascular patterns
- Benign-appearing lesions requiring definitive diagnosis

Contraindications
There are no absolute contraindications for vulvar biopsy. Relative contraindications include:

- Gross infection at site
- Coagulopathy, liver disease, anticoagulation medication use
- Allergy to local anesthetic
- Avoid biopsies on the clitoris or urethra

Table 7 Techniques for three types of vulvar biopsies

General: for all three techniques	Punch biopsy	Local resection	Shave biopsy
Consent patient and discuss risks and benefits. Risks may include infection, bleeding, inadequate sample, scarring, allergic reaction			
Eye protection should be used. Sterile gloves may be used			
Clean area with Betadine or equivalent; sterile drapes can be used			
Topical anesthetic agent may be applied prior to injecting a standard local anesthetic agent			
Using a large needle, 1–5 mL of 1–2% local anesthetic, such as lidocaine [preferably with epi]. The skin injection is done using a small needle (e.g., 25–30 gauge) to minimize pain (Eddowes 1990)			
After inserting the needle, the plunger is withdrawn to minimize risk of injecting into a vessel			
The anesthetic agent is slowly injected into the base and underneath the lesion, injecting enough to create a wheal			
	In general, the smallest punch biopsy [3 mm] that will adequately sample the lesion is used. For larger lesions, 4–5 mm biopsies are used. Multiple biopsies can be used	Larger lesions may need excisional biopsy with scalpel [i.e., 15 blade]	Elevate the lesion with a forceps, and then using either a scalpel, i.e., 15 blade, or curved scissors, use a single sweeping stroke to remove the lesion [or cut lesion with scissors with curved tips pointed upward]
	Punch biopsy is firmly placed against the skin, encompassing the entire lesion when possible and then rotated with a constant firm pressure both clockwise and counterclockwise until penetration through the skin to the base of the lesion. There is a change in tension as the punch	The lesion is grasped with forceps for stabilization or elevation. The scalpel is used to cut entirely around the lesion, generally including a margin around the entire lesion including the base. The incision is extended down to the base of the lesion. The specimen is held firmly with the forceps and	

(continued)

Table 7 (continued)

General: for all three techniques	Punch biopsy	Local resection	Shave biopsy
	biopsy enters the subcutaneous layer	removed using either the scalpel or Iris scissors	
	The punch is removed and the specimen grasped using forceps. [Curved Iris] scissors are used to cut the base of the biopsied tissue		
	Punch biopsies generally heal without suturing, but sutures may be considered for hemostasis	Suture closure is often used. A needle driver and suture, such as 4–0 monofilament or polyglactin, are used. Re-approximation of skin edges and lower tissue planes with one or more through and through stitches	Achieve hemostasis by pressure [or Monsel's solution]
	Monsel's solution or silver nitrate can be used [both may cause increased skin pigmentation and silver nitrate may cause scarring (Boardman and Cooper 2007)	Monsel's solution or silver nitrate can be used [both may cause increased skin pigmentation and silver nitrate may cause scarring (Boardman and Cooper 2007)	
Specimen is placed in pathology container [10% formalin]. For multiple biopsies, label each container accurately			

Approach Considerations

- Small, superficial lesions can be biopsied/removed using a shave biopsy. A shave biopsy samples the epidermis, and it may or may not include a section of the underlying dermis. Therefore, a shave biopsy may not provide information of the subcutaneous tissue. The lesion can be covered with a bandage.
- Punch biopsies can be used when the lesion is small enough for complete excision. Punch biopsies from 2 to 10 mm are available. Commonly punch biopsies from 3 to 5 mm are used.
- Large lesions, suspected inflammatory lesions, lesion suspicious for neoplasia, and ulcerated or pigmented lesions are often sampled using a punch biopsy. The punch biopsy can be used to either remove the entire specimen or take a small biopsy for diagnosis. In the latter case, the biopsy should include the edges of the lesion to get the best tissue for definitive diagnosis. Multiple punch biopsies may be necessary for larger lesion where areas appear to be different. Each biopsy should be placed in a separate container and labeled correctly.
- Larger lesions where complete excision with clear margins is desired may need excisional biopsy with suture repair.

Dressing

- The vulva is a difficult area to keep a dressing in place. Most vulvar biopsies are not covered with a dressing although a spot bandage can be used. Generally, a pad or panty liner is adequate.

Aftercare

- The patient should attempt to keep the area clean and dry, particularly after bowel movements as the biopsy site may be potentially contaminated with stool. If bleeding occurs, it can generally be stopped by direct pressure from the patient.

- 24 hours after biopsy with suture placements, showers are permitted, but hot tub baths should be avoided until healing is complete [usually about 5 days]. Area should be kept clean and dry and washed once to twice daily.
- Patients with suture placement are usually scheduled for suture removal about 7 days after the procedure if delayed absorbable suture is not used.

5 Conclusions

In-office gynecologic procedures are common office procedures that are now a mainstay of women's healthcare. Endometrial, cervical, and vulvar biopsies can be safely done in the office, and they allow the woman to quickly resume her normal activities. Many of these biopsies are done primarily to exclude the diagnosis of cancer, but additionally they are often helpful in establishing the correct diagnosis and treatment options.

References

Awwad JT, Toth TL, Schiff I. Abnormal uterine bleeding in the perimenopause. In J Fert. 1993;38:261–9.

Boardman LA, Cooper AS. Vulvar epithelial disorders and other vulvar conditions. In: Evans M, Series editor. General gynecology in the requisites in obstetrics and gynecology. Philadelphia: Mosby Elsevier; 2007. p. 415–23.

Chi CC, Kirtschig G, Baldo M, Lewis F, Wang SH, Wojnarowska F. Systematic review and meta-analysis of randomized controlled trials on topical interventions for genital lichen sclerosus. J Am Acad Dermatol. 2012;67(2):305–12.

Cooper JM. Contemporary management of abnormal uterine bleeding. Preface. Obstet Gynecol Clin N Am. 2000;27:xi–xiii.

Dajani AS, Taubert KA, Wilson W, et al. Prevention of bacterial endocarditis: recommendations by the American Heart Association. JAMA. 1997;277:22.

Del Priore G, Williams R, Harbatkin CB, Wan LS, Mittal K, Yang GC. Endometrial brush biopsy for the diagnosis of endometrial cancer. J Reprod Med. 2001;46(5):439.

Eddowes HA. Pipelle: a more acceptable technique for outpatient endometrial biopsy. Br J Obstet Gynecol. 1990;97:961–2.

Edey KA, Murdoch AE, Cooper S, Bryant A. Interventions for the treatment of Paget's disease of the vulva. Chchrane Database Ss Rev. 2013;10:CD009245.

Eva LJ. Screening and follow up of vulval skin disorders. Best Pract Res ClinObstet Gynaecol. 2012;26(2):175–88.

Ferry JA, Scully RE. Mesonephric remnants, hyperplasia, and neoplasia in the uterine cervix. A study of 49 cases. Am J Surg Pathol. 1990;14(12):1100–11.

Guido RS, Ranbour-Shakir A, Rulin MC, et al. Pipelle endometrial sampling: sensitivity in the detection of endometrial lesions. Cancer J Repro Med. 1995;40:553–5.

Gupta R, Singh S, Nigam S, Khurana N. Benign vascular tumors of the female genital tract. Int J Gynecol Cancer. 2006;16:1195–2000.

Gusdon JP. Hemangioma of the cervix: four new cases and a review. Am J Obstet Gynecol. 1965;91:204–9.

Higgins CA, Cruickshank ME. A population-based case-control study of aetiological factors associated with vulvar lichen sclerosus. J ObstetGynaecol. 2012;32(3):271–5.

Kaunitz AM, Masciello A, Ostrowski M. Comparison of endometrial biopsy with the endometrial Pipelle and Vabra aspirator. J Reprod Med. 1998;33:427.

Krapf JM, chief editor Isaacs C. Vulvovaginitis. Medscape. http://emedicine.medscape.com/article/2188931-overview. Assessed 27 Feb 2016.

Leclair C. Anesthesia for in office endometrial procedures: a review of the literature. Curr Womens Health Rep. 2002;2(6):429–33.

McElin TW, Bird CC, Reeves BD, et al. Diagnostic dilation and curettage. Obstet Gynecol. 1974;17:205.

Meniru G, Hopkins M. Abnormal uterine bleeding. In: Curtis M, Overholt S, Hopkins M, editors. Glass' office gynecology. 6th ed. Philadelphia: Lippincott Williams and Wilkins; 2006. p. 190.

Nichols TM, Fidler HK. Microglandular hyperplasia in cervical cone biopsies taken for suspicious and positive cytology. Am J Clin Pathol. 1971;56(4):424–9.

Phadins SV, Doshi JS, Ogunnalke O, Coady A, Padwick M, Sanusi FA. Cervical endometriosis: a diagnostic and management dilemma. Arch Gynecol Obstet. 2005;272:289–93.

Rodriguez GC, Yaqub N, King ME. A comparison of the Pipelle device and the Vabra aspirator as measured by endometrial denudation in hysterectomy specimens: the Pipelle device samples significantly less of the endometrial surface than the Vabra aspirator. Am J Obstet Gynecol. 1993;168:55–9.

Schlosser BJ. Contact dermatitis of the vulva. Dermatol Clin. 2010;28(4):697–706.

Shaco-Levy R, Bean SM, Vollmer RT, Jewell E, Jones EL, Valdes CL, et al. Paget disease of the vulva: a study of

56 cases. Eur J Obstet Gynecol Reprod Biol. 2010; 149(1):86–91.

Sierecki AR, Gudipudi DK, Montemarano N, Del Priore G. Comparison of endometrial aspiration techniques: specimen adequacy. J Repro Med. 2008;53(10):760.

Silver MM, Miles P, Rosa C. Comparison of Novak and Pipelle endometrial biopsy instruments. Obstet Gynecol. 1991;79:828–30.

Stovall TG, Ling FW, Morgan PL. A prospective, randomized comparison of the Pipelle endometrial sampling device with the Novak curette. Am J Obstet Gynecol. 1991;165:1287–9.

Sweet MG, Schmidt-Dalton TA, Weiss PM. Evaluation and management of abnormal uterine bleeding in premenopausal women. Am Fam Physician. 2012;85(1): 35–43.

Thorstensen KA, Birenbaum DL. Recognition and management of vulvar dermatologic conditions: lichen sclerosus, lichen planus, and lichen simplex chronicus. J Midwifery Womens Health. 2012;57(3):260–75.

Operative Hysteroscopy

Paul P. Smith and T. Justin Clark

Abstract

In this chapter, we aim to describe contemporary operative hysteroscopy. A further aim is to provide an outline for safe and effective practice when performing such procedures by summarizing the best available evidence supplemented by the authors' own experience. More specifically, this chapter will cover the available equipment, technologies, and techniques necessary to perform a variety of hysteroscopic procedures, namely, removal of fibroids and polyps, endometrial ablation, treatment of acquired and congenital uterine abnormalities, removal of placental remnants, and sterilization. We will also discuss the role of teaching, clinical governance, and audit in improving operative hysteroscopic services.

Keywords

Hysteroscopy • Vaginoscopy • Operative hysteroscopy • Outpatient hysteroscopy • Ambulatory hysteroscopy • Office hysteroscopy • Resectoscopy

Contents

P.P. Smith • T.J. Clark (✉)
Birmingham Women's NHS Foundation Trust, Edgbaston, UK
e-mail: paul.smith@doctors.net.uk; justin.clark@bwnft.nhs.uk

© Springer International Publishing AG 2017
D. Shoupe (ed.), *Handbook of Gynecology*,
DOI 10.1007/978-3-319-17798-4_53

1   Introduction

In 1869, the first successful diagnostic and operative hysteroscopy was performed when Pantaleoni used a cystoscope and candlelight to treat an endometrial polyp causing postmenopausal bleeding. Then in 1907, Charles David was the first to describe a lens system that allowed uterine cavity visualization. Yet, it was not until 1943 that Forestiere's cold light source and Hopkin's rod lens were combined to form the endoscopes that have become the basis for today's hysteroscopy.

With advances in technology and techniques, hysteroscopy has taken over from dilatation and curettage to become the gold-standard procedure for investigation and treatment of pathologies in the uterine cavity. It has the advantage of being able to visualize the uterine cavity directly and can sometimes allow simultaneous treatment to be performed. A large number of procedures can now be performed hysteroscopically. These include fibroid resection, polyp removal, sterilization, removal of chronically retained products of conception (RPOC), adhesiolysis, septoplasty, and endometrial ablation. Hysteroscopic surgery is minimally invasive, avoiding surgical incisions and the need for prolonged inpatient hospital stay. Furthermore, proficient operative hysteroscopy is both quick and safe. Increasingly procedures are being performed in a more convenient ambulatory or "office" setting avoiding the need for hospital admission or general anesthesia. Indeed, the concept of office-based "see-and-treat" hysteroscopy has been propagated over the last decade with simultaneous treatments being undertaken conditional upon the prior diagnostic hysteroscopy.

Although complication rates for operative hysteroscopy are low, some complications can be life threatening. It is therefore imperative that appropriate training programs are combined with an understanding of the equipment and techniques to make operative hysteroscopy a safe and efficient tool.

2   Equipment

Most operative hysteroscopes consist of an inflow channel for distension media, an outflow channel for distension media, an operating channel with a sheath to allow instrumentation, a light lead, and telescope with fiber-optic cables and a camera head (Fig. 1).

Some hysteroscopes use an angled optic that allows better visualization of the cavity. It is important to realize that when inserting the hysteroscope through the cervix, the endocervical canal is positioned at 6 o'clock if the optic is upward and 12 o'clock if the optic is downward (Fig. 2). For most hysteroscopes, the position of the light lead is the same as the location of the endocervical canal.

Light leads are fiber-optic cables that act as conduits for light between the generator and the telescope. Fiber-optic cables are prone to damage and are normally the cause of low light generated

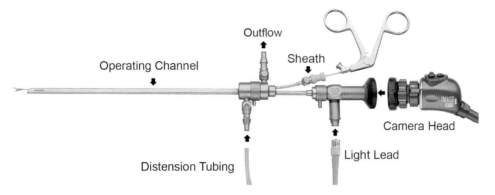

Fig. 1 Components of operative hysteroscope

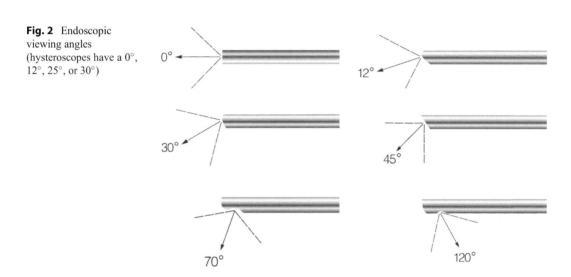

Fig. 2 Endoscopic viewing angles (hysteroscopes have a 0°, 12°, 25°, or 30°)

by the telescope. Looking for dark spots at the end of the cable can assess this.

3   Patient Preparation

An important part of patient preparation is adequate counseling about the rationale for the procedure and what it involves. The patient experience is important to describe especially for those women undergoing office-based procedures without general anesthesia. Potential complications and the expected clinical outcomes need to be discussed in a frank manner. Patient information leaflets are an essential component in preoperative counseling because they support verbal information given to further ensure that patients are adequately informed and prepared for their hysteroscopic procedure.

4   Technique

Although not always practical, hysteroscopy should be performed in the first half of the menstrual cycle when the endometrium is at its thinnest. Pregnancy should be ruled out before all cases begin. When positioning patient for hysteroscopic procedures, the patient should be in the lithotomy position with the buttocks slightly over the edge of the operating table.

4.1 Prevention of Cervical Trauma and Perforation

There is evidence to suggest the hysteroscopic procedures under direct vision are more accurate than dilatation and curettage (Loffer et al. 2000; Valle 1981). Not only should procedures under direct vision be done in preference to blind procedures for the purpose of accuracy but also for safety reasons. As further advances are made resulting in miniaturization of equipment, the need for blind dilatation, which risks uterine trauma, will also be reduced.

Cervical trauma and patient discomfort can be reduced by using the thinnest hysteroscopic equipment available and the "no touch" or vaginoscopic technique. The vaginoscopic technique is achieved by guiding the hysteroscope into the uterus under direct vision without using any potentially painful instrumentation. The easiest way to do this is to enter the vagina allowing the distension media to fill the cavity and follow the posterior wall of the vagina down into the posterior fornix. The hysteroscope is then maneuvered into the cervix above and pushed through the cervical canal into the uterus. The vaginoscopic technique can only be used for hysteroscopes less than six millimeters in diameter.

The administration of oral or vaginal prostaglandins such as misoprostol prior to operative procedures has been researched and has shown that spontaneous cervical dilatation is increased but with no decrease in complications (Cooper et al. 2011a). There are inconsistent results of the benefits of osmotic dilatators such as laminaria prior to operative procedures.

5 Distension Media

The technique of hysteroscopy requires a distension medium to be instilled into the uterine cavity to allow visualization of the uterine cavity enabling both the diagnosis and surgical treatment of intrauterine pathology. A variety of distension media can be used including liquids such as glycine, dextran, sorbitol, water and normal saline, and gases such as carbon dioxide. Comparisons of normal saline to carbon dioxide as distension media have shown no difference in pain or visualization, although procedures done with normal saline were found to be significantly faster (Cooper et al. 2011b). However, carbon dioxide is infrequently used nowadays because special insufflation equipment is needed and its use is restricted to simple diagnosis. The plethora of new therapeutic hysteroscopic systems requires fluid distension media to continuously irrigate the uterine cavity removing blood and tissue debris thereby providing a clear operative picture.

The use of isotonic fluid normal or "physiological" saline is the preferred fluid media for operative hysteroscopic procedures because inadvertent fluid overload does not lead to severe osmotic imbalance (hypervolemic hyponatremia) (Berg et al. 2009). Mechanical technologies such as tissue removal systems can be used in normal saline. When it comes to operative procedures using electrical energy, the type of distension media is dictated by whether monopolar or bipolar electrical circuits are being used. Bipolar electrodes require conductive, electrolytic solutions such as normal saline (285 mOsm/L) or Ringer's lactate (279 mOsm/L), while procedures using monopolar electrodes need nonconductive, hypo-osmolar, nonionic solutions such as glycine 1.5% (200 mOsm/L) or sorbitol 3% (165 mOsm/L).

The new generation of bipolar electrodes is generally safer than monopolar electrodes because they do not affect serum osmolality or sodium levels. However, all solutions can cause complications from intravascular absorption of large volumes of fluid into the circulatory system. Excessive fluid absorption is most likely with prolonged hysteroscopic procedures using larger diameter endoscopes with continuous irrigation of fluid or where blood vessels within the myometrium are opened. Thus, particular care is required with resection of the endometrium (transcervical resection of the endometrium – TCRE) and hysteroscopic myomectomy (transcervical resection of fibroids – TCRF). Serious complications arising from expansion of the extracellular fluid volume with the potential to generate fluid overload, pulmonary edema, include acute pulmonary edema, cerebral edema, and cardiac failure. Therefore, it is important to accurately measure the input and output of fluid during operative hysteroscopy so that significant fluid deficits can be recognized and managed promptly. While delivery of the distension medium can be safely and effectively achieved using simple gravity or pressure bags, automated pressure delivery systems facilitate the creation of a constant intrauterine pressure and accurate fluid deficit surveillance. The American Association of Gynecologic Laparoscopy (AAGL) guidelines recommend that when fluid deficits with a nonelectrolyte solution reach 1500 or 2500 mL with normal saline, the procedure should be brought to a halt (Loffer et al. 2000).

6 Hysteroscopic Treatment of Fibroids

6.1 Submucous Fibroids

Fibroids or leiomyomas are benign overgrowths of the smooth muscle layer of the uterus. They remain the most common indication for hysterectomy. Submucous fibroids are those that protrude into the uterine cavity. They account for 5% of all fibroids. Submucous fibroids are associated with pain, bleeding, infertility, and recurrent miscarriage. The most established classification system for submucous fibroids was developed by Wamsteker and the European Society of Gynecologic Endoscopy (ESGE) and accepted by the International Federation for Obstetrics and Gynecology (FIGO) (Munro et al. 2011). This nomenclature states that if the submucous fibroid is entirely intracavitary, i.e., attached to the uterine cavity sidewall by only a small stalk, they are classified as type 0; if a portion of the fibroid is intramural, then they are type 1 if less than 50% is intramural and type 2 if more than 50% is intramural.

Submucosal fibroids can be selectively removed hysteroscopically, which is particularly useful in women who want to preserve their fertility and avoid the complications of laparoscopic or laparotomic surgery. Types 0 and 1 are suitable for hysteroscopic resection. Removal of type 2 fibroids is more challenging because risks of perioperative bleeding, incomplete removal, and uterine trauma are significantly greater. Furthermore, the need for repeated hysteroscopic or other surgical interventions are greater to treat ongoing abnormal bleeding symptoms compared with type 0 and 1 fibroids (Vercellini et al. 1999). Another classification system has been developed to describe additional prognostic features related to submucous fibroids; in addition to depth of myometrial penetration, the STEPW classification records the size, topography (location), and extension of the base in relation to the uterine wall (Lasmar et al. 2012) .

Hysteroscopic removal is mostly done with resectoscopy, i.e., electrosurgical resection using a modified urological resecting loop. More recently, hysteroscopic morcellators, now termed tissue removal systems, have been introduced offering simultaneous mechanical cutting and tissue aspiration, and these technologies appear to be gaining increasing popularity (van Dongen et al. 2008). Some surgeons did use laser hysteroscopic myomectomy in the past, but the laser units are associated with high capital and running costs and have largely been abandoned now.

6.2 Endometrial Preparation

It is common practice to give medication to suppress the endometrium and shrink fibroids prior to surgery. It is thought that this improves visualization by thinning the endometrium and helps to ensure complete removal of the fibroid. The use of gonadotropin-releasing hormone analogues (GnRHa) 3–4 months prior to surgery does reduce fibroid size and corrects anemia prior to surgery (Lethaby et al. 2001). However, data supporting the benefits of endometrial downregulation prior to operative hysteroscopy are conflicting, and currently there are no randomized controlled studies showing surgical removal, and clinical outcomes are improved by this practice (Kamath et al. 2014). Recent work has shown that the selective progesterone receptor modulator, ulipristal acetate, is an effective alternative to reduce fibroid size and induce amenorrhea prior to fibroid surgery with fewer side effects than GnRHa (Donnez et al. 2012a, b). However, as with GnRHa, data supporting improved outcomes with hysteroscopic myomectomy are lacking.

It is important to assess the size and the degree of intramural involvement before embarking on medication to shrink the fibroids, to effectively counsel the patient and plan appropriate surgery. Transvaginal ultrasound is now common in the evaluation of women with gynecological problems, but on its own, it is not accurate enough to adequately describe protrusion of the fibroids into the endometrial cavity. The advent of the 3D ultrasound and saline infusion sonography has been shown to improve accuracy (de Kroon et al. 2003; Lee et al. 2006). Ultrasound is useful to describe the distance between the intramural component and the serosa, which can help the surgeon prevent perforation of the uterus during hysteroscopic treatment. Hysteroscopy provides the best method for assessing the degree of protrusion into the endometrial cavity and the suitability for surgery. With the advent of outpatient hysteroscopy, this can be done without subjecting the patient to general anesthesia.

6.3   Hysteroscopic Equipment for Removal of Fibroids

Hysteroscopic resectoscopes are versatile tools that consist of a movable cauterization electrode usually in the form of a loop (Fig. 3). Originally the resectoscopes used a monopolar electrode, but advances in technologies have led to the development of equally effective bipolar resectoscopes that have the increased safety advantage of using isotonic distension media with reduced risk of serious complications arising from fluid overload and hypervolemic hyponatremia

6.4   Technique

The first step is to identify all the uterine cavity landmarks, and these should continue to be visualized throughout the procedure. The surgeon should be familiar with their equipment and technology especially the angle of the offset lens, energy modality, and distension media management. The amount of fluid deficit considered reasonable, which will depend upon its nature and the patients' medical comorbidities, should be discussed between the surgical team and the anesthetist prior to commencing the procedure.

6.4.1   Electrosurgical Resection

For electrosurgical resection, the loop electrode should be extended beyond the fibroid. The activated electrode is then drawn toward the surgeon by either moving the entire hysteroscope or closing the electrode or a combination of these two movements. Usually a blended or pure cut current set at 120 W cutting is adequate. The activated electrode should never be pushed away from the surgeon as this can cause perforation. Cutting into the myometrium should be avoided, particularly near the cornua and cervix where it is at its thinnest and bleeding or uterine perforation may occur. The degree of magnification and extension of the loop from the distal lens should be adjusted according to the location of the fibroid or area

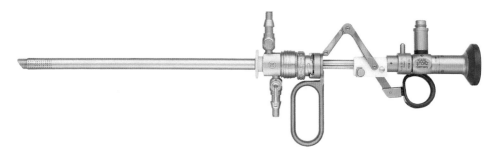

Fig. 3 Resectoscope

being resected, e.g., a higher degree of magnification (proximity of the distal lens) is needed when resecting fibroid tissue near the fundus or cornua.

One of the main disadvantages of electrosurgical resection of submucous fibroids is that as the fibroid is progressively debulked, "chips" of fibroid tissue are generated, which compromise visualization and impede the free movement of the loop electrode. One strategy to combat the impact of these fibroid chips is to push them toward the fundus to keep the view clear until enough are generated to obscure the visual field. A variety of techniques are then used to remove the chips, which include using a curette and polyp forceps or closing the inactivated resectoscope loop thus catching the chips. Also, the resectoscope can be removed from its outer sheath allowing the chips to traverse the cervical canal through the sheath.

The fibroid should be resected until it is level with the endometrium. Spontaneous uterine contractions as well as fluctuations in intrauterine pressure, e.g., increasing and decreasing the distension media pressure, can help push some of the intra-myometrial component of a grade 1/2 fibroid into the uterine cavity allowing safer resection under direct vision. Mechanical undermining of the intramural fibroid component with the passive inactivated electrode or with a firmer specially designed hook can achieve the same thing. This latter surgical approach has been described as adopting a "cold knife" technique (Mazzon et al. 2016). As the intramural extension of the capsule is reached, the myometrial sinuses are exposed which can lead to bleeding and increased and sometimes rapid intravascular absorption of fluid.

The production of fibroid chips can be avoided if grade 0 fibroids are removed en bloc by cutting through the basal attachment to the uterine side wall with miniature bipolar electrodes such as Versapoint® bipolar electrosurgical system (Gynecare™; Ethicon Inc., New Jersey, USA). These electrodes can be passed down the operating channel of a standard continuous flow operating hysteroscope, and detachment of the grade 0 fibroid can be rapidly achieved. However, given the shape and small size of the electrode, they are not generally suitable for fundally located

lesions. Moreover, blind removal of the fibrous specimen from the uterine cavity is not always possible. In these cases, the fibroid will often be left in situ and subsequently degenerate and pass.

Another alternative to reduce the production of fibroid chips is the vaporization electrode. The first vaporizing electrode developed by CIRCON ACMI was the VaporTrode® Grooved Bar. Using the Grooved VaporTrode® and higher wattage, the device is able to vaporize tissue in contact with the electrode (Brooks 1995).

6.4.2   Tissue Removal Systems

Hysteroscopic tissue removal systems appear to have overcome the most frustrating problem with resectoscopes by avoiding the generation of tissue chips. This makes fibroid removal easier to learn than traditional electrosurgical resections (van Dongen et al. 2008). Tissue removal systems use a simultaneous mechanical cutting and tissue retrieval set up that maintains better views while operating. The tissue removal systems consist of a bespoke operating 0° hysteroscope with an operating channel through which a disposable cutting hand piece comprising two rotating hollow metal tubes with a small aperture distally. This is attached to an external suction tubing. A generator provides the electrical energy to rotate the mechanical tissue removal system.

Before the device is inserted, it is important to make sure the window lock is closed when it is not activated. Once the fibroid requiring removal is identified, the window should be aimed toward the top of the fibroid, and the tissue will be sucked inside the window and shaved. As with electrosurgical resectoscopes, the strategy for fibroid removal using these systems is to start on the periphery and move closer to the myometrium. The technique is to position the opening near the pathology, which is then sucked into the opening. Rotation of the inner metal tube then shaves away the pathology. Afterward, the pathology is sucked through the device and trapped in a tissue collector. Gentle pressure is applied with minimal movement of the hysteroscope to ensure the base of the fibroid is removed. To prevent blood and debris obscuring the visual field, it is important to keep the device activated to ensure these products will be sucked into the window. The first of these systems was the TRUCLEAR™ (Smith & Nephew, Andover, MA) which has been followed by a similar product by Hologic (Bedford, MA, USA) called Myosure™ and Karl Storz (Tuttlingen, USA) called Integrated Bigatti Shaver (IBS). More recently the SYMPHION™ (Boston Scientific, Natick, MA) has been produced which combines a tissue removal system with bipolar radio-frequency energy.

7   Hysteroscopic Polypectomy

7.1   Endometrial Polyps

Endometrial polyps are benign overgrowths of endometrium that project into the uterine cavity. Generally they are pedunculated and are attached to the uterus by an elongated pedicle, but sometimes they are sessile and have a large flat base (Fig. 4).

They can be distinguished from submucous fibroids because they are soft and can be indented by the hysteroscope, and they move with the distension media. They often have a pink-red appearance similar to endometrium, but less vascular polyps can appear pale-gray. The specific hysteroscopic appearance of polyps will vary according to the relative make up of stroma, glands, and blood vessels. Endometrial polyps

are common with a prevalence of around 10% in women undergoing a diagnostic hysteroscopy (Clark and Gupta 2005). Most gynecologists recommend the removal of endometrial polyps because of their association with malignant and premalignant conditions (van Dijk et al. 2012; Timmermans et al. 2008). The incidence of polyps and risk of malignancy increases with age.

Hysteroscopic visualization allows a subjective assessment of the nature of polyps, but it can also be used to direct biopsies to increase diagnostic accuracy (Birinyi et al. 2004). Indeed, hysteroscopy has the added advantage of allowing simultaneous treatment of detected endometrial polyps. Depending on the local resources and expertise that is available, polypectomy can invariably be performed in the office setting without general anesthesia (Cooper et al. 2015). Hysteroscopic techniques utilizing both miniature mechanical and electrosurgical technologies allow polyp removal under direct vision reducing the risk of incomplete removal and uterine trauma. This represents a shift in management because until recently polyps were often removed blindly using dilation and curettage (D&C) or using large diameter electrosurgical resecting loops under general anesthesia.

7.2   Hysteroscopic Equipment for Removal of Polyps

Hysteroscopic polypectomy began with a range of mechanical instruments that could be passed down the operating channel of the hysteroscope including graspers, biopsy cups, and scissors (Bettocchi et al. 2004; Nathani and Clark 2006; Timmermans and Veersema 2005). However, these instruments are flimsy, making it difficult to remove large pathology, and there have been some studies showing problems with bleeding (Clark and Gupta 2005; Garuti et al. 2008). The resectoscope was the first electrosurgical instrument described for removing endometrial polyps, but these are large diameter instruments necessitating the use of general anesthesia and potentially traumatic, blind cervical dilatation. It is well recognized that polyps are softer than fibroids such

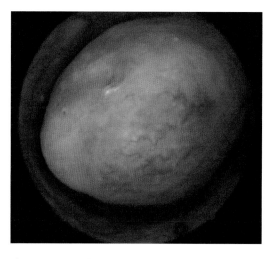

Fig. 4 Endometrial polyp as seen at hysteroscopy

that newer miniature electrosurgical instrumentation such as bipolar electrodes [e.g., Versapoint™ bipolar electrosurgical system (Gynecare, Ethicon, Somerville, NJ, USA)] and monopolar snares have been developed that obviate the need for large diameter hysteroscopes and blind cervical dilatation.

The bipolar electrodes have been demonstrated in observational series to be feasible and safe (Clark et al. 2002a; Kung et al. 1999; Vilos 1999) and have snares. The latter technology is less widely used (Timmermans and Veersema 2005). The previously mentioned hysteroscopic morcellator devices or tissue removal systems, TRUCLEAR™ (Smith & Nephew™, Andover, MA, USA) and Myosure™ (Hologic™, Marlborough, MA USA), are utilized for polypectomy as well as myomectomy. Randomized trials have shown that when compared to electrosurgical devices, tissue removal systems which allow simultaneous tissue cutting and retrieval are quicker to learn, less painful, more acceptable, faster, and more likely to completely remove polyps (van Dongen et al. 2008; Smith et al. 2014a).

7.3 Technique

7.3.1 Electrosurgery

Resecting Loops

The main drawback to the use of large diameter resectoscopes is the need for cervical dilatation and regional or general anesthesia. As with resecting submucous fibroids, the loop is extended beyond the focal lesion and then is activated and drawn toward the operator by closing the loop using the trigger or moving the whole resectoscope or a combination of both methods. The softer, less vascular nature of endometrial polyps in comparison to submucous fibroids makes them much easier to remove. They are rapidly resected either in pieces after a few passes off the resecting loop or en bloc with a sweep of the resecting loop at the polyp base where it attached to the uterine side wall. Occasionally, the inactivated loop can be deployed as a simple snare, closing the extended loop to mechanically detach the polyp from its attachment. Retrieval from the already dilated cervical canal of compressible, glandular polyps is usually achieved under vision by trapping the tissue within the withdrawn loop and end of the hysteroscope and removing the whole unit along the cervical canal.

Bipolar Electrical Resection with Miniature Electrodes

The cutting point of the bipolar electrode works by vaporization. High-temperature Ohmic heating in the immediate vicinity of the active electrode boils the saline to create a vapor pocket. This has the advantage of minimizing bleeding by cauterization of blood vessels. The initial bipolar miniature electrodes were the Versapoint™ electrodes (Fig. 5) that were designed to be used with a bespoke small-diameter operating hysteroscope. This "Versascope™," subsequently modified and renamed the "Alphascope™," is a small-diameter 0° semirigid hysteroscope incorporating a rotating cuff to manipulate the orientation of the bipolar electrodes and other ancillary instruments which have been passed down the expandable disposable outer sheath. The bipolar electrodes can, however, fit down any standard continuous flow operating 30° hysteroscope incorporating a

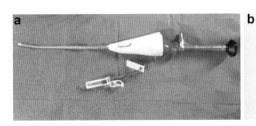
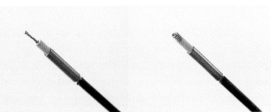

Fig. 5 Alphascope™ and Versapoint™ bipolar electrodes (**a**) twizzle electrode; (**b**) spring electrode

1.6 mm operating channel, making them highly versatile instruments. In contrast to the formal resectoscopes, use of smaller diameter electrosurgical operating set ups minimizes the need for traumatic cervical dilatation. Indeed, the development of the Versapoint™ electrode as a more effective cutting tool compared with flimsy mechanical graspers and scissors was one of the main technologies to shift polypectomy to an office setting.

Once a polyp has been diagnosed, the bipolar electrode is passed down the operating channel of a standard rigid operating hysteroscope. However, if using the Alphascope with its expandable plastic working channel, it is advisable to insert it into the uterine cavity without the electrode in the operating channel. This is because the Alphascope is narrower without the electrode and the operating channel also acts as the outflow so it is harder to clear the turbid fluid at the beginning of the procedure unless it is empty. However, for selected cases such as fundal polyps, it may be beneficial to insert the electrode at the beginning so that the twizzle tip can be bent across the camera lens to create a cutting hook and then allow entry into the uterine cavity. The main drawback of the miniature electrodes is the ability to manipulate them, as the cutting surface is small and fixed in contrast to electrosurgical loops.

When cutting a polyp using an Alphascope, there are three techniques that can be used. The first is to fix the electrode and hysteroscope but swivel the sheath using the rotating cuff creating an arc, which is particularly effective at cutting sidewall polyps. The second is to fix the sheath and hysteroscope and move the electrode in and out. The last technique is to fix the electrode and sheath and then move the hysteroscope and electrode as one instrument. If using the bipolar electrode down a rigid operating 30° hysteroscope, the orientation of the electrode can be altered by moving the light cable and hence the position of the distal offset lens. It is important that with all the techniques, the electrode is not activated when it is going toward the direction of the fundus, as this could lead to perforation and damage. The activated electrode should be withdrawn toward the operator, and when approaching attachments at the fundus and especially the thinner cornual aspects of the uterine side wall, higher magnification is required by ensuring the electrode is close to the distal lens.

The exact technique chosen to cut the polyp will depend on the operator preference, size, and position of the polyp. In the author's opinion, as polyps are compressible and feasible for removal in an office setting, the most efficient technique is to remove the polyp en bloc by cutting its basal attachment to the uterine side wall. This is easiest if the polyps are nonfundal and located on the anterior, posterior, or lateral sidewalls. Sometimes it may be necessary to bisect the polyps if they are large and located fundally so as to access the base. Other operators prefer to cut the polyp into segments, but this is time-consuming and either creates chips of tissue, which may obscure visualization within the cavity or repeated insertions and withdrawal of the hysteroscope. Removing the polyp in one piece avoids these problems, but the larger tissue specimen is harder to remove along the narrow cervical canal.

A variety of biopsy cups, grasping forceps, and snares are available that can be passed down the operating channel to remove the polyp fragments from the cavity. Leaving a small attachment between the polyp and the sidewall will make it easier to grab and stop it swirling around from the inflow of saline. If the polyp is completely detached, then turning off the fluid inflow and gently pushing the polyp using the opened forceps to pin it against the fundus can be used to then take a substantial "bite" of tissue. Others prefer to use inactivated snares to grasp the specimen. To give the greatest chance of traversing the cervical canal without the polyp becoming detached, a good degree of purchase on the polyp by having it firmly grasped should be ensured, and the largest part of the polyp should be brought proximally over the distal lens and then the whole unit moved slowly move backward down the endocervical canal. If this does not work because the polyps are large and fibrous or the cervical canal is narrow, then it may be necessary to break the polyp up under vision although this is rarely possible given its mobility within the cavity. More often the cervix will need to be dilated up to H6–8 and the hysteroscope and graspers inserted again. Blind retrieval using large polyp forceps should be avoided where possible.

7.3.2 Mechanical

Scissors and Grasping Forceps

Cold scissor resection can be performed using similar equipment as above to detach endometrial polyps. Scissors have the advantage of not producing bubbles that can impede the visual field, and they are also reusable. However, they are fragile, become blunt over time, and are difficult to manipulate. In contrast to the bipolar electrodes, they create bleeding and cannot cut through more fibrous polyps.

Tissue Removal Systems

The TRUCLEAR™ and Myosure™ tissue removal systems have been described in the preceding section on submucous fibroids (Figs. 6 and 7). These technologies can be used for removing uterine polyps. However, in contrast to submucous fibroids, the softer tissue constituting polyps makes them amenable to morcellation using systems with less cutting power (Myosure REACH, LITE & CLASSIC). In the case of TRUCLEAR, a much smaller diameter system is available, the OD TRUCLEAR system with a 2.9 mm rotary cutting

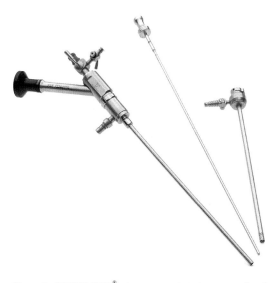

Fig. 6 TRUCLEAR® hysteroscopic tissue retrieval system

blade. The outer diameter is 5.6 mm, and it is a continuous flow system aiding visualization even in the presence of significant tissue debris and bleeding. If the outflow sheath is removed, outflow is then provided by the negative pressure, which draws saline through the aperture and along the hollow activated device. The outer diameter is then reduced to 5 mm, which is advantageous in the office setting, and vaginoscopy is more feasible.

The technique for morcellation is similar to removing fibroids. The distal aperture incorporating the cutting edges of the rotating inner and outer hollow tubes should be embedded in the polyp tissue and not visible. As polyps are mobile in a fluid distension media, they will be seen to move when the device is in contact with the tissue, simultaneously cutting and aspirating material. Movement of the device should be kept to a minimum. Small rotations of the hand piece to redirect the cutting window are all that is generally required. As the polyp base is reached, more exaggerated vertical or horizontal movements of the hand piece will lever the cutting window up against the uterine side wall. The ease of use of these systems and short learning curve compared to traditional resectoscopy was highlighted in a recent randomized control trial (RCT) (van Dongen et al. 2008). A recent RCT showed that the TRUCLEAR tissue removal system was quicker, less painful, and more acceptable and successful compared with Versapoint™ electrosurgery for the office removal of endometrial polyps (Smith et al. 2014b).

8 Endometrial Destruction for Abnormal Uterine Bleeding

8.1 Endometrial Destruction

Heavy menstrual bleeding is one of the commonest reasons patient consult with their gynecologist. There is an increasing range of medical therapies, but most have a hormonal basis for action. Some women do not like taking hormones long term, while others suffer from side effects, and these problems can limit the application of medical therapies. Traditionally, after medical

Fig. 7 Myosure®
hysteroscopic tissue
retrieval system

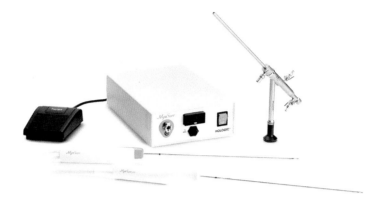

therapies had failed, definitive treatment with hysterectomy was used, but this has the morbidity and mortality associated with a major surgery. Moreover, patient preference studies have shown that women put a high value avoiding hysterectomy and retaining their uterus. Endometrial destruction techniques, i.e., ablation and resection of the endometrium, provide a cheaper, safer alternative to hysterectomy. The first-generation hysteroscopic techniques include laser ablation, rollerball ablation, and transcervical resection of the endometrium (TCRE). The costs of laser equipment were prohibitive so that electrosurgical resection with cutting loops and/or rollerball ablation using roller ball electrodes became the preeminent technique. When comparing TCRE to with rollerball ablation, there is no evidence of difference in rates of complication or re-intervention (Lethaby et al. 2005).

The second-generation techniques were then developed. These semiautomated technologies utilized the principle of controlled, global thermal destruction of the endometrium but without the requirement for enhanced operative hysteroscopic skills. They also aimed to reduce complications, particularly those of uterine trauma and fluid overload. While evidence supports their enhanced feasibility and safety, they are generally less flexible being restricted to use in regular-shaped cavities without submucous fibroids or congenital anomalies. There have been many different devices that have come to market with some no longer in use. The most prevalent devices are based upon the application to the endometrial surface of impedance-controlled radio-frequency energy

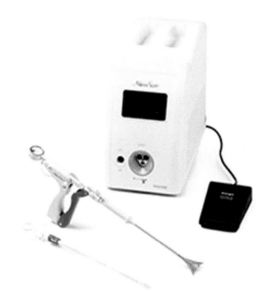

Fig. 8 The NovaSure radio-frequency ablation system (an example of a semiautomated, global, second-generation endometrial ablation device)

(NovaSure™ Fig. 8) or conducted heat from fluid within a pressurized balloon [Thermachoice™ (Gynecare™; Ethicon™ Inc., NJ, USA); Cavaterm™(Wallsten Medical SA, Lausanne, Switzerland); Thermablate™ (Gynecare™, NJ , USA)]. The Genesys HTA™(Boston Scientific) is a hydrothermal ablation method that uses heated saline and allows for visualization of the endometrial cavity during the ablation procedure. It allows for ablation of larger and irregularly shaped endometrial cavities.

The main drawback of uterine sparing endometrial ablation in comparison to hysterectomy is that it cannot guarantee amenorrhea. Around 10% of patients who have endometrial ablation will go on to have a further intervention usually in the form of a hysterectomy (Peeters et al. 2013; Smith et al. 2014a). Research looking at prognostic factors have found that large uterine cavities (>9 cm), preoperative dysmenorrhea, and younger age (<45 years) are associated with a higher chance of failure (El-Nashar et al. 2009). The reasons for hysterectomy are not always confined to persistent or recurrent abnormal uterine bleeding as some women develop cyclical pain thought to be a result of iatrogenic adenomyosis or hematometra.

8.2   Equipment

8.3   Technique of Transcervical Resection of the Endometrium and Endometrial Electrocoagulation

The first-generation techniques are all done under hysteroscopic vision. This has the advantage of allowing treatment in the presence of small fibroids, endometrial polyps, uterine abnormalities, or a large cavity. Unfortunately, these techniques require more time and higher skill levels and use distension media that can lead to complications of fluid overload and electrolyte imbalances.

The technique used for transcervical resection of the endometrium (TCRE) is similar to that used for fibroid resection, while endometrial electrocoagulation makes use of a rollerball electrode instead of a loop electrode. The rollerball electrode is easier to learn and does not generate tissue chips. The rollerball cannot be used to simultaneously treat other causes of heavy menstrual bleeding such as fibroids and requires the endometrium to be thin.

It is important to visualize all the landmarks before starting, and it can also be useful to mark the point near the endocervix that you wish to resect or ablate before starting. This is because when the activated electrode is drawn toward the surgeon, it is easy to go beyond the area you wish to resect/ablate. It is important to take a systematic

approach to treatment of the cavity. The cornual and fundal areas are technically the most difficult areas to treat and are resected by moving the entire hysteroscope using a forward-facing loop or rollerball. Drawing the activated electrode toward the surgeon treats the anterior and posterior walls by either moving the entire hysteroscope or closing the electrode or a combination of these two movements.

The complications of TCRE are similar to fibroid resection. The most serious complication is uterine perforation. This can be minimized by using the rollerball particularly in the cornual and fundal areas. Other serious complications include fluid overload, primary hemorrhage, and gas embolism from the bubbles produced by the electrode entering an open vessel. An important cause for treatment failure is a hematometra. It usually presents as cyclical menstrual pain after TCRE. The diagnosis is made when ultrasound or MRI shows a fluid-filled cavity. Treatment is with either hysterectomy or cervical dilatation and drainage. If drainage is attempted, then this may need to be done under ultrasound guidance due to the dense intrauterine adhesions that can form after resection.

8.4   Technique for Second-Generation Endometrial Ablation

Rates of satisfaction are consistently high for second-generation techniques, and they are now an established alternative to hysterectomy. The three most commonly used second-generation devices reported in the literature utilize energy applied via thermal balloons, bipolar radio-frequency electricity, and microwave energy. A network meta-analysis showed that bipolar radio frequency and microwave ablative devices are more effective than thermal balloon and free-fluid ablation in the treatment of heavy menstrual bleeding in terms of inducing amenorrhea (Daniels et al. 2012). However, while a new small microwave device has been introduced (Minitouch™), these data relate to the original larger diameter Microsulis™ system that has now been taken off the market for commercial rather than clinical reasons. Longer-term data comparing bipolar radio frequency and thermal balloon devices have shown no difference in re-intervention rates or health-related quality of life (Kleijn et al. 2008; Smith et al. 2014a). Table 1 summarizes the types and features of currently available ablative technologies.

9 Hysteroscopic Treatment of Acquired Uterine Abnormalities

9.1 Intrauterine Adhesions

Intrauterine adhesions are defined by scar tissue between the uterine walls. This is also called Asherman's syndrome. It was thought that it occurred following excessively vigorous curettage of the endometrium in a recently pregnant or pregnant uterus. However, it can occur after an infection of the uterus or uterine surgery. Patients rarely present with cyclical pain due to trapped menses but more commonly with amenorrhea and infertility. Hysteroscopy is the gold standard for accurate diagnosis and assessment of intrauterine adhesions. A hysterosalpingogram can also be screening test and has the advantage of being able to assess tubal patency in patients with infertility problems.

The type and extent of intrauterine adhesions have been classified according to Valle and Sciarra (Table 2). Other classification systems such as the American Fertility Society classification exist (Valle and Sciarra 1988).

9.2 Technique

Various different techniques can be employed to restore the size and shape of the uterine cavity. Where there are filmy adhesions only, balloon

Table 1 Description of currently available second-generation endometrial ablation devices and outcome data

Device	Mode of action	Source of information	Treatment duration	Heavy bleeding rate (%)	Amenorrhea rates (1 year) (%)	Satisfaction rates (1 year) (%)
Electrical						
NovaSure	Fan-shaped bipolar radio-frequency electrode	(Smith et al. 2014a)	90 s	8	56	93
Thermal balloon						
Thermablate	Balloon with heated glycine	(Penninx et al. 2016)	128 s	21	23	69
Cavaterm	Balloon with heated glycine	(Brun et al. 2006; Hawe et al. 2003)	10 min	3–7	33–36	81–93
Free-flowing saline						
Hydrothermablation	A closed system is formed with the cavity to deliver heated saline directly to the endometrium	(Corson 2001; Penninx et al. 2011)	10 min	14–18	24–38	79
Microwave						
Minitouch	Microwave energy via an induction loop placed in the uterine cavity	(Tas and Van Herendael 2014)	60 s	Not available	84	Not available

Table 2 Classification system for intrauterine adhesions

Mild	Filmy adhesions composed of basal endometrium, producing partial or complete uterine cavity occlusion
Moderate	Fibromuscular adhesions that are characteristically thick and still covered by endometrium. They may bleed on division, partially or totally
Severe	Composed of connective tissue with no endometrial lining and likely to bleed upon division, partially or totally occluding the uterine cavity

distension and insertion of intrauterine contraceptive devices have been described as non-hysteroscopic techniques. Hysteroscopic techniques have the advantage of being performed under direct vision, and various methods have been employed depending on the severity of the intrauterine adhesions. These include blunt or sharp adhesiolysis, using mechanical methods, laser instrument, and electrosurgical instruments. Simple distension of the uterine cavity during diagnostic hysteroscopy has also been described for adhesiolysis of filmy adhesions.

In some patients, landmarks remain obscure and entry into the uterus may not be possible. In these patients, it is necessary to perform simultaneous laparoscopy, fluoroscopy, or ultrasound to reduce the risk of perforation. Ultrasound is more useful for patients with lower segment scarring that have a normal upper segment. With laparoscopic guidance, the light source of the laparoscope is reduced so that the light from the hysteroscope can be observed through the uterus to locate its position and minimize the risk of uterine perforation. A uniform glow of the uterus is reassuring, while focused light indicates impending perforation. With complex cases, the risk of intravasation of the distension media is increased so, as with all operative hysteroscopy, careful fluid balance monitoring is required.

Increased uterine cavity size can be achieved by myometrial scoring with scissors or a Colling's knife electrode. Drawing the resectoscope from the fundus toward the isthmus with the knife electrode continuously activated makes the myometrial incisions. The Colling's knife electrode is used at a power setting of 100 W at pure cutting current. This is repeated around eight times so that equally spaced incisions are made around the complete radius of the uterine cavity and it opens up like an accordion. Myometrial scoring has also been described using miniature bipolar electrodes in an attempt to increase the capacity of a hypoplastic or T-shaped uterus (Di Spiezio Sardo et al. 2015).

Various postoperative interventions have been described to try and reduce the likelihood of recurrence of adhesions. Insertion of inert intrauterine devices or Foley balloon catheters has been used in an attempt to help maintain separation of the uterine walls. Postoperative estrogen therapy is thought to promote endometrial overgrowth and re-epithelialization of the scarred surface. Steroids have been advocated to reduce the inflammatory response as well as antibiotics to prevent endometritis. Repeated postoperative office hysteroscopy with mechanical lysis of new, filmy adhesions, prior to them becoming fibrous, until no new adhesions form has recently been reported (Yang et al. 2016).

9.3 Retained Products of Conception

Chronically retained products of conception (RPOC) or placental remnants can occur after miscarriage, termination of pregnancy, vaginal deliveries, and cesarean deliveries. Retained products of conception can be associated with short-term problems such as infection, abdominal pain, and uterine bleeding. Long-term problems include the formation of intrauterine adhesions. The most common treatment for RPOC is dilation with suction, blunt, or sharp curettage. However, for RPOC beyond 6 weeks' duration, hysteroscopic alternatives are emerging which facilitate focused and complete removal under direct vision, potentially reducing the risk of uterine trauma and intrauterine adhesions.

9.4 Technique

The techniques described include use of a cold (inactivated) resection loop to mechanically remove RPOC by entrapment of tissue between the loop, and the hysteroscope and repeated removal and insertion of the resectoscope until the cavity is empty. The use of tissue removal systems to selectively remove tissue under direct vision has been reported and seems well suited to this task as electrosurgical energy is not needed and tissue can be simultaneously cut away and extracted avoiding repeated insertion and removal of the hysteroscope (Hamerlynck et al. 2013; Smorgick et al. 2014). There is a lack of evidence to suggest that the hysteroscopic technique is superior to blind surgical evacuation at the moment. Nevertheless, in selected cases such as previous failed surgery or where there are known structural abnormalities, the hysteroscopic approach may be appropriate. Research is required to help guide best practice.

10 Hysteroscopic Treatment of Congenital Uterine Anomalies

10.1 Uterine Septum

Hysteroscopic septoplasty describes the resection of an intrauterine septum that is a Müllerian duct anomaly. The uterus and fallopian tubes are formed as the paramesonephric ducts fuse caudally in early embryonic life forming the fallopian tubes, uterine cavity, and upper third of the vagina. During the fusion of the paramesonephric ducts, a septum is formed in the uterine cavity that is usually reabsorbed by 20 weeks of gestation. Failure of the reabsorption process results in a septate uterus, which can be either partial or complete and in severe cases can extend to involve the cervix and the top of the vagina. This can be distinguished from a bicornuate uterus, in which there is failure of the fusion of the paramesonephric ducts, because there is no effect on the uterine body.

Hysteroscopic resection of the intrauterine septum has superseded conventional abdominal approaches to metroplasty that included the John's or Tompkin's technique. Not only do hysteroscopic procedures reduce the morbidity compared to the abdominal approach, but they also produce superior reproductive outcomes. Because the integrity of the uterine cavity is not breeched, hysteroscopic procedures avoid the risks of uterine rupture during labor.

10.2 Technique

The principle of septoplasty is to divide the septum along the midpoint rather than excise the septum. The tissue is usually fibroelastic, so does not bleed. Division can be done using electrosurgery using either the Versapoint™ electrode or resectoscopic division using a Colling's knife electrode. Mechanical division can be achieved using scissors. Electrosurgical and mechanical techniques can be combined. More rarely laser such as Nd:YAG can be used. Whichever technique is used, the operator has to take special care to determine the depth and direction of cutting, especially as the division of the septum often requires hysteroscopic movements toward the fundus that increase the risk of perforation. To try and reduce the risk of the perforation, the operator should not aim to create a cavity that is arcuate. Depth of cutting can be further assessed with either simultaneous ultrasound or laparoscopy. With laparoscopy, the intensity of the light source is reduced so that the intensity of light from the hysteroscope can be monitored. If the uterus glows in a uniform manner, it is presumed that the risk of perforation is low. Laparoscopy also has the advantage of keeping bowel away from the uterus but is not as accurate as ultrasound for assessing the depth of myometrium. However, if preoperative radiological imaging with either 2D/3D ultrasound or MRI clearly distinguishes a septate uterus from a bicornuate uterus, then a purely hysteroscopic approach is feasible. The operator should look out for soft, trabeculated, pink myometrial tissue as opposed to the pale, smooth, fibroelastic septal tissue to ascertain when the limits of the septum in relation to the uterine fundus has been reached. Bleeding is not a reliable indicator of reaching myometrial tissue as the high inflow pressures of distending media may tamponade such bleeding. If both cornual recesses can be visualized with the hysteroscope at the level of the internal os and the sound length is at least 7 cm, then an adequate uterine cavity has been restored following septoplasty.

Hysteroscopic metroplasty to restore the shape of the hypoplastic or "T"-shaped uterus has been reported by scoring the myometrium with activated miniature bipolar electrodes in an attempt to increase the uterine capacity (Di Spiezio Sardo et al. 2015). The electrodes can also be used to create outflow channels in non-communicating rudimentary uterine horns with the aid of ultrasound or laparoscopic guidance. Foley catheters can then be hysteroscopically placed to allow fistulization to occur creating permanent outflow tract.

11   Hysteroscopic Sterilization

Since the introduction of hysteroscopic sterilization, it has steadily increased in popularity, although more recently the US Food and Drug Administration (FDA) has required the device manufacturer, Bayer, to conduct a post-marketing surveillance study to compare adverse events with Essure™ with those seen with tubal ligation due to complaints from some patients and recent re-intervention data (Mao et al. 2015). The benefits of hysteroscopic sterilization are that it avoids the abdominal route, it allows a quicker return to normal activities, and it can be performed without general anesthesia. These advantages make hysteroscopic sterilization a good option for women who want to avoid, or have contraindications, general anesthesia and abdominal surgery. The most commonly applied technique is Essure™, which involves the placement of a 4 cm expanding spring into the fallopian tubes (Fig. 9). New warnings must be printed on the labels of the implantable sterilization device Essure™ after reports of serious side effects.

The reported rates of successful bilateral placement vary between 81% and 98% with higher success rates in studies published since 2007 (la Chapelle et al. 2015). Following successful bilateral placement, confirmation of correct placement rates is between 90% and 100% (la Chapelle et al. 2015). Hysteroscopic sterilization with the Essure™ system is an effective method of contraception. In a case series of 4306 procedures, a total of seven women (0.16%) became pregnant. Of these seven, three ignored advice to refrain from intercourse before assessment for satisfactory placement, bringing the pregnancy rate after establishing correct placement to 0.09% (Povedano et al. 2012).

Reported serious complications are rare, and in the largest series reported to date of over 4000 procedures, the most common adverse event was vasovagal reaction, which occurred in around 2% of cases. Expulsion of the micro-insert occurred in 0.4% of women, although this occurred before the 3-month follow-up in most cases. In three cases, the micro-inserts were erroneously placed in the myometrium (0.06%), and in two other cases, there was asymptomatic migration into the abdominal cavity (0.04%). The migrated devices were left in the abdominal cavity. There were also two cases of pelvic inflammatory disease (0.02%). Longer-term complications included two allergies to nickel (0.04%) and one woman who had persistent abdominal pain (0.02%) (Povedano et al. 2012). Because the incidence of nickel allergy is so low, it has been removed as contraindication to placement. Nevertheless, it is good practice to tell patients that the micro-inserts do contain small amounts of nickel, but it is unlikely to be clinically significant. It is more difficult to treat longer-term complications which often require coil removal via an abdominal route. This can be complicated because the micro-insert may be lodged in surrounding structures and can conduct electrical energy making removal difficult.

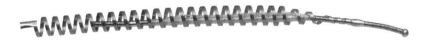

Fig. 9 Essure™ micro-insert

A recent US cohort study compared 8048 patients undergoing hysteroscopic sterilization with over 40,000 undergoing laparoscopic sterilization between 2005 and 2013, and they found, at 1 year after surgery, the risk of unintended pregnancy was around 1% and comparable between techniques. However, around 1 in 50 women undergoing hysteroscopic sterilization required reoperation to complete, reverse, or rectify complications arising from the procedure compared with 1 in 500 women undergoing laparoscopic sterilization (Mao et al. 2015). While the convenience of office-based hysteroscopic sterilization will be attractive to many women, they also need to be informed of the reoperation data to help them decide which sterilization procedure is most appropriate for them.

11.1 Equipment

11.2 Essure Technique

Prior to the procedure, nonsteroidal anti-inflammatory drugs (NSAIDs) are given to reduce tubal spasm, although evidence for this practice is not strong (Chern and Siow 2005; Nichols et al. 2006). There is no need to routinely give antibiotics during hysteroscopic sterilization.

The introducer provided is inserted to prevent retrograde leakage of distension fluid along the working channel into the working channel of the hysteroscope, which is then inserted through the cervical canal under direct vision to access the uterine cavity. This can usually be achieved vaginoscopically without the need for vaginal instrumentation or local anesthesia unless the woman is nulliparous or undergone cesarean sections or cone biopsies of the cervix. Both tubal ostia need to be visualized before beginning the procedure. This is best done by gently rotating the hysteroscope to allow the offset lens to look in each lateral direction.

The first micro-insert delivery catheter is then fed along the working channel and the offset lens of the hysteroscope closely aligned with the selected tubal ostia (Fig. 10). Close proximity of the distal hysteroscope to the tubal ostia aids precise passage of the device minimizing the risk of tubal spasm. The rigid hysteroscope can also act to splint the fragile micro-insert, preventing it bending if tubal resistance is encountered. With gentle forward movements, the micro-insert is passed into and along the tube until the black positioning marker on the insertion catheter is flush with the ostia (Fig. 11). The surgeon or assistant then retracts the outer catheter by rotating the thumbwheel until it will no longer rotate. Using careful movements, the gold marker on the micro-insert should then be aligned just outside of the tubal ostia (Fig. 12). Pressing the button on the handle deploys the micro-insert. Rotating the thumbwheel again until it will no longer rotate retracts the inner catheter. Ideally three to eight expanded coils should be seen in the uterine cavity (Fig. 13).

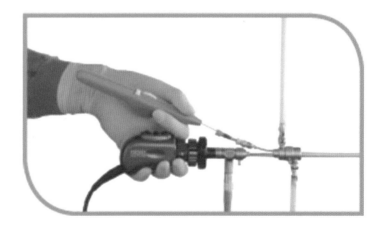

Fig. 10 Essure™ **hysteroscopic system of sterilization**; with the help of an introducer, the Essure catheter goes down the operating channel of a hysteroscope to allow deployment of the Essure insert in the fallopian tube

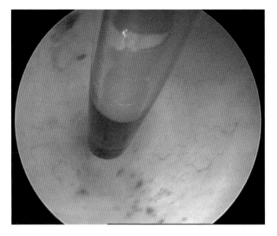

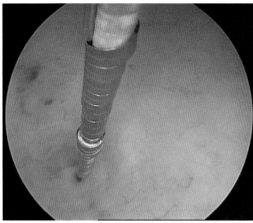

Fig. 11 Placement of the Essure™ micro-insert into the tubal ostia; the catheter tip is advanced into the fallopian tube until the black marker reaches the ostia

Fig. 12 Placement of the Essure™ micro-insert into the tubal ostia; the catheter is retracted, and the black positioning marker disappears. The gold band must be located just outside the ostium before the insert is detached

11.3 Confirmation of Correct Placement

The main disadvantage of hysteroscopic sterilization compared to laparoscopic sterilization is that it is not immediately effective; at least 3 months is required before tubal fibrosis and occlusion occur for the procedure to be effective. During this time, the woman needs to use alternative forms of contraception. After 3 months, post-procedure imaging is required to check for placement and occlusion. In the USA, the FDA requires a hysterosalpingogram for all patients with Essure™ sterilization to confirm tubal occlusion. In Europe, X-ray and transvaginal ultrasound are accepted, less invasive alternative radiological confirmation tests to confirm satisfactory device placement. Confirmation of the correct location has been reported to correlate well with effectiveness (Veersema et al. 2005).

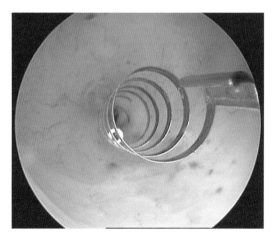

Fig. 13 Placement of the Essure™ micro-insert into the tubal ostia; the catheter tip is advanced into the fallopian tube until the black marker reaches the ostia. Once the catheter is withdrawn, three to eight coils should be seen outside the ostium

12 Hysteroscopic Tubal Occlusion for the Treatment of Hydrosalpinges

Essure can be considered in women who require tubal occlusion prior to in vitro fertilization (IVF) as treatment for hydrosalpinges. Although there may be some concern regarding the effect of a

foreign body on embryo implantation, there appears to be tissue encapsulation of the device after implantation. Several small studies have reported pregnancies from IVF following sterilization with Essure. A retrospective review of all pregnancies reported after Essure in situ in the Netherlands, including unintentional (failed Essure procedures) and those that were intentional, resulting from off-label use of Essure micro-inserts for hydrosalpinx closure before in vitro fertilization, intracytoplasmic sperm injection with embryo transfer, or in vitro fertilization with embryo transfer after regret of sterilization (Veersema et al. 2014). Of the 8 unintended pregnancies and 18 intended pregnancies, all resulted in birth of a full-term healthy baby. So it appears unlikely that the presence of intratubal micro-inserts interferes with implantation and the developing amniotic sac and fetus.

12.1 Technique

The technique is as described previously for Essure hysteroscopic sterilization. Some operators advocate more distal placement of the micro-inserts so that no more than three trailing coils are within the uterine cavity. In the presence of a unilateral hydrosalpinx, a single device placement only is required.

13 Hysteroscopic Tubal Cannulation

Tubal catheterization is a technique used to treat a proximal fallopian tube blockage (PTB) diagnosed following hysterosalpingogram (HSG). It is thought that the narrow and thick, less ciliated proximal segment of the fallopian tube is particularly prone to obstruction, initially by material that can flow back from the uterus, and then in the luteal phase of the cycle by secretions produced locally. As PTB generally occurs in otherwise undamaged tubes, tubal catheterization can potentially successfully re-cannulize the tube.

Data for hysteroscopic treatment of PTB is scarce especially in the ambulatory setting. Tubal catheterization is reported to be successful in approximately 50% of patients (10), and 20–40% of these women have been reported to become pregnant either spontaneously or after ovulation induction or intrauterine insemination (Robinson et al. 2013).

13.1 Equipment

The tubal catheterization system is shown in Fig. 14. The cannula and guidewire fit down the standard 5Fr-working channel of an operating hysteroscope. Procedures can be performed in both the inpatient and outpatient setting.

13.2 Technique for Tubal Cannulation

The radiological procedure of selective salpingography and tubal catheterization has

Fig. 14 Tubal catheter system for hysteroscopic tubal cannulation of proximal tubal occlusions

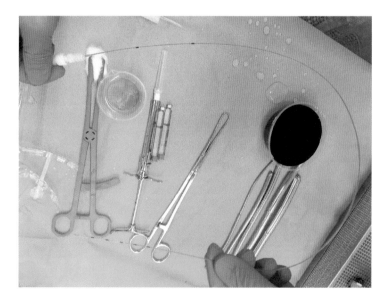

been adapted for use under direct hysteroscopic vision thereby avoiding exposure to ionizing radiation. A 5–5.5 mm 30° continuous flow operative hysteroscope is inserted. A fine catheter is passed down the 5-7Fr working channel of the hysteroscope and guided toward the tubal ostium. The catheter is pushed gently under vision into the tubal ostium and methylene blue dye instilled via a syringe, through the lumen of the catheter. If this does not overcome the obstruction, i.e., the catheter cannot be passed into the tubal ostium or retrograde spill of dye is noted despite forward instillation pressure, a guidewire is railroaded through the lumen of the catheter. The guidewire is pushed gently into the cornual portion of the tube and the instillation of dye repeated.

Hysteroscopic tubal cannulation can also be done in theater as a day case under laparoscopic guidance and a dye test performed at the end of the procedure to assess tubal patency. In the ambulatory hysteroscopy setting, confirmation that PTB has been overcome can be inferred by ease of passage dye without retrograde spill, pre- and post-procedure transvaginal pelvic ultrasound (TVS) to look for free fluid within the pelvis, and hysterosalpingo-contrast sonography scanning or follow-up HSG arranged to confirm restoration of tubal patency.

Risks of the procedure include pelvic infection and uterine trauma. Excessive forward pressure must be avoided, especially if using a fine guide wire, as this risks tubal perforation. This complication should be suspected where the patient experiences acute, sharp, localized pain as the serosal surface of the uterus is breached. The risk of tubal perforation during the procedure is approximately 2%.

14   Outpatient Procedures

Initially hysteroscopy was developed as an inpatient procedure, but advances in equipment, in particular the reduction in size of optics, have allowed first diagnostic and now a range of minor operative procedures in the outpatient setting (Clark and Gupta 2005; Clark et al. 2002b, Kremer et al. 2000). Outpatient hysteroscopy, ambulatory hysteroscopy, and office hysteroscopy all describe procedures that are done without general anesthetic and avoid admission to hospital. Women value the convenience of an immediate diagnosis and treatment. Not only is office treatment well-accepted and convenient, but it also has been shown to be more cost effective (Cooper and Clark; Moawad et al. 2014).

14.1   Equipment and Technique

Office hysteroscopy has the potential to perform the following minor hysteroscopic procedures without the need to readmit the patient to hospital:

- Localization and removal of a missed intrauterine contraceptive devices
- Endometrial polypectomy
- Resection of small type 0 submucous fibroid/office preparation of partially intramural myomas (OPPIuM) – mucosal incision
- Minor adhesiolysis (filmy adhesions)
- Endometrial ablation using second-generation devices
- Outpatient sterilization
- Tubal catheterization

The equipment and operative techniques have been provided in the preceding sections. One of the biggest challenges in office hysteroscopy is pain relief. National, evidence-based guidelines have been published for best practice when conducting office hysteroscopy to minimize adverse outcomes and optimize the patient experience (Clark et al. 2011). As with any procedure that involves the instrumentation of the uterus, this can be associated with pain, anxiety, and embarrassment. Thus, in addition to a gentle, atraumatic, proficient, and expeditious surgical approach utilizing small-diameter instrumentation, communication with the patient becomes paramount, and this can be promoted by having a member of staff dedicated to providing reassurance and support in what has been termed the vocal-local. In women without contraindications, analgesia should be taken 1 h before the procedure to reduce postoperative pain. Conscious sedation with inhalational agents such as nitrous oxide may be useful in patients who are very anxious. There is not sufficient evidence to recommend routine use of cervical preparation, but all women who require cervical dilation should receive local anesthetic.

15 Safety of Operative Hysteroscopy

15.1 Complications

All procedures have risks of complications, and hysteroscopic procedures are no exception. There are general risks associated with anesthesia, and there are risks associated with the specific procedure. With hysteroscopic procedures, there are particular risks of inserting and activating electrosurgical, thermal, or mechanical instruments within the uterus, and there are risks associated with the distension media. Insertion of the instruments is often made more difficult because of the cervical dilatation needed to accommodate the larger diameter operating instruments. Intravasation of distension media is also more of a problem due to longer operating times and opening up of deep myometrial vessels during resection of type 1 and 2 submucous fibroids. Other perioperative complications include hemorrhage, cervical trauma, uterine perforation, and electrosurgical burns. Postoperative endometritis or ascending pelvic infection can occur although the routine use of prophylactic antibiotics is not recommended (Van Eyk et al. 2012; Thinkhamrop et al. 2007). Rare late complications can include intrauterine adhesions, uterine rupture, and hematometra after endometrial destruction techniques.

In a prospective multicenter study of 13,600 women looking at complications of hysteroscopic procedures, diagnostic procedures had significantly fewer complications (0.13%) than operative procedures (0.28%). The most common complication for operative procedures was uterine perforation (0.76%). Four cases of perforation resulted in heavy bleeding that required treatment by laparoscopy (n = 2), laparotomy (n = 1), or

hysterectomy (n = 1). Fluid overload, defined as the absorption of more than 1500 mL of distension media with clinical consequences for the patient, occurred in 0.2% of operative procedures. Four of the five cases occurred during fibroid resection and one during an endometrial resection. The operative procedure associated with most complications was adhesiolysis, risk of complication 4.5%, compared to the least risky operative procedure polypectomy, risk of complication 0.4% (Jansen et al. 2000).

Using good equipment and attaining surgical proficiency through adequate training and an appropriate caseload in clinical practice as well as considering the potential causes of operative difficulties can minimize complications. Possible causes for common problems during operative hysteroscopy include:

- Difficulty with dilation of cervix – scar tissue, acutely anteverted or retroverted uterus, formation of a false passage
- Poor vision – inadequate distension, out of focus, debris (increase suction, open outflow, clear blocked suction holes)
- Bleeding during hysteroscopy – low distension pressure, inefficient coagulation, cutting too deeply
- Rapid fluid absorption – high distension pressure, transecting deep myometrial vessels, uterine perforation

15.2 Case Selection

Case selection is important to minimize complications, particularly when learning new techniques. For example, when learning fibroid resection, it is advisable to master the resection of small type 0 or 1 submucous fibroids attached to the uterine sidewalls before moving onto larger, deeper type 2 or fundal fibroids. Theoretically type 2 fibroids can be hysteroscopically resected if they are not transmural. However, there are some cases that even experienced surgeons should not attempt. Although counterintuitive, the highest complication rates were in those surgeons performing >50 procedures. This may be because the more experienced surgeons are doing the most difficult cases, but it also emphasizes the importance of audit and careful consideration before procedures are performed (Jansen et al. 2000).

Not only is it important to consider the complexity of the case but also pain relief and embarrassment with procedures done in the ambulatory setting without anesthesia. Various strategies can be employed to reduce pain, but some patients will find these procedures very embarrassing or painful, and it can be difficult to predict. Important clues can be gained by how the patient has tolerated other uterine procedures such as endometrial biopsies or diagnostic hysteroscopy. If dilation of the cervix is needed, local anesthetic should be used. Analgesia and antiemetics can also be given prior to the procedure. It is important to have a low threshold for stopping the procedure in the ambulatory setting.

16   Teaching

National training bodies, such as the Royal College of Obstetricians and Gynaecologists (RCOG) and American Association of Gynecologic Laparoscopists (AAGL), are providing structured training and accreditation packages for hysteroscopic training. The RCOG has provided a list of procedures stratified by complexity and therefore risk (Table 3).

Operative hysteroscopy skills are difficult to learn, and structured training and mentorship is required for competencies to be achieved. The rapid increase in the number of procedures done while patients are awake along with decreased training hours has led to legal and ethical concerns about training on real patients. Many minimally invasive training programs around the world have tried to tackle this by incorporating training outside the operating room. There are models and computerized simulators that are now available to help performance. However, the application of hysteroscopic models appears to have lagged behind the use of their laparoscopic counterparts.

Table 3 RCOG classification of operative hysteroscopy levels

Level 1	Diagnostic hysteroscopy with target biopsy Removal of simple polyps Removal of intrauterine contraceptive device
Level 2	Proximal fallopian tube cannulation Minor Asherman's syndrome Removal of pedunculated fibroid (type 0) or large polyp
Level 3	Division/resection of uterine septum Major Asherman's syndrome Endometrial resection or ablation Resection of submucous fibroid (type 1 or type 2) Repeat endometrial ablation or resection

Despite this, a wide variety of models have been used although few of them have been validated. Animal tissues such as pig bladders have been used as "wet" models. Pig bladders can be used to simulate endometrial ablation, and by using stitches, they can also be used to simulate polyp and septum resection (Hiemstra et al. 2008). Animal hearts have also been used to simulate endometrial ablation and resection. Training on vegetables offers a cheaper and more readily available method. Reports of peppers and squash being used to practice biopsy and tissue removal have been stated (Hiemstra et al. 2008; Kingston et al. 2004).

Training using plastic models or box trainers has been shown to improve resident performance (Burchard et al. 2007). Tactile skills can be improved performing abstract tasks such as removal of pin from the sidewall of plastic uterus, or models with fake pathology for resection have been made (Burchard et al. 2007).

Virtual reality simulators create a safe and controlled environment, but more importantly, they create standardized environments that allow the objective performance of the trainee. The VirtaMed HystSim™ (Hysteroscopic Surgery Simulator System) (Zurich, Switzerland) is the only hysteroscopic simulator available, and it has a large number of stored cases and pathologies with different levels of difficulty. The disadvantage of the simulator is the high cost and the lack of haptic feedback.

17 Clinical Governance and Audit

An important part of clinical governance is risk management. Periodic assessment of infection control, staff training, equipment condition, patient information leaflets, and local protocols should be performed.

Audit is an essential tool to improve and maintain standards especially when setting up new services. Areas suggested for audit include:

- Complications of hysteroscopic surgery (e.g., uterine perforation, fluid overload, infection, vasovagal reactions, heavy bleeding, and cervical trauma)
- Failure rates of operative hysteroscopy
- Standards of documentation
- Use of perioperative and postoperative analgesia
- Patient satisfaction in terms of pain experienced, acceptability, and quality of services

18 Future Developments

In the past, new developments in operative hysteroscopy have been dominated by miniaturization of equipment. With an increasing number of procedures being performed in the office setting, it is likely that future developments will also focus on miniaturization. Essential to the miniaturization of equipment are improvements in optics and exciting developments are expected from optical chip technology in hysteroscopy, such as the Invisio Digital Hysteroscope (GyrusACMI/Olympus, Tokyo, Japan). Portability is also becoming increasingly important such that hysteroscopy can be performed in a variety of community settings. The Endosee® office hysteroscopy system incorporates a disposable inflow cannula light lead and camera and a reusable lightweight handset incorporating a tiny touch LCD screen. Other similar and totally disposable systems are likely to be developed or ones compatible with smart devices to provide imaging and data recoding.

One of the biggest challenges in hysteroscopy is to improve pain relief and acceptability of procedures in the outpatient setting. Not only is research needed to improve the technology, but also research is needed to optimize technique and patient selection. The further refinement of tissue removal systems and evaluations of how they compare with bipolar electrosurgery for polyps and fibroids will be forthcoming. The Symphion™ system (Boston Scientific) is a new, tissue removal system utilizing radio-frequency energy and direct intrauterine fluid pressure monitoring.

For endometrial ablation, future developments will focus on improvements to existing technologies, such as miniaturization, portability, disposability and shortened treatment times, and the development of new technologies with utilizing a variety of previously tried and new energies such as cryotherapy, microwave energy, and steam.

The main disadvantage of hysteroscopic sterilization is that women need to find an alternative form of contraception for at least 3 months while the fibrosis and occlusion of the tubes occur. Even after 3 months, occlusion will not occur in 1–12% of women (Duffy et al. 2005; Levie and Chudnoff 2006; Sinha et al. 2007). Future developments will focus on techniques that will occlude the tubes in such a way as to provide immediate contraception.

19 Conclusion

Operative hysteroscopy has an increasing role in the management of uterine problems causing abnormal uterine bleeding and reproductive failure and can be used to provide sterilization. Treatments have shown to be safe, effective, and an acceptable replacement to more invasive surgery such as hysterectomy, and this is increasingly the case with the development of new operative hysteroscopic technologies such as tissue removal systems and bipolar electrosurgery. There has been an increasing movement, driven by the miniaturization, feasibility, and portability of new endoscopic technologies as well as patient expectations, toward performing procedures, while patients are awake in an office setting. This helps to reduce cost and complications of general anesthesia. Surgeons undertaking operative hysteroscopic procedures should ensure they have a sufficient caseload to maintain their skills and audit performance and outcome. Best practice guidelines should help inform practice. In addition, valid and structured training and accreditation packages for hysteroscopic training need to be implemented and keep pace with contemporary technologies and the evolving evidence.

20 Cross-References

▶ Basic Management of Infertility
▶ Diagnosis and Management of the Cancer of the Uterus
▶ Laparoscopic Hysterectomy
▶ Laparoscopic Myomectomy: Best Practices
▶ Management of Abnormal Uterine Bleeding: Later Reproductive Years
▶ Management of Pelvic Pain, Dyspareunia, and Endometriosis
▶ Management of Recurrent Pregnancy Loss
▶ Management of Uterine Fibroids
▶ Pathology of the Uterine Corpus
▶ Treatment of Gynecological Congenital Anomalies

References

Berg A, Sandvik L, Langebrekke A, Istre O. A randomized trial comparing monopolar electrodes using glycine 1.5% with two different types of bipolar electrodes (TCRis, Versapoint) using saline, in hysteroscopic surgery. Fertil Steril. 2009;91:1273–8.

Bettocchi S, Ceci O, Nappi L, Di Venere R, Masciopinto V, Pansini V, Pinto L, Santoro A, Cormio G. Operative office hysteroscopy without anesthesia: analysis of 4863 cases performed with mechanical instruments. J Am Assoc Gynecol Laparosc. 2004;11:59–61.

Birinyi L, Daragó P, Török P, Csiszár P, Major T, Borsos A, Bacskó G. Predictive value of hysteroscopic examination in intrauterine abnormalities. Eur J Obstet Gynecol Reprod Biol. 2004;115:75–9.

Brooks PG. Resectoscopic myoma vaporizer. J Reprod Med. 1995;40:791–5.

Brun J-L, Raynal J, Burlet G, Galand B, Quéreux C, Bernard P. Cavaterm thermal balloon endometrial ablation versus hysteroscopic endometrial resection to treat menorrhagia: the French, multicenter, randomized study. J Minim Invasive Gynecol. 2006;13:424–30.

Burchard ER, Lockrow EG, Zahn CM, Dunlow SG, Satin AJ. Simulation training improves resident performance in operative hysteroscopic resection techniques. Am J Obstet Gynecol. 2007;197:542.e1–4.

Chern B, Siow A. Initial Asian experience in hysteroscopic sterilisation using the Essure permanent birth control device. BJOG Int J Obstet Gynaecol. 2005;112:1322–7.

Clark TJ, Gupta JK. Handbook of outpatient hysteroscopy: a complete guide to diagnosis and therapy. CRC Press, London, UK; 2005.

Clark TJ, Cooper NAM, Kremer C. Best Practice in Outpatient Hysteroscopy. Best Practice in Outpatient Hysteroscopy: Green Top Guideline 59. RCOG/BSGE Joint Green Top Guideline. RCOG 2011 https://www.rcog.org.uk/globalassets/documents/guidelines/gtg59hysteroscopy.pdf

Clark TJ, Godwin J, Khan KS, Gupta JK. Ambulatory endoscopic treatment of symptomatic benign endometrial polyps: feasibility study. Gynaecol Endosc. 2002a;11:91–7.

Clark TJ, Bakour SH, Gupta JK, Khan KS. Evaluation of outpatient hysteroscopy and ultrasonography in the diagnosis of endometrial disease. Obstet Gynecol. 2002b;99:1001–7.

Cooper NAM, Barton PM, Breijer MC, Caffrey O, Opmeer BC, Timmermans A, Mol BWJ, Khan KS, Clark TJ. NIHR HTA Project: 09/63/01 - Cost-effectiveness of diagnostic strategies for the management of abnormal uterine bleeding (heavy menstrual bleeding and postmenopausal bleeding): Model based economic evaluation. Health Technol Assess 2014;18:1-201. (https://www.journalslibrary.nihr.ac.uk/hta/hta18240#/abstract)

Cooper NAM, Smith P, Khan KS, Clark TJ. Does cervical preparation before outpatient hysteroscopy reduce women's pain experience? A systematic review. BJOG Int J Obstet Gynaecol. 2011a;118:1292–301.

Cooper NAM, Smith P, Khan KS, Clark TJ. A systematic review of the effect of the distension medium on pain during outpatient hysteroscopy. Fertil Steril. 2011b;95:264–71.

Cooper NAM, Clark TJ, Middleton L, Diwakar L, Smith P, Denny E, Roberts T, Stobert L, Jowett S, Daniels J, et al. Outpatient versus inpatient uterine polyp treatment for abnormal uterine bleeding: randomised controlled non-inferiority study. BMJ. 2015;350:h1398.

Corson SL. A multicenter evaluation of endometrial ablation by Hydro ThermAblator and rollerball for treatment of menorrhagia. J Am Assoc Gynecol Laparosc. 2001;8:359–67.

Daniels JP, Middleton LJ, Champaneria R, Khan KS, Cooper K, Mol BWJ, Bhattacharya S, International Heavy Menstrual Bleeding IPD Meta-analysis Collaborative Group. Second generation endometrial ablation techniques for heavy menstrual bleeding: network meta-analysis. BMJ. 2012;344:e2564.

de Kroon CD, de Bock GH, Dieben SWM, Jansen FW. Saline contrast hysterosonography in abnormal uterine bleeding: a systematic review and meta-analysis. BJOG Int J Obstet Gynaecol. 2003;110:938–47.

Di Spiezio Sardo A, Florio P, Nazzaro G, Spinelli M, Paladini D, Di Carlo C, Nappi C. Hysteroscopic outpatient metroplasty to expand dysmorphic uteri (HOME-DU technique): a pilot study. Reprod Biomed Online. 2015;30:166–74.

Donnez J, Tatarchuk TF, Bouchard P, Puscasiu L, Zakharenko NF, Ivanova T, Ugocsai G, Mara M, Jilla MP, Bestel E, et al. Ulipristal acetate versus placebo for fibroid treatment before surgery. N Engl J Med. 2012a;366:409–20.

Donnez J, Tomaszewski J, Vázquez F, Bouchard P, Lemieszczuk B, Baró F, Nouri K, Selvaggi L, Sodowski K, Bestel E, et al. Ulipristal acetate versus leuprolide acetate for uterine fibroids. N Engl J Med. 2012b;366:421–32.

Duffy S, Marsh F, Rogerson L, Hudson H, Cooper K, Jack S, Hunter D, Philips G. Female sterilisation: a cohort controlled comparative study of ESSURE versus laparoscopic sterilisation. BJOG Int J Obstet Gynaecol. 2005;112:1522–8.

El-Nashar SA, Hopkins MR, Creedon DJ, St Sauver JL, Weaver AL, McGree ME, Cliby WA, Famuyide AO. Prediction of treatment outcomes after global endometrial ablation. Obstet Gynecol. 2009;113:97–106.

Garuti G, Centinaio G, Luerti M. Outpatient hysteroscopic polypectomy in postmenopausal women: a comparison between mechanical and electrosurgical resection. J Minim Invasive Gynecol. 2008;15:595–600.

Hamerlynck TWO, Blikkendaal MD, Schoot BC, Hanstede MMF, Jansen FW. An alternative approach for removal of placental remnants: hysteroscopic morcellation. J Minim Invasive Gynecol. 2013;20:796–802.

Hawe J, Abbott J, Hunter D, Phillips G, Garry R. A randomised controlled trial comparing the Cavaterm endometrial ablation system with the Nd:YAG laser for the treatment of dysfunctional uterine bleeding. BJOG Int J Obstet Gynaecol. 2003;110:350–7.

Hiemstra E, Kolkman W, Jansen FW. Skills training in minimally invasive surgery in Dutch obstetrics and gynecology residency curriculum. Gynecol Surg. 2008;5:321–5.

Jansen FW, Vredevoogd CB, van Ulzen K, Hermans J, Trimbos JB, Trimbos-Kemper TC. Complications of hysteroscopy: a prospective, multicenter study. Obstet Gynecol. 2000;96:266–70.

Kamath MS, Kalampokas EE, Kalampokas TE. Use of GnRH analogues pre-operatively for hysteroscopic resection of submucous fibroids: a systematic review and meta-analysis. Eur J Obstet Gynecol Reprod Biol. 2014;177:11–8.

Kingston A, Abbott J, Lenart M, Vancaillie T. Hysteroscopic training: the butternut pumpkin model. J Am Assoc Gynecol Laparosc. 2004;11:256–61.

Kleijn JH, Engels R, Bourdrez P, Mol BWJ, Bongers MY. Five-year follow up of a randomised controlled trial comparing NovaSure and ThermaChoice

endometrial ablation. BJOG Int J Obstet Gynaecol. 2008;115:193–8.

Kremer C, Duffy S, Moroney M. Patient satisfaction with outpatient hysteroscopy versus day case hysteroscopy: randomised controlled trial. BMJ. 2000;320:279–82.

Kung RC, Vilos GA, Thomas B, Penkin P, Zaltz AP, Stabinsky SA. A new bipolar system for performing operative hysteroscopy in normal saline. J Am Assoc Gynecol Laparosc. 1999;6:331–6.

la Chapelle CF, Veersema S, Brölmann HAM, Jansen FW. Effectiveness and feasibility of hysteroscopic sterilization techniques: a systematic review and meta-analysis. Fertil Steril. 2015;103:1516–1525.e1–e3.

Lasmar RB, Lasmar BP, Celeste RK, da Rosa DB, Depes DB, Lopes RGC. A new system to classify submucous myomas: a Brazilian multicenter study. J Minim Invasive Gynecol. 2012;19:575–80.

Lee C, Salim R, Ofili-Yebovi D, Yazbek J, Davies A, Jurkovic D. Reproducibility of the measurement of submucous fibroid protrusion into the uterine cavity using three-dimensional saline contrast sonohysterography. Ultrasound Obstet Gynecol. 2006;28:837–41.

Lethaby A, Vollenhoven B, Sowter M. Pre-operative GnRH analogue therapy before hysterectomy or myomectomy for uterine fibroids. Cochrane Database Syst Rev. 2001;2:CD000547.

Lethaby A, Hickey M, Garry R. Endometrial destruction techniques for heavy menstrual bleeding. Cochrane Database Syst Rev. 2005;4:CD001501.

Levie MD, Chudnoff SG. Prospective analysis of office-based hysteroscopic sterilization. J Minim Invasive Gynecol. 2006;13:98–101.

Loffer FD, Bradley LD, Brill AI, Brooks PG, Cooper JM. Hysteroscopic fluid monitoring guidelines. The ad hoc committee on hysteroscopic training guidelines of the American Association of Gynecologic Laparoscopists. J Am Assoc Gynecol Laparosc. 2000;7:167–8.

Mao J, Pfeifer S, Schlegel P, Sedrakyan A. Safety and efficacy of hysteroscopic sterilization compared with laparoscopic sterilization: an observational cohort study. BMJ. 2015;351:h5162.

Mazzon I, Bettocchi S, Fascilla F, DE Palma D, Palma F, Zizolfi B, DI Spiezio Sardo A. Resectoscopic myomectomy. Minerva Ginecol. 2016;68:334–44.

Moawad NS, Santamaria E, Johnson M, Shuster J. Cost-effectiveness of office hysteroscopy for abnormal uterine bleeding. JSLS. 2014 Jul-Sep;18(3). pii: e2014.00393. doi: 10.4293/JSLS.2014.00393. (https://www.ncbi.nlm.nih.gov/pmc/articles/PMC4154435/pdf/e2014.00393.pdf)

Munro MG, Critchley HOD, Fraser IS, FIGO menstrual disorders working group. The FIGO classification of causes of abnormal uterine bleeding in the reproductive years. Fertil Steril. 2011;95:2204–2208, 2208.e1–e3.

Nathani F, Clark TJ. Uterine polypectomy in the management of abnormal uterine bleeding: a systematic review. J Minim Invasive Gynecol. 2006;13:260–8.

Nichols M, Carter JF, Fylstra DL, Childers M, Essure System U.S. Post-Approval Study Group. A comparative study of hysteroscopic sterilization performed in-office versus a hospital operating room. J Minim Invasive Gynecol. 2006;13:447–50.

Peeters JAH, Penninx JPM, Mol BW, Bongers MY. Prognostic factors for the success of endometrial ablation in the treatment of menorrhagia with special reference to previous cesarean section. Eur J Obstet Gynecol Reprod Biol. 2013;167:100–3.

Penninx JPM, Herman MC, Mol BW, Bongers MY. Five-year follow-up after comparing bipolar endometrial ablation with hydrothermablation for menorrhagia. Obstet Gynecol. 2011;118:1287–92.

Penninx JPM, Herman MC, Kruitwagen RFPM, Haar AJFT, Mol BW, Bongers MY. Bipolar versus balloon endometrial ablation in the office: a randomized controlled trial. Eur J Obstet Gynecol Reprod Biol. 2016;196:52–6.

Povedano B, Arjona JE, Velasco E, Monserrat JA, Lorente J, Castelo-Branco C. Complications of hysteroscopic Essure(®) sterilisation: report on 4306 procedures performed in a single centre. BJOG Int J Obstet Gynaecol. 2012;119:795–9.

Robinson LLL, Cooper NAM, Clark TJ. The role of ambulatory hysteroscopy in reproduction. J Fam Plan Reprod Health Care. 2013;39:127–35.

Sinha D, Kalathy V, Gupta JK, Clark TJ. The feasibility, success and patient satisfaction associated with outpatient hysteroscopic sterilisation. BJOG Int J Obstet Gynaecol. 2007;114:676–83.

Smith PP, Malick S, Clark TJ. Bipolar radiofrequency compared with thermal balloon ablation in the office: a randomized controlled trial. Obstet Gynecol. 2014a;124:219–25.

Smith PP, Middleton LJ, Connor M, Clark TJ. Hysteroscopic morcellation compared with electrical resection of endometrial polyps: a randomized controlled trial. Obstet Gynecol. 2014b;123:745–51.

Smorgick N, Barel O, Fuchs N, Ben-Ami I, Pansky M, Vaknin Z. Hysteroscopic management of retained products of conception: meta-analysis and literature review. Eur J Obstet Gynecol Reprod Biol. 2014;173:19–22.

Tas B, Van Herendael B. Long-Term outcomes with mini-touch endometrial ablation in an office setting without anaesthesia. J Minim Invasive Gynecol. 2014;21:S147.

Thinkhamrop J, Laopaiboon M, Lumbiganon P. Prophylactic antibiotics for transcervical intrauterine procedures. Cochrane Database Syst Rev. 2007;3: CD005637.

Timmermans A, Veersema S. Ambulatory transcervical resection of polyps with the Duckbill polyp snare: a modality for treatment of endometrial polyps. J Minim Invasive Gynecol. 2005;12:37–9.

Timmermans A, van Dongen H, Mol BW, Veersema S, Jansen FW. Hysteroscopy and removal of endometrial polyps: a Dutch survey. Eur J Obstet Gynecol Reprod Biol. 2008;138:76–9.

Valle RF. Hysteroscopic evaluation of patients with abnormal uterine bleeding. Surg Gynecol Obstet. 1981;153:521–6.

Valle RF, Sciarra JJ. Intrauterine adhesions: hysteroscopic diagnosis, classification, treatment, and reproductive outcome. Am J Obstet Gynecol. 1988;158:1459–70.

van Dijk LJEW, Breijer MC, Veersema S, Mol BWJ, Timmermans A. Current practice in the removal of benign endometrial polyps: a Dutch survey. Gynecol Surg. 2012;9:163–8.

van Dongen H, Emanuel MH, Wolterbeek R, Trimbos J, Jansen FW. Hysteroscopic morcellator for removal of intrauterine polyps and myomas: a randomized controlled pilot study among residents in training. J Minim Invasive Gynecol. 2008;15:466–71.

Van Eyk N, van Schalkwyk J, Infectious Diseases Committee. Antibiotic prophylaxis in gynaecologic procedures. J Obstet Gynaecol Can. 2012;34:382–91.

Veersema S, Vleugels MPH, Timmermans A, Brölmann HAM. Follow-up of successful bilateral placement of essure microinserts with ultrasound. Fertil Steril. 2005;84:1733–6.

Veersema S, Mijatovic V, Dreyer K, Schouten H, Schoot D, Emanuel MH, Hompes P, Brölmann H. Outcomes of pregnancies in women with hysteroscopically placed micro-inserts in situ. J Minim Invasive Gynecol. 2014;21:492–7.

Vercellini P, Zàina B, Yaylayan L, Pisacreta A, De Giorgi O, Crosignani PG. Hysteroscopic myomectomy: long-term effects on menstrual pattern and fertility. Obstet Gynecol. 1999;94:341–7.

Vilos GA. Intrauterine surgery using a new coaxial bipolar electrode in normal saline solution (Versapoint): a pilot study. Fertil Steril. 1999;72:740–3.

Yang J-H, Chen C-D, Chen S-U, Yang Y-S, Chen M-J. The influence of the location and extent of intrauterine adhesions on recurrence after hysteroscopic adhesiolysis. BJOG Int J Obstet Gynaecol. 2016;123:618–23.

Laparoscopic Ovarian Cystectomy

Caryl S. Reinsch

Abstract

Laparoscopy has enabled the laparoscopic gynecologic surgeon to manage many gynecologic surgical challenges in a minimally invasive manner. The laparoscopic approach has become the gold standard in the surgical management of ovarian cysts due to innovative changes in surgical instrumentation and the development of new surgical techniques. Benign ovarian cysts such as persistent and symptomatic functional ovarian cysts, corpus luteum cysts, and cystic ovarian neoplasms such as endometriomas or mature cystic teratomas are now managed as an outpatient procedure decreasing cost and recovery time to the patient. Pelvic ultrasound is the most useful imaging tool in the evaluation of an ovarian cyst. Complex ovarian cysts should be considered for removal in the symptomatic premenopausal woman and in all postmenopausal women. The decision to intervene surgically may be complicated and should be individualized for each patient. Aspiration of ovarian cysts is associated with a high rate of recurrence; therefore, cystectomy is the procedure of choice. Ovarian conservation is preferred in the premenopausal woman if at all feasible, and laparoscopic salpingo-oophorectomy is usually the procedure of choice for the postmenopausal woman.

Laparoscopic entry into the abdomen requires a detailed understanding of the vasculature of the anterior abdominal wall. Techniques may need to be altered depending on a patient's BMI (body mass index), past history of abdominal surgeries, and history of bowel obstruction or hernias. Laparoscopic removal of the ovarian cyst should facilitate intact removal and avoid intraoperative spillage.

Keywords

Laparoscopic • Ovarian • Cystectomy • Functional cyst • Endometrioma • Dermoid • Complex cyst • Simple cyst • Port placement

Contents

C.S. Reinsch (✉)
Kaiser Permanente Southern California, San Diego, CA, USA
e-mail: Caryl.S.Reinsch@kp.org

© Springer International Publishing AG 2017
D. Shoupe (ed.), *Handbook of Gynecology*,
DOI 10.1007/978-3-319-17798-4_54

1 Introduction

Laparoscopy has become a standard surgical approach for many gynecologic procedures in the last 40 years. It has now become the standard treatment of choice for surgical management of ectopic pregnancies and persistent and/or symptomatic adnexal masses and diagnosis and surgical treatment of endometriosis. The laparoscopic surgical approach has also enabled surgeons to offer minimally invasive hysterectomies.

When laparoscopy was initially utilized in gynecologic surgery, it was limited to diagnostic procedures and tubal ligations. The repertoire of the laparoscopic approach has evolved in the last 20 years as a result of the development of new innovations involving more advanced equipment, improved imaging with new camera systems, and improved expertise in surgical technique. In recent years, newer surgical approaches have developed. In particular, robotic-assisted laparoscopy and, very recently, single-port laparoscopy are gaining more popularity with laparoscopic surgeons. As with the development of any new procedures, the actual roles of these procedures in gynecologic surgery are controversial, and their role remains to be well defined.

Scientific data has consistently supported the laparoscopic approach to the adnexal mass as the preferred treatment. It has been estimated that approximately 10% of women in the United States will undergo a surgical procedure for an adnexal mass in their lifetime (Hilger et al. 2006). Laparoscopy has also been consistently shown to be associated with decreased postoperative complications such as fever, infection, postoperative pain, and blood loss. Decreased length of hospitalization and overall cost offer additional advantages compared to laparotomy

(Yuen et al. 1997; Fanfani et al. 2004; Medeiros et al. 2008).

Despite the abovementioned advantages, laparoscopy should be considered to involve similar surgical risks to laparotomy such as anesthesia risks, infection, injury to intra-abdominal and pelvic organs, and bleeding. Unique risks are also associated with the laparoscopic approach. These risks include the risk of damage to organs and vasculature with laparoscopic port placement and intravascular carbon dioxide gas insufflation with use of pneumoperitoneum to perform surgery. The use of cautery or ultrasonic energy sources also introduces another element of risk to damage to intra-abdominal structures.

1.1 Ovarian Cysts

Ovarian cysts can occur at any stage in life from fetal life through menopause. They can be symptomatic or asymptomatic and found incidentally on clinical exam or on imaging.

The most common types of benign ovarian cysts that the gynecologist encounters include functional cysts (follicular, hemorrhagic, and corpus luteum cysts), mature cystic teratomas (dermoids), endometriomas, and serous and mucinous cystadenomas (Table 1).

1.2 Functional Cysts

Most ovarian cysts develop as a result of faulty ovulation where the follicle fails to release an oocyte. Gradually, a cyst forms because the follicular cells continue to secrete fluid and the fluid accumulates. The cysts are referred to as follicular cysts, and they often resolve spontaneously and do not require surgical intervention (Nelson and Gambone 2010).

Another type of functional cyst is a corpus luteum cyst. The actual mechanism of how the cyst forms is not well understood. This cyst can become quite large and cause symptoms, may be associated with a delay of menses, and is more apt to undergo torsion due to the increased size when compared to the follicular cyst.

Table 1 Classification and characteristics of benign ovarian cysts

Functional ovarian cysts	
Follicular cyst	Common in reproductive age women
Corpus luteum cyst	Common in reproductive age women; forms when the corpus luteum fails to regress, may be hemorrhagic
Benign cystic ovarian neoplasms	
Epithelial cell tumors	Derived from mesothelial cells lining the peritoneal cavity and ovary
	Examples: serous cystadenoma, mucinous cystadenoma, endometrioma
Germ cell tumors	Derived from germ cells: may contain ectoderm, mesoderm, or endoderm
	Cystic mature teratoma dermoid cyst
Sex cord-stromal tumors	Derived from sex cords and stroma of developing gonad; may cause feminizing/virilizing effects
	Examples: granulosa-theca cell tumor, Sertoli-Leydig cell tumor

(Beckmann et al. 2006; Nelson and Gambone 2010)

1.3 Benign Cystic Ovarian Neoplasms

These cysts are usually categorized due to the cell type of origin such as surface epithelium, germ cell, or sex cord-stromal cells. The majority of these cysts are benign. At least 30% of ovarian masses in women over the age of 50 are malignant (Kinkel et al. 2005). The risk of malignancy significantly increases in the postmenopausal woman with a cystic neoplasm (Beckmann et al. 2006).

Epithelial cell tumors are thought to develop from mesothelial cells that line the ovary and peritoneal cavity. Cystic epithelial tumors account for approximately 60% of all true ovarian neoplasms. The endometrioma, serous cystadenoma, and mucinous cystadenoma fall into this category.

Serous and mucinous cystadenomas are typically thin walled, unilocular, or multilocular and can range widely in size. Mucinous cystadenomas tend to be multilocular and much larger than serous cystadenomas. The peak incidence of serous and mucinous cystadenomas is in the fourth to fifth decade. One-third of all ovarian

tumors are serous and two-thirds of those are benign. Mucinous epithelial tumors account for 10–15% of all epithelial neoplasms and 75% are benign (Goldberg 2015).

Serous tumors are bilateral 25% of the time, whereas mucinous tumors have a much lower incidence of bilaterality ranging 2–3% (ACOG 2007). The incidence of bilaterality should be taken into consideration and discussed with the patient at the time of evaluation, particularly if surgical management is required.

The origin of the endometrioma is controversial. Several investigators favor the theory that the endometrioma originates as invaginated endometrial glands on the surface of the ovary (Hughesdon 1957; PPe 1957; Nezhat et al. 1992; Brosens et al. 1994). The endometrioma tends to develop very slowly over time and tends to be moderate in size averaging 5–6 cm in size.

Endometriomas are hormonally active with the menstrual cycle. This often translates into exacerbation of symptoms just prior to and during menses for the patient. The endometrioma can also present a challenge in removal of the capsule to the surgeon. The capsules tend to be very adherent to adjacent ovarian tissue and often are only able to be partially removed which may increase risk of recurrence if ovarian conservation is desired.

Mature cystic teratomas (dermoid cysts) are also common benign cystic ovarian neoplasms. Dermoid cysts account for 10–20% of ovarian neoplasms and have an incidence of bilaterality of 8–14%. They are also the most common benign ovarian tumor in the second and third decade of life (Killackey and Neuwirth 1988). They are commonly composed of multiple cell types derived from one or more of the three germ cell layers (Hamilton 2015). They are almost always benign but can undergo malignant transformation in 0.2–2% of cases (Comerci et al. 1994; Hamilton 2015)

Historically, laparoscopic management of mature cystic teratomas was not pursued due to concerns regarding the risk of chemical peritonitis in the event of intraoperative spillage of the cyst's sebaceous contents. Recent evidence has not supported this concern. Nezhat et al. noted an incidence of 0.2% of chemical peritonitis with review of 10 years of experience (Nezhat et al. 1999) It is now very feasible to remove a dermoid cyst via laparoscopic cystectomy.

Simple ovarian cysts up to 10 cm are likely to be benign at all ages with the incidence of malignancy <1% (Modesitt et al. 2003). There is little evidence in the literature to guide practitioners on which asymptomatic cysts may be ignored or followed. The decision to proceed with surgical interventions usually is usually based upon many factors and individualized for each patient. Cysts that continue to grow or become more symptomatic are more likely to undergo surgical treatment.

2 Workup

The vast majority of pelvic masses are benign in the premenopausal woman. The initial workup should include a medical history, physical exam, serial beta-HCG, CBC, and ultrasound imaging. Depending on the presentation, physicians may also elect to check serial hematocrits and cervical cultures if a hemorrhagic cyst or abscess is suspected. Many cysts can and should be managed expectantly if infection, pregnancy, or torsion have been excluded (ACOG 2007).

Cystic ovarian masses that are symptomatic with pain, pressure, or fever often require immediate intervention such as antibiotics for a tubo-ovarian abscess, medical or surgical management for an ectopic pregnancy, or surgical management for a suspected ovarian torsion.

The postmenopausal woman with a cystic adnexal mass requires a higher index of suspicion for malignancy. The initial workup in addition to a medical history and physical exam should include transvaginal ultrasound imaging and a CA 125 level. Ultrasound findings that raise suspicions for malignancy include solid areas in the mass, excrescences, and free fluid in the abdomen and/or pelvis. The ovary is also a common site of metastases for other primary cancers such as the breast, uterus, colorectal, or gastric cancers. The additional workup of the postmenopausal woman with a suspected malignancy or complex cystic mass should include breast exam, mammogram, digital rectal exam, endometrial biopsy, and upper and lower gastrointestinal endoscopy.

There is no single presurgical evaluation, blood test, and imaging modality that can definitively determine if an adnexal mass is benign or malignant. A definitive diagnosis of the adnexal mass can only be made with surgical excision and histologic evaluation. However, as previously mentioned, the vast majority of cystic adnexal masses are benign (Valentin et al. 2006). In addition, ultrasonographic findings associated with a simple ovarian cyst, endometrioma, or dermoid cysts are quite characteristic and highly predictive of histologic diagnosis.

Many studies support that a thorough preoperative workup will decrease the possibility of performing a laparoscopy in evaluation for a malignant mass (Whiteside and Keup 2009). If a malignancy is suspected, then a laparotomy is the initial proper surgical management. Unfortunately, a CA 125 level, pelvic ultrasound, or peritoneal cytology is not sufficient to rule out a suspected malignancy. Therefore, the decision often rests on the surgeon's intraoperative evaluation and judgment at the time of laparoscopy on whether to proceed with salpingo-oophorectomy and/or laparotomy for suspected malignancy.

2.1 Imaging

Pelvic ultrasound remains the preferred imaging modality to evaluate adnexal cysts.

A simple cyst appears as a round or oval anechoic space with smooth thin walls and no solid component or internal flow on Doppler (Levine et al. 2010). Color or Doppler flow is used to evaluate a complex cyst for internal flow in solid areas or septations. The principle with Doppler flow is that new vessels within tumors have lower resistance to blood flow because of no smooth muscle in the vessel walls (Helm 2015). At this time, the current role of color Doppler in evaluation of pelvic masses remains controversial because the ranges in the values of the resistive index, pulsatility index, and maximum systolic velocity between benign and malignant masses overlap considerably (ACOG 2007).

Complex cysts typically have ultrasound findings with more than one compartment, referred to as multilocular, thickened walls, papillary projections into the cyst itself or on the surface of the ovary, or abnormal-appearing areas inside the cyst. These findings can be associated with many benign neoplasms or malignant tumors of the ovary. Ultrasound is also helpful in differentiating from other adnexal masses such as hydrosalpinges, paraovarian or tubal cysts, or leiomyomata. Transvaginal, transabdominal, or both need to be utilized to fully evaluate the entire cystic structure. Transabdominal ultrasound imaging is better in evaluating large masses and other findings associated with them such as free fluid or ascites and hydronephrosis.

Other imaging modalities such as the CT, MRI, or PET are not routinely recommended in the initial workup for a cystic mass. The MRI, however, can be very useful in evaluating pelvic masses such as pedunculated leiomyomata or masses that are not adequately evaluated with ultrasound imaging. The CT is most useful in detecting metastatic disease when malignancy is suspected on initial workup.

2.2 Serum Markers

Serum markers are not useful as a routine screening test even though CA 125 levels are elevated in 85% of patient with epithelial ovarian carcinomas. The value is normal in 50% of patient with stage 1 cancers confined to the ovary and in 20–35% of advanced stage ovarian cancer cases (Jacobs and Bast 1989; ACOG 2011). CA 125 levels are also not very specific and are also elevated in patients with some benign conditions such as pregnancy, infection, menstruation, fibroids, endometriosis, cyst rupture, renal failure, and peritoneal inflammation.

Many other potential serum markers are undergoing current research. Their role in the detection of precancer or cancer of the ovary remains yet to be determined.

The presence of at least one of the following indicators warrants consideration of referral to or consultation with a gynecologic oncologist:

Postmenopausal women: elevated CA 125 level, ascites, a nodular or fixed pelvic mass, or evidence of abdominal or distant metastasis

Premenopausal women: very elevated CA 125 level, ascites, or evidence of abdominal or distant metastasis (ACOG 2011)

3 Management

3.1 Observation

Simple functional cysts have been traditionally managed with hormonal suppression with oral contraceptives. However, recent meta-analyses have demonstrated no difference between suppression with oral contraceptives and expectant management in terms of resolution of the ovarian cyst. In premenopausal women, 70% of adnexal masses will resolve over several menstrual cycles (Curtin 1994). As a result, it is now the standard of care to observe simple ovarian cysts up to 8 cm through several menstrual cycles and follow-up ultrasound imaging for resolution (Grimes et al. 2009). Oral contraceptives are no longer recommended for suppression to facilitate resolution of ovarian cysts (ACOG 2010). Observation is generally not recommended for ovarian cysts $\geq$8 cm due to increased risk of ovarian torsion.

Postmenopausal women with asymptomatic simple ovarian cysts and a normal CA 125 level may also be followed expectantly with serial ultrasound examinations. Some data supports that in this scenario, simple cysts up to 10 cm can also be followed and observed (Bailey et al. 1998). Close follow-up care is very important because the risk of a malignant ovarian neoplasm increases from 13% in premenopausal to 45% in postmenopausal patient (McDonald and Modesitt 2006).

3.2 Surgical Intervention

Persistent and/or symptomatic simple ovarian cysts >5–10 cm in size should be considered for surgical removal. Complex ovarian cysts should be considered for surgical removal in the symptomatic premenopausal female. With the exception of simple ovarian cysts on a transvaginal ultrasound finding, most pelvic masses in postmenopausal women will require surgical intervention. The decision to intervene surgically may be complicated and involve many factors and should be individualized based on the clinical scenario and associated findings.

3.3 Laparoscopy

The use of laparoscopy is constantly expanding in gynecologic surgery. It has become the preferred surgical approach for the management of symptomatic or persistent benign ovarian cysts, depending on the experience and skill of the surgeon. This includes suspected endometriomas, hemorrhagic cysts, dermoids, functional cysts, or cystadenomas that have not resolved with expectant management or are symptomatic. Typically, endometriomas, dermoid cysts, or cystadenomas do not resolve spontaneously. Quite often, the diagnosis of a serous or mucinous cystadenoma is not made until laparoscopic evaluation and subsequent removal via cystectomy or oophorectomy.

3.4 Aspiration of Cyst

Aspiration of an ovarian cyst at the time of laparoscopy is generally not recommended unless it is used to facilitate a laparoscopic ovarian cystectomy. Even in the situation of cystectomy, this should only be carried out in an endoscopic bag to avoid spillage in the event of an unsuspected malignancy. If aspiration is solely used to manage an ovarian cyst, there is a high recurrence rate of the cyst approaching up to 65% (Mesogitis et al. 2005). In addition, there is no tissue for pathologic evaluation and malignancy cannot be ruled out. It has also not been proven more effective than expectant management (Zanetta et al. 1996).

Aspiration of ovarian cysts is contraindicated in postmenopausal women due to concerns regarding the increased potential for malignancy.

Evidence shows that there is demonstrated decrease survival of stage 1 ovarian cancer patients if spillage occurs intraoperatively compared to patients with tumors removed intact (Cuesta et al. 1994; Mizuno et al. 2003).

3.5 Laparoscopic Ovarian Cystectomy

The optimal surgical goal is to remove the entire cyst intact. The cyst should be removed inside a laparoscopic bag so that inadvertent spillage into the peritoneal cavity may be avoided. If an oophorectomy is performed, the ovary with the intact cyst should be removed contained within an endoscopic bag.

Very large benign-appearing ovarian cysts are now being managed more commonly via the laparoscopic approach. In this approach, the ovary is usually placed in an endoscopic bag and drained of excess fluid and then removed within the bag through a small incision (Eltabbakh et al. 2008). This approach obviously avoids a large laparotomy incision and facilitates a faster recovery with decreased morbidity and cost for the patient.

Ovarian conservation is generally the goal in a premenopausal woman with a benign ovarian cyst requiring surgical excision. The advantage is preservation of viable ovarian tissue and thus fertility and hormone production. Oophorectomy and possibly bilateral salpingo-oophorectomy may be elected in surgical management of a postmenopausal woman with a benign cyst. Oophorectomy may also be considered for premenopausal women who are considered for increased genetic risk for ovarian cancer.

Entry into the abdomen may be performed with several techniques. In a Cochrane review of 46 randomized controlled trials comparing various techniques, there was no advantage of using any single technique in preventing vascular or visceral complications. There is insufficient evidence to recommend on laparoscopic entry technique over another (Ahmad et al. 2008).

An understanding of the anterior abdominal wall vessels is of paramount importance to avoid injury to these vessels. There are two sets of bilateral vessels, the superficial and inferior epigastric vessels. The vessels are located an average of 5.5 cm from the midline. The lateral ports should be placed approximately 8 cm from the midline to avoid vascular injury. Transillumination of the anterior abdominal wall with the laparoscope to visualize the superficial vessels is recommended during placement of lateral ports. It is also optimal to try and visualize the inferior vessels intra-abdominally with visualization of the laparoscope whenever possible.

In patients with a history of prior abdominal surgery, there is a risk of 20% of adhesions to the anterior abdominal wall involving the omentum or bowel (Vilos et al. 2007). As a result, surgeons may elect to gain entry with any of the three following techniques: the closed entry with the Veress needle, open laparoscopy, or left upper quadrant placement at Palmer's site.

3.6 Standard Closed Entry

The Veress needle may be used to create a pneumoperitoneum prior to laparoscopic port placement. The needle is advanced into the peritoneal cavity usually through a 5 mm incision at the umbilicus. During placement of the Veress needle, the abdominal wall is elevated by using two perforating towel clamps placed just lateral to the umbilicus and lifting up during insertion or manually grasping and lifting the abdominal wall superior to the suprapubic area during insertion. The abdominal wall is elevated to maximize the distance between the abdominal wall and retroperitoneal vessels. Entry into the peritoneal cavity may be confirmed with the saline drop test and observation for pressure less than 8 mmHg during insufflation. The CO_2 gas is then insufflated into the needle to create a pneumoperitoneum. Maximum insufflation pressure is usually set at 15 mm but can be increased to 20 mm if needed and tolerated by the patient. Once this pressure is obtained, then an adequate pneumoperitoneum is obtained, and the surgeon can now proceed with umbilical primary port placement.

Hurd et al. (1991) characterized the difference in abdominal wall thickness and how it can influence laparoscopic port entry. In women with ideal body weight (body mass index, [BMI] <25 kg/m^2), the Veress needle is inserted toward the hollow of the sacrum at a 45° Fig. 1a). The retroperitoneal vessels are much closer to the abdominal wall, and there may be as little as 4 cm between the skin and these vessels in thin patients. In the obese patient (BMI >30 kg/m^2), a more vertical approach, approximately 70–80°, is necessary to enter the peritoneal cavity because of increased thickness of the abdominal wall (Fig. 1c).

Open laparoscopy may also be performed to gain entry into the abdominal cavity. There is no evidence to support that overall open entry is superior or safer than the other entry techniques (Ahmad et al. 2015).

Surgeons may elect to gain entry via the left upper quadrant in the event that periumbilical adhesions are suspected, patient has a history of umbilical hernia, or there are failed attempts at entry via the umbilicus. With this technique, the Veress needle is advanced through a 5 mm incision at Palmer's point, which is at the mid-clavicular line just beneath the lower rib margin and pneumoperitoneum created with insufflation of CO_2 gas. A 5 mm laparoscopic port is then advanced into the peritoneal cavity and confirmed with visualization with the laparoscope.

Direct laparoscopic port placement is considered safe without a pneumoperitoneum when done with disposable blunt trocars. It is also faster than the Veress needle technique and is not associated with insufflation-related injuries because proper placement is confirmed with visualization with the laparoscope prior to insufflation. This is performed while elevating the abdominal wall with perforating towel clamps or manually grasping the abdominal wall and elevating it. Elevation of the abdominal wall during trocar insertion maximizes the distance between the umbilicus and the retroperitoneal vessels. Elevation of the abdominal wall during trocar or Veress needle placement, however, does not necessarily guarantee visceral or blood vessel injury.

The initial laparoscopic port is usually placed at the umbilicus with a 5–12 mm port. The pelvis is carefully surveyed, and the ovarian cyst is

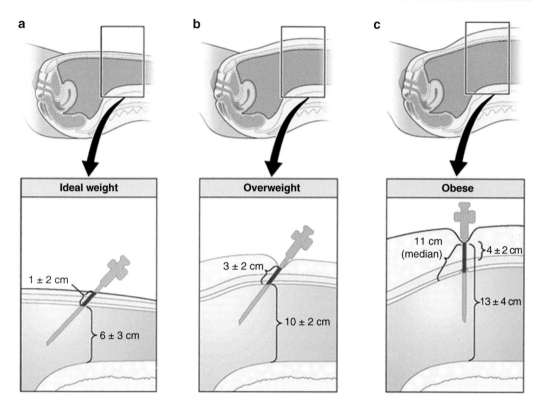

Fig. 1 Differences in umbilical trocar placement in patients with different BMIs (body mass index) (Adapted from Hurd et al. 1991)

examined for any signs that may be suggestive of malignancy such as ascites, excrescences on the surface of the ovary, and implants noted on peritoneal, liver, or diaphragm surfaces. Five millimeter ports are then placed laterally. The surgeon may opt to obtain cell washings at this time for cytology. If the cyst appears benign, then cystectomy is performed.

Cystectomy is then performed by incising the capsule of the ovary with endoshears or the surgeon's preferred laparoscopic power source. The cyst is then enucleated carefully with traction and countertraction and dissection as needed. If intraoperative rupture occurs, particularly with a dermoid cyst, the peritoneal cavity should liberally be rinsed with normal saline or Ringer's lactate that has been shown to be safe (Nezhat et al. 1999; Zanetta et al. 1999; Milingos et al. 2004).

After the cyst is removed from the ovary, an endoscopic bag is then advanced through the umbilical 10–12 mm port, and the cyst is placed in the bag. If a 5 mm umbilical port was used for initial survey, this port can be exchanged for a 10–12 mm port. The bag is then advanced up to the umbilical incision, and the port is removed while advancing the edges of the bag through the skin incision. The bag is then opened and triangulated to facilitate removal of the cyst intact if small enough or with morcellation carefully avoiding any spillage out of the bag. Prior to removal, the cyst may need to be drained while in the bag. Once the specimen is small enough, the bag is removed with the specimen through the incision. Other options for removing the specimen include a minilaparotomy or colpotomy. If colpotomy is performed, antibiotics are recommended.

If concern about the benign nature of the cyst exists, the cyst wall should be sent for frozen section at the time of removal. If malignancy is confirmed or suspected, then the procedure should be converted to a laparotomy for continued appropriate surgical management.

After removal of the bag and specimen, the 10–12 mm laparoscopic port is replaced through the umbilical incision and the camera advanced through the port. The ovary is then carefully inspected for hemostasis. Bleeding from the bed of the cyst in the ovary may require measures to obtain hemostasis. Hemostasis in the bed of the ovary at the site of the cystectomy has traditionally been accomplished with bipolar cautery. This may also be performed with use of other laparoscopic power sources or application of a hemostatic agent. Recent evidence suggests that the application of hemostatic sealants such as FloSeal (Baxter International Inc., Deerfield, IL) or Surgicel fibrillar (Ethicon, Inc., Somerville, NJ) results in improved ovarian reserve after cystectomy compared to cautery (Song et al. 2014). The edges of the ovarian capsule do not need to be reapproximated as is traditionally done with an open ovarian cystectomy. Some surgeons prefer to utilize an adhesion barrier product on the ovary to minimize postoperative adhesion formation.

The procedure is completed by irrigation of the pelvis, and a careful survey of the pelvis for hemostasis with the intraperitoneal pressure decreased to 5 mmHg. The port sites are then inspected for hemostasis. After all port sites are inspected for hemostasis, the CO_2 peritoneum is then allowed to escape through the umbilical port. Care is taken to ensure that as much gas is expressed as possible to minimize postoperative discomfort for the patient and to avoid the bowel being pushed into the incision sites as residual gas escapes. The incisions are then closed with suture, Steri-Strips, or a skin adhesive. Fascial closure is recommended for ports 10 mm or greater in size prior to skin closure to prevent subsequent development of an incisional hernia (Tonouchi et al. 2004).

Simple cysts in postmenopausal women can also be removed laparoscopically since the vast majority is benign. However, salpingo-oophorectomy is generally considered the procedure of choice.

3.7 Contraindications to Laparoscopic Ovarian Cystectomy

Absolute contraindications to ovarian cystectomy continue to be controversial. The presence of a known malignancy has traditionally been considered an absolute contraindication. As expertise increases with laparoscopy, there is currently disagreement regarding this concept. The use of laparoscopy in the setting of surgical management of malignancy continues to develop and expand. Laparoscopic staging and management of ovarian cancer have been reported (Fauvet et al. 2005; Lecuru et al. 2006). However, there are reports in the literature that suggest that laparoscopy may increase the risk of port-site metastases and intraperitoneal spread of cancer cells (Morice et al. 2004; Nagersheth et al. 2004; Ramirez et al. 2004). Continued experience will further define the role of laparoscopy in the surgical management of ovarian malignancy.

Relative contraindications have also changed over the past 30 years since laparoscopy has improved with advances in surgical technique and equipment. Previously, obese patients or patients with a history of multiple abdominal surgeries or bowel obstructions were considered not to be candidates for the laparoscopic approach. Open laparoscopy, left upper quadrant access, and the use of trocars with optical access capabilities are now widely accepted techniques for such patients.

3.8 Oophorectomy

Indications for oophorectomy as the preferred procedure are noted in the Table 2 below (Valea and Mann 2015).

Oophorectomy and most commonly laparotomy are the procedures of choice rather than cystectomy in women with an ovarian mass that is suspicious for malignancy. Oophorectomy is the preferred management for any ovarian mass that requires surgical intervention in postmenopausal women regardless of the suspicion for malignancy.

Table 2 Summary of indications for oophorectomy

Benign ovarian neoplasms not amenable to treatment
with cystectomy, enucleation, partial oophorectomy

Elective or risk-reducing salpingo-oophorectomy

Adnexal torsion with necrosis

Ovarian malignancy

Tubo-ovarian abscess unresponsive to antibiotics

Definitive treatment for endometriosis but must consider
long term health risks

Gastrointestinal or other metastatic cancers

Male pseudohermaphrodites

Valea and Mann (2015)

Laparoscopic oophorectomy is usually performed as a salpingo-oophorectomy. The infundibulopelvic ligament and the ureter are carefully identified. The ureter is easily identified through the peritoneum in most patients. If the ureter is difficult to identify, the peritoneum must be opened and dissection carried out retroperitoneally to facilitate location of the ureter. The procedure is then carried out with ligation of the infundibular pelvic ligament, the utero-ovarian ligaments, and the fallopian tube next to the cornua of the uterus. This can be performed with a variety of techniques including bipolar electrocautery, ultrasonic cutting and coagulation devices (e.g., Harmonic scalpel), bipolar vessel-sealing devices (e.g., LigaSure, EnSeal, Gyrus-PK), loop technique, or stapling devices. The ovary and fallopian tube are then placed in an endobag and brought up to the umbilical port-site incision and removed in a similar technique to the cystectomy. Cyst fluid may be carefully aspirated from the cyst while enclosed in the bag to facilitate removal through the port-site incision with care taken to avoid any spillage into the peritoneal cavity. If malignancy is suspected, morcellation of the ovary is not recommended to preserve optimal pathologic evaluation. If the ovary cannot be removed via the bag through the laparoscopic port, then a larger incision is required for safe removal.

4   Conclusion

Laparoscopic ovarian cystectomy has now evolved to become the gold standard of surgical management of benign cystic ovarian masses in premenopausal women. The development of improved laparoscopic camera systems and instruments has enabled surgeons to evolve and continually improve their laparoscopic surgical techniques. In addition, the role of minimally invasive approaches continues to gain increased acceptance with gynecologic oncologists in the management of possible malignancies.

References

ACOG Practice Bulletin No.83; Management of adnexal masses. Obstet Gynecol. 2007; 110:201–214.

ACOG Practice Bulletin No. 100; Noncontraceptive uses of hormonal contraceptives. Obstet Gynecol. 2010; 115(1):206-8.

ACOG Practice Bulletin No. 477. The role of the obstetrician-gynecologist in the early detection of epithelial ovarian cancer. Obstet Gynecol 2011; 117:742-6.

Ahmad G, Duffy JM, Phillips K, Watson A. Laparoscopic entry techniques. Cochrane Database Syst Rev. 2008;2: CD006583.

Ahmad G, Gent D, Henderson D, O'Flynn H, Phillips K, Watson A. Laparoscopic entry techniques. Cochrane Database Syst Rev. 2015;8:CD006583.

Bailey C, Ueland F, Land G, Depriest P, Gallion H, Kryscio R, et al. The malignant potential of small cystic ovarian tumors in women over 50 years of age. Gynecol Oncol. 1998;69(1):3–7

Beckmann CR, Ling F, Smith R, Laube D, Herbert W, Casanova R, Chuang A, Hueppchen N, Weiss P. Ovarian and adnexal disease. Philadelphia: Lippincott Williams & Wilkins Publishing; 2006.

Brosens IA, Puttemans P, Deprest J. The endoscopic loclization of endometrial implants n the ovarian chocolate cyst. Fertil Steril. 1994;61:1034–8.

Comerci Jr JT, Licciardi F, Bergh PA, Gregori C, Breen JL. Mature cystic teratoma: a clinicopathologic evaluation of 517 cases and review of the literature. Obstet Gynecol. 1994;84(1):22–8.

Cuesta RS d l, Goff B, Fuller AJ, Nikrui N, Eichhorn J, Rice L. Prognostic importance of intraoperative rupture of malignant ovarian epithelial neoplasms. Obstet Gynecol. 1994;84:1–7.

Curtin J. Management of the adnexal mass. Gynecol Oncol. 1994;55:542.

Eltabbakh GH, Charboneau AM, Eltabbakh NG. Laparoscopic surgery for large benign ovarian cysts. Gynecol Oncol. 2008;108(1):72–6.

Fanfani F, Fagotti A, Ercoli A, Bifulco G, Longo R, Mancuso S, et al. A prospective randomized study of laparoscopy and minilaparotomy in the management of benign adnexal masses. Hum Reprod. 2004;19: 2367–71.

Fauvet R, Boccara J, Dufournet C, Poncelet C, Darai E. Laparoscopic management of borderline ovarian tumors: results of a french multicenter study. Ann Oncol. 2005;16:403–10.

Goldber A. Benign lesions of the ovaries. Medscape, from emedicine.medscape.com/article/265548-overview.2015

Grimes DA, Jones LB, Lopez LM, Schulz KF. Oral contraceptives for functional ovarian cysts. Cochrane Database Syst Rev. 2009;2:CD006134.

Hamilton C. Cystic teratoma. Medscape. Retrieved 1 Aug 2016, 2015.

Helm C. Ovarian cysts workup. Medscape, from emedicine. medscape.com/article/255865-workup. 2015.

Hilger WS, Magrina JF, Magtibay PM. Laparoscopic management of the adnexal mass. Clin Obstet Gynecol. 2006;49(3):535–48.

Hughesdon PE. The structure of endometrial cysts of the ovary. J Obstet Gynaecol Br Emp. 1957;64(4):481–7.

Hurd WH, Bude RO, DeLancey JO, Gauvin JM, Aisen AM. Abdominal wall characterization with magnetic resonance imaging and computed tomography. The effect of obesity on the laparoscopic approach. J Reprod Med. 1991;36(7):473–6.

Jacobs I, Bast Jr RC. The CA 125 tumour-associated antigen: a review of the literature. Hum Reprod. 1989;4(1):1–12.

Killackey M, Neuwirth R. Evaluation and management of the adnexal mass: a review of 540 cases. Obstet Gynecol. 1988;71:319.

Kinkel K, Lu Y, Mehdizade A, Pelte M, Hricak H. Indeterminate ovarian mass at US: incremental value of second imaging test for characterization -meta-analysis and bayesian analysis. Radiology. 2005;236(1):236–85.

Lecuru F, Desfaux P, Camatte S, Bissery A. Impact of initial surgical access on stagina dnd survival of patients with stage 1 ovarian cancer. Int J Gynecol Cancer. 2006;16:87–94.

Levine D, Brown DL, Andreotti RF, Benacerraf B, Benson CB, Brewster WR, Coleman B, DePriest P, Doubilet PM, Goldstein SR, Hamper UM, Hecht JL, Horrow M, Hur HC, Marnach M, Patel MD, Platt LD, Puscheck E, Smith-Bindman R, U. Society of Radiologists in. Management of asymptomatic ovarian and other adnexal cysts imaged at US Society of Radiologists in Ultrasound consensus conference statement. Ultrasound Q. 2010;26(3):121–31.

McDonald JM, Modesitt SC. The incidental postmenopausal adnexal mass. Clin Obstet Gynecol. 2006; 49(3):506–16.

Medeiros LR, Rosa DD, Bozzetti MC, Rosa MI, Edelweiss MI, Stein AT, Zelmanowicz A, Ethur AB, Zanini RR. Laparoscopy versus laparotomy for FIGO Stage I ovarian cancer. Cochrane Database Syst Rev. 2008;4: CD005344.

Mesogitis S, Daskalakis G, Pialis A, Papantoniou N, Tomakos N, Dessipris N, Pantiota K, Antsaklis A. Managment of ovarian cysts with aspiration and methotrexate injection. Radiology. 2005;235:668.

Milingos S, Protopapas A, Drakakis P, Liapi A, Loutradis D, Rodolakis A, Milingos D, Michalas

S. Laparoscopic treatment of ovarian dermoid cysts: eleven years' experience. J Am Assoc Gynecol Laparosc. 2004;11(4):478–85.

Mizuno M, Kikkawa F, Shibata K, Kajiyama H, Suzuki T, Ino K. Longterm prognosis of stage 1 ovarian carcinoma. Prognostic importance of intraoperative rupture. Oncology. 2003;65:29–36.

Modesitt SC, Pavlik EJ, Ueland FR, DePriest PD, Kryscio RJ, van Nagell Jr JR. Risk of malignancy in unilocular ovarian cystic tumors less than 10 centimeters in diameter. Obstet Gynecol. 2003;102(3):594–9.

Morice P, Camatte S, Larregain-Fournier D, Thoury A, Duvillard P, Castaigne D. Port-site implantation after laparoscopic treatment of borderline ovarian tumors. Obstet Gynecol. 2004;104(5 Pt 2):1167–70.

Nagersheth N, Rahaman J, Cohen C, Gretz H, Nezhat F. The incidence of port site metastases in gynecologic cancers. JSLS. 2004;8:133–9.

Nelson AL, Gambone J. Congenital anomalies and benign conditions of the ovaries and fallopian tubes. In: Gambone J, Hacker NI, Hobel CJ, editors. Hacker and Moore's essentials of obstetrics and gynecology. Philadelphia: Saunders; 2010.

Nezhat F, Nezhat C, Allan CJ, Metzger DA, Sears DL. Clinical and histologic classification of endometriomas. Implications for a mechanism of pathogenesis. J Reprod Med. 1992;37(9):771–6.

Nezhat CR, Kalyoncu S, Nezhat CH, Johnson E, Berlanda N, Nezhat F. Laparoscopic management of ovarian dermoid cysts: ten years' experience. JSLS. 1999;3(3):179–84.

Pe H. The structure of the endometrial cysts of the ovary. J Obstet Gynaecol Br Emp. 1957;44:481–7.

Ramirez PT, Frumovitz M, Wolf JK, Levenback C. Laparoscopic port-site metastases in patients with gynecological malignancies. Int J Gynecol Cancer. 2004;14(6):1070–7.

Song T, Lee S-H, Woo Y. Additional benefit of hemostatic sealant in preservation of ovarian reserve during laparoscopic ovarian cystectomy. Hum Reprod. 2014; 29(8):1659–1665.

Tonouchi H, Ohmori Y, Kobayashi M, Kusunoki M. Trocar site hernia. Arch Surg. 2004;139(11):1248–56.

Valea F, Mann W. Oophorectomy and ovarian cystectomy. Uptodate, from http://www.uptodate.com. 2015.

Valentin L, Ameye L, Jurkovic D, Metzger U, Lecuru F, Van Huffel S, Timmerman D. Which extrauterine pelvic masses are difficult to correctly classify as benign or malignant on the basis of ultrasound findings and is there a way of making a correct diagnosis? Ultrasound Obstet Gynecol. 2006;27(4):438–44.

Vilos GA, Ternamian A, Dempster J, Laberge PY, O. The Society of and C. Gynaecologists of. Laparoscopic entry: a review of techniques, technologies, and complications. J Obstet Gynaecol Can. 2007;29(5): 433–65.

Whiteside JL, Keup HL. Laparoscopic management of the ovarian mass: a practical approach. Clin Obstet Gynecol. 2009;52(3):327–34.

Yuen P, Yu K, Yip S, Lau W, Rogers M, Chang A. A randomized porspective study of laparoscopy and laparotomy in the managment of benign ovarian masses. Am J Obstet Gynecol. 1997;177:109–14.

Zanetta G, Lissonni A, Torri V, Valle C, Trio D, Rangoni G, Mangioni C. Management of ovarian cysts with aspiration in expectant managment of simple ovarian cysts: a randomised study. BMJ. 1996;313:1110.

Zanetta G, Ferrari L, Mignini-Renzini M, Vignali M, Fadini R. Laparoscopic excision of ovarian dermoid cysts with controlled intraoperative spillage. Safety and effectiveness. J Reprod Med. 1999;44(9): 815–20.

Laparoscopic Myomectomy: Best Practices

Brianne D. Romeroso and William H. Parker

Abstract

Leiomyomas are common pelvic tumors that can cause abnormal uterine bleeding, bulk-related symptoms, and possible effects on fertility and pregnancy. Myomectomy is a surgical treatment option for women who desire uterine preservation. A laparoscopic approach provides the benefits of minimally invasive surgery while achieving similar outcomes to those of open myomectomy. Appropriate patient selection, thorough patient counseling, careful preoperative preparation, and proper surgical technique are paramount to the success and safety of this procedure.

Keywords

Fertility preservation • Fibroid • Laparoscopy • Leiomyoma • Minimally invasive • Myoma • Myomectomy • Uterine preservation

Contents

B.D. Romeroso (✉) • W.H. Parker
Department of Obstetrics and Gynecology, David Geffen School of Medicine at UCLA, Los Angeles, CA, USA
e-mail: bromeroso@mednet.ucla.edu; wparker@mednet.ucla.edu

© Springer International Publishing AG 2017
D. Shoupe (ed.), *Handbook of Gynecology*,
DOI 10.1007/978-3-319-17798-4_82

1   Introduction

Leiomyomas, also known as fibroids or myomas, are benign monoclonal smooth muscle tumors. They are the most common type of pelvic tumor in women with a reported incidence of 70–80% by the age of 50 years (Baird et al. 2003). Although many women are asymptomatic, leiomyomas can cause a variety of symptoms, resulting in significant morbidity and high economic burden. Accordingly, many treatment options, both medical and surgical, are available. Women who desire uterine preservation for fertility or other reasons often opt for myomectomy. This procedure can be performed via laparotomy (i.e., abdominal myomectomy) or by use of minimally invasive techniques. Laparoscopic myomectomy is an effective treatment option for appropriately selected patients in whom leiomyoma characteristics preclude a hysteroscopic or vaginal approach.

2   Indications for Myomectomy

The indications for myomectomy are somewhat subjective as they are based on the effects of leiomyomas on the patient's quality of life and daily activities. Many women with leiomyomas are largely asymptomatic; it is difficult to justify any intervention, surgical or otherwise, in these patients. The principal symptoms associated with leiomyomas include abnormal uterine bleeding (with or without anemia), pelvic pressure and pain (caused by uterine bulk and, occasionally, leiomyoma degeneration), urinary and gastrointestinal symptoms (e.g., urinary frequency, incontinence, hydronephrosis, and/or constipation resulting from uterine mass effect on the urinary and gastrointestinal systems), and effects on fertility and pregnancy.

Of these indications, the effects of leiomyomas on fertility and pregnancy may be the most controversial. Indeed, there are no high-quality data that prove that leiomyomas decrease fertility or increase the risk of adverse obstetric outcomes. However, the data that are available do support this notion. Retrospective studies demonstrate that endometrial cavity-distorting leiomyomas (i.e., submucosal leiomyomas or intramural leiomyomas with an intracavitary component; International Federation of Gynecology and Obstetrics [FIGO] types 0, 1, 2, and 3) are associated with decreased fertility outcomes (e.g., clinical pregnancy, implantation, and live birth rates) and that these outcomes are improved with myomectomy. Subserosal leiomyomas (FIGO types 5, 6, and 7) do not affect fertility and therefore should not be removed solely for this indication. Intramural leiomyomas that do not distort the endometrial cavity (FIGO types 3 and 4) are also associated with decreased fertility, but myomectomy has not been shown to improve outcomes (Pritts et al. 2009). The mechanism by which non-cavity distorting intramural leiomyomas affect fertility remains unclear but may be related to the influence of these leiomyomas on endometrial receptivity (Rackow and Taylor 2010).

Available data also demonstrate that leiomyomas are associated with slightly increased risks of adverse obstetric outcomes, including abnormal placentation, fetal malpresentation, preterm premature rupture of membranes (PPROM), placental abruption, preterm delivery, cesarean delivery, intrauterine fetal demise, and postpartum hemorrhage. However, the odds ratios for almost all of these outcomes are less than 2.0, indicating that the absolute risks, although statistically significant, are relatively low (Qidwai et al. 2006; Stout et al. 2010). Surgical intervention to decrease the risks of future adverse obstetric outcomes should be balanced with the risks of preconception myomectomy.

3   Benefits of Laparoscopy

The advantages of laparoscopy over laparotomy are well established and include decreased morbidity and shorter recovery. Studies show that, compared to open myomectomy, laparoscopic myomectomy is associated with increased operative time but decreased intraoperative blood loss, smaller drop in hemoglobin, decreased postoperative pain, more patients fully recovered by postoperative day number 15, and fewer overall complications. Furthermore, the incidence of major complications (e.g., hemorrhage, visceral injury, thromboembolism), new leiomyoma formation, and pregnancy was not significantly different between laparoscopic and open approaches (Jin et al. 2009). Available data also demonstrate that laparoscopic myomectomy results in less adhesive disease which may affect fertility and subsequent small bowel obstruction (Bulletti et al. 1996).

4 Patient Selection

The wide application of laparoscopic myomectomy is limited by the characteristics of leiomyomas that can be feasibly removed by this approach and the availability of gynecologic surgeons with advanced laparoscopic skills (i.e., laparoscopic suturing). The location, size, and number of leiomyomas determine whether or not a patient is a candidate for laparoscopic myomectomy, although these parameters vary with surgical expertise.

Subserosal leiomyomas (FIGO types 5, 6, and 7), especially those that are pedunculated (FIGO type 7), are the easiest to remove laparoscopically. However, completely intramural leiomyomas (FIGO types 3 and 4) can also be excised with this approach. Some surgeons feel comfortable removing submucosal leiomyomas as well, although these are more often removed with hysteroscopy, depending on their size. If only relatively small FIGO type 0, 1, or 2 leiomyomas are to be removed, then a hysteroscopic approach should be used. Anterior and fundal leiomyomas are often easier to remove than are posterior leiomyomas. Proximity to important structures such as the uterine cornua and the uterine vessels should also be considered. Performing a laparoscopic myomectomy on large and/or many leiomyomas may be time-consuming because morcellation is usually necessary. Removal of such leiomyomas may also result in increased intraoperative blood loss.

The optimal criteria for laparoscopic myomectomy have not been established and depend on the experience and skill of the surgeon. The largest study to investigate this issue included 2,050 laparoscopic myomectomies and concluded that the following leiomyoma characteristics were associated with a significant increase in major complications (e.g., hemorrhage, visceral injury, failure to complete the planned procedure): size greater than 5 cm, total number removed more than three, and intraligamentous location (Sizzi et al. 2007).

Myomectomy should be considered in any patient with symptomatic uterine leiomyomas who desire uterine preservation for the purposes of fertility or other personal reasons. Laparoscopic myomectomy should not be performed in women in whom uterine preservation is contraindicated (e.g., uterine or cervical malignancy) nor in women in whom laparoscopy is contraindicated (e.g., due to medical comorbidities).

5 Preoperative Evaluation and Preparation

5.1 History and Physical Exam

Preoperative evaluation should start with a detailed history of the patient's leiomyoma-related symptoms, such as abnormal uterine bleeding or bulk symptoms. It is important to document how these symptoms affect her quality of life and daily activities. If abnormal uterine bleeding is present, then the patient should also be asked about the presence of symptoms of anemia. The medical history should include questions regarding a personal or family history of bleeding or clotting disorders, as well as other medical comorbidities which may affect the patient's ability to tolerate general anesthesia and laparoscopic surgery.

A thorough pelvic examination should be performed. On bimanual examination, uterine size, contour, and mobility should be noted along with any other abnormal findings such as the presence of adnexal masses. A fibroid uterus is usually enlarged, irregularly contoured, and/or firm on examination. Examination findings help guide surgical planning and the need for further evaluation including imaging studies.

5.2 Laboratory Tests

As significant blood loss can occur during myomectomy, a blood type and screen as well as a complete blood count should be performed, especially if a history of anemia is present or suspected. Further evaluation for bleeding disorders such as von Willebrand disease should be performed in the presence of other suggestive symptoms or signs, such as a history of heavy menstrual bleeding since menarche.

Premenopausal women aged 45 years or older with abnormal uterine bleeding and postmenopausal women with any uterine bleeding should undergo endometrial sampling to rule out endometrial hyperplasia and malignancy. Endometrial sampling should also be performed in women younger than 45 years with a history of unopposed estrogen exposure (e.g., obesity, polycystic ovarian syndrome), failed medical management, and persistent abnormal uterine bleeding (American College of Obstetricians and Gynecologists 2012). The presence of a uterine malignancy is a contraindication to myomectomy.

5.3   Imaging Studies

Clinically significant subserosal and intramural fibroids can usually be palpated on bimanual examination. Imaging studies can be used to confirm the presence, number, location, and size of leiomyomas. They can also detect the presence of other lesions, such as adnexal masses, that may impact surgical planning. Typically, pelvic ultrasound using a combination of transabdominal and transvaginal approaches is the initial study performed as it is the most readily available and least costly imaging technique. Ultrasonography is reasonably reliable for the evaluation of smaller uteri with four or fewer leiomyomas. Saline infusion sonohysterography, during which saline is injected into the endometrial cavity to provide uterine distension, allows for better delineation of submucosal leiomyomas and their intracavitary involvement. However, ultrasound has significant operator-dependent variability, resulting in inconsistent accuracy and poor reproducibility. Furthermore, ultrasonography has a limited field of view and does not capture most anatomic landmarks, making it difficult to use its images to create a three-dimensional representation of the uterus and its adjacent anatomy (Falcone and Parker 2013).

Pelvic magnetic resonance imaging (MRI) has been shown to have superior sensitivity and reproducibility in the detection of leiomyomas when compared to other imaging modalities, including ultrasonography, saline sonohysterography, and hysteroscopy (Dueholm et al. 2001). More accurate information regarding leiomyoma number, location, and size helps determine if a laparoscopic approach is feasible for myomectomy. Furthermore, tactile sensation is limited during laparoscopy, unlike during open myomectomy in which even small leiomyomas can be palpated. MRI may help a laparoscopic surgeon localize smaller leiomyomas intraoperatively.

MRI is considered the best imaging modality for the detection of adenomyosis, a condition characterized by the presence of endometrial glands within the myometrium (Champaneria et al. 2010). Adenomyosis can mimic leiomyomas in its clinical presentation as both can cause abnormal uterine bleeding, abdominal/pelvic pain, and uterine enlargement. MRI features consistent with adenomyosis include poor definition and thickening of the junctional zone (the interface between the endometrium and the myometrium) greater than 12 mm (Gordts et al. 2008).

Pelvic MRI is also indicated if uterine sarcoma is suspected. Due to their increased vascularity, leiomyosarcomas may demonstrate increased enhancement on gadolinium-enhanced timed MRI. Elevated serum total lactate dehydrogenase (LDH) and LDH isoenzyme-3 should also raise concern for leiomyosarcoma (Goto et al. 2002). Although rapid growth of a uterine mass (i.e., increasing by 6 weeks' gestational size within 1 year) being a sign of a potential uterine sarcoma is a commonly held belief, it has been shown that this is almost never true in premenopausal women (Parker et al. 1994). Ultimately, women in whom there exists a strong preoperative suspicion for uterine sarcoma or other uterine malignancy should not undergo laparoscopic myomectomy.

5.4   Informed Consent

Preoperative informed consent should include a discussion of alternatives to myomectomy, including expectant management, medical management, interventional radiology procedures such as uterine leiomyoma embolization and magnetic resonance-guided focused ultrasound, and other surgical options. Hysterectomy should be discussed with women who are not interested in preserving fertility as quality-of-life outcomes may be better than those with myomectomy (Spies et al. 2010).

Possible complications of myomectomy should be discussed. Complications include excessive bleeding requiring blood transfusion or, in the rare situation that life-threatening bleeding occurs and is unable to be controlled with other measures, hysterectomy. Patients who plan to become pregnant should be counseled about the potential need for cesarean delivery and the risk of uterine rupture. New leiomyoma formation and recurrence or persistence of leiomyoma-associated symptoms should also be discussed. Conversion to laparotomy is a possibility with all laparoscopic procedures.

Leiomyoma morcellation, if planned, must be discussed in detail. The safety of power morcellation during laparoscopic myomectomy and hysterectomy has recently come into question by the United States Food and Drug Administration (FDA), prompted by a widely publicized case report in which morcellation was used in the presence of an undiagnosed leiomyosarcoma. After performing a limited literature review which included nine studies, the FDA concluded that 1 in 350 women undergoing hysterectomy or myomectomy for the treatment of leiomyomas is found to have an unsuspected uterine sarcoma (U.S. Food and Drug Administration 2014). Subsequent literature reviews and case series have yielded a much lower incidence, as low as 1 in 1,960 women per a meta-analysis of 133 studies (Pritts et al. 2015). Patients should be counseled about the prevalence of uterine sarcoma and the possible risks of morcellation in the setting of an undiagnosed malignancy. Other risks of morcellation, including visceral injury, should also be discussed.

The informed consent discussion should be documented in the medical record and on the surgical consent form.

5.5 Managing Preoperative Anemia

Anemia resulting from heavy menstrual bleeding is a common symptom of leiomyomas. Preoperative anemia increases the risks of blood transfusion and perioperative morbidity and mortality. Iron supplementation is often used to increase preoperative hemoglobin levels. Oral iron is first-line therapy in nonurgent situations due to its ease of administration and cost-effectiveness. However, the response is relatively slow, requiring at least 1–2 weeks before any increase in hemoglobin occurs, and patients often report gastrointestinal side effects. Intravenous iron produces a more rapid rise in hemoglobin without gastrointestinal side effects but has the potential to cause allergic reactions including anaphylaxis, although rare. Epoetin, a recombinant form of erythropoietin, a hormone that stimulates red blood cell production, can also produce more rapid correction of preoperative anemia but is more expensive than iron supplementation.

Another approach toward the management of preoperative anemia is to treat the patient's heavy menstrual bleeding while she is awaiting surgery, resulting in an increase in hemoglobin. Pharmacologic agents that can induce amenorrhea include gonadotropin-releasing hormone (GnRH) agonists, continuous combined oral contraceptive pills, and oral progesterone. Many surgeons report that, in patients with prior GnRH agonist use, leiomyoma enucleation is noticeably more difficult because the tissue plane between the leiomyoma and the myometrium becomes obscured; however, this belief has not been proven in any study.

6 Operative Technique

6.1 Anesthesia and Patient Positioning

As with most laparoscopic gynecologic procedures, the patient should be placed under general endotracheal anesthesia and in the supine or lithotomy position. Lithotomy is required if the surgeon chooses to place a uterine manipulator which can be used to improve intraoperative visualization. A uterine manipulator also allows for instillation of indigo carmine or methylene blue dye if chromopertubation is planned or to determine if the endometrial cavity is entered during the procedure. The patient should also be placed in lithotomy if concomitant hysteroscopy is performed. Tucking of the bilateral upper extremities often provides surgeons with the best access to the operative field. Adequate intravenous access should be established by the anesthesiologist before the arms are padded and tucked. Both the abdomen and the vagina are surgically prepared. An indwelling catheter is inserted into the bladder to decrease the risk of intraoperative bladder injury and to monitor urine output. The catheter can also be used to backfill the bladder should delineation of its borders become necessary.

6.2 Prophylaxis

Virtually all laparoscopic myomectomies are at least 30 minutes in duration and are therefore considered major surgeries. As such, they pose at least low to moderate risk of venous thromboembolism. Therefore, prior to induction of anesthesia, each patient should receive venous thromboembolism prophylaxis, mechanical and/or pharmacologic, tailored to her individual risk factors, or lack thereof (American College of Obstetricians and Gynecologists 2007). A benefit of laparoscopic surgery is that patients regain postoperative mobility more rapidly than after laparotomy, thereby decreasing the risk of postoperative venous thromboembolism.

Antibiotic prophylaxis is not indicated for laparoscopic procedures. The risk of surgical site infection is low in procedures during which the bowel or vagina is not entered (American College of Obstetricians and Gynecologists 2009).

6.3 Laparoscopic Port Placement

Laparoscopic port placement is based on the location and size of the leiomyomas to be removed. The initial port is often placed at the umbilicus but may also be placed in the left upper quadrant (i.e., Palmer's point) if the uterine fundus is at or above the umbilicus or if significant umbilical adhesions are anticipated. Once the initial port is placed, the laparoscope is inserted into the peritoneal cavity and the abdomen and pelvis are examined. If there are findings that preclude safe completion of a laparoscopic myomectomy such as the presence of extensive adhesive disease, then the procedure should be converted to laparotomy.

Typically, three additional laparoscopic ports are placed. To make laparoscopic suturing more ergonomic, two right-sided ports are placed if the surgeon is right-handed or two left-sided ports if the surgeon is left-handed. The first port is placed approximately 2 cm superior and medial to the anterior superior iliac spine. This port can be 12 mm in size to allow for the passage of curved needles for suturing and for the insertion of the morcellation device, if used. A second, 5 mm port is placed medial and slightly superior to the first port. Another 5 mm port is placed in the contralateral lower quadrant.

6.4 Strategies to Decrease Intraoperative Blood Loss

Intraoperative blood loss can be decreased with pharmacologic and/or mechanical intervention. Perhaps the method most commonly used during laparoscopic myomectomy is the use of vasopressin, a pharmacologic agent that causes vasoconstriction. Vasopressin is injected into the myometrium at the site of the planned uterine incision. Injection can be performed using a long needle inserted through a laparoscopic port or directly through the anterior abdominal wall. Care should be taken to avoid intravascular injection by withdrawing the plunger of the syringe to check for blood prior to injection. Even in the absence of intravascular injection, vasopressin can cause systemic hemodynamic changes and has been associated with rare cases of cardiovascular collapse and death (Falcone and Parker 2013). Clear communication should occur between the surgeon and the anesthesiologist; the surgeon should notify the anesthesiologist when vasopressin is being administered, and, in turn, the anesthesiologist should notify the surgeon of any signs of hemodynamic instability in the patient. Furthermore, a maximum dose of vasopressin should be determined prior to surgery. Although the maximum safe dose of vasopressin has not been definitively established, a total dose of 4–6 units per procedure is widely used. Dilution of the vasopressin (e.g., 20 units of vasopressin in 100 ml of normal saline) helps to limit the total dose (Frishman 2009).

Uterotonics have also been used to decrease intraoperative blood loss. Small studies have demonstrated that both vaginal dinoprostone and vaginal misoprostol significantly decrease blood loss during myomectomy; however, the latter has not been shown to decrease the risk of blood transfusion. There is no evidence that the use of oxytocin decreases intraoperative blood loss or the risk of blood transfusion (Kongnyuy and Wiysonge 2014).

Mechanical interventions, such as the use of tourniquets or clamps, can be used to decrease intraoperative blood loss by occluding the uterine blood supply from the uterine and ovarian arteries. However, it is difficult to secure a tourniquet using laparoscopic instruments. Accordingly, they are not used as often during laparoscopic myomectomy as they are during open myomectomy.

Intraoperative blood salvage (e.g., Cell Saver) may be used in procedures in which significant blood loss is anticipated, thereby avoiding allogeneic blood transfusion and its associated complications. This technology involves suction of blood from the surgical field, separation and washing of the red blood cells, and eventual reinfusion to the patient. Intraoperative blood savage is less commonly used during laparoscopic myomectomy than during open myomectomy, likely because significant blood loss is more often anticipated during the removal of leiomyomas with characteristics that require an open approach.

6.5 Uterine Incision and Leiomyoma Removal

A transverse incision is made on the uterus directly over the leiomyoma and extended deeply until the leiomyoma is clearly seen. A monopolar device such as the hook or an ultrasonic cutting and coagulating device such as the Harmonic scalpel may be used. The transverse direction allows for more ergonomic suturing of the uterine defect when compared with a vertical incision. Care should be taken to avoid the uterine cornua, the ascending uterine artery and venous plexus lateral to the uterus, and the site where the uterine artery enters the uterus at the level of the internal cervical os. The leiomyoma is grasped with a tenaculum to provide traction. A combination of traction and countertraction, blunt and sharp dissection, and/or electrosurgery is used to dissect under the pseudocapsule and separate the plane between the leiomyoma and the surrounding myometrium, thereby enucleating the leiomyoma.

6.6 Repair of Uterine Defects

As is performed during an open myomectomy, all uterine incisions are closed in one or more layers, depending on the depth of the incision. Size 0 delayed absorbable suture such as poliglecaprone (Monocryl) or polydioxanone (PDS) is often used. Polyglactin (Vicryl) is another option but has a higher friction coefficient which may cause more fraying of the suture with extracorporeal knot tying. Absorbable barbed suture may also be used to close the myometrium. This suture not only obviates the need for knot tying but also maintains tension on the myometrium, thereby facilitating laparoscopic suturing. Indeed, expeditious closure of uterine defects significantly reduces intraoperative blood loss.

6.7 Morcellation of Leiomyomas

For leiomyomas that are too large to be removed from the abdomen directly through one of the laparoscopic port sites, morcellation can be accomplished by using an electromechanical device or manually by using a scalpel. Both techniques can be performed in an uncontained fashion or in a contained fashion within an extraction bag. To decrease the risk of visceral injury, the blade of the morcellation device should be under direct laparo-scopic visualization at all times, including during its insertion and removal from the abdomen. The blade should also be directed toward the anterior abdom-inal wall as much as possible. After all leiomyomas have been morcellated, the device should be removed from the abdomen and a thorough inspec-tion of the peritoneal cavity for tissue fragments must be performed. Copious irrigation and suctioning should be used to remove blood and any smaller tissue fragments.

6.8   Closure

At the close of the procedure, hemostasis should be assured throughout the peritoneal cavity. Mea-sures to prevent adhesion formation, such as placement of adhesion barrier products (e.g., Interceed, Seprafilm), may be taken if desired. The fascia of any laparoscopic port site that is 10 mm or larger should be closed to decrease the risk of incisional hernia development (Boike et al. 1995).

7   Complications

Complications of laparoscopic myomectomy are similar to those of open myomectomy, including blood loss, infection, and adhesion formation. Complications unique to a laparoscopic approach include conversion to laparotomy and those related to trocar insertion, such as trocar-related bowel or vascular injury.

8   Postoperative Care

Laparoscopic myomectomy is typically performed as an outpatient procedure. Overnight inpatient observation may also be considered. The patient may resume her routine activities including vaginal intercourse as soon as she feels comfortable. She may return to work once she has regained sufficient strength and mobility, usually within 2 weeks. A routine postoperative outpatient visit should occur within 2–6 weeks. During this visit, details of the

surgery and pathology results are reviewed, the abdomen and incisions are examined, the uterus is evaluated for hematoma formation, and the patient is evaluated for any potential complications.

9   Outcomes

9.1   Improvement of Symptoms

Although there is currently no data regarding the rate of symptom relief following laparoscopic myomectomy, success rates may be extrapolated from data for open myomectomy, which has been reported to provide symptom relief in approxi-mately 80% of patients (Broder et al. 2002).

9.2   New Leiomyoma Formation

The rate of new leiomyoma formation at 5 and 8 years after myomectomy has been reported to be 53% and 85%, respectively. However, rates of reoperation, arguably more significant for patients, were much lower at 7% and 16%, respec-tively. Risk factors for new leiomyoma formation include multiple leiomyomas present at the time of surgery, uterine size of 13 weeks or larger, and age younger than 36 years (Yoo et al. 2007). The rate of new leiomyoma formation is not signifi-cantly different between laparoscopic myomec-tomy and open myomectomy (Jin et al. 2009).

10   Pregnancy After Myomectomy

10.1   Interval to Conception

It is recommended that patients wait at least 3 months after myomectomy before attempting to conceive. A small prospective study used serial MRI to investigate the amount of time necessary for the uterine structure to reach a stable state following myomectomy. The authors concluded that the recovery process is complete at 12 weeks in the absence of hematoma or edema formation in the myometrium on MR images (Tsuji et al. 2006).

10.2 Risk of Uterine Rupture

Although cases of uterine rupture during labor in patients with prior myomectomy have been reported, the actual risk of rupture and the factors associated with an increased risk are unknown. Myomectomy in which the endometrial cavity is entered or the myometrium is otherwise significantly compromised is thought to incur risk similar to that of a prior classical cesarean delivery, the reported incidence of which ranges from 1% to 12%. Accordingly, it is recommended that women with prior myomectomy in which the myometrium may have been significantly compromised be delivered by cesarean delivery at 36–38 weeks of gestation. Myomectomy in which only pedunculated leiomyomas (FIGO type 7) are removed is thought to incur significantly less risk of uterine rupture. Therefore, women with prior myomectomy requiring minimal or no myometrial dissection are given the option of a trial of labor (Spong et al. 2011).

It has been argued that the risk of uterine rupture following laparoscopic myomectomy is higher than that following open myomectomy, possibly due to the technical challenge of laparoscopic suturing. However, more recent studies have demonstrated that the incidence of uterine rupture following myomectomy is similar between laparoscopic and open approaches (Flyckt and Falcone 2015). Multiple-layer closure of uterine defects and prudent use of electrosurgery are recommended to limit this risk (Parker et al. 2010).

11 Conclusion

Laparoscopic myomectomy is a safe, effective, and minimally invasive alternative to open myomectomy for women with symptomatic uterine leiomyomas who desire uterine preservation. Thorough preoperative evaluation and preparation ensure that appropriate patients are selected for this surgery. Outcomes are similar to that of open myomectomy while providing the benefits of decreased morbidity and quicker recovery that are afforded by laparoscopy. The wide application of laparoscopic myomectomy is limited by certain leiomyoma characteristics and the availability of gynecologic surgeons with advanced laparoscopic skills.

12 Cross-References

▶ Laparoscopic Hysterectomy
▶ Management of Abnormal Uterine Bleeding: Later Reproductive Years
▶ Management of Uterine Fibroids

References

American College of Obstetricians and Gynecologists Committee on Practice Bulletins – Gynecology. Practice bulletin number 84: prevention of deep vein thrombosis and pulmonary embolism. Obstet Gynecol. 2007;110(2 Pt 1):429–40.

American College of Obstetricians and Gynecologists Committee on Practice Bulletins – Gynecology. Practice bulletin number 104: antibiotic prophylaxis for gynecologic procedures. Obstet Gynecol. 2009;113(5):1180–9.

American College of Obstetricians and Gynecologists Committee on Practice Bulletins – Gynecology. Practice bulletin number 128: diagnosis of abnormal uterine bleeding in reproductive-aged women. Obstet Gynecol. 2012;120(1):197–206.

Baird DD, Dunson DB, Hill MC, Cousins D, Schectman JM. High cumulative incidence of uterine leiomyoma in black and white women: ultrasound evidence. Am J Obstet Gynecol. 2003;188(1):100–7.

Boike GM, Miller CE, Spirtos NM, Mercer LJ, Fowler JM, Summitt R, et al. Incisional bowel herniations after operative laparoscopy: a series of nineteen cases and review of the literature. Am J Obstet Gynecol. 1995;172(6):1726–31. discussion 1731–3

Broder MS, Goodwin S, Chen G, Tang LJ, Costantino MM, Nguyen MH, et al. Comparison of long-term outcomes of myomectomy and uterine artery embolization. Obstet Gynecol. 2002;100(5 Pt 1):864–8.

Bulletti C, Polli V, Negrini V, Giacomucci E, Flamigni C. Adhesion formation after laparoscopic myomectomy. J Am Assoc Gynecol Laparosc. 1996;3(4):533–6.

Champaneria R, Abedin P, Daniels J, Balogun M, Khan KS. Ultrasound scan and magnetic resonance imaging for the diagnosis of adenomyosis: systematic review comparing test accuracy. Acta Obstet Gynecol Scand. 2010;89(11):1374–84.

Dueholm M, Lundorf E, Hansen ES, Ledertoug S, Olesen F. Evaluation of the uterine cavity with magnetic resonance imaging, transvaginal sonography, hysterosonographic examination, and diagnostic hysteroscopy. Fertil Steril. 2001;76(2):350–7.

Falcone T, Parker WH. Surgical management of leiomyomas for fertility or uterine preservation. Obstet Gynecol. 2013;121(4):856–68.

Flyckt RL, Falcone T. Uterine rupture after laparoscopic myomectomy. J Minim Invasive Gynecol. 2015;22(6): 921–2.

Frishman G. Vasopressin: if some is good, is more better? Obstet Gynecol. 2009;113(2 Pt 2):476–7.

Gordts S, Brosens JJ, Fusi L, Benagiano G, Brosens I. Uterine adenomyosis: a need for uniform terminology and consensus classification. Reprod BioMed Online. 2008;17(2):244–8.

Goto A, Takeuchi S, Sugimura K, Maruo T. Usefulness of Gd-DTPA contrast-enhanced dynamic MRI and serum determination of LDH and its isozymes in the differential diagnosis of leiomyosarcoma from degenerated leiomyoma of the uterus. Int J Gynecol Cancer. 2002;12(4):354–61.

Jin C, Hu Y, Chen XC, Zheng FY, Lin F, Zhou K, Chen FD, Gu HZ. Laparoscopic versus open myomectomy – a meta-analysis of randomized controlled trials. Eur J Obstet Gynecol Reprod Biol. 2009;145(1):14–21.

Kongnyuy EJ, Wiysonge CS. Interventions to reduce haemorrhage during myomectomy for fibroids. Cochrane Database Syst Rev [Internet]. 2014 [cited 2016 Feb 22]. Available from: http://onlinelibrary.wiley.com/doi/10. 1002/14651858.CD005355.pub5/abstract

Parker WH, YS F, Berek JS. Uterine sarcoma in patients operated on for presumed leiomyoma and rapidly growing leiomyoma. Obstet Gynecol. 1994;83(3):414–8.

Parker WH, Einarsson J, Istre O, Dubuisson JB. Risk factors for uterine rupture after laparoscopic myomectomy. J Minim Invasive Gynecol. 2010;17(5):551–4.

Pritts EA, Parker WH, Olive DL. Fibroids and infertility: an updated systematic review of the evidence. Fertil Steril. 2009;91(4):1215–23.

Pritts EA, Vanness DJ, Berek JS, Parker W, Feinberg R, Feinberg J, et al. The prevalence of occult leiomyosarcoma at surgery for presumed uterine fibroids: a meta-analysis. Gynecol Surg. 2015;12(3):165–77.

Qidwai GI, Caughey AB, Jacoby AF. Obstetric outcomes in women with sonographically identified uterine leiomyomata. Obstet Gynecol. 2006;107(2 Pt 1): 376–82.

Rackow BW, Taylor HS. Submucosal uterine leiomyomas have a global effect on molecular determinants of endometrial receptivity. Fertil Steril. 2010;93(6):2027–34.

Sizzi O, Rossetti A, Malzoni M, Minelli L, La Grotta F, Soranna L, Panunzi S, Spagnolo R, Imperato F, Landi S, Fiaccamento A, Stola E. Italian multicenter study on complications of laparoscopic myomectomy. J Minim Invasive Gynecol. 2007;14(4):453–62.

Spies JB, Bradley LD, Guido R, Maxwell GL, Levine BA, Coyne K. Outcomes from leiomyoma therapies: comparison with normal controls. Obstet Gynecol. 2010; 116(3):641–52.

Spong CY, Mercer BM, D'Alton M, Kilpatrick S, Blackwell S, Saade G. Timing of indicated late-preterm and early-term birth. Obstet Gynecol. 2011;118(2 Pt 1): 323–33.

Stout MJ, Odibo AO, Graseck AS, Macones GA, Crane JP, Cahill AG. Leiomyomas at routine second-trimester ultrasound examination and adverse obstetric outcomes. Obstet Gynecol. 2010;116(5):1056–63.

Tsuji S, Takahashi K, Imaoka I, Sugimura K, Miyazaki K, Noda Y. MRI evaluation of the uterine structure after myomectomy. Gynecol Obstet Investig. 2006;61(2): 106–10.

U.S. Food and Drug Administration. Safety communication: laparoscopic uterine power morcellation in hysterectomy and myomectomy [Internet]. 2014 [cited 2016 Mar 5]. Available from: http://www.fda.gov/ MedicalDevices/Safety/AlertsandNotices/ucm424443. htm

Yoo EH, Lee PI, Huh CY, Kim DH, Lee BS, Lee JK, et al. Predictors of leiomyoma recurrence after laparoscopic myomectomy. J Minim Invasive Gynecol. 2007;14(6): 690–7.

Laparoscopic Hysterectomy

Alexander Chiang, Steve Yu, and William H. Parker

Abstract

Laparoscopic hysterectomy is a minimally invasive surgical technique for removal of the uterus. It is more commonly performed than the vaginal hysterectomy. The laparoscopic approach has better outcomes compared with an abdominal hysterectomy. Laparoscopic hysterectomy can be used for treatment of abnormal uterine bleeding, uterine fibroids, pelvic pain, and premalignant and malignant gynecologic conditions involving the uterus. Alternatives to hysterectomy should always be discussed when possible and appropriate. The appropriate selection for a laparoscopic hysterectomy is largely based on the surgeon's experience and skill and the preference of the patient.

Keywords

Laparoscopic hysterectomy • Laparoscopy • Minimally invasive gynecologic surgery • Uterine fibroid • Uterine leiomyoma • Endometriosis

A. Chiang (✉) • S. Yu • W.H. Parker
Department of Obstetrics and Gynecology, David Geffen School of Medicine at UCLA, Los Angeles, CA, USA
e-mail: achiang@mednet.ucla.edu; spyu@mednet.ucla.edu; wparker@mednet.ucla.edu; wparker@ucla.edu

© Springer International Publishing AG 2017
D. Shoupe (ed.), *Handbook of Gynecology*,
DOI 10.1007/978-3-319-17798-4_83

Contents

1 Introduction

Laparoscopy is a diagnostic and therapeutic surgical procedure that uses a laparoscope attached to a video camera. The procedure is considered minimally invasive because the incisions on the abdomen are significantly smaller than the traditional open surgery. For instance, most laparoscopic instruments will fit through an opening of 5 mm. The abdomen is insufflated with carbon dioxide (CO_2) gas, which is bio-inert and non-flammable. Access into the abdomen is provided by laparoscopic ports, also known as trocars, that allow easy insertion and exchange of the camera and/or surgical instruments. The trocars also function as a valve, preventing the loss of gas during surgery. In other words, it maintains pneumoperitoneum allowing adequate visualization during the case. The first trocar inserted into the abdomen is referred to as the primary trocar. All subsequent trocars are called secondary.

Laparoscopic surgical procedures have been developed for most surgical procedures that were previously only done by laparotomy. In gynecology, laparoscopy is performed for most surgeries including, but not limited to, hysterectomy, cystectomy, oophorectomy, sterilization, salpingectomy, myomectomy, and cancer staging procedures.

Hysterectomy used to be the second most common surgical procedure after cesarean section in the 1980s to early 2000s. Currently, the numbers have declined from approximately 600,000 per year to 480,000 per year as of the latest census in 2009. Hysterectomy is now the seventh most common surgical procedure performed in the United States (Fingar et al. 2014). Many alternatives to hysterectomy, both medical and surgical, have contributed to this decline. The first laparoscopic hysterectomy was performed in 1989 (Reich et al. 1989). Since then, as surgeons have become better trained in laparoscopic surgery, there has been an increasing trend toward the use of laparoscopic hysterectomy. According to the 2009 census, approximately 20% of all hysterectomies for benign disease were performed by laparoscopy. Abdominal hysterectomy comprises approximately 56%, vaginal hysterectomy 19%, and robotic 5% of all hysterectomies (Cohen et al. 2014).

2 Types of Hysterectomy

Hysterectomies can be divided into total (removal of the cervix with the uterus) or supracervical (removal of the uterine corpus without the cervix). A supracervical hysterectomy is also called a partial or subtotal hysterectomy. In gynecologic oncology cases, radical hysterectomies (a total hysterectomy including the parametria) can also be performed to obtain wider margins.

Routes of hysterectomy include:
- Vaginal hysterectomy
- Laparoscopic or robotic-assisted laparoscopic hysterectomy
- Abdominal (open) hysterectomy

Laparoscopic hysterectomies can be subdivided into:
- Total laparoscopic hysterectomy: the uterus and cervix are removed en bloc through the vagina or morcellated (cut and removed in smaller pieces) and removed through the trocars. After removal of the cervix, the resulting vaginal cuff (the proximal opening of the vagina where the uterus was amputated) is sutured closed.
- Laparoscopic supracervical hysterectomy: the uterus is at the level of the cervix, which is left intact. The uterus must be morcellated in order to extract it or delivered through a minilaparotomy.

- Laparoscopic-assisted vaginal hysterectomy: the round and broad ligaments and possibly the adnexa (ovaries and fallopian tubes) are transected laparoscopically, and the remainder of the hysterectomy is completed vaginally as with a vaginal hysterectomy.
- Robotic-assisted laparoscopic hysterectomy: the laparoscopic camera and instruments are manipulated with a surgeon-controlled computerized robot.

3 Indications

Hysterectomies are commonly performed for abnormal uterine bleeding, pelvic pain, uterine prolapse, and premalignant or malignant conditions. According to a census in 2005, 26.9% of hysterectomies were performed with fibroids as the indication, 25.2% for abnormal uterine bleeding, 16.2% for endometriosis, and 11.7% for pelvic pain (Merrill 2008).

4 Benefits and Risks

Many of the studies assessing the benefit and risk profiles between abdominal, vaginal, and laparoscopic hysterectomies are limited by poor reporting or imprecise data. Any discussion of benefits and risks are ultimately based on the patient's wishes and surgeon's experience and skill set. The risks are generally reduced with increased experience with laparoscopic hysterectomy (usually more than 30 cases (Mäkinen et al. 2013)). In general, there are many benefits to laparoscopic hysterectomy compared to abdominal hysterectomy. The benefits include: reduction in overall morbidity, blood loss, infection, postoperative pain, length of stay in the hospital, and recovery time. Ureteral and bowel injury rates are generally equal between laparoscopic and open procedures (Mäkinen et al. 2013).

Specifically, benefits include:

- Shorter length of stay in the hospital: decreased by 1–3 days for the laparoscopic approach

compared to the abdominal approach (Aarts et al. 2015)
- Shorter recovery time: return to normal activities was 36.3 days for the abdominal approach vs 22.7 days for the laparoscopic approach (Aarts et al. 2015)
- Decreased wound infection rates: 2.4% with abdominal and 1.5% with laparoscopic (Mäkinen et al. 2013)
- Fewer thromboembolic events: 0.1% with abdominal vs 0% with laparoscopic (Mäkinen et al. 2013)
- Less significant bleeding (as measured by postoperative hemoglobin drop or need for blood transfusion): 1.6% with abdominal and 0.6% with laparoscopic (Aarts et al. 2015)

The risks of laparoscopic hysterectomy versus abdominal hysterectomy include a higher risk of:

- Vaginal cuff dehiscence (0.75% in laparoscopic hysterectomies versus 0.38% in abdominal hysterectomies (Hur et al. 2011))
- Bladder injuries (1.0% for laparoscopic hysterectomies versus 0.7% for abdominal hysterectomies (Härkki-Sirén et al. 1998; Mäkinen et al. 2013)
- Vascular injuries (1.6% for laparoscopic hysterectomies versus 0.9% for abdominal hysterectomies (Aarts et al. 2015)
- Increased operating time: 30 min more for laparoscopic hysterectomy (Aarts et al. 2015)

When comparing laparoscopic hysterectomy with vaginal hysterectomy, there is no overall statistically significant difference except a longer operating time for laparoscopic hysterectomy of about 17 min (Aarts et al. 2015).

Increased risks with a laparoscopic hysterectomy have been associated with larger uterine size (or mass) >250–300 g, increased body mass index (or degree of obesity), pelvic adhesive disease such as endometriosis or prior abdominal surgeries, and other comorbidities (e.g., cardiopulmonary disease), or increased concern for malignancy. Consideration and management strategies for these conditions will be further discussed later in this chapter.

5 Alternatives

Since the late 1990s, viable alternatives to hysterectomy have been further developed due to improvements in medical and surgical therapies.

It is noteworthy that many women with uterine leiomyoma do not need any treatment. Expectant management of fibroids causing nonlife-threatening bleeding or pelvic pressure has been underappreciated. There is some evidence that expectant management is a viable alternative based on several factors including the impact of symptoms such as bleeding or pain on a woman's quality of life and patient age (Reiter et al. 1992). Some women may find their symptoms improve or resolve with menopause.

For patients with pelvic organ prolapse, pelvic floor therapy and pessary usage may provide improvement in symptoms and allow patients to avoid surgery.

5.1 Medical Therapy

Nonhormonal medical treatments are available for abnormal uterine bleeding, symptomatic fibroids, adenomyosis, and endometriosis. A common medication regimen includes high-dose nonsteroidal anti-inflammatory drugs (NSAIDs) such as ibuprofen or naproxen taken orally to minimize bleeding and pain. NSAIDs can decrease heavy menstrual bleeding from adenomyosis, fibroids, and ovulatory dysfunction and decrease pelvic pain from endometriosis, adenomyosis, and fibroids. Two proteins that mediate coagulation in the endometrium are prostacyclins and thromboxane A2, and their relative levels allow a homeostatic effect for control of bleeding. Prostacyclins inhibit vasoconstriction and the platelet aggregation effect of thromboxane A2. NSAIDs indirectly inhibit prostacyclin synthesis and thus increase the relative effect of thromboxane A2 causing vasoconstriction and platelet aggregation at the site of the uterine endometrial and myometrial vasculature. This leads to attenuation of heavy menstrual bleeding. Additionally with fibroids, endometriosis, and adenomyosis, the anti-inflammatory effects of NSAIDs also block the cytokine cascade of inflammation that causes pain.

Another effective nonhormonal treatment for heavy menstrual bleeding is tranexamic acid (Lysteda), an antifibrinolytic agent that can reduce heavy menstrual bleeding by 26–54% (Milsom et al. 1991). In comparative studies, this medication was more effective than NSAIDs, but not as effective as a levonorgestrel intrauterine system (LNG-IUS) (Milsom et al. 1991). This drug has been used in Sweden since the 1960s for heavy menstrual bleeding and is widely available and affordable in Canada and Europe. It has been available in the United States since the FDA approval in 2009. It has not gained wide popularity due to its high cost. The safety of this medication has been widely studied, and it does not seem to increase the risk of thrombosis; however it is not recommended to use tranexamic acid in conjunction with birth control pills. Tranexamic acid is a safe alternative to hormonal medical management in patients who have contraindications to hormones, such as breast cancer, but also desire to avoid surgery.

Gonadotropin-releasing hormone (GnRH) agonists such as Lupron Depot can be used in cases of symptomatic fibroids, adenomyosis, endometriosis, and ovulatory dysfunction by suppressing ovarian function and decreasing hormonal stimulation of these conditions. This treatment is limited due to the side effects of pharmacologically induced menopause, including hot flashes, vaginal dryness, and headaches and is thus only a temporary solution, usually when the patient is transitioning to menopause or preparing for surgery.

Another hormonal treatment option for both dysmenorrhea and heavy menstrual bleeding is progesterone-only medication such as norethindrone or medroxyprogesterone. These synthetic progestins can cause an attenuation of growth of the endometrial lining and minimize fibroid-related heavy menstrual bleeding. A similar effect can be seen with the LNG-IUS, also known as the Mirena intrauterine device (IUD) in the United States. This device is placed inside the uterine cavity, and the slowly released levonorgestrel decidualizes the endometrium with subsequent decreased heavy menstrual bleeding or dysmenorrhea. The advantage of the LNG-IUS is that it has a long-acting effect up to 5 years and has minimal systemic progesterone-related side effects such as nausea, bloating, breast tenderness, appetite stimulation, or bone mineral density loss. For younger women not currently desiring fertility, this would have the added benefit of a highly effective, reversible, long-acting contraception. Fibroids distorting the uterine cavity are a contraindication stipulated by the manufacturer if used for contraception due to the increased expulsion rates of 0–20% from a recent systematic review (Zapata et al. 2010). However, if the patient is highly motivated to avoid surgery, this could still be a viable option as long as the patient is counseled on all risks. Furthermore, the patient should also be informed that any progesterone-only method has the risk of causing breakthrough spotting or bleeding, which may also be equally undesired compared with heavy menstrual bleeding. A comparative 10-year study done in Finland in the 2000s showed that for women with heavy menstrual bleeding, 46% of those initially randomized to an IUD ultimately underwent a hysterectomy due to continued symptoms. Satisfaction measured by standardized questionnaires was similarly improved in both the IUD and hysterectomy groups over the first 5 years but returned to baseline for both groups between 5 and 10 years (Heliövaara-Peippo et al. 2013).

5.2 Surgical Therapy

Endometrial ablation is a minimally invasive procedure for the treatment of abnormal uterine bleeding. The general principle involves the use of a heating element to ablate the endometrium, which produces menstrual blood. There are many different devices that have been developed. The procedure usually takes less than 10 min to perform. Endometrial ablation is a popular choice for many patients since it does not require any incisions and the recovery is almost instantaneous. The general contraindications for this procedure include suspected malignancy or malignancy, desire for future childbearing, and a large uterus.

Uterine artery embolization (UAE) is performed by an interventional radiologist. The idea is to occlude the blood supply to the fibroid, causing ischemic degeneration. Over time, the fibroid or fibroids reduce(s) in size, resulting in reduction of uterine bleeding and pain. Uterine artery embolization has been shown to be effective in short- and long-term follow-up studies with 95% of women who underwent this procedure noting a significant improvement of fibroid-related symptoms and quality of life after 3 years. However, 29% of women developed post-procedure amenorrhea, and 14.4% underwent an additional invasive procedure such as hysterectomy (9.8%), myomectomy (2.8%), and a repeat UAE (Goodwin et al. 2008). After 5 or more years, 75% of women who underwent UAE reported normal or improved bleeding, while 20% had undergone an additional invasive procedure (Walker and Barton-Smith 2006). Contraindications include size and types of fibroids (e.g., pedunculated or intracavitary fibroids) and desire for future childbearing. The safety of this procedure with regard to subsequent future fertility and pregnancy is limited by small case series and conflicting results. Slightly increased rates of miscarriage, malpresentation, preterm delivery, and postpartum hemorrhage have been reported (Homer and Saridogan 2010).

Myomectomy is also an alternative to hysterectomy for symptomatic fibroids and can be performed hysteroscopically, laparoscopically, or abdominally depending on the location and size of the fibroid(s). Traditionally, this is performed in women of reproductive age desiring to preserve fertility; however, the rates of myomectomy have increased since the 1990s in women no longer desiring future fertility. In addition to the preservation of the uterus, myomectomy has an additional benefit compared to hysterectomy. The main blood supply to the ovary is the ovarian artery, which is a direct branch from the aorta. However, some of the ovarian blood supply arises from the uterus. Therefore, after a hysterectomy, about 10% of women undergo menopause 2–3 years before their expected natural time. This iatrogenic effect is not observed after a myomectomy (Farquhar et al. 2005).

6 Surgical Planning

6.1 Preoperative Workup

A thorough medical, surgical, gynecologic, and obstetric history should first be obtained. Any comorbidities that may impact the ability to tolerate surgery should be evaluated and properly assessed. A careful physical examination should be performed with attention to uterine size and shape when considering feasibility of a laparoscopic approach and need for morcellation. Furthermore, the location of potential fibroids specifically in the cervix or posterior lower uterus should be identified as this may make the uterus more difficult to remove. Prior surgical scars and the absence of uterine mobility should be assessed as indicative of possible adhesive disease. Obesity can also alter the ability to successfully complete a surgical procedure, and thus any excessive abdominal pannus should be noted.

Imaging can be very helpful in the majority of hysterectomies. A pelvic ultrasound is generally useful for evaluation of a fibroid uterus and any concomitant adnexal pathology that may also need to be addressed at the time of surgery. Magnetic resonance imaging (MRI) may sometimes help with diagnosis of atypical fibroids or help determine if morcellation should be attempted if leiomyosarcoma is suspected based on imaging. Imaging is not helpful in determining the severity or extent of endometriosis or adhesive disease.

Tissue evaluation with an endometrial biopsy may be necessary for patients at risk for uterine malignancy. Preoperative knowledge of malignancy would change the planning of the surgery by involving a gynecologic oncologist who would perform staging procedures, such as lymph node sampling. A recent pap smear to ensure there is no concomitant cervical cancer is also recommended according to the current American College of Obstetrics and Gynecology (ACOG) guidelines.

The minimum laboratory evaluation should include a complete blood count in cases of acute or chronic abnormal uterine bleeding. A basic metabolic panel should be considered if an obstructive uropathy is suspected from a large pelvic mass. Any additional labs may be necessary depending on other comorbid conditions.

7 Patient-Specific Risk Factors

7.1 Obesity

Laparoscopy can be safely performed on obese patients. The increased degree of difficulty in obese patients can be decreased with robotic-assisted laparoscopy, but this may not improve operating time or costs. Attention to patient positioning with extra cushioning along the joints and extremities is advised. The degree of tilt in the Trendelenburg position may be limited due to increased weight and pressure of the abdominal pannus on the chest compromising the ability to adequately ventilate. This is compounded by the fact that pneumoperitoneum pressures may need to be increased in obese patients in order to improve intra-abdominal visualization. Anti-slip padding and straps should be used to prevent sliding of the patient in the Trendelenburg position. Entry into the abdominal cavity for insufflation via a Veress needle or a direct optical entry technique is still considered easiest at the umbilicus where the distance from the skin into the abdominal cavity is the shortest. An open Hasson entry technique may not be feasible without a larger incision due to the depth of the subcutaneous fat. Central obesity also increases the distance to the aorta, and thus a $90°$ entry angle will increase successful entry into the abdomen. Longer trocars may be needed depending on the degree of obesity.

7.2 Uterine Size and Contour

The size of the uterus not only plays an important role in determining the route of hysterectomy, but with laparoscopic hysterectomy, large uteri over

16 weeks in size may make visualization of the anterior lower uterine segment and parametria difficult. Limited visualization can prohibit adequate access to the uterine vessels for ligation. An appropriate uterine manipulator and usage of a single tooth tenaculum in the assistant's laparoscopic port may facilitate further caudal and contralateral manipulation of the uterus off the pelvic side wall to improve visualization of the adnexa and uterine vessels. Any fibroids that distort the uterine anatomy such as cervical, broad ligament, or posterior fibroids may preclude completion of a hysterectomy due to limited visualization and access to the uterine vessels or bladder flap. Laparoscopic myomectomy, if feasible, may be necessary prior to completion of the hysterectomy.

7.3 Abdominal and/or Pelvic Adhesive Disease

Prior abdominal surgeries, such as cesarean sections and/or myomectomies, and endometriosis or a history of a prior abdominal infection, such as ruptured appendicitis, may increase the degree of adhesive disease and thus increase the risks of injury to adjacent bowel, bladder, or adnexal organs. Usually, a safe route of entry is at Palmer's point, located approximately 3 cm inferior to the left costal margin along the midclavicular line. If this site of entry is desired, placement of an oral-gastric or nasogastric tube is highly advised in order to decompress the stomach and move the associated small gastric vessels away from the site of entry.

7.4 Concern for Malignancy

If there is a high index of suspicion for a gynecologic malignancy and if the uterus is too large to be extracted through the vagina, then laparoscopic hysterectomy should be avoided. In other words, tissue extraction by morcellation should not be performed if malignancy is suspected. There should be a high level of suspicion if a fibroid increases in size in a postmenopausal woman.

8 Preoperative Preparation

8.1 Prior to the Day of Surgery

A preoperative medical clearance may be needed for significant comorbid conditions. The patient should have an adequate NPO status, usually 8 hours prior to the surgery. In cases of anemia due to abnormal uterine bleeding, an adequate hematocrit level should be achieved with iron supplementation or a blood transfusion perioperatively in cases of acute hemorrhage. Bowel preparation is not necessary, although this is controversial as some surgeons find it beneficial for visualization.

8.2 On the Day of Surgery

The patient is placed under general anesthesia to manage ventilation, while the abdomen is insufflated and the patient is in the Trendelenburg position. Adequate mechanical, pharmacologic, or a combination of both types of thromboprophylaxis should be given. Obese patients have a higher risk of thromboembolism. Antibiotics should be given prior to the start of the case. Typical regimens include a third-generation cephalosporin, such as cefazolin or cefoxitin, or in case of penicillin allergy, clindamycin and gentamicin or metronidazole with either gentamicin or a fluoroquinolone.

The patient should be positioned in a low lithotomy position on the table with antiskid or anti-slippage pads and careful cushioning to avoid neurologic injury but still allow for surgeon position and access to the vagina. The sacrum should be near the end of the operating table. Tucking the arms to the sides of the patient allows more mobility for the surgeon. The anesthesiologist should be notified to ensure adequate access to IV lines and the blood pressure cuff. In patients with a high risk of blood loss or a low starting hematocrit level, a second large bore IV access should be considered. The chest above the level of the nipples is often strapped or taped to the bed in order to minimize cephalad slippage of the patient while in the Trendelenburg position. Caution must be taken to ensure that the chest strap or taping allows adequate ability to ventilate while under general anesthesia.

A uterine manipulator should be placed for manipulation of the uterus during surgery. This facilitates visualization during surgery, displaces the ureter laterally when ligating and transecting the uterine artery, and delineates the cervicovaginal junction when amputating the uterus and cervix away from the vagina. A bladder catheter should be placed to decompress the bladder.

9 Procedure

Most hysterectomies can be performed with three trocars (the primary and one secondary trocar on each side of the abdomen). Attention should first be focused on what is commonly referred to as the triple pedicles of the uterus. These structures include the round ligament, the utero-ovarian ligament, and the fallopian tube. The triple pedicles should be individually ligated and transected. There are numerous disposable and reusable surgical instruments that can perform this function.

Visualization of the ureters should be done early in the case, before abrasion of the peritoneum makes identification more difficult. Small incisions can be made in the peritoneum above the ureters to help with later identification, if necessary. The next step is to serially ligate and transect the broad ligament to the level of the isthmus of the uterus. At this level, the bilayers of the broad ligament should be separated into its anterior and posterior leaflets. Careful dissection should be made anteriorly to dissect the bladder away from the lower uterine segment and the cervix. It is imperative to develop the vesicovaginal space to adequately repair the vaginal cuff during the later steps of the surgery. After the bladder is safely dissected away from the isthmus of the uterus, the uterine artery should be further isolated by dissecting the posterior leaf of the broad ligament. Once the uterine artery is isolated, it should be ligated and transected. It is very important to clamp the uterine artery perpendicular to the cervix at the level of the cervical os. This practice, adopted from the widely performed abdominal hysterectomy, will minimize ureteral injury.

Once the uterine artery is transected from the isthmus of the uterus, the next step is to dissect down the cardinal ligament until the lateral fornix of the vagina is reached. It is critical to stay medial to the transected uterine artery and dissect the cardinal ligament parallel to the cervix. Again, this practice will minimize the risk of ureteral injury and also prevent unnecessary blood loss.

After the cardinal ligament is dissected to the lateral fornix of the vagina, the same steps should be taken on the contralateral side. Once this is performed, then the uterus is ready for amputation. The colpotomy can be cumbersome and challenging to perform in many cases because the cervicovaginal junction may be difficult to delineate. However, the use of some of the newer disposable uterine manipulators, which outline the cervicovaginal junction circumferentially, can make this task relatively simple. Once the cervicovaginal junction is clearly identified, then the colpotomy can be performed with monopolar cautery, bipolar cautery hook, or harmonic scalpel. Regardless of energy source used, it is crucial to minimize thermal injury during this step to minimize the risk of vaginal cuff dehiscence.

If the amputated uterus can be extracted from the vagina, then it is advisable to keep the uterus in the vagina to retain pneumoperitoneum if the vaginal cuff is going to be repaired laparoscopically. The vaginal cuff can be repaired by interrupted sutures or by running a continuous suture. Both techniques are acceptable. With both techniques, it is crucial to take at least 1 cm of full thickness purchase of the pubocervical fascia to reapproximate the vaginal cuff. This is only possible by taking the time and diligence to dissect the bladder off of the upper vagina in order to adequately develop the vesicovaginal junction.

10 Operative Considerations

10.1 Types of Uterine Manipulators

Generally, the type of uterine manipulator depends on personal preference due to experience or familiarity of use. Some uterine manipulators are reusable while others are disposable. Many manipulators have cups that clearly delineate the vaginal fornices and thus the cervicovaginal junction. This makes the colpotomy much easier. Some have built-in pneumo-occluder balloons that trap the CO_2 in the abdominal cavity when the colpotomy is made. Others have various mechanisms to allow greater degrees of freedom of movement.

10.2 Choice of Abdominal Entry (Peritoneal Access) Technique

There are three common techniques for entering the abdominal cavity: Hasson open entry, closed entry with a Veress needle, and closed entry with direct optical entry.

The open entry (Hasson) technique is performed by making a periumbilical incision on the skin and dissecting until the fascia is reached. The fascia is then grasped with a Kocher clamp, and the fascia and underlying peritoneum is entered with scissors. Sutures are placed on both sides of the fascia and anchored to the trocar.

The Veress needle technique involves using a hollow-bore needle to directly enter the peritoneal cavity. This is a blind technique that relies on haptic feedback and audible "clicks" as the needle penetrates the fascia and peritoneum. The "clicks" are produced by the recoil of the spring-loaded safety obturator as it traverses the fascia and peritoneum. Intraperitoneal placement is confirmed by the free passage of saline through the needle and low starting intraperitoneal pressure confirmed by the insufflator machine. Once access is confirmed, the abdomen is fully insufflated with carbon dioxide gas.

The direct optical entry technique is performed using specialized optical trocars with a transparent tip. The obturator of the trocar has an opening that allows for direct insertion of the laparoscope. The peritoneal cavity is then entered with direct visualization. The major advantage of this technique compared to the Veress needle technique is lower rates of failed entry (Larobina and Nottle 2005).

The latest meta-analysis in 2012 has concluded that major complications for all entry techniques are similar. There was no advantage of open versus closed entry techniques in reduction of vascular or visceral injury contrary conventional wisdom. There was an increased rate of failed entry with the Veress needle. Lastly, there was quicker entry time with the direct optical entry technique. (Ahmad et al. 2012)

10.3 Placement of Ports

The location for port placement is determined by the size of the uterus, the concern for underlying adhesive disease, the presence of any abdominal wall hernias, and the surgeon's preference. The primary port is usually placed intra- or peri-umbilically with bilateral secondary ports placed just lateral to the rectus muscles and inferior epigastric vessels. The location of the inferior epigastric vessels is generally delineated by using an imaginary line extending superiorly along the anterior abdominal wall from the insertion of the round ligaments at the inguinal canal. Staying lateral to this imaginary line avoids injury to the inferior epigastric vessels. Transillumination from the peritoneal cavity does not reveal these epigastric vessels but instead reveals superficial vessels in the skin. These superficial vessels may be inadvertently lacerated during port placement leading to superficial hematomas and thus should also be avoided. In cases of suspected abdominopelvic adhesive disease, Palmer's point can be used for the primary port, as described in the previous section.

10.4 Selection of Instruments

With any surgery, the availability and usage of appropriate instruments facilitates the ease, speed, and safety of surgery. A 0° laparoscope is typically used to start. A 30° laparoscope is recommended for visualization around a large uterine body: anteriorly during the creation of the bladder flap, laterally for access to the uterine vasculature and ligaments, and posteriorly to aid visualization of the cervicovaginal junction during colpotomy. Typically, a vessel-sealing device and a cutting device are needed. There are many devices that perform one or both of these functions, but the advantages and limitations of specific devices are beyond the scope of this chapter. Generally, a bipolar vessel sealer with a cutting feature capable of ligation and transection of the ligaments, vessels, and peritoneal layers and a monopolar electrosurgical device to perform the colpotomy are sufficient. A suction irrigator is necessary for clearing away any blood and to ensure that no uterine or fibroid tissue fragments remain after morcellation. An array of grasping tools, both penetrating and blunt, are also required to manipulate the uterus, adnexa, or bowel. In case of morcellation of a large uterus or in a supracervical hysterectomy, a morcellator is commonly used to facilitate removal of the uterine corpus and cervix, as long as malignancy is not suspected.

10.5   Minimizing Risk of Ureteral Injury

The most common complication in laparoscopic hysterectomy is injury to the urinary tract. The ureters can be easily injured for all types of hysterectomy, especially laparoscopic hysterectomy. Knowledge of the anatomic course of the ureter is vital to avoid direct or indirect injury to the ureter. Injury may occur when ligating and transecting the infundibulopelvic ligaments and vessels, the uterine arteries, the cardinal ligaments, and the uterosacral ligaments. With laparoscopy, visualization of the ureter is much easier due to the magnified optics, illumination, and insufflation of the abdominal cavity. The ureter is commonly identified transperitoneally at the lateral pelvic side wall as it courses inferiorly and medially toward and lateral to the uterosacral ligaments. It can also be located overlying and crossing the bifurcation of the common iliac vessels or at the pelvic brim just lateral to the insertion of the infundibulopelvic ligament and vessels. If scarring of the peritoneum from prior pelvic infection, surgery, or endometriosis is noted, a retroperitoneal entry and dissection starting with the transection of the round ligament will allow identification

of the ureter along its course. In rare cases, a complete ureterolysis may be required.

During ligation of the uterine artery, the uterine manipulator cup is pushed in a cephalad direction to create tension at the cervicovaginal junction. This increases the distance between the uterine artery and ipsilateral ureter to minimize direct injury or indirect thermal injury to the ureter. Currently the recommendation by the American Association of Gynecologic Laparoscopists (AAGL) recommends cystourethroscopy after laparoscopic hysterectomy at the surgeon's discretion. However, their recommendation stops short of recommending routine use in all laparoscopic hysterectomy procedures due to insufficient evidence of benefit for detecting all urinary tract injuries. Further discussion of management of ureteral injury is discussed below.

10.6   Minimizing Risk of Bladder Injury

Adequate visualization of the bladder peritoneal fold is necessary, and using a 30° laparoscope may facilitate this. When skeletonizing the uterine artery, the anterior and posterior leaflets of the broad ligament are typically separated with the anterior layer incised medially to create the bladder flap. In the case of adhesions from endometriosis or pelvic infection or scarring from prior surgery (such as a cesarean section), careful attention to the underlying cervical and vaginal vasculature as well as the bladder vascular pillars is necessary to avoid persistent oozing of blood that can obscure the surgical field. One technique to minimize this is to tent the bladder using a grasper or to backfill the bladder with air or saline to demarcate the borders of the bladder dome. Blunt dissection using an atraumatic grasper, a probe, or an electrosurgical instrument can gently separate the bladder from the anterior lower uterine segment, cervix, and vagina. If scarring is dense, sharp dissection using laparoscopic scissors or careful monopolar coagulation just superior or at the level of the bladder flap will further dissect deeper into the lower uterus or cervix, which can facilitate separation of the bladder adhesion. Lateral transection of the round ligament can also provide access to the bladder flap. Another technique is a posterior approach where the cardinal ligament and uterine vessels are first transected, allowing access to the plane of pubocervical fascia, and thus entry to the vagina is made posteriorly to the scarred bladder adhesion.

Further discussion of management of bladder injury is described below.

10.7 Techniques to Identify the Uterine Artery

Gentle separation of the anterior and posterior leaflets of the broad ligament should allow for skeletonization of the uterine artery. If prior scarring is noted, anatomy may be distorted. Additional techniques to locate the uterine artery include retroperitoneal dissection of the internal iliac artery to locate the origin of the uterine artery. Traction on the medial umbilical fold will identify the origin of the obliterated umbilical vessels from the uterine artery. The ureter can be found directly below this insertion point.

10.8 Approaches to Closure of the Vaginal Cuff

The closure of the vaginal cuff can be done vaginally after removal of the amputated uterus and cervix specimens or before removal of the specimens if the specimen is too large to remove vaginally and morcellation is planned. The closure of the vaginal cuff can also be performed laparoscopically with intracorporeal or extracorporeal knot tying. Deciding which route of closure is based on surgeon experience, preference, and patient factors such as age, parity, and obesity. Extensive electrosurgical desiccation at the cuff site should be avoided. Ideally, at least a 1 cm margin of tissue should be incorporated to

minimize cuff dehiscence. Transvaginal closure of the cuff has been shown in retrospective studies to have a lower risk of cuff dehiscence, although this has not been evaluated with randomized prospective studies (Uccella et al. 2012).

10.9 Concomitant Removal of the Fallopian Tubes and/or Ovaries

The risks and benefits for removal of the fallopian tubes and/or ovaries at the time of hysterectomy should be discussed preoperatively with the patient. There are increasingly numerous studies showing that the fallopian tube may be the origin of ovarian, fallopian, and primary peritoneal cancer. Thus, concomitant removal of the fallopian tube at the time of hysterectomy is becoming more common (Przybycin et al. 2010). Removal of the ovaries at the time of hysterectomy depends on the indication of the hysterectomy, age of the patient, and any concomitant adnexal pathology. Without indication for removal, ovaries should be left in situ as numerous studies have shown benefit for morbidity and mortality in retaining the ovaries. (Parker et al. 2013)

11 Complications

11.1 Bladder Injury

If bladder injury is suspected, instillation of the bladder with sterile milk or methylene blue diluted in saline can identify extravasation of colored fluid. A bubble test can also be performed by insufflating the bladder with air after filling the pelvis with saline above the level of the bladder. If there is a bladder injury, then bubbles can be visualized from the injured site. After repair of the bladder, a Foley catheter should be placed for 1–2 weeks to decompress the bladder and facilitate the bladder healing. If the trigone is injured, careful assessment for ureteral kinking or injury must also be performed following repair.

11.2 Ureteral Injury

Identification and prophylactic measures as described above are key to minimizing ureteral injury. Cystourethroscopy should be performed if ureteral injury is suspected. If ureteral injury is identified, intraoperative consultation with a urologist is recommended in case ureteral stents, reanastomosis, or resection may be necessary. Thermal spread injuries from electrosurgery are insidious and may present 7–10 days after the time of trauma. Awareness of this potential complication and careful attention to nonspecific complaints in the postoperative period are required to make this diagnosis.

11.3 Bowel Injury

Identification of possible bowel injury is the first step to treatment. The type of repair necessary depends on the type of bowel injury. Injuries often arise from laparoscopic instruments, resulting in sharp puncture or thermal damage. Superficial serosal injuries may be oversewn with excellent results. However, repair of enterotomies depends on size of the defect and the location within the gastrointestinal tract. The repair may be done with primary closure or may require a bowel resection with primary reanastomosis. Intraoperative consultation with a general or colorectal surgeon is recommended.

12 Postoperative Management

Most studies show improved recovery with enhanced recovery regimens including early ambulation for prevention of venous thrombotic events and discontinuation of bladder catheterization immediately after surgery or early during the postoperative recovery period to prevent catheter-associated urinary tract infections. Furthermore, early enteral feeding and minimization of overall

intravenous fluids to decrease risk of ileus can also expedite recovery (Kalogera et al. 2013).

The decision for same-day discharge or discharge after 1–2 days depends on surgeon comfort level, institutional guidelines, availability of outpatient follow-up, patient comfort, difficulty of the surgery, and types and severity of comorbidities. Studies have shown that same-day discharge can be safe and cost-effective (Khavanin et al. 2013), however at the risk of slightly increased rates of reevaluation within 60 days (4% for outpatient postoperative care vs 3.6% for inpatient) (Khavanin et al. 2013) and risk of decreased reported quality of life at 2 and 4 days post-operation (Kisic-Trope et al. 2011).

12.1 Common Postoperative Complaints

Informing the patient preoperatively of the likely healing process following surgery can often alleviate patient concerns. Most common postoperative complaints can be addressed with expectation management. The patient should be informed of the duration and degree of vaginal spotting or bleeding. Right shoulder pain due to irritation of the phrenic nerve in the right diaphragm from the carbon dioxide gas and blood should also be discussed. The phrenic nerve innervates both the right diaphragm and right shoulder. The patient should be made aware of expected soreness or bruising at the incision sites. Face and upper body swelling due to prolonged Trendelenburg position may also be expected. Subcutaneous emphysema or crepitus can also occur due to insufflation of carbon dioxide gas in the subcutaneous tissue which then tracks along the subcutaneous plane.

13 Conclusion

Laparoscopic hysterectomy is a minimally invasive procedure that is rapidly growing in popularity compared to other routes of hysterectomy. It is important to counsel patients about the risks, alternatives, and benefits inherent to this procedure.

Successful outcomes are associated with surgeon experience, awareness of pitfalls, timely identification of complications, and active postoperative management.

14   Cross-References

▸ Diagnosis and Management of Delayed Postoperative Complications in Gynecology: Neuropathy, Wound Complications, Fistulae, Thromboembolism, Pelvic Organ Prolapse, and Cuff Complications
▸ Gynecologic History and Examination of the Patient
▸ Management of Abnormal Uterine Bleeding: Later Reproductive Years
▸ Management of Uterine Fibroids
▸ Pathology of the Uterine Corpus
▸ Robotic Surgery in Gynecology: Indications, Advantages, Avoiding Complications
▸ Vaginal Hysterectomy: Indications, Avoiding Complications

References

Aarts JW, Nieboer TE, Johnson N, Tavender E, Garry R, Mol BW, Kluivers KB. Surgical approach to hysterectomy for benign gynaecological disease. Cochrane Database Syst Rev. 2015;8:CD003677. doi:10.1002/14651858.CD003677.pub5.

Ahmad G, O'Flynn H, Duffy JMN, Phillips K, Watson A. Laparoscopic entry techniques. Cochrane Database Syst Rev. 2012;2:CD006583. doi:10.1002/14651858.CD006583.pub3.

Cohen SL, Vitonis AF, Einarsson JI. Updated hysterectomy surveillance and factors associated with minimally invasive hysterectomy. JSLS. 2014;18(3). https://www.ncbi.nlm.nih.gov/pmc/articles/PMC4208898/.

Farquhar CM, Sadler L, Harvey SA, Stewart AW. The association of hysterectomy and menopause: a prospective cohort study. BJOG. 2005;112:956–62.

Fingar K, Stocks C, Weiss AJ, Steiner CA. Most frequent operating room procedures performed in U.S. hospitals, 2003–2012. [Internet] 2014. [Updated 2014 Dec; cited 2016 Feb 23] Available from: https://www.hcup-us.ahrq.gov/reports/statbriefs/sb186-Operating-Room-Procedures-United-States-2012.jsp

Goodwin SC, Spies JB, Worthington-Kirsch R, Peterson E, Pron G, Li S, Myers ER, Fibroid Registry for Outcomes Data (FIBROID) Registry Steering Committee and Core Site Investigators. Uterine artery embolization for treatment of leiomyomata: long-term outcomes from the FIBROID Registry. Obstet Gynecol. 2008;111(1):22.

Härkki-Sirén P, Sjöberg J, Tiitinen A. Urinary tract injuries after hysterectomy. Obstet Gynecol. 1998;92(1):113.

Heliövaara-Peippo S, Hurskainen R, Teperi J, Aalto AM, Grénman S, Halmesmäki K, Jokela M, Kivelä A, Tomás E, Tuppurainen M, Paavonen J. Quality of life and costs of levonorgestrel-releasing intrauterine system or hysterectomy in the treatment of menorrhagia: a 10-year randomized controlled trial. Am J Obstet Gynecol. 2013;209(6):535.e1.

Homer H, Saridogan E. Uterine artery embolization for fibroids is associated with an increased risk of miscarriage. Fertil Steril. 2010;94(1):324.

Hur HC, Donnellan N, Mansuria S, Barber RE, Guido R, Lee T. Vaginal cuff dehiscence after different modes of hysterectomy. Obstet Gynecol. 2011;118(4):794.

Kalogera E, Bakkum-Gamez JN, Jankowski CJ, Trabuco E, Lovely JK, Dhanorker S, Grubbs PL, Weaver AL, Haas LR, Borah BJ, Bursiek AA, Walsh MT, Cliby WA, Dowdy SC. Enhanced recovery in gynecologic surgery. Obstet Gynecol. 2013;122(2 Pt 1):319–28.

Khavanin N, Mlodinow A, Milad MP, Bilimoria KY, Kim JY. Comparison of perioperative outcomes in outpatient and inpatient laparoscopic hysterectomy. J Minim Invasive Gynecol. 2013;20(5):604–10.

Kisic-Trope J, Qvigstad E, Ballard K. A randomized trial of day-case vs inpatient laparoscopic supracervical hysterectomy. Am J Obstet Gynecol. 2011;204(4):307.e1.

Larobina M, Nottle P. Complete evidence regarding major vascular injuries during laparoscopic access. Surg Laparosc Endosc Percutan Tech. 2005;15(3):119.

Mäkinen J, Brummer T, Jalkanen J, Heikkinen AM, Fraser J, Tomás E, Härkki P, Sjöberg J. Ten years of progress – improved hysterectomy outcomes in Finland 1996–2006: a longitudinal observation study. BMJ Open. 2013;3:e003169. doi:10.1136/bmjopen-2013-003169.

Merrill RM. Hysterectomy surveillance in the United States, 1997 through 2005. Med Sci Monit. 2008;14(1):CR24–31.

Milsom I, Andersson K, Andersch B, Rybo G. A comparison of flurbiprofen, tranexamic acid, and a levonorgestrel-releasing intrauterine contraceptive device in the treatment of idiopathic menorrhagia. Am J Obstet Gynecol. 1991;164(3):879.

Parker WH, Feskanich D, Broder MS, Chang E, Shoupe D, Farquhar CM, Berek JS, Manson JE. Long-term mortality associated with oophorectomy compared with ovarian conservation in the nurses' health study. Obstet Gynecol. 2013;121(4):709–16.

Przybycin CG, Kurman RJ, Ronnett BM, IeM S, Vang R. Are all pelvic (nonuterine) serous carcinomas of tubal origin? Am J Surg Pathol. 2010;34(10):1407–16.

Reich H, DeCaprio J, McGlynn F. Laparoscopic hysterectomy. J Gynecol Surg. 1989;5:213.

Reiter R, Wagner P, Gambone J. Routine hystectomy for large asymptomatic uterine leiomyomata: a reappraisal. Obstet Gynecol. 1992;79:481.

Uccella S, Ceccaroni M, Cromi A, Malzoni M, Berretta R, De Iaco P, Roviglione G, Bogani G, Minelli L, Ghezzi F. Vaginal cuff dehiscence in a series of 12,398 hysterectomies: effect of different types of colpotomy and vaginal closure. Obstet Gynecol. 2012;120(3):516–23.

Walker WJ, Barton-Smith P. Long-term follow up of uterine artery embolisation – an effective alternative in the treatment of fibroids. BJOG. 2006;113(4):464.

Zapata LB, Whiteman MK, Tepper NK, Jamieson DJ, Marchbanks PA, Curtis KM. Intrauterine device use among women with uterine fibroids: a systematic review. Contraception. 2010;82(1):41.

Robotic Surgery in Gynecology: Indications, Advantages, Avoiding Complications

John P. Lenihan Jr.

Abstract

The use of computers to assist surgeons in the operating room has been an inevitable evolution in the modern practice of surgery. Robotic assisted surgery has been evolving now for over two decades and has finally matured into a technology that has caused a monumental shift in the way gynecologic surgeries are performed. Prior to robotics, the only minimally invasive options for most gynecologic procedures including hysterectomies were either vaginal or laparoscopic approaches. However, even with over 100 years of vaginal surgery experience and more than 20 years of laparoscopic advancements, most gynecologic surgeries in the United States were still performed through an open incision. That changed in 2005 with the introduction of the da Vinci Surgical Robot™ for gynecology. Over the last decade, the trend across the country has now dramatically shifted to less open and more minimally invasive procedures. Robotic assisted procedures now include not only hysterectomy but also most all other commonly performed gynecologic procedures including myomectomies, pelvic support procedures, and reproductive surgeries. This success however has not been without controversies particularly around costs and complications. The evolution of computers to assist surgeons and make minimally invasive procedures more common is clearly a trend that is sustainable. It is now incumbent on surgeons, hospitals, and medical societies to determine the most cost-efficient and productive use for this technology.

Keywords

Robotic assisted surgery • Hysterectomy • Myomectomy • Credentialing and privileging

Contents

J.P. Lenihan Jr. (✉)
Department of Obstetrics and Gynecology, University of Washington School of Medicine, Medical Director of Robotics and Minimally Invasive Surgery, MultiCare Health System, Tacoma, WA, USA
e-mail: john.lenihan@multicare.org

© Springer International Publishing AG 2017
D. Shoupe (ed.), *Handbook of Gynecology*,
DOI 10.1007/978-3-319-17798-4_55

1   Introduction

Robotic surgery is actually surgery performed by a skilled surgeon with the assistance of a computer utilizing a remote **telesurgery** platform (Herron and Michael Marohn 2007). Remote surgery has been a dream for the last century. In the late 1980s, DARPA (Defense Advanced Research Projects Agency) funded a remote surgery program targeted for the battlefield. Researchers at Stanford University (Stanford Research Institute or SRI), developed early technology around tele-presence. Many civilian companies and labs worked on robotics such as IBM who developed remote center technology, MIT who developed cable-driven technology for low friction manipulators, and Computer Motion who developed the first surgical robot, ZEUS. In 1990, researchers at SRI formed a company that licensed these technologies and started the long process of turning a good idea into a product. They merged with their primary competitor at the time, Computer Motion and formed Intuitive Surgical (Sunnyvale, CA), the developer of the **da Vinci Surgical Robotic System**™. This system was the only commercially available robot from the late 1990s to 2015. Today, other manufacturers are entering the marketplace with new novel robotic systems.

2   Early Days

Initially, the surgical robot was designed for battlefield use with predominantly vascular capabilities. However, urologists soon found the robot was a great surgical approach to prostate cancer surgery, and the commercial version took off. Lonnie Smith, the first CEO of Intuitive Surgical, said that, initially, the company "aimed for the heart but hit the prostate instead." In June 2005, the FDA approved the da Vinci Robot™ for use by gynecologists. Because hysterectomies are the second most common surgery done in the United States, it didn't take long for GYN to surge to the top of the robotic surgery adoption curve. The initial robot, the "standard system, evolved" to an "S" model with improved high-definition 3-D vision and easier docking technology. In 2010, the "Si" next-generation model was introduced. It had a more flexible bedside cart (the actual robot) as well as improved technology that allowed the development and use of newer instruments such as vessel sealers, staplers, as well as new imaging modalities such as infrared and fluorescence. It also was the platform for the first robotic single-site technology that allowed surgeons to perform single-site surgery with the help of the computer to make it less challenging for surgeons who were used to operating in a 2-D laparoscopic world. The latest robot model was introduced in 2014: the "Xi." This robotic platform is designed for complex multi-quadrant abdominal surgery such as cancer surgery (Figs. 1, 2, 3 and 4). Future platforms for Single Port™ surgery from Intuitive Surgical and from competitors such as Trans-Enterix (Alf-X™) and Titan Medical (Sport™) will bring welcome competition to this market and lead to more innovation that will ultimately benefit surgeons and patients (Figs. 5 and 6).

3   Single Site

Reduced port laparoscopic surgery has been a goal of most minimally invasive surgeons since the dawn of laparoscopy. The drawbacks of fewer ports decreased the ability of the surgeon to utilize instruments in a typical comfortable fashion to dissect tissue and particularly to sew. Single-site techniques such as single-incision laparoscopic surgery (SILS), laparo-endoscopic single-site (LESS), and single-site surgery (SSS) have been reported since the 1990s, but these have been slow to catch on with most gynecologic surgeons

Fig. 1 Original DaVinci™ Standard Robotic Surgical System

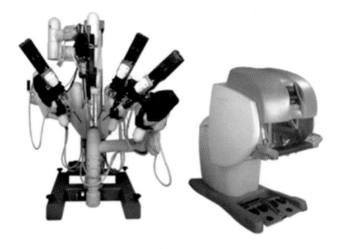

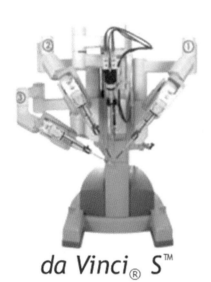

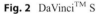

Fig. 2 DaVinci™ S

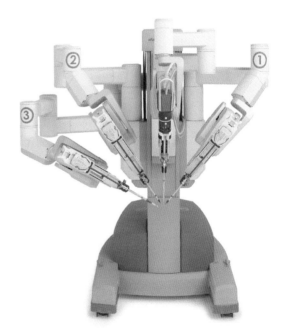

Fig. 3 DaVinci™ Si

primarily due to the long learning curves and the requirement for exceptional innate ability to perform laparoscopy. In 2014, Intuitive Surgical released a modification of their Si robot that allowed surgery to be performed robotically through a single site. This four channel port housed the camera, an accessory channel, and two non-wristed robotic instruments. The robotic microprocessors converted the surgeon's hand control to operate the left arm instrument with the surgeon's right hand, which was now on the patient's right side, and vice versa. This allowed the surgery to proceed like normal robotic surgery and not require "cross vision" which was typical of straight stick single-site laparoscopy. Recently in 2015, a wristed needle driver was added to this platform making suturing more like traditional robotics. Future developments are aiming to increase the mobility and articulation of the instruments as well as the camera flexibility to provide a more ergonomic and standardized procedure.

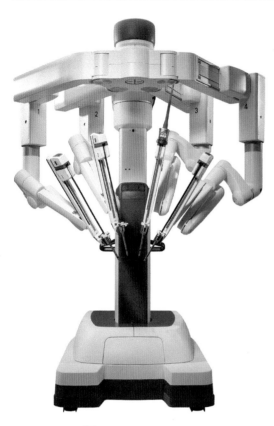

Fig. 4 DaVinci™ Xi

4 Robotic Advantages

The computer-assisted enhancement of robotics has many advantages over straight stick laparoscopy. The most significant advantage acknowledged by most all surgeons is the advantage to see the operative field in **high-definition 3-D** with a stable camera platform controlled by the surgeon. Additional advantages include wristed instruments with **articulation** that goes beyond the normal ability to manipulate instruments, scaled motion to allow for more precise movements, and a significant **ergonomic** benefit of being able to sit comfortably in a console rather than standing upright at the bedside trying to watch a remote video monitor while moving rigid instruments into small spaces. Disadvantages of robotic surgery pointed out by many include the loss of **haptic feedback** (touch), which many surgeons feel is integral to being a good surgeon. Another drawback is limited ability to communicate with the OR team while the surgeon is task focused in the robotic console. Team training with **"cockpit communication"** techniques employed by the aviation industry helps to minimize this limitation. That being said, many surgeons who did not feel comfortable performing hysterectomies or other complex gynecologic procedures with traditional laparoscopy have

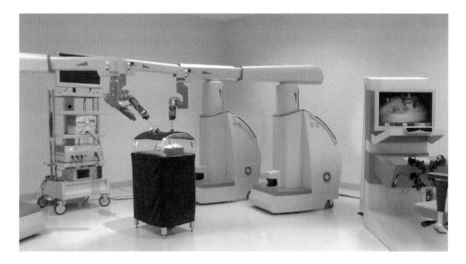

Fig. 5 TransEnterix Alf-X Robotic platform

Fig. 6 Titan Medical Sport™ Robotic System

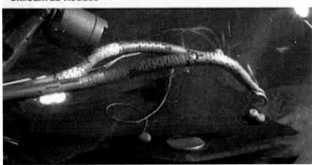

found the robot to be an enabling device allowing them to convert open procedures to minimally invasive operations.

As robotic technology evolves, there are now enhancements to the robot that provide even more advantages to the surgeon. The Si and Xi robots have the capability of visualizing **infrared** without additional equipment. This enables surgeons to see infrared ureteral catheters (Stryker Infra-Vision™), which may help to identify ureters in the face of complex pathology and thereby prevent an inadvertent ureteral injury. **Fluorescence imaging** utilizing dyes that fluoresce with laser stimulation such as indocyanine-green dye (ICG Dye) have proven useful in identifying sentinel lymph nodes, aberrant blood vessels, and even endometriosis implants, again enabling surgeons to see structures that might otherwise not be visible with the naked eye. Future developments being studied now include improved single-port capabilities, "GPS" guidance for surgeons using overlayed imaging technology such as ultrasound and MRI, and even remote co-surgery using internet-connected consoles to allow expert surgeons in academic centers to operate with primary surgeons in their local facilities.

5   Gynecology Adoption

Initially, the robot seemed most useful for enabling surgeons to perform complex minimally invasive procedures more easily for the surgeon than most surgeons could perform with laparoscopy. Laparoscopy is a minimally invasive technique that has been utilized by gynecologists since the mid-

1970s. In the 1980s, surgeons started attempting more complex procedures requiring dissection and sewing, and in 1989, Dr. Harry Reich reported the first total laparoscopic hysterectomy (Reich 1989). In 2003, Dr. Arnold Advincula reported an initial series of robotic myomectomies which at the time were typically accomplished by almost all gynecologists as an open procedure (Advincula et al. 2004). Subsequently, after the da Vinci Robot™ was approved for gynecology surgeons, many reports were published evaluating it as a new tool compared to laparoscopy (Advincula and Song 2007). **Learning curves** were defined as being more extensive than was initially suspected, and early adoption associated with complications was reported in national media, prompting the legal profession to become interested in robotic surgery and advertise for patients injured by the robot (Carreyrou 2010). It became clear that while robots were enabling, they didn't substitute for good surgical technique and judgment. Based on this, professional societies sought to provide guidance for the proper utilization of this expensive technology as well as recommendations for training and credentialing (ACOG technology assessment in obstetrics and gynecology No. 6: robot-assisted surgery 2009; AAGL Guidelines: Guidelines for Privileging for Robotic-Assisted Gynecologic Laparoscopy 2014).

The rapid adoption of computer-assisted telesurgery by gynecologists had led to a dramatic change in the route of hysterectomy in the United States. Traditionally, rates of abdominal hysterectomy surgery have been very high approaching 60–70% (CDC-MMWR 2002; Jacobsen et al. 2006). The minimally invasive approaches to hysterectomy seemed to be stuck at 25% for several

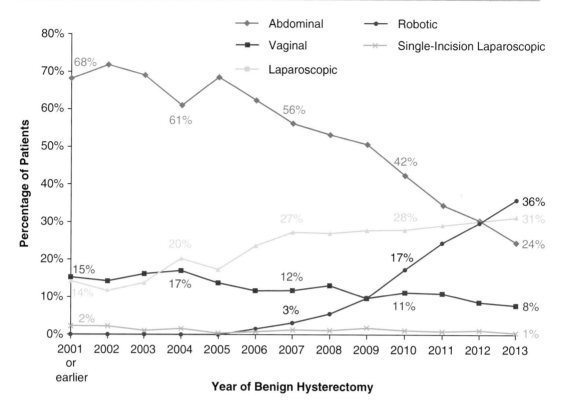

Fig. 7 Changing trends in types of hysterectomies performed in the USA

decades for the vaginal approach and less than 15% for the laparoscopic approach (CDC-MMWR 2002; Jacobsen et al. 2006). With the adoption of robotic hysterectomy in 2005, the rate of TAH has dropped across the country to <40% (Wright et al. 2013a) (Fig. 7).

There have been many controversies regarding robotic surgery, however, mostly based on the high cost of the surgical robots. Many medical societies are now pushing to limit the robot to skilled surgeons performing complex surgeries and to encourage most gynecologists in the communities to use less expensive minimally invasive approaches such as vaginal or laparoscopic hysterectomy (Rardin 2014; Advincula 2014).

6   Hysterectomy

Hysterectomy is one of the most common surgical procedures performed in the United States. While the numbers of hysterectomies have fallen over

the last decade due to a variety of other less-invasive options for managing abnormal uterine bleeding, hysterectomy is still considered the definitive treatment for many gynecologic conditions and has a high satisfaction rate among patients when compared to other simpler but often less-effective treatments (Pinion et al. 1994; Dickersin et al. 2007). Initial reports by experienced laparoscopic surgeons who started to perform robotic assisted surgeries showed that similar outcomes could be achieved compared to laparoscopic procedures but that operative times were often much longer. The **learning curve** to become proficient for experienced expert gynecologic surgeons has been shown to be between 50 and 100 cases (Lenihan et al. 2008; Seamon et al. 2008; Payne and Dauterive 2008). Gynecologic oncologists have reported extensive data showing the advantages of robotic surgery for complex cancer surgeries (Bell et al. 2008; Estape et al. 2009; Sert and Abeler 2011). Initially, these surgeries were limited to **endometrial cancers** with pelvic lymph node staging, but now there are many series showing excellent results compared to laparoscopic and traditional open surgeries for cancers requiring para-aortic node dissection, radical hysterectomies for **cervical cancer,** and even **ovarian cancer** staging procedures (Magrina et al. 2011).

The role of robotic surgery in benign hysterectomy has been more debated based primarily around **cost issues**. Many studies have shown increased costs associated with robotic surgery over other forms of hysterectomy. One well-publicized study used a large national payor inpatient database and showed that for low-volume surgeons (average <12 procedures per year), quality outcomes with robotics were not different than with laparoscopic surgery but that the cost for robotic cost surgery was higher. This study was done, however, when almost all of the robotic surgeons were still in the early stages of their learning curves. Also, capital costs of the robot were factored in but not laparoscopic equipment capital costs. And finally, this study evaluated surgeons who only performed on average ten cases per year (Wright et al. 2013b).

More recent publications comparing costs among experienced high-volume robotic surgeons have shown that these differences return to negligible once surgeons are through their learning curves (Lim et al. 2016).

Additional studies have looked at outcomes for robotic hysterectomies in patients with very large uteri who would typically not be candidates for laparoscopic or vaginal surgery and would in most instances require a traditional open procedure. These studies showed again excellent outcomes with a minimally invasive approach in the hands of experienced surgeons (Payne et al. 2010).

7   Myomectomy

The da Vinci Robot has wristed instruments with five degrees of motion similar to a surgeon's natural wrist motion. This allows surgeons to overcome one of the most difficult tasks associated with traditional "straight stick" laparoscopy:

sewing. Removing fibroids is a sewing intensive surgical procedure, hence, one for which the robot is ideally suited. Minimally invasive myomectomy was an uncommon procedure prior to the development of the da Vinci Robot. Despite three randomized trials showing the superiority of laparoscopic myomectomy over open myomectomy, less than 3% of gynecologic surgeons performed laparoscopic myomectomies on at least 50% of their patients (Gargiulo 2011). Being able to use multiple instrument arms and wristed instruments of the robot enabled surgeons to perform myomectomies with multiple layer myometrial closures comparable to what could be achieved in an open procedure. Multicenter trials have reported excellent outcomes both for the procedure itself as well as for **subsequent pregnancies**. In a large series by Pitter et al., 107 women out of 872 myomectomies over a 5 year period conceived 127 pregnancies and 92 deliveries. Uterine rupture occurrence was minimal (one patient), and adhesions were found in 11% at the time of cesarean section (Pitter et al. 2013). Most robotic myomectomy procedures experienced minimal blood loss with a same-day discharge and rapid return to normal activities (Advincula et al. 2011; Ascher-Walsh and Capes 2010; Barakat et al. 2011).

8   Sacrocolpopexy and Pelvic Suport Procedures

A sacrocolpopexy is another sewing intensive surgery that requires precise dissection techniques as well as excellent sewing skills. Laparoscopic sacrocolpopexy (SCP) was shown in the late 1990s to have excellent outcomes comparable to open procedures (Ross and Preston 2005). But like myomectomy, this procedure required an advanced skill set for any surgeon who wanted to perform this surgery with traditional straight stick laparoscopy. The da Vinci Robot™ was utilized by early pioneers to perform mesh sacrocolpopexies with or without hysterectomy. These initial procedures had long operative times, especially while the surgeons were early in their learning curves; however outcomes were comparable (Geller et al. 2008). One randomized controlled sacrocolpopexy trial was done that also showed longer operative times but similar length of stay and outcomes (Paraiso et al. 2011). This study however compared expert laparoscopic surgeons with surgeons who had done less than ten robotic surgeries, so the learning curve effect was not taken into account. Subsequent publications have shown improved operative times and improved outcomes with experienced surgeons who do a high volume of these procedures (Ploumidis et al. 2014). Recent controversies surrounding the use of synthetic mesh in pelvic organ prolapse repairs have shown a lower incidence of mesh erosion with sacrocolpopexy than with vaginally placed mesh used for anterior and posterior repairs. Almost all of the Female Pelvic Medicine and Reconstructive Surgery (FPMRS) fellowships across the country now teach robotic approaches to sacrocolpopexy to their fellows (Occhino et al. 2013).

8.1   Endometriosis and Chronic Pelvic Pain

Patients who suffer from endometriosis can have more complex pathology and adhesions than patients with cancer. Traditionally, most surgeons performing diagnostic laparoscopy for **chronic pelvic pain** patients have limited options for dealing with extensive endometriosis and inflammatory adhesions based on the limitations of traditional laparoscopy and the surgeon's innate abilities. Most experts now recommend aggressive surgical excision of endometriosis implants and adhesions in patients with advanced and chronic disease (Hart et al. 2005; Shakiba et al. 2008). Meta-analyses have shown no benefit to surgery in patients with early-stage disease when comparing surgery to medical therapy for the treatment of pain, although there has been some benefit if **infertility** is considered (Giudice 2010; John and Hummelshoi 2013). Another potential advantage of robotics over traditional laparoscopy for treating endometriosis is associated with the enhanced high-definition 3-D vision afforded by the robotic system which may give surgeons an increased ability to recognize endometriotic

lesions with this enhanced visual capability. The use of laser-enhanced dyes that identify vascular lesions has also been studied recently to increase the ability of surgeons to recognize endometriosis (Lue et al. 2015). This technology, called Firefly by Intuitive Surgical, is not yet approved by the FDA for this purpose and is still under IRB approved investigations. There have also been reports of surgeries to transect pelvic nerves, such a presacral neurectomies, to help with chronic central pelvic pain and dysmenorrhea in younger patients wishing to preserve fertility (Kapetanakis et al. 2012). The dissection of the presacral space is challenging with regard to identifying the major vessels as well as the nerves in this area. The enhanced visual capabilities of the da Vinci Robot along with the wristed and scaled motion of the instruments allow for this dissection to be done by surgeons who are not comfortable working in this space with traditional laparoscopic instruments.

8.2   Reproductive Surgery

The da Vinci Robot™ has been used by reproductive surgical specialists to try and restore normal anatomy in patients requesting future childbearing. The ability to lyse **adhesions** carefully and gently, similar to laparoscopy, has shown better outcomes when compared to open surgery. Some authors have reported series of tubal reanastamosis after prior tubal ligation to restore fertility with good outcomes (Falcone et al. 1999; Dharia Patel et al. 2008). While this technique facilitates excellent repairs with good results based on the enhanced 3-D high-definition vision and micro dexterity associated with the robot, these procedures have not been widely adopted due primarily to costs as well as the availability of other successful fertility techniques such as in vitro fertilization (IVF).

8.3   Ovarian Cysts

Use of the robot has also proven helpful in the management of complex and large ovarian cysts such as **dermoid cysts** (benign cystic teratomas) as well as other benign and even malignant neoplasms (Magrina et al. 2009). The robot enables many surgeons to enucleate the cysts and preserve the ovary compared to those surgeons simply removing the ovary with laparoscopy. The use in functional and hemorrhagic cysts has not been widely adopted based primarily on the fact that most surgeons can manage those problems more easily conservatively without surgery or with traditional laparoscopic approaches. Also, since many of these procedures are emergencies, many surgeons do not have the availability of a robot late in the day after normal OR hours.

9 Special Populations

Obesity is becoming epidemic in the United States with dramatic increases in obese and very obese populations across the country over the last decade. Surgery in obese patients has been demonstrated through the years to have higher risks and complications related to wound healing, ventilation, and anesthesia problems and management of common comorbid medical conditions in the intra- and postoperative phases (Early 1995). An ideal surgery for a morbidly obese patient would allow the surgeon to operate in a precise fashion with comfortable ergonomics and would also reduce wound complications and other risks associated with bariatric patients. This definition fits robotics.

Many studies have shown the clear benefits of robotic surgery in this population (Scheib et al. 2011; Gehrig et al. 2008). Many of these studies have involved malignant hysterectomies, which require more extensive surgery including lymph node dissection, particularly challenging in the laparoscopic environment. With the adoption of robotic surgery, many programs have seen a significant increase in the numbers of obese patient who are now able to have a minimally invasive procedure; and in addition, most authors report significantly reduced or even no **conversions to open** which were common in at least half of patients prior to robotics (Veljovich et al. 2008).

9.1 Complications

As with many new technologies, it didn't take long for the robot to attract the attention of malpractice attorneys. While initially promoted as enabling technology by Intuitive Surgical, the manufacturer of the da Vinci Robot ™, it soon became clear that new surgeons were attempting much more difficult and challenging surgeries than they ever would have tried with traditional laparoscopy. It is also clear that many new surgeons did not fully accept the learning curve of 50–100 cases, which led them to tackle more complex cases than they were prepared for in their early adoption of robotic surgery. This has led to the recognition of an increase in robotic surgery injuries occurring in the early years after initial approval by the FDA in 2005 (AndoniN et al. 2008; Manoucheri et al. 2014).

In retrospective studies, the reported incidence of complications for robotic surgery is 2–10%, and the complications identified include bowel, vascular, bladder, ureteral, and nerve injuries. Incidence of complications for robotic surgery is lower than for open surgery; but outcomes were no different in a retrospective comparison of perioperative outcome for robotic versus laparoscopic hysterectomy (Patzkowsky et al. 2013).

9.2 Direct and Indirect Injuries

Complications of robotic surgery can occur as a result of malfunction of the robotic system, surgeon inexperience and poor technique, improper patient positioning, and other unrelated factors such as trocar injuries. The incidence of robotic system failure during surgical procedures has been reported to be 2.4% for robotic general surgical procedures and 4.5% for robotic urologic and gynecologic procedures (Patzkowsky et al. 2013; Kim et al. 2009; Agcaoglu et al. 2012; Finan and Rocconi 2010). Reported injuries can be broken down into robot-caused (direct) and robot-associated (indirect) injuries. Direct injuries are injuries to other structures such a bowel laceration caused by the surgeon tearing the bowel serosa with one of the robotic arms or energy related injuries such as a thermal burn to the bowel or a vessel caused by electricity sparking from the robotic instrument to that structure. Delayed thermal injuries from the heat generated by cautery can result in late tissue necrosis of the ureter, bowel serosa, or other vulnerable structures.

Indirect injuries are injuries related to the use of the robot such as vaginal hysterectomy **cuff dehiscence**. Cuff separation and cuff dehiscence are well-known complications of any hysterectomy. Newer studies have reported an increased incidence of dehiscence after both laparoscopic and robotic surgeries (Koo et al. 2013; Uccella et al. 2012). No specific cause has been identified, but many experts feel it is a combination of tissue desiccation from the use of cautery on the tissue and closing the cuff with suture bites that are too small but seem large to the surgeon based on the magnified vision provided by the robot. No specific suture or method of closure has been identified as being more at risk for this problem. Many prudent surgeons are now, however, using delayed absorbable sutures as well as restricting their patients from vaginal activity or sexual relations for 6–8 weeks after surgery. Barbed delayed absorbable horizontal running sutures are commonly used for cuff closure.

9.3 Preventing Complications

Often, many factors contribute to surgical complications. This is particularly true for surgeons who utilize robotics. Working in the surgeon console remote from the patient's bedside, surgeons must have excellent **communication** with the other members of the operating room team. A good example of this is in preventing a lost suture needle. An excellent technique for preventing missed communication has been developed by the aviation industry called "cockpit communication." This technique requires the copilot or other crew member to state the communication back to the pilot. For example: "Landing gear down?" "Landing gear down." An operating room example would be: "Needle out?" "Needle out." Having the first assist or surgical techs reply back to the surgeon after every query using this technique is an excellent safety measure.

Another issue is **task saturation** by the surgeon. Often, a surgeon can get so focused on the dissection and process of the surgery that they lose track of the time in the operating room. Having a patient immobilized in unusual positions such as Trendelenburg position for prolonged periods of time can lead to numerous problems such as neuropathy, facial edema, and respiratory difficulties (Scheib et al. 2011). Many institutions have adopted second "**time-outs**" after a designated period of time such as 4 h and then every 2 h after that (Song et al. 2013). This helps get the entire team communicating as to the status of the patient and helps the surgeon and the team decide if they can safely continue or should consider converting to a different approach.

The most common cause of direct robotic complications, however, is that the surgeon is not prepared for the pathology that they find at the time of surgery. Poor exposure, inadequate instrumentation, and failure to plan for unusual emergencies all play a role in most complications. **Surgical planning** and preparation is the single most important step a surgeon can take to minimize complications (Gawande 2011). There are many courses available every year through university medical schools, societies such as the American Association of Gynecologic Laparoscopists (AAGL)-Advancing Minimally Invasive Gynecology Worldwide, and even industry sponsored advanced and master's sourses which focus on new techniques, complex anatomy, and proper patient selection for the robotic approach.

10 Training, Credentialing, and Privileging

Initial training pathways were developed by Intuitive Surgical that focused on how to operate the robot. Typically, these training classes involved a computer-based learning module, hands-on practice with operating and docking the robot, and a pig or cadaver lab or equivalent. Proctored cases were required although the numbers varied and there was no standard pathway or recommendation. Subsequently, learning curve studies were published showing that in the hands of accomplished laparoscopic surgeons, learning curves for robotic surgery were much longer than was originally thought (Lenihan et al. 2008; Seamon et al. 2008; Payne and Dauterive 2008). Recent studies have demonstrated that for gynecologic oncologists and urogynecologists, the learning curve to become proficient was over 91 cases (Woelk et al. 2013).

Recently, the national news media such as the Wall Street Journal has reported on robotic surgery complications that have now brought the whole issue of training and credentialing into focus (Carreyrou 2010). Hospitals are also being sued for failing to provide adequate oversight. In July 2015, the State of Washington Supreme Court upheld a lower court decision in *Taylor v. Intuitive Surgical* that hospitals had the primary responsibility to oversee training and privileging of surgeons, not surgical device manufacturers such as Intuitive Surgical (Estate of Fred Taylor v. Intuitive Surgical Inc. n.d.; Ostrom 2013).

Many highly reliable industries such as aviation and nuclear energy have systems in place to train and verify competency on an ongoing basis. Most hospitals do not have such systems. Surgeons are automatically recredentialed every year based on lack of serious adverse events. The aviation industry uses a model based on standardized initial training, progressing from simple activities to more complex activities as one becomes more experienced, continued certification based on numbers of procedures done such as takeoffs and landings (currency), and annual or biannual proficiency testing done with either check rides with a check-pilot examiner or passing simulation exercises or both. This aviation based model was adopted by the in March 2014 as a recommendation for Initial and Ongoing Privileging and Certification for Robotic Surgery (AAGL Guidelines: Guidelines for Privileging for Robotic-Assisted Gynecologic Laparoscopy 2014; Lenihan 2011, 2014). It focuses on standardized training pathways, requiring surgeons to only do basic cases initially, utilize simulation on a regular basis, and set a minimal number of cases per year to maintain privileges at 20. Many hospitals have chosen to use lower annual surgical currency numbers due to pressure from low-volume surgeons who still wish to offer robotics to their patients. Others have pointed out that currency numbers insure higher volume but do not always correlate with skill or patient outcomes despite many articles correlating better outcomes with higher volume surgeons (Wallenstein et al. 2012). Recently, innovative robotic surgeons have utilized **crowdsourcing** to evaluate technical skills and surgical judgment by reviewing robotic surgical videos, (www.csats.com) (Lendvay and Kowalski 2015). This innovative approach is more objective and has the potential to replace currency numbers with actual graded assessments of technical skill and judgment insuring that hospitals meet the legal and Joint Commission requirements of oversight of their surgeons.

Robotic surgery training at the residency and fellow level presents additional challenges. Obstetrics and gynecology residents are required by American Board of Obstetrics and Gynecology (ABOG) to have performed at least 70 hysterectomies prior to completing their training programs in order to qualify for board certification. Hysterectomy rates have declined dramatically in the United States over the last decade due to a number of causes, and many programs are not able to meet this number. In addition, residency directors are challenged with which approaches to teach their residents. Shorter residency work week and hour restrictions limit time available for training. This contributes to resident perception of not feeling competent to perform minimally invasive procedures after graduation without additional training (Burkett et al. 2011).

The **residency training network** (RTN) was developed in 2012 by a group of robotic surgeons who were residency program coordinators. This group developed standardized teaching models for training future robotic surgeons. It relies heavily on simulation to teach psychomotor skills and requires its students to become proficient by passing these exercises prior to considering them adequately trained to perform robotic surgery. Cognitive training is also being developed to teach anatomy and surgical steps in procedures such as hysterectomy. Currently, there are over 70 residency training programs that are members of this network. More information can be found at www.robotictraining.org.

11   Summary and Conclusions

Robotic assisted gynecologic surgery is a significant technological advancement that utilizes computers to help surgeons become more successful at offering their patients a minimally invasive approach to almost all gynecologic conditions. There have been controversies regarding this approach, primarily focused on increased costs without significant benefits when compared to laparoscopic or vaginal surgeries in the hands of expert surgeons. These are real issues especially in our current health-care system, and the costs of robotic surgery need to be addressed by hospitals and medical societies. It is up to individual hospital systems to determine the most cost-effective ways to use robotic surgery and to encourage surgeons to use less costly methods when possible on patients who qualify for those approaches (Rardin 2014; Advincula 2014). Current cost studies however have looked at direct costs and have not accounted for the most part in cost savings due to reductions in open surgeries as well as decreased conversions and short term readmissions. A retrospective study by Martino et al. measured procedure-related **readmissions** within 30 days of discharge after benign hysterectomy in 2554 patients in an academic hospital system. Patient's undergoing robotic assisted laparoscopic hysterectomy (RALH) had a significantly lower chance of readmission <30 days after surgery when compared to laparoscopic, abdominal (open), and vaginal approaches. They also experienced shorter length of stay (LOS), lower estimated blood loss (EBL), and significant cost savings associated with readmission when compared to non-robotic approaches (Martino et al. 2014). Under the Affordable Care Act (ACA), environment, hospitals, and surgeons are paid for better outcomes and penalized for complications. This type of information should clearly be factored into future analyses of the relative value of robotic surgery (Liberman et al. 2012).

Complications initially were thought to be higher with robotic surgeries, but with increasing experience, these seem to be equivalent to other techniques and have been associated more commonly with low-volume surgeons as well as with surgeons who are in the early stage of their learning curves. Robotic surgery is still in its relative infancy compared to other surgical approaches. As technology advances, computer-assisted robotic surgery will continue to advance and provide enabling benefits to both surgeons and to their patients in the future. There is a significant need to create prospective studies and registries in order to further assess best practices, costs, and outcomes so that future surgeons will be better prepared with good data to make appropriate choices for how to deliver surgical care to their patients.

References

AAGL Guidelines: Guidelines for Privileging for Robotic-Assisted Gynecologic Laparoscopy. J Minim Invasive Gynecol. 2014;21(2).

ACOG technology assessment in obstetrics and gynecology No. 6: robot-assisted surgery. Obstet Gynecol. 2009;114:1153–5.

Advincula A. Editorial: robotics in gynecology. Is the glass half empty or half full? Obstet Gynecol. 2014;123:3–4.

Advincula AP, Song A. The role of robotic surgery in gynecology. Curr Opin Obstet Gynecol. 2007;19:331–6. doi:10.1097/GCO.0b013e328216f90b.

Advincula AP, Song A, Burke W, Reynolds KR. Preliminary experience with robot-assisted laparoscopic myomectomy. J Minim Invasive Gynecol. 2004;11(4):511–8.

Advincula AP, Xu X, Goudeau S, Ransom SB. Robotic-assisted, laparoscopic, and abdominal myomectomy: a comparison of surgical outcomes. Obstet Gynecol. 2011;117(2, part 1):256–65.

Agcaoglu O, Aliyev S, Taskin HE, et al. Malfunction and failure of robotic systems during general surgical procedures. Surg Endosc. 2012;26:3580–3.

AndoniN S, Okeke Z, Okeke DA. Device failures associated with patient injuries during robot-assisted laparoscopic surgeries: a comprehensive review of FDA MAUDE database. Can J Urol. 2008;15(1):3912–6.

Ascher-Walsh CJ, Capes TL. Robotic assisted laparoscopic myomectomy is an improvement over laparotomy in women with limited numbers of myomas. J Minim Invasive Gynecol. 2010;17:306–10.

Barakat EE, Bedaiwy MA, Zimberg S, MNutter B, Nosseir M, Falcone T. Robotic assisted laparoscopic and abdominal myomectomy: a comparison of surgical outcomes. Obstet Gynecol. 2011;117(2, Pt 1):256–65.

Bell MC, Torgenson J, Seshadri-Kreaden U, Suttle AW, Hunt S. Comparison of outcomes and costs for endometrial cancer staging via traditional laparotomy, standard laparososcopy and robotic technique. Gynecol Oncol. 2008;111:407–11.

Burkett D, Horwit J, Kennedy V, Murphy D, Graziano S, Kenton K. Assessing current trends in resident hysterectomy training. Female Pelvic Med Reconstr Surg. 2011;17(5):210–4. doi:10.1097/SPV.0b013e3182309a22.

Carreyrou J. Surgical robot examined in injuries. *The Wall Street Journal*. 2010. http://www.wsj.com/articles/SB10001424052702304703104575173952145907526. Accessed 16 Dec 2015.

CDC-MMWR: Hysterectomy Surveillance-1994-99 July, 2002/51 (SS05); 1–8.

Dharia Patel SP, Steinkampf MP, Whitten SJ, Malizia BA. Robotic tubal anastomosis: surgical technique and cost effectiveness. Fertil Steril. 2008;90(4):175–1179.

Dickersin K, Munro M, Clark M, for the Surgical Treatments Outcomes Project for Dysfunctional Uterine Bleeding (STOP-DUB) Research Group, et al. Hysterectomy compared with endometrial ablation for dysfunctional uterine bleeding: a randomized controlled trial. Obstet Gynecol. 2007;110:1279–89. doi:10.1097/01.AOG.0000292083.97478.3.

Early HW. Complications of abdominal and vaginal hysterectomy in obese women. OB-GYN Surv. 1995;50(11):795.

Estape R, Lambrou N, Diaz R, Estape E, Dunkin N, Rivera A. A case matched analysis of robotic radical hysterectomy with lymphadenectomy compared with laparoscopy and laparotomy. Gynecol Oncol. 2009;113:357–61.

Estate of Fred Taylor v. Intuitive Surgical Inc., 09-2-03136-5, Superior Court. State of Washington, Kitsap County (Port Orchard). n.d.

Falcone T, Goldberg J, Garcia-Ruiz A, Margossian H, Stevens L. Full robotic assistance for laparoscopic tubal anastamosis: a case report. J Laparosc Adv Surg Technol. 1999;9(1):107–13. doi:10.1089/lap.1999.9.107.

Finan MA, Rocconi RP. Overcoming technical challenges with robotic surgery in gynecologic oncology. Surg Endosc. 2010;24:1256–60.

Gargiulo AR. Fertility preservation and the role of robotics. Clin Obstet Gynecol. 2011;54(3):431–48.

Gawande A. The checklist Manifesto: how to get things right. New York: Henry Holt & Company; 2011.

Gehrig PA, Cantrell LA, Shafer A, Abaid LN, Mendivil A, Boggess JF. What is the optimal minimally invasive surgical procedure for endometrial cancer staging in the obese and morbidly obese woman? Gynecol Oncol. 2008;111:41–5.

Geller EJ, Siddiquiu NY, Barnett JC, Visco AG. Shot term outcomes of robotic sacrocolpopexy compared with abdominal sacrocolpopexy. Obstet Gynecol. 2008;112:1201–6.

Giudice LC. Endometriosis. N Engl J Med. 2010;362:2389–98. doi:10.1056/NEJMcp1000274.

Hart RJ, Hickey M, Maouris P, Buckett W, Garry R. Excisional surgery versus ablative surgery for ovarian endometriomas. Cochrane Database Syst Rev. 2005;3:CD004992.

Herron DM, Michael Marohn M. The SAGES-MIRA Robotic Surgery Consensus Group3: a consensus document on robotic surgery. 2007. http://www.sages.org/publications/guidelines/consensus-document-robotic-surgery/. Accessed 16 Dec 2015.

Jacobsen, et al. Hysterectomy for benign indications. Obstet Gynecol. 2006;107:1278–83.

John NP, Hummelshoi L. Consensus on current management of endometriosis. Hum Reprod. 2013;28(6):1552–68.

Kapetanakis V, Jacob K, Klauschie J, Kho R, Magrina J. Robotic presacral neurectomy – technique and results. Int J Med Rob Comput Assist Surg. 2012;8(1):73–6. doi:10.1002/rcs.438.

Kim WT, Ham WS, Jeong W, et al. Failure and malfunction of da Vinci Surgical systems during various robotic surgeries: experience from six departments at a single institute. Urology. 2009;74:1234–7.

Koo YJ, Kim DY, Kim JH, Kim YM, Kim YT, Nam JH. Vaginal cuff dehiscence after hysterectomy. Int J Gynaecol Obstet. 2013;122(3):248–52. doi:10.1016/j.ijgo.2013.04.004.

Lendvay TS, Kowalski T. Crowd sourcing to assess surgical skills. JAMA Surg. 2015;150(11):1–2. doi:10.1001/jamasurg.2015.2405.

Lenihan JP. Navigating credentialing, privileging, and learning curves in robotics with an evidence and experienced-based approach. Clin Obstet Gynecol. 2011;54(3):382–90. doi:10.1097/GRF.0b013e31822b47e2.

Lenihan J. Flight plan for robotic surgery credentialing: new AAGL guidelines. OBG Manag. 2014;26(11):44–8.

Lenihan JP, Kovanda C, Seshadri-Kreaden U. What is the learning curve for robotic assisted gynecologic surgery? J Minim Invasive Gynecol. 2008;15:589–94.

Liberman D, Trinh QD, Jeldres C, Zorn K. Is robotic surgery cost-effective: yes. Curr Opin Urol. 2012;22(1):61–5. doi:10.1097/MOU.0b013e32834d543f.

Lim PC, Crane JT, English EJ, et al. Outcomes of robotic assisted hysterectomy from experienced robotic surgeons. Int J of Gynecol Obstet. 2016;133(3):359–364.

Lue JR, Pyrzak A, Allen J. Improving accuracy of intraoperative diagnosis of endometriosis: role of firefly in minimal access robotic surgery. J Minim Access Surg. 2015. http://www.journalofmas.com/preprintarticle.asp?id=158969;type=0. Accessed online 22 Dec 2015.

Magrina JF, Espada M, Munoz MR, Noble BN, Kho RM. Robotic adnexectomy compared with laparoscopy for adnexal mass. Obstet Gynecol. 2009;114(3):581–4.

Magrina JF, Zanagnolo V, Noble BN, Kho RM, Magtibay P. Robotic approach for ovarian cancer: perioperative and survival results and comparison with laparoscopy and laparotomy. Gynecol Oncol. 2011;121:100–5.

Manoucheri E, Fuchs-Weizman N, Cohen SL, Wang KC, Einarsson J. MAUDE: analysis of robotic-assisted gynecologic surgery. 2013. J Minim Invasive Gynecol. 2014;21(4):592–5. doi:10.1016/j.jmig.2013.12.122.

Martino MA, Berger EA, McFetridge JT, et al. A comparison of quality outcome measures in patients having a hysterectomy for benign disease: robotic vs. non-robotic approaches. J Minim Invasive Gynecol. 2014;21:389–39.

Occhino JA, Myer EL, Singh R, Gebhart JB. Surgical and non-surgical education practices in female pelvic medicine and reconstructive surgery fellowships within the United States. Open J Obstet Gynecol. 2013;3 No.4 article # 33234, 8 pages. doi:10.4236/ojog.2013.34A004.

Ostrom C. Failed robotic surgery focus of Kitsap trial. *Seattle Times*. www.seattletimes.com/html/localnews/2020918732_robottrialxml.html. Published May 3, 2013. Accessed 22 Dec 2015.

Paraiso MF, Jelovsek JE, Frick A, Chen CC, Barber MD. Laparoscopic compared with robotic sacrocolpopexy for vaginal prolapse: a randomized controlled trial. Obstet Gynecol. 2011;118:1005–13.

Patzkowsky KE, As-Sanie S, Smorgick N, et al. Perioperative outcomes of robotic versus laparoscopic hysterectomy for benign disease. JSLS. 2013;17:100–6.

Payne TN, Dauterive FR. A comparison of total laparoscopic hysterectomy to robotically assisted hysterectomy: surgical outcomes in a community practice. J Minim Invasive Gynecol. 2008;15:286–91.

Payne TN, Dauterive FR, Pitter MC, Giep HN, Giep BN, Grogg TW, Shanbour KA, Goff DW, Hubert HB. Robotically assisted hysterectomy in patients with large uteri: outcomes in five community practices. Obstet Gynecol. 2010;115:535–42. doi:10.1097/AOG.0b013e3181cf45ad.

Pinion SB, Parkin DE, Abramovich DR, Naji A, Alexander DA, Russell IT, Kitchener HC. Randomised trial of hysterectomy, endometrial laser ablation, and transcervical endometrial resection for dysfunctional uterine bleeding. BMJ. 1994;309. doi:10.1136/bmj.309.6960.979.

Pitter MC, Gargiulo AR, Bonaventura LM, Lehman JS, Srouji SS. Pregnancy outcomes following robot-assisted myomectomy. Hum Reprod. 2013;28:99–108. doi:10.1093/humrep/des365.

Ploumidis A, Spinoit AF, De Naeyer G, Schatteman P, Gan M, et al. Robot-assisted sacrocolpopexy for pelvic organ prolapse: surgical technique and outcomes at a single high-volume institution. Eur Urol. 2014;65(1):138–45.

Rardin CR. The debate over robotics in benign gynecology. Am J Obstet Gynecol. 2014;210(5):418–22. doi:10.1016/j.ajog.2014.01.016.

Reich H. New techniques in advanced laparoscopic surgery. Baillieres Clin Obstet Gynaecol. 1989;3(3): 655–81.

Ross JW, Preston M. Laparoscopic sacrocolpopexy for severe vaginal vault prolapse: five year outcome. J Minim Invasive Gynecol. 2005;12(3):221–6.

Scheib S, et al. Laparoscopy in the morbidly obese: physiologic considerations and surgical techniques to optimize success. J Minim Invasive Gynecol. 2011;21:180–96.

Seamon LG, Cohn DE, Richardson DL, et al. Robotic hysterectomy and pelvic-aortic lymphadenectomy for endometrial cancer. Obstet Gynecol. 2008;112:1207–13.

Sert MB, Abeler V. Robot-assisted laparoscopic radical hysterectomy: comparison with total laparoscopic hysterectomy and abdominal radical hysterectomy; one surgeon's experience at the Norwegian Radium Hospital. Gynecol Oncol. 2011;121:600–4.

Shakiba K, Bena JF, McGill KM, Minger J, Falcone T. Surgical treatment of endometriosis: a 7-year follow-up on the requirement for further surgery. Obstet Gynecol. 2008;111(6):1285–92.

Song JB, Vemana G, Mobley JM, Bhayani SB. The second "time-out": a surgical safety checklist for lengthy robotic surgeries. Patient Saf Surg. 2013; 7(1):19–21.

Uccella S, Ceccaroni M, Cromi A, Malzoni M, Berretta R, De Iaco P, Roviglione G, Bogani G, Minelli L, Ghezzi F. Vaginal cuff dehiscence in a series of 12,398 hysterectomies: effect of different types of colpotomy and vaginal closure. Obstet Gynecol. 2012;120(3): 516–23.

Veljovich DS, Paley PJ, Drescher CW, Everett EN, Shah C, Peters WA. Robotic surgery in gynecologic oncology: program initiation and outcomes after the first year with comparison with laparotomy for endometrial cancer staging. Am J Obstet Gynecol. 2008;198(6):679 e9–10.

Wallenstein MR, et al. Effects of surgical volume on outcomes for laproscopic hysterectomy for benign conditions. Obstet Gynecol. 2012;119(4):710–6.

Woelk JL, Casiano ER, Weaver AL, Gostout BS, Trabuco EC, Gebhart JB. The learning curve of robotic hysterectomy. Obstet Gynecol. 2013;121(1):87–95. doi:10.1097/AOG.0b013e31827a029e.

Wright JD, Herzog TJ, Tsui J, Ananth CV, et al. Nationwide trends in the performance of inpatient hysterectomy in the United States. Obstet Gynecol. 2013a;122 (2 0 1):233–41. doi:10.1097/AOG.0b013e318299a6cf.

Wright JD, Anath CV, Lewin SN, et al. Robotically assisted vs. laparoscopic hysterectomy among women with benign gynecologic disease. JAMA. 2013b;309:689–98.

Minimally Invasive Procedures for Incontinence and Lower Urinary Tract Disorders: Indications and Avoiding Complications

Begüm Özel

Abstract

Stress urinary incontinence is a common condition affecting women. When conservative therapy is unsuccessful in relieving symptoms, several minimally invasive options exist for the surgical management of stress incontinence. Women with stress incontinence symptoms, post-void residual less than 150 ml, negative urinalysis, a positive cough stress test, no pelvic organ prolapse beyond the hymen, and urethral hypermobility are candidates for an anti-incontinence procedure without preoperative urodynamic testing. The retropubic and transobturator mid-urethral sling procedures have an efficacy of approximately 85% and low rate of complications. The transobturator approach avoids passage into the retropubic space and minimizes the risk of bladder, bowel, and major vessel injury but is associated with higher rate of neurologic symptoms. Postoperative voiding dysfunction after the mid-urethral sling is low and can be managed with sling loosening in the first few weeks after surgery or simple sling transection later in the postoperative period. The mid-urethral slings have been shown to have similar efficacy to the Burch colposuspension. The retropubic mid-urethral sling appears to be more successful in women with Valsalva leak point pressure ≤ 60 cm H_2O and maximum urethral closure pressure ≤ 20 cm H_2O. The laparoscopic Burch colposuspension offers an alternative to the mid-urethral sling for women who are already having a laparoscopic procedure or who wish to avoid the use of permanent mesh. A maximum urethral closure pressure ≤ 20 cm H_2O is generally considered contraindication to a Burch colposuspension procedure. Outcomes appear to be similar to the open Burch colposuspension and mid-urethral sling.

Keywords

Mid-urethral sling • Transobturator sling • Retropubic sling • Laparoscopic colposuspension • Laparoscopic Burch

Contents

B. Özel (✉)
Division of Female Pelvic Medicine and Reconstructive Surgery, Department of Obstetrics and Gynecology, Keck School of Medicine, University of Southern California, Los Angeles, CA, USA
e-mail: ozel@usc.edu; Begum.Ozel@med.usc.edu

© Springer International Publishing AG 2017
D. Shoupe (ed.), *Handbook of Gynecology*,
DOI 10.1007/978-3-319-17798-4_56

679

1 Introduction

Urinary incontinence is a common condition among women. Estimates of prevalence vary depending on the definition used, the question asked, and the patient population, but in a racially diverse sample of noninstitutionalized women over the age of 20 in the United States, almost 50% of women reported symptoms of urinary incontinence (Dooley et al. 2008).

Over 250,000 anti-incontinence operations are performed in the United States each year (Haya et al. 2015). Minimally invasive therapies for stress urinary incontinence fall into two categories: the mid-urethral sling and the laparoscopic colposuspension. Ulmsten and colleagues first described the minimally invasive mid-urethral sling in 1996 (Ulmsten et al. 1996). The transobturator sling was introduced in 2001 (Delorme 2001). The retropubic and transobturator mid-urethral sling procedures have now become the most commonly performed procedure for stress urinary incontinence; approximately two-thirds of anti-incontinence procedures in the United States are mid-urethral slings, and the rate

is as high as 98% in Sweden (Haya et al. 2015). Laparoscopic retropubic colposuspension was first described in the early 1990s (Taylor and Tsokos 1993), but the procedure has been less widely adopted by surgeons, most likely because it is more technically challenging than the mid-urethral sling procedure. However, it offers a minimally invasive option for women who prefer to avoid the use of a permanent implant.

2 Indications for Surgery

Surgery for stress incontinence is indicated in women bothered by these symptoms, who request treatment, and when more conservative therapies have been unsuccessful. Stress incontinence is defined as the complaint of involuntary loss of urine on effort or physical exertion (such as sporting activities) or on sneezing or coughing (Haylen et al. 2010). Conservative therapies shown to be effective include pelvic floor exercises, with or without biofeedback or pelvic floor physical therapy, timed voiding, fluid management, and weight loss in overweight and obese patients. Even moderate weight loss can be effective. In a randomized trial comparing a 6-month weight-loss program with a structured education program in overweight and obese women with urinary incontinence, women in the 6-month weight-loss program had a mean weight loss of 8.0% (7.8 kg) and a reduction in weekly incontinence (mostly stress urinary incontinence) of 47% compared to 1.6% (1.5 kg) and 28% in the structured education program, respectively ($p < 0.001$) (Subak et al. 2009).

Urodynamic stress incontinence is the involuntary leakage of urine during filling cystometry, associated with increased intra-abdominal pressure, in the absence of a detrusor contraction. However, urodynamic testing is not mandatory before planning on surgery for stress incontinence. In women with uncomplicated stress incontinence, urodynamic testing has not been shown to improve the outcome of surgical intervention (Nager et al. 2012). Uncomplicated stress urinary incontinence is defined as post-void residual urine volume less than 150 mL, negative urinalysis, a positive cough stress test result, and no pelvic organ prolapse beyond the hymen. It is important to demonstrate objective evidence of stress incontinence. This can be done with a cough stress test in which the patient is asked to cough with a full bladder, initially in lithotomy position and then in standing position if no leak is demonstrated in lithotomy. It may be necessary to retrograde fill the bladder if the patient does not have a full bladder. If leak cannot be demonstrated with a cough stress test or if the patient has an elevated post-void residual volume, urodynamics is indicated.

Lack of urethral hypermobility is a relative contraindication to most anti-incontinence procedures as a higher rate of failure has been demonstrated (Richter et al. 2011). Urethral hypermobility is generally defined as a resting angle or displacement angle of the urethra–bladder neck with maximum Valsalva of at least 30° from the horizontal (Zyczynski et al. 2007).

The Burch colposuspension has been shown to have a higher failure rate in women with maximum urethral closure pressure ≤20 cm H_2O (Sand et al. 1987), and this would generally be considered a contraindication to the procedure, whether performed via an open abdominal incision or laparoscopically. Low leak point pressure ≤60 cm H_2O, however, does not appear to be a risk factor for failure of the Burch colposuspension (Hsieh et al. 2001).

3 Mid-urethral Sling

The mid-urethral sling was originally described in 1996 by Ulmsten and colleagues. The tension-free tape (TVT; Gynecare, Ethicon Women's Health and Urology, Somerville, New Jersey, USA) was first introduced in the United States in 1998. The TVT introduced several modifications to the traditional bladder neck slings resulting in a revolutionary change to the management of stress urinary incontinence. These modifications were (1) mid-urethral placement (rather than at the bladder neck), (2) no suture fixation of the sling mesh, (3) no tension placed on the urethra, and (4) minimal dissection. The transobturator sling offered a lower risk of certain complications by

avoiding significant retropubic passage of the needle.

4 Retropubic Mid-urethral Sling

4.1 Technique

The retropubic mid-urethral sling (Fig. 1) is most commonly performed as a bottom-up procedure as originally described by Ulmsten and colleagues (1996). There are slight variations in technique depending on the sling kit utilized, and it is important to be familiar with the product available. All of the currently available sling kits use a loosely woven, monofilament polypropylene sling mesh with pore size greater than 75 µm. This type of mesh allows for tissue ingrowth and fibrosis, allowing the mesh to be incorporated into the surrounding tissues as well as allowing for

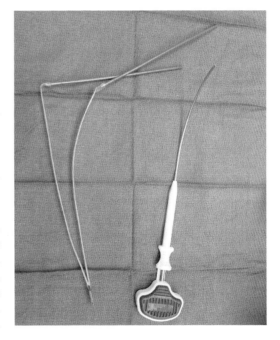

Fig. 1 Photo of a retropubic mid-urethral sling (Advantage Fit sling, Boston Scientific, Natick, MA, USA). The polypropylene sling is covered by a plastic sheath. The sling is attached to the needle for passage. The plastic sheaths allow for easy movement of the sling through the tissue and prevent contamination of the sling before insertion; they are removed once the sling is adjusted below the urethra

migration of macrophages and other leukocytes for infection surveillance.

For the retropubic mid-urethral sling, the patient is placed in low to moderate dorsal lithotomy with an 18 or 20 French Foley catheter to drain the bladder. Two 0.5 cm skin incisions are made just above the pubic bone, i.e., suprapubic, about 2 cm from the midline (Fig. 2a). The skin may be infiltrated with local anesthetic prior to making these incisions. Retropubic hydrodissection is then performed. Saline or local anesthetic may be used (Fig. 3). This is done by starting at the previously made skin incisions and passing an 18 gauge spinal needle along the back of the pubic symphysis until the needle touches the endopelvic fascia. Location of the needle tip is confirmed with a hand in the vagina palpating lateral to the urethra. 20–50 cc of saline (or local anesthesia) is injected on each side. Saline or local anesthetic is also injected along the anterior vaginal wall below the urethra. A sagittal incision no more than 1.5 cm long starting at 1 cm proximal to the urethral meatus is made with a #15 scalpel blade. Lateral periurethral tracks are made with the Metzenbaum scissors. Care should be taken to keep the dissection to full thickness of the vaginal wall. The vaginal dissection should be carried out until the tip of the Metzenbaum scissors touches the interior portion of the inferior pubic ramus. The bladder is emptied, and the rigid catheter guide is inserted into the channel of the Foley catheter (Fig. 4). The tip of the catheter is then pushed toward the posterior lateral wall of the bladder opposite to

the intended trocar passage. When passing the right side, the tip of the catheter should be directed toward the left side and vice versa. On the right side, the left hand should hold the trocar handle, and the right hand should be used to control initial insertion of the device. The position of the hands is reversed for the other side. The needle tip is then placed into the vaginal incision. The right index finger is placed under the anterior vaginal wall, just lateral of the suburethral incision. The needle tip is directed horizontally until the urogenital diaphragm is perforated; sometimes a "pop" is felt. This initial push should occur with the palm of the vaginal hand, the hand on the handle being there to ensure stability. At this point, the needle is directed more upward, staying immediately behind the pubic bone, and the trocar handle is dropped. The needle should be aimed toward the previously made skin incisions, and care should be taken not to rotate the handle. There will be resistance once the rectus fascia is reached. At this point, the vaginal hand is removed, and taking care not to rotate the needle, the needle is pushed up through the fascia, muscle, and skin with the hand on the handle. The plastic tip is grasped and the metal guide/needle is removed. The procedure is repeated on the left side. The bladder and urethra are diverted to the patient's right. The right hand now is used to hold the handle, and the left hand is placed vaginally.

Cystourethroscopy with a 70° rigid cystoscope should then be performed to ensure bladder integrity. There are different ways to adjust the mesh,

Fig. 2 Markings demonstrate location of suprapubic incisions (**a**) and groin incisions (**b**) for the retropubic and transobturator slings, respectively

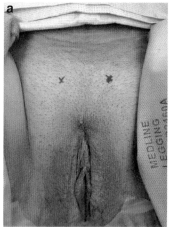
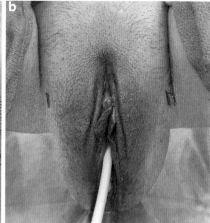

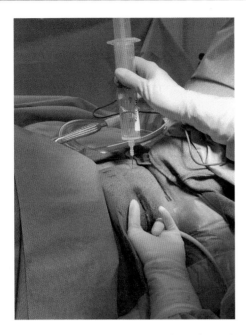

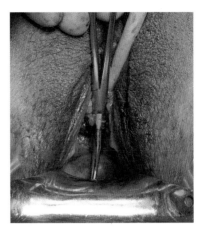

Fig. 5 Adjusting the sling. A small instrument, such as a Kelly clamp, should then be placed between the mesh and the urethra to ensure that the sling does not tighten further during removal of the plastic sheaths

Fig. 3 Retropubic hydrodissection with saline or local anesthetic. An 18 gauge spinal needle is passed along the back of the pubic symphysis until the needle touches the endopelvic fascia. Location of the needle tip is confirmed with a hand in the vagina palpating lateral to the urethra. 20–50 cc of saline (or local anesthesia) is injected on each side

Once the plastic sheaths are removed, the vaginal wall incision should be closed with 2-0 or 3-0 delayed absorbable suture, and the skin incisions may be closed with 4-0 monofilament absorbable suture or Dermabond (Ethicon Endosurgery, Inc., Cincinnati, OH). A postoperative voiding trial is mandatory.

The SPARC (Astora Women's Health, LLC, Eden Prairie, MN, USA) differs from the other retropubic slings in that the SPARC needles are inserted through two 0.5 cm incisions just above the symphysis pubis (top-down route). The exit point for the SPARC needles is through the midline vaginal incision. A finger in the vaginal incision guides the exit of the needle.

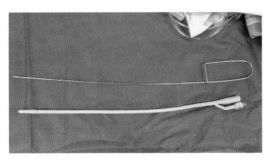

Fig. 4 Rigid catheter guide and Foley catheter

including using an intraoperative cough test as discussed below, but it is important that the mesh is adjusted loosely below the urethra and does not place tension on the urethra. It is often helpful again to have an 18 or 20 French Foley catheter in place when adjusting the sling. A small instrument, such as a Kelly clamp, should then be placed between the mesh and the urethra to ensure that the sling does not tighten further during removal of the plastic sheaths (Fig. 5).

5   Anesthesia and the Cough Stress Test for the Retropubic Mid-urethral Sling

In the initial description of the TVT, Ulmsten described performing the procedure under conscious sedation and local anesthesia and with the use of an intraoperative cough test to adjust the sling. However, this posed a challenge with some patients who either did not do well with this type of anesthesia or had relative contraindications. Surgeons initially began looking into the use of regional anesthesia as an alternative to conscious sedation and local anesthesia. This allowed the intraoperative cough test to be performed and arguably allowed the patient better anesthesia. Wang and Chen randomized 73 women having the TVT procedure to conscious sedation and local anesthesia versus epidural anesthesia (Wang and Chen 2001). Intraoperative cough test was performed in both groups. At a minimum of 12 months of follow-up, there was no difference in subjective or objective outcome. Adamiak and colleagues randomized 103 women having the TVT to conscious sedation and local anesthesia versus spinal anesthesia. Intraoperative cough test was again performed in both groups. They found no difference in subjective outcome 6 months postoperatively (Adamiak et al. 2002). Similarly Liapis and colleagues randomized 86 women having a TVT to conscious sedation and local anesthesia versus epidural anesthesia and found no difference in objective outcome at 12 months (Liapis et al. 2007). However, regional anesthesia has been suggested as a risk factor for early voiding dysfunction. Women who had regional anesthesia had an increased odds (adjusted odds ratio, 4.4; 95% confidence interval, 1.9–10.2) of acute postoperative urinary retention compared with women receiving conscious sedation with local anesthesia or general anesthesia (Wohlrab et al. 2009), and there is concern that the pelvic floor muscle paralysis as a result of regional anesthesia may lead to overtightening of the sling, especially when intraoperative cough test is used to adjust the sling.

Moore and colleagues specifically addressed the question of the cough test intraoperatively in a randomized study of 92 women having the TVT procedure using conscious sedation and local anesthesia for both groups (Moore et al. 2012). Their primary outcome was the proportion of women had a successful voiding trial within 24 h of catheter removal/clamping, and they found no significant difference between both groups. As a secondary outcome, they looked at 24 h pad test and validated quality-of-life questionnaires 12 months postoperatively and found no significant difference between the two groups.

Over time many surgeons began performing the procedure under general anesthesia. While there are no randomized trials, multiple retrospective studies have found no difference in efficacy or complications with general anesthesia versus conscious sedation and local anesthesia or regional anesthesia (Centinel et al. 2004; Ghezzi et al. 2005; Lo et al. 2003; Low et al. 2004; Murphy et al. 2003). Murphy and colleagues prospectively examined a cohort of 170 women having the TVT procedure; anesthesia type was selected at the discretion of the operating surgeon (Murphy et al. 2003). At a median follow-up of 32 months, with 132 (84.6%) of women responding, they found a significantly greater improvement in stress incontinence symptoms as reported by a validated questionnaire in women who had conscious sedation and local anesthesia versus general anesthesia. However, the data was confounded by the fact that only two surgeons performed all of the procedures, with one surgeon performing almost all the cases under general anesthesia.

The use of local anesthesia as an adjunct to general anesthesia for postoperative pain was examined in a randomized trial of 42 women having a SPARC sling under general anesthesia (Dunivan et al. 2011). The primary outcome, 2 h postoperative visual analogue scale score, was significantly lower in the group that received intraoperative injection of 0.125% bupivacaine along the retropubic path of the sling when compared to the control group (1.9 vs. 2.6 out of 10.0, respectively; $p = 0.05$). There was no difference in the outcome of the voiding trial; in the bupivacaine group, 15/19 (79%) subjects versus 12/19 (63%) in the control group failed the voiding trial (RR 1.25, 95% CI 0.83–1.89). Success rates were not examined in this study.

6   Retropubic Mid-urethral Sling Compared to Open Burch Colposuspension

Ward and Hilton performed the landmark trial comparing the TVT sling with the retropubic colposuspension proving comparable efficacy for the retropubic mid-urethral sling and the retropubic colposuspension (Ward and Hilton 2002). In this multicenter trial, 344 women with urodynamic stress incontinence were randomized to the TVT sling versus the retropubic colposuspension. The primary outcome measure was objective cure of stress incontinence based on a negative 1 h pad test (<1 g change in weight) and a negative stress test on urodynamic testing. At 6 months of follow-up, a negative 1 h pad test was recorded in 128 (73%) patients in the TVT group and 109 (64%) in the colposuspension group. There was no evidence of urodynamic stress incontinence in 142 (81%) patients after the TVT procedure and 114 (67%) after the colposuspension. Objective cure, as defined above, was found in 115 (66%) patients in the TVT group and 97 (57%) in the colposuspension group ($p = 0.099$, Cochran-Mantel-Haenszel test; 95% confidence interval for difference in cure -4.7 to 21.3%). Of the 98 women who had TVT and 79 who had the colposuspension who returned for 5-year follow-up (Ward and Hilton 2008), a negative 1 h pad test was recorded in 58 (81%) women in the vaginal tape group and in 44 (90%) women in the colposuspension group at 5 years. A last observed result carried forward analysis was carried out, in which pad test data from the last available follow-up visit were imputed to substitute missing data. On this basis, the cure rates at 5 years were 75% for TVT and 69% for colposuspension (OR 1.32 [95% CI 0.82–2.12]).

7 Bottom-Up Versus Top-Down Retropubic Sling

When examining the more commonly performed retropubic bottom-up route to the top-down route, subjective cure is higher with the bottom-up route (RR 1.10, 95% CI 1.01 to 1.19; three trials, 477 women) (Ford et al. 2015).

8 Complications of Retropubic Mid-urethral Sling

Certain complications are inherent to the retropubic mid-urethral sling because of blind passage of the needle. Trocar cystotomy occurs in about 5% of cases; with previous pelvic surgery, especially prior to retropubic colposuspension, the risk increases to as high as 31% (Haab et al. 2001). Obesity appears to be protective (Lovatsis et al. 2003). Intraoperative cystotomy does not appear to affect the outcome of surgery and can be managed with short-term (1–3 days) catheterization (La Sala et al. 2006). However, perforation of both the small bowel and the large bowel has been reported as has injury to the external iliac vessels (Aslam and Denman 2013; Castillo et al. 2004; Fourie and Cohen 2003; Leboeuf et al. 2004; Meschia et al. 2002; Sivanesan et al. 2007; Zilbert and Farrell 2001). Careful technique is essential to minimize the risk of these types of complications. The potential for these types of catastrophic and life-threatening complications made it attractive to find an alternate route of sling placement.

9 Transobturator Sling

9.1 Technique

The outside-in transobturator sling is the most common approach to the procedure. The bladder is emptied before beginning. A large caliber Foley catheter can be helpful to have in place to help identify the urethra during the procedure. The dissection is started with an anterior vaginal wall incision at the mid-urethra (Fig. 6). The vaginal wall can be infiltrated with saline if desired for hydrodissection. Similar to the retropubic mid-urethral sling, the incision usually begins about 1 cm proximal to the urethral meatus and is made to have a length of 1.5–2 cm. The vaginal wall is then incised, and the lateral periurethral tracks are made with the Metzenbaum scissors. It is important that the vaginal dissection be carried out until the tip of the Metzenbaum scissors touches the interior portion of the inferior pubic ramus. To make the skin incisions, first palpate the edge of the ischiopubic ramus; identify the adductor longus tendon insertion to the pubic ramus; then move down along the edge of the ischiopubic ramus to approximately the level of the clitoris. Mark this site just lateral to the bony edge

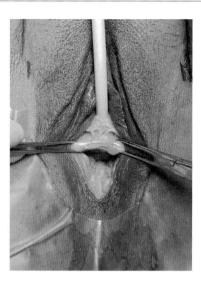

Fig. 6 Location of anterior vaginal wall incision. Allis clamps are used to hold the vaginal epithelium so that an incision can be made at the level of the mid-urethra, starting 1 cm proximal to the urethral meatus

bilaterally and then make stab incisions with a #15 scalpel blade.

The helical needle is grasped with the contralateral hand. A catheter guide can be placed through the Foley catheter to divert the bladder and urethra to the contralateral side. When passing the helical needle on the left side, the needle should be initially be placed in the previously made skin incisions, perpendicular to the skin, and the index finger of the left hand should be placed in the vaginal incision until the bone is palpable. The thumb from the left hand should be on the outside curve of needle to control the needle movement as it perforates the obturator membrane and muscle. The needle is then pushed in through the obturator membrane and muscle until a "pop" is felt, i.e., until resistance against needle stops. The needle shaft and handle are then positioned at a 45° angle to the patient's vertical axis and close to body and rotated along the posterior surface of the ischial pubic ramus and toward the left index finger that is in the vaginal incision. The index finger will meet the needle tip as it moves around the pubic ramus. If the needle tip cannot be located, then the needle should not be advanced and its position reassessed. It may need to be withdrawn to just behind the pubic

ramus and advanced again. It is important at this point to check for perforation at the lateral vaginal sulcus before attaching the mesh. The mesh is then attached to the needle tip and pulled through. The procedure is repeated on the other side.

Cystourethroscopy with a 70° rigid cystoscope is performed at this point to ensure bladder integrity. There are different ways to adjust the mesh, including using an intraoperative cough test, but it is important that the mesh is adjusted loosely below the urethra and does not place tension on the urethra. It is often helpful again to have an 18 or 20 French Foley catheter in place when adjusting the sling. A small instrument, such as a Kelly clamp, should then be placed between the mesh and the urethra to ensure that the sling does not tighten further during removal of the plastic sheaths.

Once the plastic sheaths are removed, the vaginal wall incision should be closed with 2-0 or 3-0 delayed absorbable suture, such as Vicryl, and the skin incisions can be closed with Dermabond. A postoperative voiding trial is mandatory.

The inside-out technique is used by the TVT-Obturator (Gynecare, Ethicon, Johnson & Johnson, Somerville, NJ, USA). The dissection is the same as above. The safety-winged guide that comes with the kit is inserted into the dissected track and just through the obturator membrane. The helical passer is inserted inward along the winged guide until a "pop" is felt through the obturator membrane with the helical passer. At this point, it is important to immediately stop insertion of the helical passer once tactile feel confirms the membrane has been penetrated. Remove the guide. Reposition the handle of the helical passer by dropping it toward the midline until the handle is nearly vertical to the floor. Rotate the helical passer and hug the ischiopubic ramus, until the skin is tented. Make skin incision at the point where the tip of the helical passer tents the skin. Grasp the exposed tip with a clamp. Stabilize the tube near the urethra and remove the helical passer with a reverse rotation of the handle. Pull the plastic tube completely through the skin until the mesh appears. Repeat the procedure on the other side, perform cystoscopy, and adjust the sling as indicated above.

10 Retropubic Versus Transobturator Sling

The trial of mid-urethral slings (TOMUS) was a multicenter, randomized equivalence trial comparing outcomes with retropubic and transobturator mid-urethral slings in women with stress incontinence (Richter et al. 2010). The primary outcome was treatment success at 12 months according to both objective criteria (a negative stress test, a negative pad test, and no retreatment) and subjective criteria (self-reported absence of symptoms, no leakage episodes recorded, and no retreatment). The investigators found no significant difference in objective (82.4 vs. 79.6% for retropubic vs. transobturator sling) or subjective (62.4 vs. 56.0% for retropubic vs. transobturator sling) cure rate between the two groups. The median estimated blood loss and operative time were both significantly higher in the retropubic sling than in the transobturator sling group (estimate blood loss, 50 ml vs. 25 ml, $p < 0.001$; operative time, 30 min vs. 25 min, $p < 0.001$). There were 15 (5%) bladder perforations in the retropubic sling group and none in the transobturator group, whereas vaginal perforations were more common with the transobturator sling (4.3% vs. 2%, transobturator vs. retropubic sling, respectively). Voiding dysfunction requiring surgery, use of catheter, or both were seen in 2.7% in women who had the retropubic sling versus none of the women who had a transobturator sling

($p = 0.004$). Neurologic symptoms were more common in the transobturator sling (9.4% vs. 4%, transobturator vs. retropubic sling, $p = 0.01$). Among 68% of women with 5-year follow-up, treatment success at 5 years was 7.9% greater after retropubic compared to transobturator sling (51.3% vs. 43.4%, 95% CI −1.4, 17.2); however, a greater proportion of women in the transobturator group reported they were "very much better" or "much better" at 5 years (88% vs. 77%, $P = 0.01$) (Kenton et al. 2015).

Results from a recent meta-analysis of 17 studies involving 2,995 women (Seklehner et al. 2015) are shown in Table 1. Both the objective and subjective cures were slightly better for the retropubic approach. Bladder perforation and excess bleeding were also more common with the retropubic approach. However, neurologic symptoms were more commonly seen in the transobturator sling. Operative time was about 5 min longer in the retropubic approach; however, the authors attribute that to the fact that most of the studies used the original Gynecare TVT sling, which required two separate cystoscopy evaluations, while most currently utilized retropubic sling kits require only one cystoscopy after passing the needles on both sides.

In contrast, the Cochrane working group included 81 trials that evaluated 12,113 women; 55 trials with 8,652 women compared the retropubic to the transobturator sling (Ford et al. 2015). The short-term (up to 1 year) subjective

Table 1 Outcome of retropubic and transobturator mid-urethral sling

	Retropubic	Transobturator	Odds ratio
Objective cure	86.8%	83.4%	1.35 (95% CI 1.10–1.67, $p = 0.005$)
Subjective cure	76.4%	72.9%	1.24 (95% CI 1.04–1.49, $p = 0.02$)
Bladder perforation	3.2%	0.2%	5.72 (95% CI 2.94–11.12, $p < 0.0001$)
Excess bleeding	3.2%	1.1%	2.65 (95% CI 1.54–4.59, $p = 0.0005$)
Vaginal perforation	0.9%	3.6%	0.29 (95% CI 0.15–0.56, $p = 0.0002$)
Neurological symptoms	3.5%	9.4%	0.35 (95% CI 0.25–0.5, $p < 0.0001$)
Mesh exposure	2.5%	2.6%	0.97 (95% CI 0.63–1.48, $p = 0.97$)
Infection	6.6%	5.4%	1.21 (95% CI 0.79–1.57, $p = 0.28$)
LUTS	9.7%	8.9%	1.04 (95% CI 0.72–1.5, $p = 0.83$)
Urinary retention	6.3%	4%	1.54 ($p = 0.07$) (95% CI not given)
Operative time (min)	28.3	23.4	1.38 (95% CI0.88–1.89, $p < 0.0001$)

LUTS lower urinary tract symptoms (Seklehner et al. 2015)

cure rates were similar, ranging from 62 to 98% for the transobturator and 71 to 97% for the retropubic sling, respectively (RR 0.98, 95% CI 0.96–1.00; 36 trials, 5,514 women). Short-term objective cure rates were also similar (RR 0.98, 95% CI 0.96–1.00; 40 trials, 6,145 women). In the long term, subjective cure rates ranged from 43% to 92% in the transobturator group and from 51% to 88% in the retropubic group.

The rate of bladder perforation was lower with the transobturator sling (0.6% vs. 4.5%; RR 0.13, 95% CI 0.08–0.20; 40 trials, 6,372 women), and postoperative voiding dysfunction was less common after the transobturator sling (RR 0.53, 95% CI 0.43–0.65; 37 trials, 6,200 women).

The Cochrane working group found that the rate of groin pain postoperatively was higher with the transobturator sling (6.4% vs. 1.3%; RR 4.12, 95% CI 2.71–6.27; 18 trials, 3,221 women), while suprapubic pain was lower with the transobturator sling (0.8% vs. 2.9%; RR 0.29, 95% CI 0.11–0.78). The overall rate of vaginal tape exposure or extrusion was not significantly different between the two approaches – 2.4% with the transobturator sling and 2.1% for the retropubic sling (RR 1.13, 95% CI 0.78–1.65; 31 trials, 4,743 women).

The TOMUS trial (Richter et al. 2010) found no significant difference in success rate between transobturator and retropubic slings when they looked at women with lower Valsalva leak point pressure or maximal urethral closure pressure values. However, several studies have noted a higher failure rate in these women. In a retrospective cohort analysis, a cutoff point of 42 cm H_2O for preoperative maximum urethral closure pressure was identified as predictor of success (Miller et al. 2006). The relative risk of postoperative urodynamic stress incontinence 3 months after surgery in women with a preoperative maximum urethral closure pressure (MUCP) of 42 cm or less H_2O was 5.89 (1.02–33.90, 95% confidence interval) when the transobturator sling was compared with the retropubic sling (Miller et al. 2006). Schierlitz and colleagues performed a randomized controlled trial comparing the transobturator sling to the retropubic sling in women with stress urinary incontinence and intrinsic sphincter deficiency,

which was defined as either a maximum urethral closure pressure of 20 cm H_2O or less or a pressure rise from baseline required to cause incontinence (Δ Valsalva or cough leak point pressure) of 60 cm H_2O or less (Schierlitz et al. 2008). Of the 138 women who had follow-up urodynamics at 6 months after surgery, 14 of 67 (21%) in the retropubic sling group had stress incontinence demonstrated during repeat urodynamic assessment compared with 32 of 71 (45%) in the transobturator sling group ($p = 0.004$). Nine of 67 women (13%) in the transobturator sling group requested further surgical treatment to correct SUI compared with 0 of 71 (0%) in the retropubic group. The retropubic sling appears to be more effective in women with stress incontinence with low MUCP or leak point pressures.

11 Voiding Dysfunction After Mid-urethral Sling

The rate of voiding dysfunction, incomplete bladder emptying, elevated post-void residuals, or difficulty emptying the bladder is generally low after the mid-urethral sling and is reported in about 4% of women (Glavind and Shim 2015; Klutke et al. 2001; Moore and Paraiso 2005; Ozel et al. 2004). The sling can be released in the early postoperative period (within 3 weeks) with successful resolution of voiding dysfunction and with the majority of women maintaining continence (Glavind and Shim 2015; Price et al. 2009). To release the sling in the early postop period, before tissue fibrosis has fully taken place, the anterior vaginal incision can be opened by releasing the sutures and the sling identified and pulled down with gentle traction. Ideally this should be done between 7 and 14 days after surgery if the patient has persistent difficulty emptying the bladder, incomplete emptying, or elevated post-void residual volume. If the sling is not released in the early postop period, sling transection can be very successful in treating voiding dysfunction, but with recurrent incontinence rates as high as 60% (Viereck et al. 2013). Simple division or incision of the sling carries lower risk of recurrent stress incontinence (Agnew et al. 2012; Rardin et al.

2002). The simplest way to incise the sling is to make a vaginal incision in the midline along the anterior vaginal wall and then dissecting to one side or the other. The sling can be easily identified lateral to the urethra with less risk of urethral injury (Long et al. 2004). The sling can then be transected. Early transection (within 1 year of surgery) appears to result in greater improvement in lower urinary tract symptoms than delayed transection (South et al. 2009).

12 Laparoscopic Retropubic Colposuspension (Burch)

12.1 Technique

As in any laparoscopic procedure, it is important that the open procedure is closely mimicked without significant modification in technique. The use of mesh and staple modification of the colposuspension has been shown to be significantly less effective than the open Burch or the laparoscopic Burch using sutures (Ankardal et al. 2005). The retropubic space can be approached via an extraperitoneal or intraperitoneal dissection. The extraperitoneal approach is generally reserved for women who do not require other intraperitoneal procedures. The presence of prior pelvic incisions, especially a low transverse incision, may also hinder the ability to utilize this approach. The advantage of the extraperitoneal approach is that it avoids the risk of intra-abdominal injury and intraperitoneal adhesions. In the extraperitoneal approach, the space of Retzius can be easily dissected with a balloon or with a finger and pneumodissection. However, there is a risk of increased absorption of CO_2 leading to pneumothorax. For the intraperitoneal approach, the bladder is retrograde filled to about 300 ml of normal saline with or without methylene blue to facilitate identification of the bladder. The anterior peritoneum is then incised, and sharp and blunt dissection is used to enter the space of Retzius. The bladder is drained. Two number 0 braided delayed absorbable sutures (such as Vicryl; Ethicon Endosurgery, Inc., Cincinnati, OH) on a CT-2 needle are passed through the endopelvic fascia/vaginal wall about 2 cm lateral to the urethra and bladder, one at the level of the bladder neck and one at the level of the mid-urethra; these stitches are then passed through Cooper's ligament on the ipsilateral side (Tanagho modification) (Tanagho 1976). A figure-of-eight suture can be used to ensure that a good purchase of tissue has been obtained. Some authors place a third stitch on each side. The knots are tied extracorporeally with a hand in the vagina used to elevate the anterior vaginal wall. Gel foam can be placed between the sutures to promote fibrosis and improve hemostasis. Some authors prefer the use of permanent sutures such as number 0 braided polyester suture (Ethibond, Ethicon Endosurgery, Inc., Cincinnati, OH) rather than the traditional delayed absorbable suture. Cystourethroscopy with a 70° rigid cystoscope is mandatory to confirm integrity of the bladder wall and ureteral patency. The peritoneal defects are then closed sequentially using 2-0 polyglactin 910 sutures (Vicryl; Ethicon Endosurgery, Inc., Cincinnati, OH) in a figure-of-eight intracorporeal surgical slipknot technique.

13 Laparoscopic Burch Compared to Open Burch

The laparoscopic Burch appears to have similar efficacy with the open Burch colposuspension, but there are no long-term studies. Carey and colleagues compared the laparoscopic Burch to the open Burch in a randomized trial of 200 women with urodynamic stress incontinence with maximum urethral closure pressure greater than or equal to 20 cm H_2O (Carey et al. 2006). Operating time was significantly shorter in the open Burch group compared to the laparoscopic Burch group (42 min vs. 87 min, $p < 0.0001$). Estimated blood loss was significantly greater in the open Burch group compared to the laparoscopic Burch group (170 ml vs. 126 ml, $p = 0.03$). Urodynamic stress incontinence at 6 months of follow-up was found in 22% of women in the open Burch group and 28% in the laparoscopic Burch group ($p = 0.22$). At 24 months of follow-up, 30% of the open Burch group and 37% of the laparoscopic Burch group reported occasional or frequent stress incontinence symptoms ($p = 0.38$).

In the Cochrane review of open Burch versus the laparoscopic Burch, no significant differences in subjective and objective cure rate was found (Lapitan et al. 2009). The meta-analyses of data available at less than 1 year (RR 0.98, 95% CI 0.80–1.20) and between 1 and 5 years (RR 0.91, 95% CI 0.77–1.06) did not show any significant differences in subjective incontinence rates between the two groups. When looking at objective outcomes, there was again no significant difference at less than 1 year (RR 0.87, 95% CI 0.62–1.21) and between 1 and 5 years (RR 0.91, 95% CI 0.77–1.06).

14 Laparoscopic Burch Compared to Mid-urethral Sling

When compared to the mid-urethral sling, the laparoscopic Burch again shows comparable efficacy, but long-term outcome data is limited. When the laparoscopic Burch was compared to the mid-urethral sling in the Cochrane review (Dean et al. 2006), there was no statistically significant difference in the reported subjective cure rates between laparoscopic colposuspension and mid-urethral sling procedures within 18 months (RR 0.91, 95% CI 0.80–1.02). This finding remained at longer-term follow-up (4–8 years); the TVT had similar subjective cure rates as laparoscopic colposuspension (RR 1.18, 95% CI 0.36–3.81). However, laparoscopic colposuspension procedures had statistically significantly lower objective cure rates (RR 0.88, 95% CI 0.81–0.95), but there was a wide variety of definitions used for objective cure rate. Urodynamic testing was used to assess objective cure in three studies and showed no difference between the two procedures (RR 0.91, 95% CI 0.80–1.03). There was no difference in the perioperative complication rates between laparoscopic colposuspension and mid-urethral sling procedures (RR 0.99, 95% CI 0.60–1.64). However, laparoscopic surgery took significantly longer than the mid-urethral sling surgery, by an average of 20 min (mean difference 20.31 min, 95% CI 16.75–23.86).

Paraiso and colleagues performed a randomized controlled trial comparing the laparoscopic Burch colposuspension to the TVT (Paraiso et al. 2004). Women with urodynamic stress incontinence with abdominal leak point pressure greater than or equal to 60 cm H_2O and urethral hypermobility were included. The primary outcome was objective cure defined as no leakage during postoperative urodynamic studies. Seventy-two women were randomized. There was a higher rate of urodynamic stress incontinence at 1-year follow-up in the laparoscopic Burch group compared to the TVT group (18.8% vs. 3.2%; RR 1.19, 95% CI 1.00–1.42, $p = 0.056$). The laparoscopic Burch group had significantly longer operating time (101 min vs. 42 min for laparoscopic Burch vs. TVT sling, $p < 0.001$). However, at longer-term follow-up, in which 74% of the participants were seen at least 4 years after surgery, 58% of the laparoscopic Burch group and 48% of the TVT group reported any urinary incontinence after surgery (RR 1.19; 95% CI 0.71–2.00).

15 Conclusion

Several minimally invasive surgical options exist for women who have failed conservative therapy for stress urinary incontinence.

16 Cross-References

▶ Urinary Incontinence: Diagnosis, Treatment, and Avoiding Complications

References

Adamiak A, Milart P, Skorupski P, Kuchnicka K, Nestorowicz A, Jakowicki J, Rechberger T. The efficacy and safety of the tension-free vaginal tape procedure do not depend on the method of analgesia. Eur Urol. 2002;42(1):29–33.

Agnew G, Dwyer PL, Rosamilia A, Edwards G, Lee JK. Functional outcomes for surgical revision of synthetic slings performed for voiding dysfunction: a retrospective study. Eur J Obstet Gynecol Reprod Biol. 2012;163(1):113–6.

Ankardal M, Milsom I, Stjerndahl JH, Engh ME. A three-armed randomized trial comparing open Burch colposuspension using sutures with laparoscopic colposuspension using sutures and laparoscopic colposuspension using mesh and staples in women with stress urinary incontinence. Acta Obstet Gynecol Scand. 2005;84(8):773–9.

Aslam MF, Denman MA. Delayed diagnosis of vascular injury with a retropubic midurethral sling. Obstet Gynecol. 2013;122(2 Pt 2):444–6.

Carey MP, Goh JT, Rosamilia A, Cornish A, Gordon I, Hawthorne G, Maher CF, Dwyer PL, Moran P, Gilmour DT. Laparoscopic versus open Burch colposuspension: a randomised controlled trial. BJOG. 2006;113(9):999–1006.

Castillo OA, Bodden E, Olivares RA, Urena RD. Intestinal perforation: an infrequent complication during insertion of tension-free vaginal tape. J Urol. 2004;172(4):1364.

Cetinel B, Demirkesen O, Onal B, Akkus E, Alan C, Can G. Are there any factors predicting the cure and complication rates of tension-free vaginal tape? Int Urogynecol J Pelvic Floor Dysfunct. 2004;15(3):188–93.

Dean NM, Ellis G, Wilson PD, Herbison GP. Laparoscopic colposuspension for urinary incontinence in women. Cochrane Database Syst Rev. 2006; (3):CD002239.

Delorme E. Transobturator urethral suspension: mini-invasive procedure in the treatment of stress urinary incontinence in women. Prog Urol. 2001;11:1306–13.

Dooley Y, Kenton K, Cao G, Luke A, Durazo-Arvizu R, Kramer H, Brubaker L. Urinary incontinence prevalence: results from the National Health and Nutrition Examination Survey. J Urol. 2008;179(2):656–61.

Dunivan GC, Parnell BA, Connolly A, Jannelli ML, Horton BJ, Geller EJ. Bupivacaine injection during midurethral sling and postoperative pain: a randomized controlled trial. Int Urogynecol J. 2011;22(4):433–8.

Ford AA, Rogerson L, Cody JD, Ogah J. Mid-urethral sling operations for stress urinary incontinence in women. Cochrane Database Syt Rev 2015; (7):CD006375.

Fourie T, Cohen PL. Delayed bowel erosion by the tension-free vaginal tape. Int Urogynecol J. 2003;14:362–4.

Ghezzi F, Cromi A, Raio L, Bergamini V, Triacca P, Serati M, Kuhn A. Influence of the type of anesthesia and hydrodissection on the complication rate after tension-free vaginal tape procedure. Eur J Obstet Gynecol Reprod Biol. 2005;118(1):96–100.

Glavind K, Shim S. Incidence and treatment of postoperative voiding dysfunction after the tension-free vaginal tape procedure. Int Urogynecol J. 2015;26(11):1657–60.

Haab F, Sananes S, Amarenco G, et al. Results of the tension-free vaginal tape procedure for the treatment of type II stress urinary incontinence at a minimum follow up of 1 year. J Urol. 2001;165:159–62.

Haya N, Baessler K, Christmann-Schmid C, de Tayrac R, Dietz V, Guldberg R, Mascarenhas T, Nussler E, Ballard E, Ankardal M, Boudemaghe T, JM W, Maher CF. Prolapse and continence surgery in countries of the Organization for Economic Cooperation and Development in 2012. Am J Obstet Gynecol. 2015;212(6):755.e1–e27.

Haylen BT, et al. An International Urogynecological Association (IUGA)/International Continence Society (ICS) joint report on the terminology for female pelvic floor dysfunction. Neurourol Urodyn. 2010;29:4–20.

Hsieh GC, Klutke JJ, Kobak WH. Low valsalva leak-point pressure and success of retropubic urethropexy. Int Urogynecol J Pelvic Floor Dysfunct. 2001;12(1):46–50.

Jelovsek JE, Barber MD, Karram MM, Walters MD, Paraiso MF. Randomised trial of laparoscopic Burch colposuspension versus tension-free vaginal tape: long-term follow up. BJOG. 2008;115(2):219–25. discussion 225.

Kenton K, Stoddard AM, Zyczynski H, Albo M, Rickey L, Norton P, Wai C, Kraus SR, Sirls LT, Kusek JW, Litman HJ, Chang RP, Richter HE. 5-year longitudinal follow up after retropubic and transobturator mid urethral slings. J Urol. 2015;193(1):203–10.

Klutke C, Siegel S, Carlin B, Paszkiewicz E, Kirkemo A, Klutke J. Urinary retention after tension-free vaginal tape procedure: incidence and treatment. Urology. 2001;58(5):697–701.

Lapitan MC, Cody JD, Grant A. Open retropubic colposuspension for urinary incontinence in women. Cochrane Database Syst Rev 2009; (4):CD002912.

LaSala CA, Schimpf MO, Udoh E, O'Sullivan DM, Tulikangas P. Outcome of tension-free vaginal tape procedure when complicated by intraoperative cystotomy. Am J Obstet Gynecol. 2006;195(6):1857–61.

Leboeuf L, Mendez LE, Gousse AE. Small bowel obstruction associated with tension-free vaginal tape. Urology. 2004;63(6):1182.

Liapis A, Bakas P, Creatsas G. Assessment of TVT efficacy in the management of patients with genuine stress incontinence with the use of epidural vs intravenous anesthesia. Int Urogynecol J Pelvic Floor Dysfunct. 2007;18(10):1197–200.

Lo TS, Lin CT, Huang HJ, Chang CL, Liang CC, Soong YK. The use of general anesthesia for the tension-free vaginal tape procedure and concomitant surgery. Acta Obstet Gynecol Scand. 2003;82(4):367–73.

Long CY, Lo TS, Liu CM, Hsu SC, Chang Y, Tsai EM. Lateral excision of tension-free vaginal tape for the treatment of iatrogenic urethral obstruction. Obstet Gynecol. 2004;104(6):1270–4.

Lovatsis D, Gupta C, Dean E, Lee F. Tension-free vaginal tape procedure is an ideal treatment for obese patients. Am J Obstet Gynecol. 2003;189(6):1601–4. discussion 1604–5.

Low SJ, Smith KM, Holt EM. Tension free vaginal tape: is the intra-operative cough test necessary? Int Urogynecol J Pelvic Floor Dysfunct. 2004;15(5): 328–30.

Meschia M, Busacca M, Pifarotti P, De Marinis S. Bowel perforation during insertion of tension-free vaginal tape (TVT). Int Urogynecol J Pelvic Floor Dysfunct. 2002;13(4):263–5. discussion 265.

Miller JJ, Botros SM, Akl MN, Aschkenazi SO, Beaumont JL, Goldberg RP, Sand PK. Is transobturator tape as effective as tension-free vaginal tape in patients with borderline maximum urethral closure pressure? Am J Obstet Gynecol. 2006;195(6):1799–804.

Moore C, Paraiso MF. Voiding dysfunction after the tension-free vaginal tape procedure. Curr Urol Rep. 2005;6(5):356–9.

Moore KH, Shahab RB, Walsh CA, Kuteesa WM, Sarma S, Cebola M, Allen W, Wang YA, Karantanis E. Randomized controlled trial of cough test versus no cough test in the tension-free vaginal tape procedure: effect upon voiding dysfunction and 12-month efficacy. Int Urogynecol J. 2012;23(4):435–41.

Murphy M, Heit MH, Fouts L, Graham CA, Blackwell L, Culligan PJ. Effect of anesthesia on voiding function after tension-free vaginal tape procedure. Obstet Gynecol. 2003;101(4):666–70.

Murphy M, Culligan PJ, Arce CM, Graham CA, Blackwell L, Heit MH. Is the cough-stress test necessary when placing the tension-free vaginal tape? Obstet Gynecol. 2005;105(2):319–24.

Nager CW, Brubaker L, Litman HJ, Zyczynski HM, Varner RE, Amundsen C, et al. A randomized trial of urodynamic testing before stress-incontinence surgery. Urinary Incontinence Treatment Network. N Engl J Med. 2012;366:1987–97.

Ozel B, Minaglia S, Hurtado E, Klutke CG, Klutke JJ. Treatment of voiding dysfunction after transobturator tape procedure. Urology. 2004;64(5):1030.

Paraiso MF, Walters MD, Karram MM, Barber MD. Laparoscopic Burch colposuspension versus tension-free vaginal tape: a randomized trial. Obstet Gynecol. 2004;104(6):1249–58.

Price N, Slack A, Khong SY, Currie I, Jackson S. The benefit of early mobilisation of tension-free vaginal tape in the treatment of post-operative voiding dysfunction. Int Urogynecol J Pelvic Floor Dysfunct. 2009; 20(7):855–8.

Rardin CR, Rosenblatt PL, Kohli N, Miklos JR, Heit M, Lucente VR. Release of tension-free vaginal tape for the treatment of refractory postoperative voiding dysfunction. Obstet Gynecol. 2002;100(5 Pt 1):898–902.

Richter HE, Albo ME, Zyczynski HM, Kenton K, Norton PA, Sirls LT, Kraus SR, Chai TC, Lemack GE, Dandreo KJ, Varner RE, Menefee S, Ghetti C, Brubaker L, Nygaard I, Khandwala S, Rozanski TA, Johnson H, Schaffer J, Stoddard AM, Holley RL, Nager CW, Moalli P, Mueller E, Arisco AM, Corton M,

Tennstedt S, Chang TD, Gormley EA, Litman HJ. Urinary Incontinence Treatment Network. Retropubic versus transobturator midurethral slings for stress incontinence. N Engl J Med. 2010;362(22):2066–76.

Richter HE, Litman HJ, Lukacz ES, Sirls LT, Rickey L, Norton P, et al. Demographic and clinical predictors of treatment failure one year after midurethral sling surgery. Urinary Incontinence Treatment Network. Obstet Gynecol. 2011;117:913–21.

Sand PK, Bowen LW, Panganiban R, Ostergard DR. The low pressure urethra as a factor in failed retropubic urethropexy. Obstet Gynecol. 1987;69(3 Pt 1): 399–402.

Schierlitz L, Dwyer PL, Rosamilia A, Murray C, Thomas E, De Souza A, Lim YN, Hiscock R. Effectiveness of tension-free vaginal tape compared with transobturator tape in women with stress urinary incontinence and intrinsic sphincter deficiency: a randomized controlled trial. Obstet Gynecol. 2008;112(6): 1253–61.

Seklehner S, Laudano MA, Xie D, Chughtai B, Lee RK. A meta-analysis of the performance of retropubic mid urethral sling versus transobturator mid urethral slings. J Urol. 2015;193:1–7.

Sivanesan K, Abdel-Fattah M, Ghani R. External iliac artery injury during insertion of tension-free vaginal tape: a case report and literature review. Int Urogynecol J Pelvic Floor Dysfunct. 2007;18(9):1105–8.

South MM, Wu JM, Webster GD, Weidner AC, Roelands JJ, Amundsen CL. Early vs late midline sling lysis results in greater improvement in lower urinary tract symptoms. Am J Obstet Gynecol. 2009;200(5):564. e1–5.

Subak LL, Wing R, West DS, Franklin F, Vittinghoff E, Creasman JM, et al. Weight loss to treat urinary incontinence in overweight and obese women. PRIDE Investigators. N Engl J Med. 2009;360:481–90.

Tanagho EA. Colpocystourethropexy: the way we do it. J Urol. 1976;116:751–3.

Taylor JD, Tsokos N. Retroperitoneal laparoscopic surgery for stress incontinence. Lancet. 1993;342 (8886–8887):1564–5.

Ulmsten U, Henriksson L, Johnson P, Varhos G. An ambulatory surgical procedure under local anesthesia for treatment of female urinary incontinence. Int Urogynecol J Pelvic Floor Dysfunct. 1996;7(2):81–5. discussion 85–6.

Viereck V, Rautenberg O, Kociszewski J, Grothey S, Welter J, Eberhard J. Midurethral sling incision: indications and outcomes. Int Urogynecol J. 2013;24(4): 645–53.

Wang AC, Chen MC. Randomized comparison of local versus epidural anaesthesia for tension-free vaginal tape operation. J Urol. 2001;165:1177–80.

Ward K, Hilton P, United Kingdom and Ireland Tension-free Vaginal Tape Trial Group. Prospective multicentre randomised trial of tension-free vaginal tape and colposuspension as primary treatment for stress incontinence. BMJ. 2002;325(7355):67.

Ward KL, Hilton P, UK and Ireland TVT Trial Group. Tension-free vaginal tape versus colposuspension for primary urodynamic stress incontinence: 5-year follow up. BJOG. 2008;115(2):226–33.

Wohlrab KJ, Erekson EA, Korbly NB, Drimbarean CD, Rardin CR, Sung VW. The association between regional anesthesia and acute postoperative urinary retention in women undergoing outpatient midurethral sling procedures. Am J Obstet Gynecol. 2009;200(5): 571.e1–5.

Zilbert AW, Farrell SA. External iliac artery laceration during tension-free vaginal tape procedure. Int Urogynecol J Pelvic Floor Dysfunct. 2001;12(2):141–3.

Zyczynski HM, Lloyd LK, Kenton K, Menefee S, Boreham M, Stoddard AM. Correlation of Q-tip values and point Aa in stress-incontinent women. Urinary Incontinence Treatment Network (UITN). Obstet Gynecol. 2007;110:39–43.

Part VIII

Gynecologic Operative Procedures
(Begüm Özel)

Vaginal Hysterectomy: Indications, Avoiding Complications

Begüm Özel

Abstract

Vaginal hysterectomy is believed to have been first successfully performed in 1813. Most women requiring a hysterectomy are candidates for the vaginal approach, and it should always be considered as first-line approach to hysterectomy. Both the American Congress of Obstetrics and Gynecology and the American Academy of Gynecologic Laparoscopists recommended vaginal hysterectomy whenever possible. Previous cesarean delivery and obesity are not contraindications to the vaginal approach; in fact the vaginal approach may be preferred in these patients. Paracervical vasopressin has been shown to decrease blood loss during vaginal hysterectomy, although the difference may not be clinically significant. Preemptive oral gabapentin and preemptive local anesthesia reduce post-op pain. Vaginal salpingoo-phorectomy and salpingectomy can be accomplished in the majority of patients. Unless vaginal apical suspension is planned, a modified McCall-type culdoplasty should be performed to prevent enterocele formation and to reattach the uterosacral ligaments to the vaginal cuff. In randomized trials, women returned to normal activities sooner after vaginal compared to abdominal hysterectomy and have less wound infections, urinary tract infections, and febrile episodes after a vaginal versus abdominal hysterectomy. Compared to laparoscopic-assisted vaginal hysterectomy or total laparoscopic hysterectomy, vaginal hysterectomy has shorter operating time, hospital stay, and cost. Complications occur in about 5% of cases, with the most common complications being cuff infection/abscess and dissection cystotomy. Cuff infection/abscess complicates about 1.2% of case, while dissection cystotomy occurs in roughly 0.5% of cases. Ureteral injury is relatively rare, but pelvic organ prolapse increases the risk of this complication.

Keywords

Hysterectomy • Vaginal • Laparoscopic • Cost • Complications • Vaginal hysterectomy

Contents

B. Özel (✉)
Division of Female Pelvic Medicine and Reconstructive Surgery, Department of Obstetrics and Gynecology, Keck School of Medicine, University of Southern California, Los Angeles, CA, USA
e-mail: ozel@usc.edu; Begum.Ozel@med.usc.edu

© Springer International Publishing AG 2017
D. Shoupe (ed.), *Handbook of Gynecology*,
DOI 10.1007/978-3-319-17798-4_69

1   Background

The first report of a vaginal hysterectomy was for a gangrenous prolapsed uterus, reported by Soranus of Ephesus in 120 AD; however, it involved transection of the bladder and ureters (Sutton 2010). A second well-documented case was of Faith Howard, a peasant woman who grew tired of her prolapsed uterus and amputated it with a sharp knife; unfortunately she also suffered subsequently from "water passing from her insensible day and night" (Sutton 1997). In 1813, Conrad Lagenbeck of Gottingen performed the first planned and successful surgical vaginal hysterectomy (Sutton 1997).

Today hysterectomy is one of the most commonly performed surgical procedures. Roughly 600,000 hysterectomies are performed annually in the United States. Both the American Congress of Obstetricians and Gynecologists the American Association of Gynecologic Laparoscopists recommend vaginal hysterectomy as the preferred route of hysterectomy for benign indications (ACOG 2009; AAGL 2011). Despite this, there has been a decline in the percentage of hysterectomies performed vaginally in the United States, from 24.8% in 1998 to 16.9% in 2012 (Desai 2015).

A major challenge to vaginal hysterectomy is inadequate training. In a recent survey of fellowship program directors, only 20% of graduating obstetrics and gynecology residents starting fellowship in female pelvic medicine and reconstructive

surgery were deemed competent to independently perform a vaginal hysterectomy (Guntupalli et al. 2015). In 2010, a survey of graduating residents found that one third felt unprepared to perform a vaginal hysterectomy independently, and only 27.8% of graduating residents reported being "completely prepared." In comparison, only 5.6% and 19.5% of graduating residents felt unprepared to independently perform abdominal hysterectomies and laparoscopic hysterectomies, respectively (Burkett et al. 2011). In another survey of graduating senior resident, 90% stated that they would perform vaginal hysterectomy in the future and 75% felt adequately trained. Residents were more likely to feel comfortable performing the procedure independently if they had performed more than 20 vaginal hysterectomies (odds ratio [OR], 10.2; 95% CI, 3.3–30.9; $P < 0.0001$) and if they learned vaginal morcellation techniques (OR, 5.1; 95% CI, 1.5–17.8; $P = 0.01$) (Antosh et al. 2011).

There has been a decrease in the number of vaginal hysterectomies performed by residents during training, despite no change in the total number of hysterectomies being performed over the 4-year residency training. The mean number of hysterectomies performed by residents was 118.1 cases in 2008–2009 and 116.1 cases in 2011–2012 ($p = 0.16$); however, the number of vaginal hysterectomies performed went from 34.9 cases to 19.4 cases during the same time period, representing a 40% decrease ($p < 0.001$; 95% CI, 14.3–16.7) (Washburn et al. 2014).

One reason behind this is believed to be an increase in laparoscopic and robotic hysterectomies. Between 2007 and 2010, the rate of robotic hysterectomy increased from 0.5% to 9.5%, and the rate of laparoscopic hysterectomy increased from 24.3 to 30.5% in 441 hospitals in the United States (Wright et al. 2013b). In another study of 1440 hysterectomies performed at four academic medical centers, the proportion of hysterectomies performed via the vaginal route decreased from 42.5% before the introduction of the robot to the medical centers to 30.5% after the robot ($p < 0.0001$) (Jeppson et al. 2015).

The vaginal hysterectomy remains the most minimally invasive technique for the surgical removal of the uterus, with the advantage of quickest recovery, lowest complications, and best cosmesis. It is also the most cost effective among the various approaches to hysterectomy with an average cost savings of $2200 per hysterectomy (Woelk et al. 2014). Total laparoscopic hysterectomy costs on average $3500 more per case and robotic hysterectomy more than $5000 more per case than vaginal hysterectomy (Dayaratna et al. 2014).

2   Indications and Patient Selection

Most common benign indications for hysterectomy are leiomyoma, abnormal uterine bleeding, endometriosis, benign ovarian neoplasm, and pelvic organ prolapse (Wright et al. 2013a). The most common indication for a vaginal hysterectomy is uterine prolapse, which in 2005 accounted for 62% of cases (Clarke-Pearson and Geller 2013). With appropriate patient selection, vaginal hysterectomy can be performed for any benign indication.

Kovac described guidelines to determine if a patient was a vaginal hysterectomy candidate and applied them in a resident clinic (Fig. 1) (Kovac et al. 2002). The first determination is whether the uterus is accessible vaginally. This determination was made with the following criteria: the uterus is deemed accessible transvaginally if the vagina is >2 fingerbreadths in width at the apex or if the uterus is at least stage 1 when the Valsalva maneuver is performed. If there was adequate vaginal access, then uterine size was taken into consideration. If the uterus was estimated to be less than 12 weeks or 280 gm, then a vaginal approach was appropriate. Although other formulas exist, the simplest and easiest to remember formula to estimate uterine weight is $0.52 \times$ length $\times$ width $\times$ depth based on ultrasound measurements (Goldstein et al. 1988). If the clinical history or pelvic examination indicated possible extrauterine disease (endometriosis, pelvic inflammatory disease, ovarian disease, or chronic pelvic pain), laparoscopic assistance was performed to confirm the presence and the extent of extrauterine pathologic condition

accurately and whether operative laparoscopy would permit vaginal hysterectomy to be performed. Consideration was also given to the appropriateness and ability to perform uterine size reduction techniques, such as morcellation, myomectomy, or coring. Using these criteria, 92% of planned vaginal hysterectomies could be accomplished vaginally in a resident clinic population (Kovac et al. 2002). There were no conversions from vaginal hysterectomy to abdominal hysterectomy due to findings on laparoscopy; the remainder of the cases was performed abdominally or with laparoscopic assistance.

Vaginal hysterectomy may be appropriate in women with uterus >12 weeks without an increased rate of complications (Cho et al. 2014; Fantania et al. 2014; Sahin 2007). However, mean operating time was significantly longer in the uteri $\geq$280 gm than in the <280 gm (69.4 ± 24.4 versus 108.2 ± 41.2 min, $p < 0.0001$). There was also a higher rate of hemorrhage as defined as a fall in hemoglobin value of >4 g/100 mL. (8.43% versus 1.2%) in women with uteri $\geq$280 gm (Sahin 2007).

Although there is some data suggesting that women with two or more prior cesarean deliveries may be at higher risk of bladder injury with a vaginal hysterectomy (Duong and Patterson 2014), prior cesarean delivery does not contraindicate a vaginal hysterectomy (Purohit et al. 2013; Unger and Meeks 1998), and a history cesarean delivery is known to be a risk factor for bladder injury regardless of the route of hysterectomy (Rooney et al. 2005).

Obesity is not a contraindication, and vaginal hysterectomy remains the procedure of choice in obese women who are having a hysterectomy (Harmanli et al. 2011; Muffly and Kow 2014; Sheth 2010).

3   Contraindications

There are contraindications to a vaginal hysterectomy which include cervical cancer, endometrial hyperplasia, or malignancy when morcellation would be necessary; concern for leiomyosarcoma when morcellation would be necessary; large

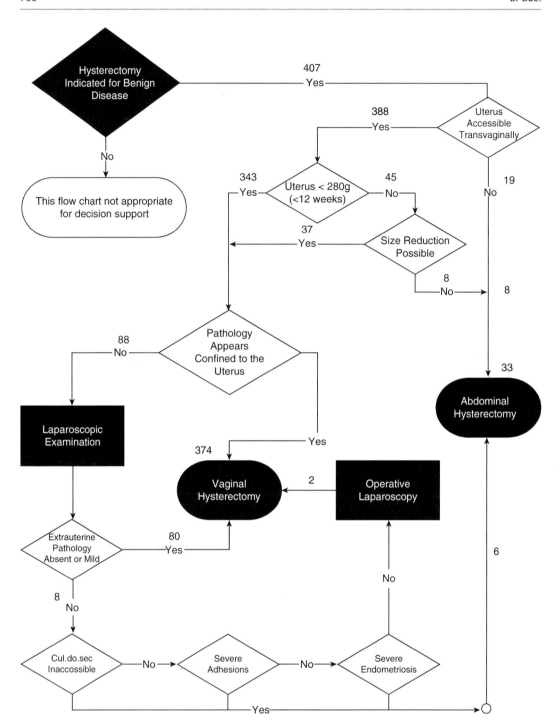

Fig. 1 Determining the route of hysterectomy (Reprinted from Kovac et al. (2002), with permission from Elsevier)

ovarian mass, especially when there is concern for malignancy; and large cervical leiomyoma when the uterine vessels cannot be accessed. Severe pelvic adhesions, obliterated cul-de-sac, and very large uterine size are all relative contraindications.

4 Technique

4.1 Vaginal Prep

Vaginal preparation with povidone iodine or chlorhexidine solution is routinely performed to decrease infectious morbidity. Use of saline to prep the vaginal has been shown to increase infectious morbidity in the early post-op period (Kjolhede et al. 2011). Culligan and colleagues found that 4% chlorhexidine gluconate with 4% isopropyl alcohol was more effective than povidone iodine in decreasing the bacterial colony counts that were found in the operative field for vaginal hysterectomy (Culligan et al. 2005).

4.2 Antimicrobial Prophylaxis

It is standard of care to provide perioperative antimicrobial prophylaxis in all hysterectomy cases. First-generation cephalosporins, such as cefazolin, are as effective as second- or third-generation cephalosporins and are less expensive. They are also less likely to induce bacterial beta-lactamase response. In women who are penicillin allergic, alternatives include clindamycin or metronidazole plus a fluoroquinolone (ciprofloxacin or levofloxacin) or gentamicin. Repeat dosing is recommended after 3 h of when estimated blood loss is greater than 1500 ml. Antibiotics should not be continued past 24 h postoperatively.

4.3 Patient Positioning

Optimal position will result in both excellent exposure and minimize the risk of patient injury. The patient is positioned in high dorsal lithotomy in boot-type or candy cane stirrups. It is important to avoid hyperflexion or external rotation of the hips to prevent stretch injury to the sciatic nerve and compression injury to the femoral nerve which passes under the ilioinguinal ligament in the groin. It is important to place the legs in the position that they will be in during the case before draping to ensure that there is no hyperflexion at the hip when the legs are raised to high lithotomy.

The peroneal nerve is also at risk during lithotomy, and care should be made to prevent bowing out of the knee which can cause stretch injury during the use of candy cane stirrups. The nerve can also be subject to compression injury with boot-type stirrups. Extra padding should be used if needed. The posterior tibial nerve is stretched with ankle dorsiflexion and can also be at risk when the foot is in candy cane stirrups. Consideration should be given to positioning the patient in stirrups when she is awake if she has any issues with pain or limiting mobility of her lower extremities.

It is helpful to use a foam egg crate on the table and place the patient directly on the foam egg crate to minimize sliding up on the bed with Trendelenburg. The patient should be placed in Trendelenburg at the start of the case to allow for visualization and to move small bowel out of the cul-de-sac. The patient should be positioned on the operating table so that her buttocks are over the edge of the cutout in the table. This will help when retractors are used.

4.4 Vasopressin

A dilute vasopressin solution may be injected paracervically to reduce blood loss during vaginal hysterectomy. When vasopressin is injected into tissue, it has a vasoconstrictive effect that is produced by the contraction of smooth muscle cells in vessels. This effect lasts less than an hour and the half-life is 10–20 min. Kammerer-Doak and colleagues conducted a randomized controlled trial of 117 women who received paracervical vasopressin versus saline during vaginal hysterectomy; 8 mL of vasopressin (20 units/100 mL normal saline solution) is injected into the submucosa circumferentially around the cervix in six small wheals at the 1, 3, 5, 7, 9, and 11 o'clock positions (Kammerer-Doak et al. 2001). They found that estimated blood loss (312 ± 222 mL vs. 446 ± 296 mL; $p = 0.006$) and change in hemoglobin and hematocrit levels (2.1 ± 1.4 gm vs. 2.9 ± 1.4 gm; $p = 0.02$; and $6.7\% \pm 3.4\%$ vs. $8.5\% \pm 3.8\%$; $p = 0.01$; vasopressin versus normal saline solution, respectively) were significantly less in the vasopressin group.

There was no significant difference in infection rates; in fact, the normal saline solution group had a higher rate of infection (7.3%) compared with the vasopressin group (1.6%; relative risk, 4.51; 95% CI, 0.52–39.14; $p = 0.19$). In another randomized controlled trial, 20 mL (8 units) of dilute vasopressin solution (20 units of vasopressin in 50 mL of normal saline) was injected in 5 mL increments at 2, 4, 8, and 10 o'clock circumferentially around the cervix at the cervicovaginal junction. The use of vasopressin injected paracervically resulted in significantly less blood loss (145.3 mL compared with 266.4 mL control; $p = 0.022$). However, there was no difference in postoperative hematocrit, but there was a significant difference in the increase in mean blood pressure at 5 min after injection (10.4 for the vasopressin group compared with 2.5 for the control group, $p = 0.043$) as well as an increase in patient-controlled anesthesia usage postoperatively (Ascher-Walsh et al. 2009).

5   Preemptive Techniques to Minimize Postoperative Pain

Gabapentin is a gamma-aminobutyric acid (GABA) analogue that has been shown to be effective in the treatment of neuropathic pain; its use has been studied perioperatively to decrease post-op pain and requirements. The mechanism of action is unknown since it does not appear to interact with GABA receptors. Rorarius and colleagues performed a double-blind randomized study of 1200 mg of gabapentin versus 15 mg of oxazepam 2.5 h before surgery in women undergoing elective vaginal hysterectomy (Rorarius et al. 2004). They found that women treated with gabapentin needed approximately 40% less doses of fentanyl than women in the control group. The women who received gabapentin also had significantly less nausea. There were no differences in medication related side effects.

The use of preemptive local anesthesia in vaginal hysterectomy may be beneficial in terms of postoperative pain. O'Neal and colleagues conducted a small randomized controlled trail of 20 women; one group received paracervical injection of 0.5% bupivacaine with epinephrine, while the other group received saline injections (O'Neal et al. 2003). Pain scores were lower in the bupivacaine group ($p = 0.03$). Total morphine and patient-controlled analgesia morphine was significantly less in patients receiving bupivacaine ($p = 0.01$ and 0.04). There was no difference in estimated blood loss or length of hospital stay. Long and colleagues compared paracervical injection of 20 mL of 0.5% bupivacaine with 1:200,000 epinephrine to placebo in a randomized controlled trial of 90 women having a vaginal hysterectomy and found that the mean total dose of narcotic within the first 24 h was 30% lower for the bupivacaine group than the placebo group ($p = 0.009$), and pain on the visual analogue scale was significantly lower at 30 min and 3 h postoperatively with no difference at 12 and 24 h (Long et al. 2009).

A randomized controlled trial using ropivacaine in a modified paracervical block before prior to incision found that this significantly reduced both pain at rest up to 8 h and pain with coughing and movement up to 4 h after surgery (Hristovska et al. 2014). The median time until first ambulation was significantly shorter in the ropivacaine group, and the use of post-op analgesics was significantly less in the ropivacaine group. In this study ropivacaine 0.50% or saline 30 mL was injected before incision as a modified paracervical block; 5 mL was injected through the vaginal fornices at 2, 4, 6, 8, 10, and 12 o'clock at 2 cm depth while the needle was retracted, and 2 mL was injected in each resection line (uterosacral and cardinal ligaments and the adnexal corners) close to the suture.

5.1   Surgical Steps

The bladder is initially drained, and a Foley catheter is left in place but clamped during the case. This allows for intermittent bladder drainage, as well as allowing the surgeon to palpate the Foley balloon to identify the bladder. Lastly, since the bladder is not continuously drained, an incidental cystotomy should be easy to identify because of the drainage of urine through the cystotomy site.

A weighted speculum is placed in the vagina. A Heaney retractor can be used to retract the anterior vaginal wall to visualize the cervix. The cervix is grasped with a double tooth Jacobs' tenaculum or Lahey clamp. Traction and counter traction throughout the case are important to increase the distance between the clamps and the ureters.

An incision is made in the full thickness of the vagina around the cervix either with cautery or with a knife. This incision should be made just at the point that the vaginal rugae appear anteriorly and laterally and a few millimeters proximal to this point posteriorly. The posterior peritoneal reflection is then identified and grasped with tissue forceps and entered sharply with curved Mayo scissors. At this point, either a Heaney retractor or a long weighted speculum can be inserted though the posterior colpotomy.

The bladder is then dissected off the anterior cervix with Metzenbaum scissors (Fig. 2). The anterior peritoneal reflection appears as a smooth crescent-shaped line above the level of the cervix. The Foley balloon can aid in identifying the bladder during dissection. If entry is difficult, if the uterus is small enough, a finger can be placed over the uterine fundus and the anterior peritoneal reflection palpated and identified. Otherwise, the bladder can be dissected off the cervix anteriorly, and so long as it is off the cervix, ligation of the pedicles can occur. With the resulting uterine descent, the anterior peritoneal reflection will become easier to identify. It is important not to rush to try to enter anteriorly without good visualization. Once the anterior peritoneum is entered, a Heaney or Deaver retractor can be placed into this space.

The uterosacral ligaments are then clamped, transected, and suture ligated bilaterally. The clamp is placed perpendicular to the cervix and the tissue is cut so as to leave a small amount of tissue distal to the clamp. A Heaney needle driver is useful during a vaginal hysterectomy for suturing in tight spaces. It is best to ligate this pedicle with a Heaney stitch because this pedicle will be tagged with a Kelly clamp or hemostat to help with visualization of the pedicles at the end of the case. If it is not transfixed, the suture can easily slip off.

The cardinal ligaments are then clamped, transected, and suture ligated bilaterally. When the cervix is long, it will take several bits of tissue to fully ligate this ligament. The uterine arteries are clamped, transected, and suture ligated on both sides. Again, traction and counter traction are important at this point to increase the distance between the arteries and the ureters. The anterior peritoneal reflection should be entered if it has not been entered yet.

The broad ligament is then clamped. At this point it is important not to place too much traction on the uterus since the primary support structures have been transected, and there is a risk for avulsion of the upper pedicles. The triple pedicle (round ligament, fallopian tube, utero-ovarian ligament) can be tied off with a free tie, which is held to allow for identification of this pedicle before closing, and then clamped, transected, and suture ligated.

Once the uterine arteries are ligated, it is possible to start using techniques to facilitate removal of an enlarged uterus. However, these techniques should be avoided if there is any risk for malignancy. These techniques include bivalving, which can be accompanied by morcellation, or coring of the myometrium. The latter is accomplished by circumferentially incising the myometrium beneath the serosa with a scalpel while placing the cervix on tension. This allows for delivery of the uterus in one elongated piece.

A sponge stick or moist vaginal pack can be placed in the peritoneal cavity to retract bowel

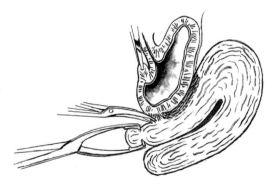

Fig. 2 Dissection of the bladder off the anterior cervix and uterus (Reprinted from Unger and Meeks (1998), with permission from Elsevier)

and allow for visualization of the pedicles. At this point there should be a tag on both the first and last pedicles so that the entire suture line can be visualized on both sides. If there is good hemostasis, the free tie on the triple pedicle can be cut. It is important to note that only the free tie should be tagged and not the ligated stitch since the traction on the stitch may cause it to come lose resulting in loss of this pedicle which can be hard to reidentify vaginally. There is little harm to the free tie coming lose because it is not a hemostatic tie.

Salpingectomy, salpingo-oophorectomy, culdoplasty, or apical suspension can be performed next. The cuff is closed with continuous locked or interrupted figure of eight stitches. The culdoplasty stitch is tied last.

5.2   Energy-Based Sealing Devices

Energy-based sealing devices are an alternative to using suture ligation for vaginal hysterectomy. In a meta-analysis, energy-based vessel-sealing devices decreased operative time by a mean of 17.2 min (seven studies, 662 patients; 95% confidence interval [CI] 7.5–27.0), blood loss by a mean of 47.7 mL (five studies, 437 patients; 95% CI 15.5–79.9), drop in hemoglobin by 0.3 g/dL (two studies, 291 patients; 95% CI 0.1–0.6), and postoperative hospital stay by 0.25 days (five studies, 554 patients; 95% CI 0.13–0.37). There was no increase in the rate of complications for energy-based vessel sealing compared with traditional suturing (Kroft and Selk 2011).

Two studies were published since that meta-analysis which both showed reduced operating time with the use of energy-based sealing devices. In a randomized study comparing using Ligasure™ Impact (LF4200) in combination with the ForceTriad™ energy platform (Covidien; Tyco Healthcare, Valleylab, CO, USA) to traditional suture ligation in 100 women, operating time was shorter in the vessel-sealing group (59.7 versus 71.3 min, $p = 0.05$); the amount of blood loss and duration of hospital stay did not differ (Lakeman et al. 2012). Pain scores after

surgery were significantly different on the evening after surgery (5.7 versus 4.5 on a scale of 0–10 for Ligasure versus traditional suture, respectively, $p = 0.03$) but were similar thereafter. Silva-Filho and colleagues compared the bipolar vessel-sealing system (Ligasure, Valleylab, Boulder, CO) with conventional suturing in a randomized trial of 90 women having a vaginal hysterectomy (Silva-Filho et al. 2009). They also found reduced operating time (29.2 ± 2.1 min vs. 75.2 ± 5 min; $p < 0.001$), as well as reduced operative blood loss (84 ± 5.9 mL vs. 136.4 ± 89.1 mL; $p = 0.001$), pain at 12 h after surgery (1.6 ± 0.4 vs. 3.6 ± 0.4; $p < 0.001$) and hospital stay (25.6 ± 0.9 h vs. 33.2 ± 1.7 h; $p < 0.001$) compared to the control group. There was no increase in complications.

The Harmonic scalpel (Ethicon Endo-Surgery, Inc., Cincinnati, OH) was compared to traditional suture ligation in a randomized trial of 40 women and was found to result in no difference in operative time, clinically significant blood loss, or analgesic requirements (Fitz-Gerald et al. 2013). Estimated blood loss was significantly less in the Harmonic scalpel group [62.63 (12.46) mL vs. 136.05 (21.54) mL; $p = 0.006$], but this did not translate into any significant differences in change in hemoglobin levels after surgery.

5.3   Vaginal Salpingo-Oophorectomy

Planned oophorectomy and/or salpingectomy do not contraindicate vaginal approach to the hysterectomy. The uterus is typically removed first, and the adnexa are then examined. It is helpful to grasp the ovary and tube with a Babcock clamp and gently pull the adnexa into the operative field to determine if the infundibulopelvic ligament can be accessed. Sometimes packing the bowel up with a moist pack can be helpful. A peon clamp can then be placed across the infundibulopelvic ligament; it is important to note that once the clamp has been placed, it should not be removed and one is committed to the salpingo-oophorectomy because removal of the clamp may result in bleeding from the vessels and retroperitoneal hematoma formation. A peon clamp is preferred because it is less traumatic. The adnexa are then transected with scissors and the pedicle ligated with a Heaney stitch using 0 delayed absorbable suture. It is not necessary or advisable to try to place a free tie around this pedicle as it may result in losing the pedicle. Vaginal salpingectomy can be accomplished in a similar manner by grasping with a Babcock clamp, placing a peon clamp across the mesosalpinx, transecting the tube, and ligating the pedicle with 0 delayed absorbable suture.

Karp and colleagues found that 65% of adnexa can be safely removed vaginally, and younger age (OR = 2.18, CI 1.1–8.4, $p < 0.001$) and shorter cervical length (OR = 4.5, CI 1.2–10.7, $p < 0.001$) were predictors of success (Karp et al. 2012). Dain also reported that younger age was associated with greater likelihood of success of vaginal salpingo-oophorectomy (Dain and Abramov 2011). Vaginal salpingectomy is possible in 65–88% of cases (Dain and Abramov 2011; Karp et al. 2012; Robert et al. 2015). However, in cases were removal of the adnexa is absolutely necessary, such as in women with complex endometrial hyperplasia or BRCA mutation, it is advisable to consider adding laparoscopic for removal of the adnexa; this will also allow for survey of the pelvis and obtaining pelvic washings in these high-risk individuals.

5.4 Culdoplasty

In the absence of other procedures to suspend the vaginal apex, such as an uterosacral or sacrospinous colpopexy, a culdoplasty is generally recommended at the time of vaginal hysterectomy to prevent formation of an enterocele and vaginal vault prolapse (Fig. 3). Cruikshank and Kovac demonstrated that a modified McCall-type culdoplasty is best at preventing enterocele after vaginal hysterectomy (Cruikshank and Kovac 1999). The modified McCall's culdoplasty not only closes the cul-de-sac to prevent an enterocele, it reattaches the transected uterosacral ligaments to the vaginal apex, thereby providing apical support to the vagina.

5.5 Cuff Closure

Two randomized studies suggest that vertical cuff closure appears to preserve vaginal length better than horizontal cuff closure. Vassallo and colleagues found in their randomized trial of 43 women that closing the cuff vertically resulted in lesser mean change in vaginal length (-0.35 +/$- 0.91$ cm) compared to horizontal closure (-1.13 +/$- 1.15$ cm) ($p = 0.01$) (Vassallo et al. 2006). In another randomized trial of 52 women without pelvic organ prolapse having a vaginal hysterectomy, at 6 weeks postoperatively, the vagina was

Fig. 3 Modified McCall culdoplasty

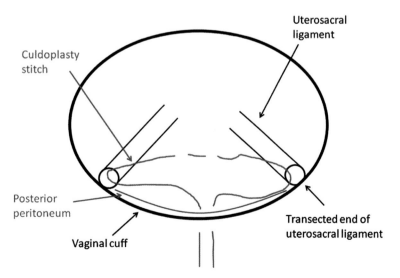

significantly shorter in the horizontal closure group (6.55 [0.89] cm vs. 7.42 (0.73) cm; $p < 0.001$) (Cavkaytar et al. 2014). However, Cruikshank and Pixley compared five different cuff closure techniques in 107 women and found no difference in vaginal length (Cruikshank and Pixley 1987). The clinical significance of this remains unclear.

The use of vault drainage has been examined in a randomized trial and found to offer no benefit (Dua et al. 2012). Likewise, peritoneal closure does not appear to be necessary (Lipscomb et al. 1996).

5.6   Post-op Care

Vaginal hysterectomy can be performed on an outpatient basis. Summit and colleagues in 1992 demonstrated that the majority of women can be discharged home within 12 h of surgery once ambulating, voiding, and tolerating a liquid diet (Summitt et al. 1992). In a more recent study, 84% of healthy (ASA I or II) women after a mean observation period of 4.6 h were discharged home post-op day 0 (Engh and Hauso 2012).

Postoperative catheterization is not mandatory but short-term catheterization is probably without significant risk. Ideally the urinary catheter should be removed within 24 h after surgery. Summit and colleagues randomized 100 women having vaginal hysterectomy to no catheter after surgery versus catheterization for 24 h after surgery (Summitt et al. 1994). Two (4%) of women without a catheter required catheterization after surgery. They found no difference in post-op febrile episodes or urinary tract infections. Also no differences were found in the incidence of positive urine cultures between the study groups at 48 h (8 vs. 14, $p = 0.227$) and 2 weeks (6 vs. 1, $p = 0.111$), respectively.

5.7   Outcomes Compared to Other Types of Hysterectomy

The American Congress of Obstetrics and Gynecology and the American Academy of Gynecologic Laparoscopists have both recommended vaginal hysterectomy whenever possible as the best route of hysterectomy.

> Recent Cochrane meta-analysis (Aarts et al. 2015) demonstrated that for women undergoing hysterectomy for benign disease, vaginal hysterectomy appears to be superior to both abdominal and laparoscopic hysterectomy and is associated with faster return to normal activities.

In this meta-analysis, 47 randomized controlled trials including 5102 women were reviewed. The majority of these studies excluded women with pelvic organ prolapse or with uterus >12–16 weeks. The Cochrane review included nine trials with 762 women comparing vaginal versus abdominal hysterectomy. Women returned to normal activities sooner after vaginal hysterectomy compared to abdominal hysterectomy (Median difference 9.5 days, 95% CI 6.4 to 12.6 days; 176 women, three trials). More women would choose a vaginal hysterectomy again when compared to an abdominal hysterectomy. There were three times as many urinary tract injuries after vaginal versus abdominal hysterectomy, although there was no statistical difference (OR 3.09, 95% CI 0.48 to 19.97, four RCTs, 439 women) (Aarts et al. 2015). There was no difference in other intraoperative complications or operative time. Hospital stay was shorter in vaginal hysterectomy compared to standard abdominal hysterectomy. Wound/abdominal wall infection (OR 0.21, 95% CI 0.04 to 1.00, three RCTs, 355 women), urinary tract infection (OR 0.59, 95% CI 0.08 to 4.61, three RCTs, 176 women), and febrile episodes or unspecified infections (OR 0.62, 95% CI 0.36 to 1.08, five RCTs, 495 women) all occurred less after VH than after AH, but there was no statistical difference.

The Cochrane group also reviewed 16 studies including 1440 women comparing vaginal hysterectomy to laparoscopic hysterectomy (including both laparoscopic-assisted vaginal hysterectomy and total laparoscopic hysterectomy). No advantage of laparoscopic-assisted vaginal hysterectomy or total laparoscopic hysterectomy over vaginal hysterectomy was demonstrated (Aarts et al. 2015). Hospital stay was 1 day shorter after vaginal hysterectomy. Women undergoing laparoscopic hysterectomy returned to work 1 day earlier than women undergoing VH, but the time to return to normal activities showed no evidence of a difference. There was no statistical difference in intraoperative or postoperative complications. Operating time is longer with a laparoscopic approach compared to vaginal hysterectomy. Although one study demonstrated lower post-op pain with laparoscopic hysterectomy (Ghezzi et al. 2010), other studies have not found similar results. Cost analysis has shown that mean total hospital charge when surgery was performed on an outpatient basis was significantly higher for laparoscopic hysterectomy compared to vaginal hysterectomy (Summit et al. 1992).

The eVALuate study was a major multicenter study that consisted of two parallel randomized trials – one that compared abdominal hysterectomy to total laparoscopic hysterectomy and the other compared vaginal hysterectomy and total laparoscopic hysterectomy (Garry et al. 2004). Included in the study were women who needed a hysterectomy for nonmalignant conditions, and excluded were those who had a second or third degree uterine prolapse, a uterine size greater than the size of a 12-week pregnancy, a medical illness precluding laparoscopic surgery, or a requirement for bladder or other pelvic support surgery. It is the largest study to date comparing vaginal and total laparoscopic hysterectomy; 504 women were enrolled in the vaginal trial. There was no difference between vaginal and total laparoscopic hysterectomy in terms of complications, pain, and length of stay. Vaginal hysterectomy had a significantly shorter operating time (46.6 versus 76.5 min for vaginal versus laparoscopic, respectively).

While most randomized trials included women with only a slightly enlarged uterus, less than 12 weeks, Sesti and colleagues conducted a randomized study of women having a hysterectomy for benign reasons with a uterus between 12 and 16 weeks in size (Sesti et al. 2014). Women were randomized to vaginal hysterectomy, laparoscopic-assisted vaginal hysterectomy, or total

laparoscopic hysterectomy; there were 36 women in each group. All surgeons were experienced in all three techniques, having performed at least 100 of each type of hysterectomy. Operating time (mean 70 min) and estimated blood loss (mean 182.8 mL) was significantly less in the vaginal hysterectomy group compared to both laparoscopic-assisted vaginal hysterectomy and total laparoscopic hysterectomy. The mean hospital discharge time was also significantly shorter after VH (50.7 h). There were no differences in complication rates.

In another study of hysterectomies for enlarged uterine size >280 g with at least one additional risk factor, previous pelvic surgery, history of pelvic inflammatory disease, moderate or severe endometriosis, concomitant adnexal masses, or indication for adnexectomy, Darai and colleagues randomized 80 women to laparoscopic-assisted vaginal hysterectomy versus vaginal hysterectomy (Darai et al. 2001). They found lower rate of complications with vaginal hysterectomy (15% with vaginal hysterectomy versus 37% with laparoscopic-assisted vaginal hysterectomy, $p < 0.05$) and shorter operating time with vaginal hysterectomy [mean operating time (range) was 108 (60–270 min) min for vaginal hysterectomy and 160 min (60–180 min) for laparoscopic-assisted vaginal hysterectomy ($p < 0.001$)]. Conversion to laparotomy was required in 3 of 40 (7.5%) women who had laparoscopic-assisted vaginal hysterectomy, compared with none in the vaginal hysterectomy group ($p < 0.05$). No difference was found in the mean uterine weight (range) between vaginal hysterectomy and LAVH groups [424 g (280–930) and 513 g (290–1560), respectively]. The study included 13 cases (32.5%) of uterine size at least 500 gm in the vaginal hysterectomy group that were successfully completed vaginally.

Wright and colleagues looked at actual patient charges for the various modes of hysterectomy and found that at their institution, Brigham and Women's Hospital, women who had a vaginal hysterectomy had the shortest operating time [mean 153 min (95% confidence interval 143.8–163.5, $p < 0.001$)] and women who had a vaginal, laparoscopic, and robotic hysterectomy had a significantly shorter hospital stay compared to those who had an abdominal hysterectomy. The mean length of stay for vaginal hysterectomy was 1.24 days. Based on this they calculated mean total patient costs and found that it was significantly lower for vaginal hysterectomy compared to other modes of hysterectomy (Wright et al. 2012); the mean cost for vaginal hysterectomy was $31,934, whereas robotic hysterectomy, the most expensive of the four modes of hysterectomy, costs $49,526.

5.8   Complications

Vaginal hysterectomy is associated with complications in 5.2% of women (Makinen et al. 2013). The most common complications are cuff cellulitis and abscess and incidental cystotomy. Surgical site infections are reported in 12 per 1000 women (Roy et al. 2014).The rate of cuff cellulitis is 0.6%, and the rate of deep/organ space surgical site infection is 1.0% after a vaginal hysterectomy (Lake et al. 2013). Bladder and ureteric injury are reported to occur at a rate of 5.1 per 1000 women and 0.4 per 1000 women, respectively (Teeluckdharry et al. 2015). In one large retrospective study where universal cystoscopy was used, the authors found that the rate of ureteral injury is higher when there is concomitant prolapse repair (0.9% versus 1.7%) (Ibeanu et al. 2009). The use of routine cystoscopy has been suggested to be cost effective if the rate of ureteral injury is greater than 2% for vaginal hysterectomy (Visco et al. 2001). The risk of vesicovaginal fistula formation is the lowest after vaginal hysterectomy for prolapse with a rate of 1 in 3861 or 0.26 per 1000 (Hilton and Cromwell 2012). The rate of bowel injury during vaginal hysterectomy ranges from 0.1% to 1.0% (Clarke-Pearson and Geller 2013). The estimated blood loss for a vaginal hysterectomy is 215–287 mL (Clarke-Pearson and Geller 2013). Urinary tract infection is reported in 3.1% of cases (Lake et al. 2013). Vaginal cuff dehiscence is lowest after vaginal hysterectomy compared to other routes of hysterectomy and is reported in 0.11% of cases (Hur et al. 2011). Pulmonary complications, defined as postoperative pneumonia, respiratory failure,

symptomatic atelectasis (requirement of intervention, such as bronchoscopy, respiratory therapy consultation, or SICU admission), or pneumothorax within 365 days of the procedure, occur in 1.2 per 1000 of women after vaginal hysterectomy (Solomon et al. 2013). Venous thromboembolism after a vaginal hysterectomy occurs in 0.2% and is less common than with abdominal hysterectomy (Swenson et al. 2015).

6   Conclusion

Vaginal hysterectomy should be considered for all women having a hysterectomy as it has been shown to be cost effective with low risk of complications.

7   Cross-References

▶ Laparoscopic Hysterectomy
▶ Management of Abnormal Uterine Bleeding: Later Reproductive Years
▶ Management of Uterine Fibroids

References

AAGL Advancing Minimally Invasive Gynecology Worldwide. AAGL position statement: route of hysterectomy to treat benign uterine disease. J Minim Invasive Gynecol. 2011;18:1–3.

Aarts JW, Nieboer TE, Johnson N, Tavender E, Garry R, Mol BW, Kluivers KB. Surgical approach to hysterectomy for benign gynaecological disease. Cochrane Database Syst Rev. 2015;8:CD003677.

American College of Obstetricians and Gynecologists. Choosing the route of hysterectomy for benign disease. ACOG Committee Opinion No. 444. Obstet Gynecol. 2009;114:1156–8.

Antosh DD, Gutman RE, Iglesia CB, Sokol AI, Park AJ. Resident opinions on vaginal hysterectomy training. Female Pelvic Med Reconstr Surg. 2011;17(6): 314–7.

Ascher-Walsh CJ, Capes T, Smith J, Michels A. Cervical vasopressin compared with no premedication and blood loss during vaginal hysterectomy: a randomized controlled trial. Obstet Gynecol. 2009;113(2 Pt 1): 313–8.

Burkett D, Horwitz J, Kennedy V, Murphy D, Graziano S, Kenton K. Assessing current trends in resident hysterectomy training. Female Pelvic Med Reconstr Surg. 2011;17(5):210–4.

Cavkaytar S, Kokanali MK, Topcu HO, Aksakal OS, Doganay M. Effects of horizontal vs. vertical vaginal cuff closure techniques on vagina length after vaginal hysterectomy: a prospective randomized study. J Minim Invasive Gynecol. 2014;21(5):884–7.

Cho HY, Park ST, Kim HB, Kang SW, Park SH. Surgical outcome and cost comparison between total vaginal hysterectomy and laparoscopic hysterectomy for uteri weighing >500 g. J Minim Invasive Gynecol. 2014; 21(1):115–9.

Clarke-Pearson DL, Geller EJ. Complications of hysterectomy. Obstet Gynecol. 2013;121(3):654–73.

Cruikshank SH, Kovac SR. Randomized comparison of three surgical methods used at the time of vaginal hysterectomy to prevent posterior enterocele. Am J Obstet Gynecol. 1999;180(4):859–65.

Cruikshank SH, Pixley RL. Methods of vaginal cuff closure and preservation of vaginal depth during transvaginal hysterectomy. Obstet Gynecol. 1987;70(1): 61–3.

Culligan PJ, Kubik K, Murphy M, Blackwell L, Snyder J. A randomized trial that compared povidone iodine and chlorhexidine as antiseptics for vaginal hysterectomy. Am J Obstet Gynecol. 2005;192(2):422–5.

Dain L, Abramov Y. Factors affecting the feasibility of bilateral salpingo-oophorectomy during vaginal hysterectomy for uterine prolapse. Aust N Z J Obstet Gynaecol. 2011;51(4):307–9.

Daraï E, Soriano D, Kimata P, Laplace C, Lecuru F. Vaginal hysterectomy for enlarged uteri, with or without laparoscopic assistance: randomized study. Obstet Gynecol. 2001;97(5 Pt 1):712–6.

Dayaratna S, Goldberg J, Harrington C, Leiby BE, McNeil JM. Hospital costs of total vaginal hysterectomy compared with other minimally invasive hysterectomy. Am J Obstet Gynecol. 2014;210:120.e1–6.

Desai VB. An update on inpatient hysterectomy routes in the United States. AJOG. 2015;213(5):742–743.

Dua A, Galimberti A, Subramaniam M, Popli G, Radley S. The effects of vault drainage on postoperative morbidity after vaginal hysterectomy for benign gynaecological disease: a randomised controlled trial. BJOG. 2012;119(3):348–53.

Duong TH, Patterson TM. Lower urinary tract injuries during hysterectomy in women with a history of two or more cesarean deliveries: a secondary analysis. Int Urogynecol J. 2014;25(8):1037–40.

Engh ME, Hauso W. Vaginal hysterectomy, an outpatient procedure. Acta Obstet Gynecol Scand. 2012;91:1293–9.

Fatania K, Vithayathil M, Newbold P, Yoong W. Vaginal versus abdominal hysterectomy for the enlarged non-prolapsed uterus: a retrospective cohort study. Eur J Obstet Gynecol Reprod Biol. 2014;174: 111–4.

Fitz-Gerald AL, Tan J, Chan KW, Polyakov A, Edwards GN, Najjar H, Tsaltas J, Vollenhoven B. Comparison of ultrasonic shears and traditional suture ligature for vaginal hysterectomy: randomized controlled trial. J Minim Invasive Gynecol. 2013;20(6):853–7.

Garry R, Fountain J, Mason S, Hawe J, Napp V, Abbott J, Clayton R, Phillips G, Whittaker M, Lilford R, Bridgman S, Brown J. The eVALuate study: two parallel randomised trials, one comparing laparoscopic with abdominal hysterectomy, the other comparing laparoscopic with vaginal hysterectomy. BMJ. 2004;328 (7432):129.

Ghezzi F, Uccella S, Cromi A, Siesto G, Serati M, Bogani G, Bolis P. Postoperative pain after laparoscopic and vaginal hysterectomy for benign gynecologic disease: a randomized trial. Am J Obstet Gynecol. 2010;203(2):118.e1–8.

Goldstein SR, Horii SC, Snyder JR, Raghavendra BN, Subramanyam B. Estimation of nongravid uterine volume based on a nomogram of gravid uterine volume: its value in gynecologic uterine abnormalities. Obstet Gynecol. 1988;72(1):86–90.

Guntupalli SR, Doo DW, Guy M, Sheeder J, Omurtag K, Kondapalli L, Valea F, Harper L, Muffly TM. Preparedness of obstetrics and gynecology residents for fellowship training. Obstet Gynecol. 2015;126(3):559–68.

Harmanli OH, Dandolu V, Isik EF, Panganamamula UR, Lidicker J. Does obesity affect the vaginal hysterectomy outcomes? Arch Gynecol Obstet. 2011;283(4): 795–8.

Hilton P, Cromwell DA. The risk of vesicovaginal and urethrovaginal fistula after hysterectomy performed in the English National Health Service – a retrospective cohort study examining patterns of care between 2000 and 2008. BJOG. 2012;119(12):1447–54.

Hristovska AM, Kristensen BB, Rasmussen MA, Rasmussen YH, Elving LB, Nielsen CV, Kehlet H. Effect of systematic local infiltration analgesia on postoperative pain in vaginal hysterectomy: a randomized, placebo-controlled trial. Acta Obstet Gynecol Scand. 2014; 93(3):233–8.

Hur HC, Donnellan N, Mansuria S, Barber RE, Guido R, Lee T. Vaginal cuff dehiscence after different modes of hysterectomy. Obstet Gynecol. 2011;118(4):794–801.

Ibeanu OA, Chesson RR, Echols KT, Nieves M, Busangu F, Nolan TE. Urinary tract injury during hysterectomy based on universal cystoscopy. Obstet Gynecol. 2009;113:6–10.

Jeppson PC, Rahimi S, Gattoc L, Westermann LB, Cichowski S, Raker C, Lebrun EW, Sung VW, Fellows' Pelvic Research Network of Society of Gynecologic Surgeons. Impact of robotic technology on hysterectomy route and associated implications for resident education. Am J Obstet Gynecol. 2015;212(2): 196.e1–6.

Kammerer-Doak DN, Rogers RG, Johnson Maybach J, Traynor Mickelson M. Vasopressin as an etiologic factor for infection in gynecologic surgery: a randomized double-blind placebo-controlled trial. Am J

Obstet Gynecol. 2001;185(6):1344–7. discussion 1347–1348

Karp DR, Mukati M, Smith AL, Suciu G, Aguilar VC, Davila GW. Predictors of successful salpingo-oophorectomy at the time of vaginal hysterectomy. J Minim Invasive Gynecol. 2012;19(1):58–62.

Kjølhede P, Halili S, Löfgren M. Vaginal cleansing and postoperative infectious morbidity in vaginal hysterectomy. A register study from the Swedish National Register for Gynecological Surgery. Acta Obstet Gynecol Scand. 2011;90(1):63–71.

Kovac SR, Barhan S, Lister M, Tucker L, Bishop M, Das A. Guidelines for the selection of the route of hysterectomy: application in a resident clinic population. Am J Obstet Gynecol. 2002;187(6):1521–7.

Kroft J, Selk A. Energy-based vessel sealing in vaginal hysterectomy: a systematic review and meta-analysis. Obstet Gynecol. 2011;118(5):1127–36.

Lake AG, McPencow AM, Dick-Biascoechea MA, Martin DK, Erekson EA. Surgical site infection after hysterectomy. Am J Obstet Gynecol. 2013;209(5):490.e1–9.

Lakeman M, The S, Schellart R, Dietz V, ter Haar J, Thurkow A, Scholten P, Dijkgraaf M, Roovers J. Electrosurgical bipolar vessel sealing versus conventional clamping and suturing for vaginal hysterectomy: a randomised controlled trial. BJOG. 2012;119: 1473–82.

Lipscomb GH, Ling FW, Stovall TG, Summitt Jr RL. Peritoneal closure at vaginal hysterectomy: a reassessment. Obstet Gynecol. 1996;87(1):40–3.

Long JB, Eiland RJ, Hentz JG, Mergens PA, Magtibay PM, Kho RM, Magrina JF, Cornella JL. Randomized trial of preemptive local analgesia in vaginal surgery. Int Urogynecol J Pelvic Floor Dysfunct. 2009;20(1): 5–10.

Mäkinen J, Brummer T, Jalkanen J, Heikkinen AM, Fraser J, Tomás E, Härkki P, Sjöberg J. Ten years of progress – improved hysterectomy outcomes in Finland 1996–2006: a longitudinal observation study. BMJ Open. 2013;3(10):e003169.

Muffly TM, Kow NS. Effect of obesity on patients undergoing vaginal hysterectomy. J Minim Invasive Gynecol. 2014;21(2):168–75.

O'Neal MG, Beste T, Shackelford DP. Utillity of preemptive local anesthesia in vaginal hysterectomy. Am J Obstet Gynecol. 2003;189(6):1539–41. discussion 1541–1542

Purohit RK, Sharma JG, Singh S, Giri DK. Vaginal hysterectomy by electrosurgery for benign indications associated with previous cesarean section. J Gynecol Surg. 2013;29(1):7–12.

Robert M, Cenaiko D, Sepandj J, Iwanicki S. Success and complications of salpingectomy at the time of vaginal hysterectomy. J Minim Invasive Gynecol. 2015;22(5): 864–9.

Rooney CM, Crawford AT, Vassallo BJ. Is previous cesarean section a risk for incidental cystotomy at the time of hysterectomy? A case-controlled study. Am J Obstet Gynecol. 2005;193:2041.

Rorarius M, Mennander S, Suominen P, Rintala S, Puura A, Pirhonen R, Salmelin R, Haanpaa M, Kujansuu E, Yli-Hankala A. Gabapentin for the prevention of postoperative pain after vaginal hysterectomy. Pain. 2004;110:175–81.

Roy S, Patkar A, Daskiran M, Levine R, Hinoul P, Nigam S. Clinical and economic burden of surgical site infection in hysterectomy. Surg Infect. 2014; 15(3):266–73.

Sahin Y. Vaginal hysterectomy and oophorectomy in women with 12–20 weeks' size uterus. Acta Obstet Gynecol Scand. 2007;86(11):1359–69.

Sesti F, Cosi V, Calonzi F, Ruggeri V, Pietropolli A, Di Francesco L, Piccione E. Randomized comparison of total laparoscopic, laparoscopically assisted vaginal and vaginal hysterectomies for myomatous uteri. Arch Gynecol Obstet. 2014;290(3):485–91.

Sheth SS. Vaginal hysterectomy as a primary route for morbidly obese women. Acta Obstet Gynecol Scand. 2010;89(7):971–4.

Silva-Filho AL, Rodrigues AM, Vale de Castro Monteiro M, da Rosa DG, Pereira e Silva YM, Werneck RA, Bavoso N, Triginelli SA. Randomized study of bipolar vessel sealing system versus conventional suture ligature for vaginal hysterectomy. Eur J Obstet Gynecol Reprod Biol. 2009;146(2):200–3.

Solomon ER, Muffly TM, Barber MD. Common postoperative pulmonary complications after hysterectomy for benign indications. Am J Obstet Gynecol. 2013;208(1):54.e1–5.

Summitt Jr RL, Stovall TG, Lipscomb GH, Ling FW. Randomized comparison of laparoscopy-assisted vaginal hysterectomy with standard vaginal hysterectomy in an outpatient setting. Obstet Gynecol. 1992; 80(6):895–901.

Summitt Jr RL, Stovall TG, Bran DF. Prospective comparison of indwelling bladder catheter drainage versus no catheter after vaginal hysterectomy. Am J Obstet Gynecol. 1994;170(6):1815–8. discussion 1818–1821

Sutton C. Hysterectomy: a historical perspective. Baillieres Clin Obstet Gynaecol. 1997;11:1–22.

Sutton C. Past, present and future of hysterectomy. J Minim Invasive Gynecol. 2010;17(4):421–35.

Swenson CW, Berger MB, Kamdar NS, Campbell Jr DA, Morgan DM. Risk factors for venous thromboembolism after hysterectomy. Obstet Gynecol. 2015;125(5): 1139–44.

Teeluckdharry B, Gilmore D, Flowerdew G. Urinary tract injury at benign gynecologic surgery and the role of cystoscopy: a systematic review and meta-analysis. Obstet Gynecol. 2015;126:1161. E pub ahead of print

Unger JB, Meeks GR. Vaginal hysterectomy in women with history of pervious cesarean delivery. AJOG. 1998;179:1473–8.

Vassallo BJ, Culpepper C, Segal JL, Moen MD, Noone MB. A randomized trial comparing methods of vaginal cuff closure at vaginal hysterectomy and the effect on vaginal length. Am J Obstet Gynecol. 2006;195(6): 1805–8.

Visco AG, Taber KH, Weidner AC, Barber MD, Myers ER. Cost-effectiveness of universal cystoscopy to identify ureteral injury at hysterectomy. Obstet Gynecol. 2001;97(5 Pt 1):685–92.

Washburn EE, Cohen SL, Manoucheri E, Zurawin RK, Einarsson JI. Trends in reported resident surgical experience in hysterectomy. J Minim Invasive Gynecol. 2014;21(6):1067–70.

Woelk JL, Borah BJ, Trabuco EC, Heien HC, Gebhart JB. Cost differences among robotic, vaginal, and abdominal hysterectomy. Obstet Gynecol. 2014;123 (2 Pt 1):255–62.

Wright KN, Jonsdottir GM, Jorgensen S, Shah N, Einarsson JI. Costs and outcomes of abdominal, vaginal, laparoscopic and robotic hysterectomies. JSLS. 2012;16:519–24.

Wright JD, Herzog TJ, Tsui J, Ananth CV, Lewin SN, Lu YS, Neugut AI, Hershman DL. Nationwide trends in the performance of inpatient hysterectomy in the United States. Obstet Gynecol. 2013a;122 (201):233–41.

Wright JD, Ananth CV, Lewin SN, Burke WM, Lu YS, Neugut AI, Herzog TJ, Hershman DL. Robotically assisted vs. laparoscopic hysterectomy among women with benign gynecologic disease. JAMA. 2013b; 309(7):689–98.

Pelvic Organ Prolapse: Diagnosis, Treatment, and Avoiding Complications

Christina Dancz and Morgan Elizabeth Fullerton

Abstract

Pelvic organ prolapse (POP) is defined as the descent of one or more of the anterior vaginal wall, posterior vaginal wall, the uterus (cervix), or the apex of the vagina (vaginal vault or cuff scar after hysterectomy). Prolapse is extremely common and is one of the leading reasons for surgery in the United States.

The main symptom of prolapse is the sensation of bulge or pressure in the vagina. Severe prolapse may interfere with successful urination, defecation, or sexual function. Prolapse diagnosis is usually based on physical exam, though several formal staging systems exist. Asymptomatic or minimally symptomatic prolapse may not require any intervention. Patients with significant bother may elect to use a plastic device (pessary) to hold their prolapsed organs in place, or they may elect for surgery. There are a variety of surgical procedures for prolapse, depending on the patient's health, preferences, degree, and location of prolapse.

C. Dancz (✉)
University of Southern California, Los Angeles, CA, USA
e-mail: christina.dancz@med.usc.edu

M.E. Fullerton
Department of Obstetrics and Gynecology, University of Southern California, Los Angeles, CA, USA
e-mail: morgan.fullerton@med.usc.edu

Keywords

Pelvic organ • Prolapse • Pessary • Surgery

Contents

© Springer International Publishing AG 2017
D. Shoupe (ed.), *Handbook of Gynecology*,
DOI 10.1007/978-3-319-17798-4_70

1   Introduction

Pelvic organ prolapse (POP) is defined as the descent of one or more of the anterior vaginal wall, posterior vaginal wall, uterus (cervix), or apex of the vagina (vaginal vault or cuff after hysterectomy) (Haylen et al. 2010). POP is estimated to affect 3.3 million women in the United States alone, and the number of women affected is projected to increase by nearly 50% by 2050 (Wu et al. 2009). Prolapse is one of the most common reasons for surgery in the United States and is projected to increase from 166,000 surgeries annually in 2010 to 245,970 in 2050 (Wu et al. 2011).

The most common symptom of prolapse is the sensation or discomfort of vaginal or uterine tissue prolapsing from the vagina and between the legs (Fig. 1). Severe prolapse may be associated with sexual complaints and urinary symptoms such as voiding difficulty, bladder outlet obstruction, and detrusor overactivity (Romanzi et al. 1999). It is rare that prolapse will cause significant morbidity or mortality, but it is commonly associated with sexual, urinary, and defecatory

symptoms that may interfere with activities of daily living and affect quality of life. It is not uncommon for women to digitally reduce their prolapse (splint) in order to urinate or defecate. In extreme cases, obstructed urination may result in obstructive uropathy causing hydronephrosis and even progressing to renal failure (Sudhakar et al. 2001).

Many patients with prolapse will elect for conservative management or go without treatment altogether (Culligan 2012). Conservative management strategies include pelvic floor muscle training and pessaries. A variety of surgical options are available, depending on the type and degree of prolapse, as well as patient preference and comorbidities. The necessity of hysterectomy at the time of prolapse repair is controversial, as is the need for mesh or graft to augment native tissue repairs.

2   Anatomy/Pathophysiology

Pelvic organ prolapse is the result of disruption of one or more of the supports that normally hold the pelvic organs in place. There are three primary supports of the uterus and upper vagina: 1) the cardinal/uterosacral ligament complex, 2) the lateral/paravaginal attachments of the endopelvic fascia, and 3) the perineal membrane (DeLancey 1992).

2.1   Level 1: The Cardinal and Uterosacral Ligament Complex

First, a note on terminology: Although the cardinal and uterosacral ligaments are commonly described as ligaments, true ligaments attach bone to bone, while the cardinal and uterosacral "ligaments" are more of a condensation of fibrous tissue, collagen, muscle, and nerves.

The cardinal ligament stretches between the base of the uterus and the lateral wall of the pelvis, thereby preventing inferior movement of the

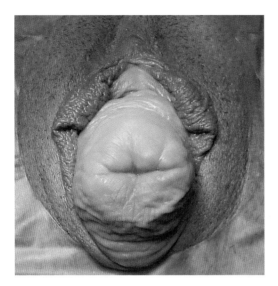

Fig. 1 Pelvic organ prolapse (Photograph courtesy of Dr. Begüm Özel)

uterus. The uterosacral ligament connects the lateral edge of the uterus to the anterior surface of the sacrum, which prevents the uterus from being displaced inferiorly and anteriorly (Drake et al. 2008).

These ligaments may be disrupted through surgical or obstetric trauma. However, it is more common that these ligaments are intact, but stretched out by consistent downward traction of the uterus and vagina. Similarly, collagen vascular disorders may be associated with lengthening and stretching of these ligaments and result in pelvic organ prolapse.

2.2 Level 2: The Endopelvic Fascia

Another note on terminology: The "endopelvic fascia" is not a true fascial layer, rather a condensation of areolar and connective tissue; however, it will hereafter be referred to as "fascia."

The endopelvic fascia is essentially the tendinous insertion of the levator ani complex where it attaches on the arch of the pelvis. This tendinous arch (arcus tendineus fascia pelvis) runs from the bottom of the pubic symphysis to the ischial spine on either side. Injury to this fascial layer or

disruption of these lateral attachments is commonly seen after childbirth, even in the absence of a perineal laceration and is thought to be one of the primary causative factors for pelvic organ prolapse.

2.3 Level 3: The Perineal Body

The perineal body is the third and most distal level of support. This layer is made up of the superficial perineal muscles that form the anterior urogenital triangle (bulbocavernosus, ischiocavernosus, and transverse perineal). Within the triangle is a confluence of connective tissue that provides additional support to the vulva and lower vagina. Disruption of this layer may occur during childbirth, or due to chronic traction of the uterus and vagina due to defects in the upper two levels of support.

3 Risk Factors

The causes of prolapse are multifactorial. There are some genetic risk factors; a family history of prolapse is associated with increased risk, as is Caucasian race and Hispanic ethnicity, when compared to Asian and African Americans. The most common risk factors include vaginal childbirth, increasing age, and increasing body mass index. Vaginal childbirth is strongly associated with anatomic disruption of the pelvic organ supports, and pregnancy is associated with laxity/stretching of the pelvic floor ligaments. Increasing age is thought to be associated with changes in the collagen composition of the ligamentous supports, leading to increased risk of prolapse. Body mass index is likely a risk factor for prolapse due to chronic increases in abdominal pressure and straining. In fact, other causes of chronic increase in abdominal pressure have also been associated with prolapse (constipation, chronic cough) (Koelbl et al. 2013).

Although there have not been any proven effective strategies to reduce risk, it is reasonable to think that weight loss, reduction of heavy lifting, treatment of constipation, modification of obstetric risk factors, and pelvic floor physical therapy may be effective in preventing the development or progression of pelvic organ prolapse.

4 Diagnosis

4.1 Patient History

As pelvic organ prolapse is rarely associated with significant morbidity or mortality, the most important principle in prolapse evaluation is assessing the degree of bother for the patient. The most effective strategy in managing prolapse is to allow the patient to express what aspect of the prolapse bothers her most. This allows the practitioner to tailor treatment plans to the patients' needs and wishes, rather than focusing on the anatomic outcomes that may or may not reflect successful treatment for the patient.

The most specific complaint of women with pelvic organ prolapse is the sensation of bulge or pressure in the vagina. This sensation may be difficult to distinguish from the sensation of pressure in the lower abdomen. Low abdominal pressure is often nonspecific, and, in the absence of vaginal pressure, is unlikely to be due to prolapse. Urinary, defecatory, and sexual symptoms are also common and should be evaluated in women with prolapse.

4.2 Physical Exam

Pelvic organ prolapse can almost always be evaluated completely with physical exam. Ancillary radiologic testing is rarely indicated. A comprehensive physical exam is indicated when considering any surgical intervention for pelvic organ prolapse. A complete evaluation should include: basic sensory testing, visual inspection of the external genitalia and cervix, bimanual and rectovaginal examination and visual assessment of prolapse with Valsalva. Additional testing for incontinence may be indicated in patients with

urinary or fecal incontinence and some advocate testing for occult incontinence in women with prolapse considering surgical intervention.

4.3 Sensory Exam

Sensation to the vulva and perineum is primarily provided by the pudendal nerve, a branch of the S2–S4 nerve root. Intact sensation to the inner thigh and perineum to light touch and pinprick confirms function of the pudendal nerve to the cerebral cortex. The anal wink reflex or clitoral reflex requires an intact levator ani and pudendal nerves, as well as connection to the cerebral cortex. The anal wink may be checked by gently stroking perianally with the soft edge of a cotton swab; a positive test will result in contraction of the external anal sphincter. The clitoral reflex may be checked by gently squeezing the clitoris and looking for contraction of the pelvic floor. Both of these tests are specific but not sensitive, meaning that a positive test confirms intact nerves, but the absence of the reflex is not diagnostic of neurologic disruption.

4.4 Pelvic Exam

A careful speculum, bimanual, and rectovaginal exam is important to look for other etiologies of bulge in the vagina and to screen for cervical, vaginal, and vulvar cancers. The presence of prolapse does not increase the risk for any type of cancer, but prolapse may exist concomitantly with other gynecologic conditions, and these need to be ruled out.

Careful evaluation of the degree of prolapse must be documented for all patients with complaints of prolapse. The maximum amount of prolapse that can be elicited should be documented. This usually requires the patient to perform Valsalva or cough and may require the patient to stand in order to demonstrate the maximum descent of her prolapse. Often, it is appropriate to separate a speculum and use the lower half to reduce the compartment not being evaluated. The posterior wall may be reduced in order to completely see and evaluate the anterior wall, and vice versa.

There are a variety of staging systems that have been proposed for prolapse. The most common are the Baden-Walker grading system and the Pelvic Organ Prolapse Quantification (POP-Q) staging system (Bump et al. 1996), which have been developed and endorsed by the International Continence Society and the International Urogynecological Association (Haylen et al. 2010).

The Baden-Walker grading system divides the vagina into three compartments: anterior, apical, and posterior. The anterior compartment consists of the upper vagina between the cervix and urethra and generally corresponds to the area just under the bladder and urethra. The apical compartment is the upper vagina and cervix, while the posterior compartment is the pelvic floor between the cervix and perineal body. Each compartment is considered separately and the maximum descent of each compartment evaluated. Prolapse in the upper half of the vagina is considered grade 1, in the lower half of the vagina is grade 2, coming out halfway is grade 3, and completely everted is considered grade 4 (Table 1). Such a grading system is easy to understand and remember and is often used by gynecologists to document the degree of prolapse (Baden and Walker 1992).

In an effort to further quantify prolapse and to describe and compare treatment outcomes,

Table 1 Baden-Walker grading system for pelvic organ prolapse

Grade of Prolapse	Extent of prolapse in relationship to the hymen
Grade 0	Normal position for each respective site
Grade 1	Descent halfway to the hymen
Grade 2	Descent to the hymen
Grade 3	Descent halfway past the hymen
Grade 4	Maximum possible descent for each site

the POP-Q examination was developed. This technique is more complicated to learn, but is more quantitative and uses clear anatomic landmarks. It uses 9 points. All points of the POP-Q are measured in cm, relative to the hymen. Inside of the body are negative values, and outside of the body are measured as positive values. GH, PB, and TVL are measured at rest. The remainder of the points should be measured with the maximum prolapse elicited. Prolapse may be elicited with patient on Valsalva maneuver, with standing, or both (Table 2).

5 Complications of Prolapse

Significant complications from untreated pelvic organ prolapse are rare. The most common complications include vaginal abrasions, bleeding, and urinary retention. In rare cases, the prolapse may become so edematous that it is difficult or impossible to reduce – an incarcerated prolapse.

Vaginal abrasions or ulcerations with bleeding may be avoided with reduction of prolapse, either surgically or with pessary (Fig. 2). Vaginal abrasions related to atrophy may be treated with topical estrogen cream. Occasionally, the vaginal epithelium is so dry and irritated that additional treatment with Vaseline or vitamin A and D ointment is necessary.

Symptoms of urinary retention may be treated with reduction of prolapse. A recent study showed that in women with stage 3–4 prolapse, the prevalence of hydronephrosis was up to 55% (Dancz et al. 2015; Hui et al. 2011). Therefore, in women who decline intervention, it may be indicated to screen for retention with post-void residual, creatinine level, and renal ultrasound.

Prolapse that is traumatized, usually from a fall or other inadvertent harsh manipulation of the prolapse, may become edematous and irreducible. These may usually be reduced with adequate pain control and gentle, consistent pressure. The fundus must be gently aimed into the body in order to return the uterus to the pelvis.

Table 2 POP-Q staging system for pelvic organ prolapse

Aa – anterior wall 3 cm proximal to the urethral meatus (range, −3 to +3)	Ba – anterior wall Most distal part of the anterior wall	C – cervix or cuff Most distal descent of cervix/vaginal cuff
gh – genital hiatus Mid-urethral meatus to the posterior fourchette	pb – perineal body Posterior fourchette to the mid-anus	tvl – total vaginal length Greatest depth of the vagina when prolapse is reduced
Ap – posterior wall 3 cm proximal to the hymenal remnant (range, −3 to +3)	Bp – posterior wall Most distal part of the posterior wall	D – posterior fornix (omitted if there is no cervix)

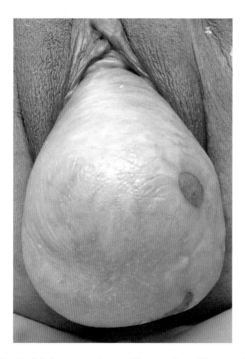

Fig. 2 Pelvic organ prolapse with ulcerations (Photograph courtesy of Dr. Begüm Özel)

6 Nonsurgical Management of Prolapse

6.1 Pessary

Pessaries are devices of various shapes and sizes that are placed in the vagina to reduce pelvic organ prolapse and restore normal anatomy. Pessary use can be temporary or long term. It provides immediate relief from pelvic organ prolapse symptoms, but requires some maintenance. Long-term pessary use may be an alternative to surgery in women with multiple comorbidities or in women who prefer to avoid surgical risks (Culligan 2012). Pessary use has been shown to be as effective as surgery in improving patients' symptoms of prolapse including bowel complaints, bladder complaints, sexual function, and overall quality of life (Abdool et al. 2011).

6.1.1 Fitting of Pessary

The success of pessaries lies in a proper fitting. Pessaries can be successfully fitted 60–90% of the time (Clemons et al. 2004; Lone et al. 2011). When a pessary is successful at the 4-week point, most women continue to use a pessary at 5 years (Lone et al. 2011). When choosing a pessary, the provider needs to consider the stage of pelvic organ prolapse, the size of vaginal vault, and the ability of the patient to manage their own pessary. The goal is to find the smallest pessary that effectively treats their prolapse symptoms. Initial fitting may require a trial of several different pessary types and/or sizes to adequately and comfortably reduce their prolapse (Culligan 2012).

Ring with support pessaries (Fig. 3) is widely available and the most commonly used (Cundiff et al. 2000). The initial choice of pessary size should be based on the examiner's bimanual exam and appreciation of the width of the vaginal canal (Culligan 2012). Once the exam is performed, the provider should identify an appropriate size and shape pessary. The pessary should be placed by the provider and tested by the patient. Initial tests for correct sizing can be performed by having the patient cough or stand with the pessary in place. If it stays in place, then the patient should attempt a Valsalva maneuver while sitting. If the

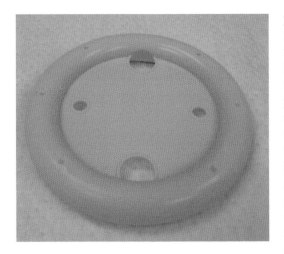

Fig. 3 Ring with support pessary

pessary continues to remain in place with these measures and is comfortable, it is likely the correct size. The patient should also be able to ambulate and urinate with the pessary in place. Well-fit pessaries should not be felt by the patient.

Once a pessary is successfully fit, the patient should return for close follow-up. Typically the patient is given a return appointment in 1–2 weeks to make sure the pessary continues to comfortably reduce the patient's prolapse and allows for normal daily functions (Trowbridge and Fenner 2007). At this time, if the patient is uncomfortable or has lost the pessary with activity, this is an opportunity to change pessary size or type. This visit also provides a good opportunity to educate a motivated patient on how to remove and clean her pessary so that she can manage her pessary at home. Once a patient is comfortable and has learned to manage her pessary, she can then be followed every 3–6 months. She is instructed to remove and clean the pessary with soap and water approximately once a week. If the patient is comfortable, but cannot change her own pessary, she should be seen every 2–3 months for outpatient exchange by her provider (Culligan 2012; Trowbridge and Fenner 2007).

6.1.2 Types of Pessaries

There are two general categories of pessaries – support and space filling. Support pessaries typically sit between the pubic symphysis and cally sit between the pubic symphysis and

posterior fornix. They reduce prolapse by elevating the superior vagina and often have perforations that allow the escape of vaginal secretions. Examples of support pessaries are the ring, ring with support, Gehrung, and Hodge. Space-filling pessaries work by elevating the prolapse and maintaining the normal anatomic position by creating a barrier within the vagina that is larger than the genital hiatus. The cube pessary (Fig. 4) may be used for refractory cases, as it stays in place by creating suction to the vaginal walls. A commonly used option is the Gellhorn pessary, (Fig. 5) which acts both as suction and barrier (Cundiff et al. 2000). A randomized crossover trial showed no difference in patient satisfaction or symptom relief from the ring versus Gellhorn pessary (Cundiff et al. 2007).

The ring with support pessary is relatively easy to place/remove and is well tolerated by patients (Cundiff et al. 2000). If the ring with support does not work, the next choice is typically the Gellhorn. If neither of these work, chances of successful prolapse management with pessary are unlikely (Culligan 2012). A variety of other pessaries may be used, each with slightly different features. Overall, these pessaries are typically more difficult for patients to manage (Culligan 2012; Trowbridge and Fenner 2007). The inflatoball (Fig. 6) is an option for women with stage 3 or 4 pelvic organ prolapse who desire the ability to manage their pessary at home. It is more easily placed and removed by the patient compared to a Gellhorn or donut pessary because it can be inflated after insertion and deflated prior to removal, though the stem does protrude from the vagina and may cause discomfort for the patient (Trowbridge and Fenner 2007).

Pessaries are generally made of surgical-grade silicone; therefore, patients with latex allergies may use them without concern. Over time, the silicone may develop some discoloration. The structural integrity of the pessary is not affected, and discolored pessaries may be used indefinitely. The inflatoball pessary (Fig. 6) is the only pessary that is made of rubber. The rubber material in the inflatoball pessary may absorb a slight odor, and the rubber may dry out over time. Inflatoball pessaries should be checked and replaced periodically.

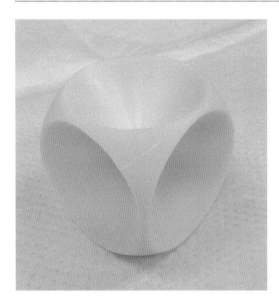

Fig. 4 Cube pessary

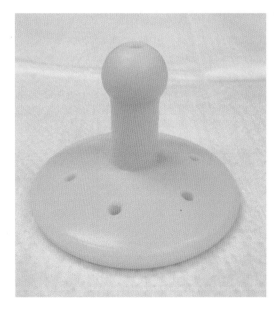

Fig. 5 Gellhorn pessary

6.1.3   Complications

Reported complication rates from pessaries vary, but in a large study of over a thousand women, 88.5% had no complications (Hanson et al. 2006). The most commonly reported complications are vaginal discharge, vaginal ulcerations, and abrasions. It is normal for women to have increased vaginal discharge with a pessary in place, but there is concern for infection if they report itching, foul odor, or burning sensation. With a pessary in place, the vaginal flora is altered, and women are more predisposed to bacterial vaginosis (Alnaif and Drutz 2000). A vaginal wet prep will distinguish between bacterial vaginosis and physiologic discharge and should be used prior to administration of antibiotics. If the patient is bothered by the physiologic vaginal discharge, it may be alleviated by more frequent removal and cleaning of the pessary.

Vaginal ulcerations or abrasions due to local pressure effects are also common and typically occur if the pessary is left in place over time. Symptoms of vaginal ulcerations or abrasions include discharge, odor, and bleeding. If the patient can change it herself, the pessary may be removed for a few hours or overnight and replaced. At each follow-up visit, a speculum exam should be performed to evaluate for the presence of any ulcerations or abrasions. The patient should also be instructed to make an appointment if she notices any vaginal bleeding. Vaginal abrasions and ulcerations may be treated with removal of the pessary for a few weeks, and use vaginal estrogen cream on a daily basis for a short-term course (Clemons et al. 2004; Trowbridge and Fenner 2007). The patient should be followed regularly until the ulceration has resolved, and then the pessary may be replaced with continued use of vaginal estrogen cream two to three times a week (Trowbridge and Fenner 2007).

Another potential side effect of pessary is urinary incontinence. Typically, it is the reduction of prolapse and return of normal anatomic positioning of the urethra that may unmask occult incontinence or worsen existing incontinence. In cases with incontinence, a specific incontinence pessary (incontinence ring, incontinence dish, or incontinence dish with support) may be used. The incontinence pessaries have an additional knob to provide support at the urethrovesical junction (Trowbridge and Fenner 2007).

Severe complications with pessary are rare. Pessary impaction can occur if a pessary is in place for a prolonged period of time without removal. There have been case reports of severe complications from

Fig. 6 Inflatoball pessary

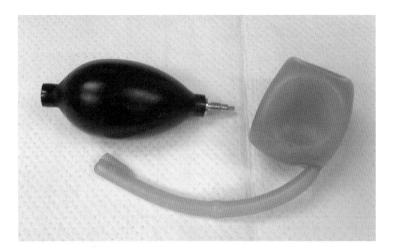

pessaries, including impaction of or erosion into the urethra, rectum, or cervix (Figs. 7 and 8). Potential for compression of the urethra should be evaluated at pessary placement; anyone who cannot urinate should have the pessary removed and a smaller one placed. Obstructed voiding may lead to urinary retention, infection, and urosepsis (Wheeler et al. 2004). Rectal compression can lead to obstructed defecation or bowel obstruction (Roberge et al. 2001). Some pessaries are designed with a central space, through which the cervix may prolapse and become incarcerated (Thubert and Deffieux 2014). There are case reports of pessaries left in situ for years that then erode into the bladder or rectum (Arias et al. 2008; Rogo-Gupta et al. 2012).

These severe complications may be avoided with regular pessary removal and replacement. It is also reasonable to advise patients to confide in a family member or close friend of the presence of the pessary. In case of accident or incapacitation, someone should be aware the pessary should be removed at least once every 3 months.

7 Pelvic Floor Muscle Training

Pelvic floor muscle training has been suggested as management for mild to moderate prolapse. It consists of both sessions with a trained therapist to assess muscle strength and teach exercises for muscle strengthening and regimented exercise programs for the patient to complete at home. The goal of pelvic floor muscle training is to increase muscle volume and thereby diminish the size of the levator hiatus and provide improved structural support for the pelvic organs (Bø 2006). A prospective randomized trial demonstrated that with regimented pelvic floor muscle training over the course of 6 months, women with up to stage 3 pelvic organ prolapse were able to symptomatically and objectively improve their pelvic organ prolapse (Braekken et al. 2010). That study also demonstrated increased muscle thickness, elevated location of the bladder and rectum, and decreased hiatal size with the regimented exercises. Similar improvement in symptoms and reduction of prolapse have been reported in women with training as brief as 14 weeks with improved symptoms and up to stage 2 improvement of pelvic organ prolapse as measured by the POP-Q, though the majority showed no change or reduction of stage 1 of pelvic organ prolapse (Hagen et al. 2009; Stüpp et al. 2011). Limitations of this course of therapy are patient motivation and access to trained therapists.

8 Surgical Management

A variety of surgical treatments are available for pelvic organ prolapse. The choice of surgery depends on many factors including compartment of prolapse, severity of prolapse, patient health and overall treatment goals, prior surgeries, and

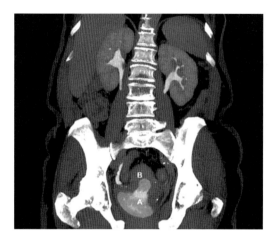

Fig. 7 Computed tomography (*CT*) of intravesical pessary demonstrating a Gellhorn pessary (*A*) located in the bladder (*B*) (Originally published in Rogo-Gupta L, Le NB, Raz S. Foreign body in the bladder 11 years after intravaginal pessary. Int Urogynecol J 2012; 23:1311–1313; with kind permission of © Springer Science+Business Media. All Rights Reserved)

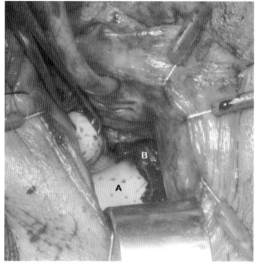

Fig. 8 Intraoperative image of pessary (*A*) within the bladder (*B*) (Originally published in Rogo-Gupta L, Le NB, Raz S. Foreign body in the bladder 11 years after intravaginal pessary. Int Urogynecol J 2012; 23:1311–1313; with kind permission of © Springer Science+Business Media. All Rights Reserved)

surgeon preference. Graft or mesh augmentation may be considered in select cases. The surgical techniques used for pelvic organ prolapse can broadly be categorized by compartment: anterior, apical, and posterior.

9 Anterior Prolapse

The anterior compartment is the most common site of pelvic organ prolapse and the most difficult to repair. Anatomic and symptomatic outcomes after surgical repair are generally good, but when prolapse recurs, it is most commonly in the anterior compartment.

10 Anterior Colporrhaphy

The mainstay of surgical management of anterior prolapse is the anterior colporrhaphy (Fig. 9). During this procedure, a transverse incision is made at the apex of the anterior vagina (if concurrent hysterectomy is performed, then the anterior colpotomy site may be used). The anterior vagina is then put on traction using Allis clamps, to essentially evert the anterior wall (or ceiling of the vagina). Using

Metzenbaum scissors, the anterior vaginal epithelium is undermined to separate it from the underlying muscularis. This epithelium is then incised in a linear fashion from the apex of the vagina to approximately 3–4 cm below the urethral meatus. Allis clamps or Pratt-Smith clamps may be placed on the cut edge of the epithelium, and the epithelium dissected off the underlying muscularis. This dissection is extended laterally to the pelvic sidewall. The underlying muscularis is then plicated with a series of U stitches of 0 polyglactin suture. These stitches should be placed along the junction of where the epithelium has been dissected off the muscularis, taking care that the tissue plicated is the muscularis and not the vaginal epithelium. While these sutures are tied down, the underlying prolapsed tissue is reduced. The result is a midline reduction of the anterior prolapse. The excess vaginal epithelium is then trimmed, and the epithelium is plicated in the midline using 2–0 polyglactin suture.

Studies on the success of prolapse repair are difficult to compare, as different outcomes are often reported. Symptomatic success does not necessarily require anatomic success, and often

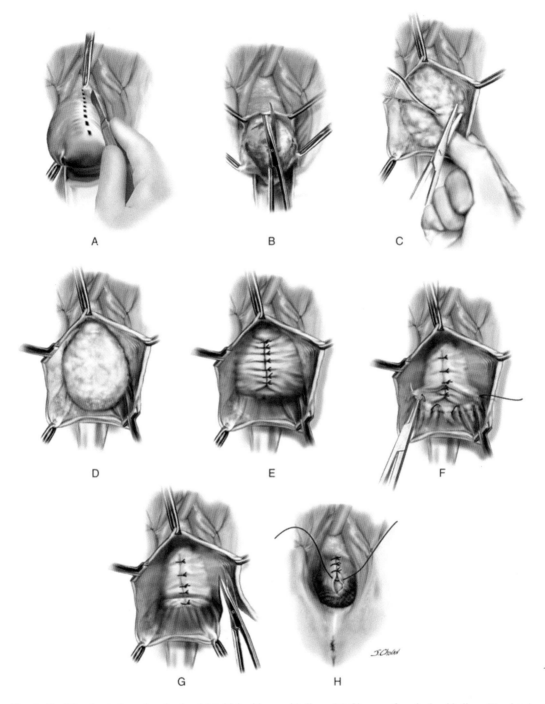

Fig. 9 Traditional anterior colporrhaphy. (**a**) Initial midline anterior vaginal wall incision. (**b**) Midline incision is extended. (**c**) Sharp dissection of the bladder off the vaginal wall. (**d**) The bladder has been mobilized off the vagina. (**e**) Initial plication layer is placed. (**f**) Second plication layer is placed. (**g**) Trimming of excess vaginal epithelium. (**h**) Closure of vaginal epithelium (Reprinted from Surgical Management of Pelvic Organ Prolapse, 1st Edition, Maher CF, Karram M. Surgical Management of Anterior Vaginal Wall Prolapse, p117–137, with kind permission from Elsevier)

both are reported as separate measures. In general, the reported success rates of anterior colporrhaphy range from 80% to 100% in retrospective series, though in prospective studies, the rates are much lower (30–55%) (Menefee et al. 2011; Nguyen and Burchette 2008; Weber et al. 2001).

Multiple procedures have been developed to try to improve anatomic and symptomatic outcomes of anterior colporrhaphy. Variations on the anterior colporrhaphy include the paravaginal (or ultralateral) repair, site-specific repair, anterior colporrhaphy with mesh augmentation, and anterior colporrhaphy with graft augmentation. Several studies have compared reoperation rates, as well as anatomic and symptomatic outcomes between these procedures. In general, anatomic outcomes are slightly better using mesh or graft augmentation, but the symptomatic outcomes and reoperation rates are the same between procedures (Maher et al. 2013).

10.1 Vaginal Paravaginal Repair

Some surgeons advocate an ultralateral approach to anterior colporrhaphy, referred to as a vaginal paravaginal repair (Fig. 10). The paravaginal repair is based on the theory that prolapse may be caused by a detachment of the underlying muscularis from its lateral attachments to the arcus tendineus fascia pelvis (ATFP). This technique involves opening the anterior vaginal wall, similar to the dissection used in a traditional anterior colporrhaphy as described above. The vaginal epithelium is dissected off the underlying muscularis farther laterally than for a traditional anterior colporrhaphy, and the paravaginal space is developed between the obturator internus muscle and the vaginal muscularis layer. This space is extended along the ischiopubic rami using palpation in order to identify the ischial spines and the ATFP. The ATFP runs between the pubic symphysis and the ischial spine on either side. The ATFP is palpated and then visualized using Breisky-Navratil retractors. Upon clear identification of the ATFP, three to six sutures of 0 polyglactin suture are placed through the ATFP. These sutures may be held if a concomitant anterior colporrhaphy or apical suspension is being performed. The sutures through the ATFP are then brought through the muscularis tissue close to the midline, so that the muscularis is brought up and laterally toward the ATFP. The stitch is then carried to the underside of the vaginal epithelium. This technique obliterates the paravaginal space and essentially brings the epithelium, the muscularis, and the ATFP into close approximation. The excess vaginal epithelium is trimmed, and the vaginal epithelium is reapproximated in the midline.

This technique has a high success rate (67–100%), which is tempered by complications including bilateral ureteric obstruction, retropubic hematomas, abscesses, and transfusion (Maher et al. 2013). This procedure may be performed abdominally or laparoscopically, but requires a high degree of surgical skill, and efficacy data is limited.

10.2 Site-Specific Repair

An additional variation of the anterior colporrhaphy is a site-specific repair. The concept behind this repair is that although some cases of anterior prolapse are due to complete separation of the muscularis from its lateral attachments, other cases of anterior prolapse are due to specific defects in the muscularis. When these defects are sought out and identified during anterior colporrhaphy, they should be repaired individually. A midline plication may be performed at the same time as a site-specific repair.

10.3 Graft and Mesh Augmentation

Due to the relatively high failure rates of prolapse repairs, there has been significant interest in augmenting repairs with synthetic or biologic materials. Although mesh and graft augmentation has been used with wide success in the hernia repair literature, vaginal augmentation has been more controversial. Generally, mesh or graft augmentation may be considered for patients who fail a native tissue repair.

The technique for the placement of synthetic mesh or biologic graft is essentially the same. Several companies have developed prefabricated meshes to fit the various vaginal compartments.

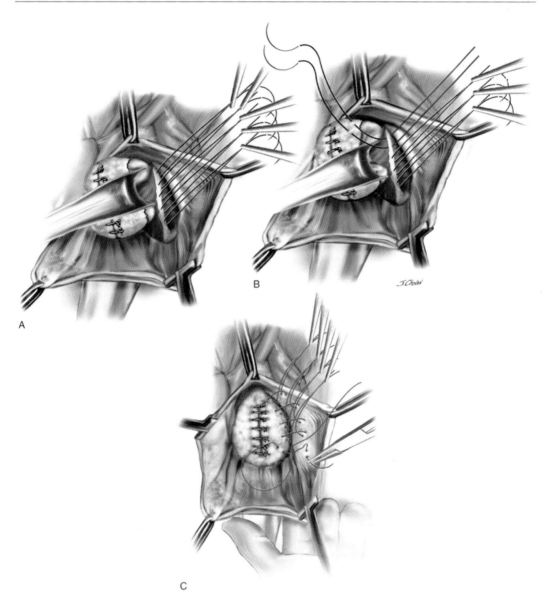

Fig. 10 Vaginal paravaginal repair. (**a**) Numerous sutures are passed through the arcus tendineus fascia pelvis (*white line*). (**b**) Each suture is passed through the edge of the detached fascia. (**c**) Each suture is passed through the vaginal wall excluding the epithelium (Reprinted from Surgical Management of Pelvic Organ Prolapse, 1st Edition, Maher CF, Karram M. Surgical Management of Anterior Vaginal Wall Prolapse, p117–137, with kind permission from Elsevier)

These mesh kits vary in size and shape of the mesh, as well as the introducer to fix the mesh to the vaginal tissues. Many of the kits use a trocar introducer to fix the apical portion of the mesh to the sacrospinous ligament, and the lateral or distal portion of the mesh may be sutured to the ATFP (as described above for a paravaginal repair) or may be trocar guided through the obturator space.

When a kit is not used, the mesh or graft may be cut to fit the patient's anterior vaginal wall. The vaginal wall is incised in the midline, taking care to dissect full thickness through the vaginal muscularis down to the bladder. This is in contrast to the anterior colporrhaphy, where the vaginal epithelium is split from the underlying muscularis. After dissection of the epithelium and muscularis off the bladder, the graft/mesh is placed loosely under the tissue and sutured to the ATFP laterally. The overlying vagina is not trimmed and is then reapproximated in the midline.

10.4 Types of Grafts

10.4.1 Biologic Grafts

Biologic grafts may be used as an alternative to synthetic mesh grafts. Biologic graft options include:

Autograft – graft material is harvested from the patient herself. Generally it is taken from the rectus sheath or fascia lata. The use of autologous fascia has the advantage of lower risk of infection and host rejection. The size of the graft is generally 6–8 cm long and 4 cm wide. The harvest of an autologous fascial graft of this size may be associated with significant morbidity and is rarely used. It may be considered in patients with contraindications to mesh (Cormio et al. 2015).

Allograft – fascial material is harvested from donor or cadaveric tissue. Several small studies have demonstrated success rates ranging from 81% to 100%, with acceptable complication rates, though the only randomized controlled trial failed to show an improvement over traditional anterior colporrhaphy. Concerns regarding prior transmission and residual antigenicity resulting in host-graft reactions have limited the acceptance of allograft materials for prolapse repair.

Xenograft – Porcine dermis, porcine small intestine submucosa, bovine pericardium, or bovine dermis. Xenografts have been used in the anterior compartment with mixed results. One study retrospectively compared anterior colporrhaphy, porcine dermis, and polypropylene graft, with the porcine dermis significantly less effective than the other two treatments,

with a 21% rate of vaginal extrusion of the porcine dermis. Other groups have found much better success rates, with graft extrusion rates of 1–17% (Maher et al. 2013). A Cochrane meta-analysis found that when graft was used to augment the anterior compartment, the objective failure rate was higher than when no graft was used (Maher et al. 2013).

Overall, some advocate biologic grafts as an alternative to synthetic mesh, although no subjective benefit has been reported by patients, and the complication rates are similar to synthetic meshes. Biologic grafts should be considered in patients who refuse synthetic meshes or those with contraindications to synthetic mesh. Synthetic mesh is contraindicated in patients who have had a prior mesh complication and those who desire future fertility (as the synthetic meshes do not stretch). Biologic grafts may be preferred to synthetic meshes in patients with impaired wound healing such as those with prior pelvic irradiation. Both meshes and grafts should be used with caution in patients with chronic pelvic pain, endometriosis, painful bladder syndrome, vulvodynia, and other vulvar pain disorders.

11 Transvaginal Mesh for Anterior/Apical Prolapse

Starting in 2004, a variety of prepackaged kits were introduced to augment prolapse repair in the vagina (Figs. 11 and 12). These kits use a variety of techniques to augment the anterior, apical, and posterior compartments. There is reasonable evidence to support that anatomic outcomes in the anterior and apical compartments are improved relative to native tissue repairs (Maher et al. 2013). However, there is no difference in patient subjective improvement, quality of life measures, or reoperation rates for prolapse. The improvement in anatomic outcomes comes at the cost of increased complications related to the mesh, with mesh erosion rates reported up to 25% (Maher et al. 2013). The consequences of mesh

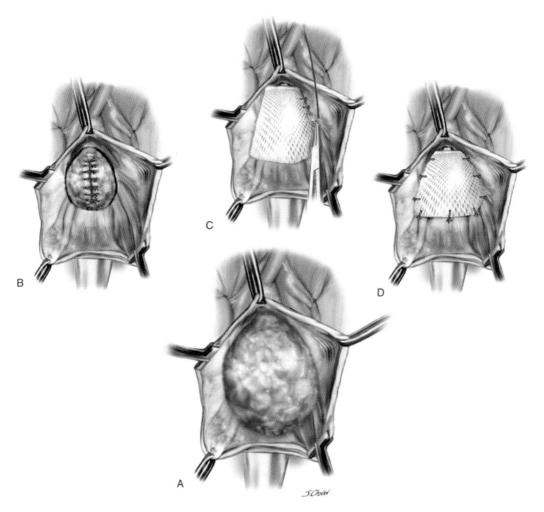

Fig. 11 Mesh augmentation of anterior wall prolapse repair. (**a**) Anterior prolapse is visualized. (**b**) Midline plication is completed. (**c–d**) Self-styled mesh is sutured in place (Reprinted from Surgical Management of Pelvic Organ Prolapse, 1st Edition, Maher CF, Karram M. Surgical Management of Anterior Vaginal Wall Prolapse, p117–137, with kind permission from Elsevier)

complications can be significant and often result in reoperation. These findings prompted the FDA to release an alert about transvaginal mesh placement in 2011. The alert essentially states that mesh may improve outcomes, but the complications in most cases outweigh the benefits. However, it is important to note that no transvaginal mesh has been recalled and that in selected patients who are appropriately counseled, transvaginal mesh augmentation may be preferred to more invasive, abdominal procedures.

11.1 Concomitant Hysterectomy

The role of concomitant hysterectomy for anterior prolapse is controversial. The uterus, if normal and not significantly prolapsed, may be left in situ during anterior colporrhaphy. However, anterior prolapse rarely occurs in isolation and is most commonly associated with apical (uterine) prolapse. Support of the apex is important to creating a durable and effective repair of the anterior wall (Hsu et al. 2008; Rooney et al. 2006). Many of the

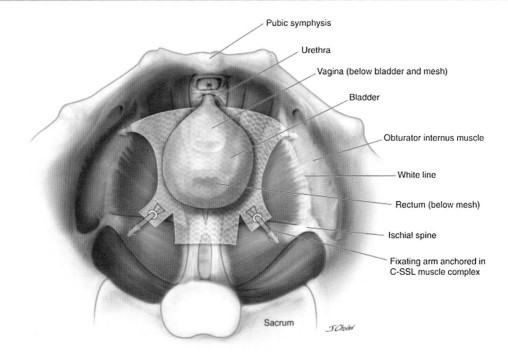

Pubic symphysis

Urethra

Vagina (below bladder and mesh)

Bladder

Obturator internus muscle

White line

Rectum (below mesh)

Ischial spine

Fixating arm anchored in
C-SSL muscle complex

Sacrum

Elevate mesh, anterior placement
(pelvic view from above)

Fig. 12 Transvaginal mesh kit for anterior/apical prolapse. The elevate incisionless mesh (American Medical Systems) is bilaterally anchored to the sacrospinous ligament and obturator internus muscle near the distal end of the arcus tendineus fascia pelvis (Reprinted from Surgical Management of Pelvic Organ Prolapse, 1st Edition, Maher CF, Karram M. Surgical Management of Anterior Vaginal Wall Prolapse, p117–137 (2013); with kind permission from Elsevier)

apical suspension techniques described below can be adapted to leave the uterus in situ. The decision to remove the uterus must be approached by the physician in consultation with the patient and take into account the patient's comorbidities, degree of prolapse, and preferences, as well as the surgeon's experience with the surgical procedures.

12 Apical Prolapse

Apical prolapse includes descent of the uterus and the vault after prior hysterectomy. Apical prolapse repairs generally have good results, and there are a variety of approaches to apical prolapse. Apical repairs can broadly be categorized into vaginal, abdominal, and obliterative approaches. Abdominal repairs may be performed via laparotomy, laparoscopy, or robotically.

13 Vaginal Approach for Apical Prolapse

13.1 Mayo/McCall Culdoplasty

One of the most common procedures for apical suspension, the Mayo/McCall culdoplasty, is often performed at the time of vaginal hysterectomy for non-prolapse indications. There are a number of variations, but there are several key steps to the Mayo/McCall culdoplasty (Fig. 13). After removal of the uterus, the vaginal cuff is examined for hemostasis. The vaginal cuff is transfixed to the cut edges of the uterosacral ligaments in order to suspend the cuff within the vagina. One to three sutures are placed through the uterosacral ligament as high as possible. Sequential bites are taken superficially across the peritoneum overlying the rectum until the opposite uterosacral

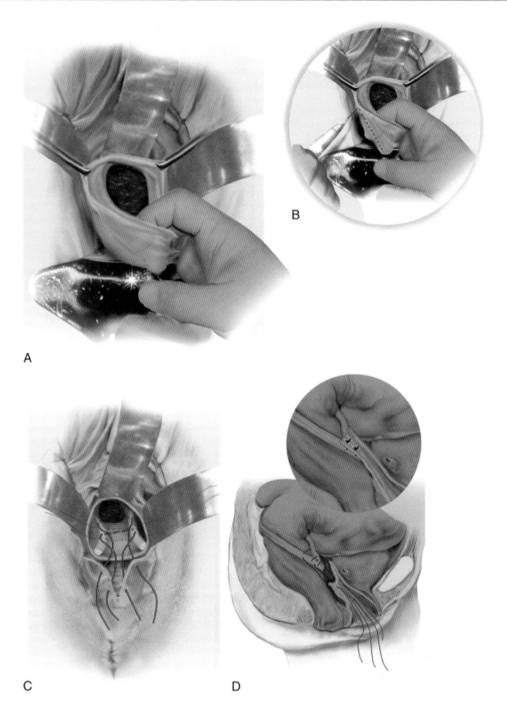

Fig. 13 Modified McCall culdoplasty. (**a**) The cul-de-sac is palpated and excessive peritoneum and posterior vaginal wall are noted. (**b**) A wedge of tissue (*dotted line*) is excised to decrease the caliber of the upper portion of the posterior vaginal wall. (**c**) External McCall stitches are placed in the traditional fashion. (**d**) Tying these sutures obliterates the cul-de-sac, supports the vaginal cuff, and increases posterior vaginal wall length (Reprinted from Urogynecology and reconstructive pelvic surgery, 4th Edition, Karram MM, Ridgeway BM, Walters MD. Surgical treatment of vaginal apex prolapse, p360–382. (2015); with kind permission from Elsevier)

ligament is sutured. When tied down, the uterosacral ligaments are plicated in the midline, and the posterior cul-de-sac is obliterated. Variations on this procedure are commonly performed, but outcome data is limited. The few retrospective studies available show success rates of up to 85%, with reoperation rates ranging from 0% to 14% (Barber and Maher 2013).

14 Uterosacral Ligament Suspension

14.1 Technique

Much of the support of the uterus comes from the cardinal/uterosacral ligament complex (Level 1 support). Uterosacral ligament suspension uses the patient's own ligaments to suspend the vaginal cuff above the level where the uterus has been amputated (Fig. 14). After the uterus is removed, the cuff is examined for hemostasis (if hysterectomy is not performed, the vaginal apex is grasped and incised). The ischial spines are identified and palpated intraperitoneally. The cut edge of the uterosacral ligament is grasped with Allis clamps on either side (at approximately 5:00 and 7:00 on the clockface). Traction allows for palpation of the uterosacral ligaments. Several sutures of permanent or delayed absorbable suture are placed through the uterosacral ligament at the level of the ischial spine. This procedure is repeated on the opposite side. The distal edge of the uterosacral ligaments is then plicated in the midline to obliterate the cul-de-sac. The highest delayed absorbable suture is placed full thickness through the posterior vaginal wall. If necessary, an anterior colporrhaphy may be performed. The vagina is trimmed and closed with 0 or 2-0 absorbable suture. After closure of the vagina, the uterosacral sutures are tied down on either side with suspension of the vault. Abdominal and laparoscopic approaches to this procedure have also been described.

14.2 Outcomes and Complications

Outcomes after uterosacral ligament suspension are generally good, with anatomic success ranging from 81% to 98%, and symptomatic improvement in 82–100% of patients (Margulies et al. 2010). In a recent large, prospective, randomized, controlled trial, the composite outcome of anatomic success and subjective success and lack of reoperation were reported to be 59.2% (Barber et al. 2014). The most commonly identified complication is ureteral injury or kinking, which should be looked for and identified intraoperatively. Ureteral kinking can be managed by removal of the offending suture and usually requires no further intervention. The incidence of ureteral injury or kinking ranges from 1% to 11% (Margulies et al. 2010) with most studies reporting a low incidence. However, intraoperative cystoscopy is highly recommended to ensure ureteral patency.

15 Sacrospinous Ligament Fixation

15.1 Technique

The sacrospinous ligaments extend from the ischial spines to the lower portion of the sacrum and coccyx and should be palpated prior to initiation of the procedure. The vagina is typically fixed unilaterally to the sacrospinous ligament, though bilateral fixations have been described. The posterior vaginal wall is incised in the midline and the vaginal epithelium dissected off the rectovaginal fascia. If an enterocele is encountered, it should be dissected off the posterior vaginal wall and closed with a high purse-string suture. The dissection of the epithelium off the rectovaginal fascia is extended laterally to identify the arcus tendineus fascia pelvis. The perirectal space is identified in this area by using blunt or sharp dissection and by mobilizing the rectum medially. The ischial spine is identified, and the

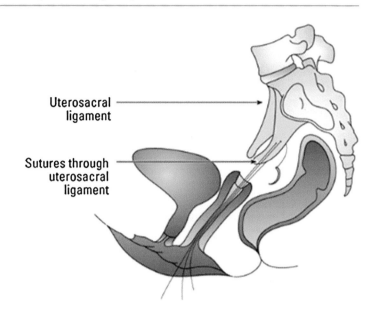

Fig. 14 Uterosacral ligament suspension. The vaginal cuff is fixed to the cut uterosacral ligaments on either side at the level of the ischial spines (Originally published in Cvach K, Dwyer P. Surgical management of pelvic organ prolapse: abdominal and vaginal approaches. World J Urol 2011;30 (4):471–7; with kind permission of Springer Science+Business Media. All Rights Reserved)

Uterosacral ligament

Sutures through uterosacral ligament

sacrospinous ligament is palpated dorsal and medial to the ischial spine. Once the ligament is identified, a rectal exam should be performed to confirm that no inadvertent injury has occurred. A suture is then passed through the sacrospinous ligament. The position of the ligament makes this suture passage difficult, and a variety of instruments have been designed to facilitate passage of the suture through the sacrospinous ligament. Commonly used techniques include the long-handled Deschamps ligature carrier, the Miya Hook, or proprietary instruments such as the Capio Suture device (Boston Scientific) (Figs. 15 and 16) or the Nichols-Veronikis ligature carrier (Cooper).

15.2 Outcomes and Complications

Overall, outcomes for sacrospinous ligament fixation are similar to uterosacral ligament suspension. A large randomized trial compared the two and found no significant difference in composite outcome of 60.5% at 2 years (composite outcome combines: anatomic success and subjective success and no reoperation) (Barber et al. 2014). The

most commonly reported complication of sacrospinous ligament fixation is buttock pain, which is seen in 12.4% of cases (Barber et al. 2014). Such pain is usually self-limiting and should resolve completely by 6 weeks postoperatively. Additional rare but serious intraoperative complications have been reported, including hemorrhage (0.2%) and rectal injury (0.4%) (Sze and Karram 1997). Hemorrhage may result from laceration of the inferior gluteal vessels, the hypogastric venous plexus, or the internal pudendal vessels. If a rectal injury occurs, it can usually be repaired transvaginally.

16 Alternative Vaginal Approaches

Several procedures have been described for the suspension of the vaginal vault, with or without hysterectomy. The most notable of which are the levator myorrhaphy and the iliococcygeus fascial suspension.

The technique for the levator myorrhaphy involves a wide plication of the levator muscles and fixation of the vaginal cuff to the plicated

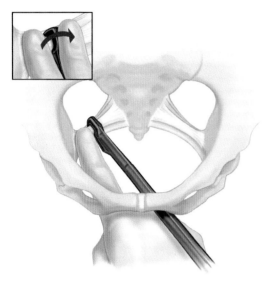

Fig. 15 Suture device for sacrospinous ligament fixation. The sacrospinous ligament is palpated at the level of the ischial spine. The suture device is placed medial to the operator finger, and the suture is passed through the ligament (Image reproduced with kind permission from Boston Scientific)

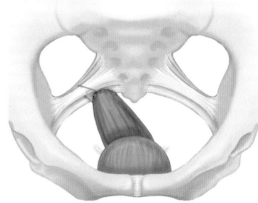

Fig. 16 Sacrospinous ligament fixation. The apex of the vagina is fixed unilaterally to the sacrospinous ligament (Image reproduced with kind permission from Boston Scientific)

muscles (Francis and Jeffcoate 1961). Packing is placed in the rectum to avoid narrowing of the rectum. Comparative studies to uterosacral ligament suspension have shown no difference in anatomic success or subjective outcomes; however, the total vaginal length was shorter after levator myorrhaphy (7.9 vs. 8.9 cm, $p = 0.04$) (Natale et al. 2010).

Iliococcygeus fascial suspension is also known as the Inmon technique (Inmon 1963). It is used to suspend the vaginal apex to the iliococcygeus fascia just below the ischial spine. The initial studies describing the procedure reported a case series of 152 patients. In that initial series, four intraoperative complications occurred (one rectal and one bladder laceration and two cases of hemorrhage requiring transfusion) (Shull et al. 1993; Meeks et al. 1994).

Retrospective reviews have shown that iliococcygeus fascial suspension is similar in outcomes to abdominal procedures and sacrospinous ligament fixation (Barber and Maher 2013). However, there are no randomized trials that evaluate this technique.

17 Abdominal Approach to Apical Prolapse

17.1 Sacral Colpopexy

Sacral colpopexy has been shown to be effective and durable for the correction of apical prolapse. Traditionally, sacral colpopexy is performed via laparotomy; however, laparoscopic and robotic approaches are also commonly used.

Regardless of approach, the basic steps of the procedure stay the same (Fig. 17). The peritoneal cavity is entered, and if indicated, hysterectomy is performed and the cuff is closed. The vagina is elevated using a sponge stick, probe, or end-to-end anastomosis sizer. The bladder is dissected off of the anterior vagina. Attention is then turned to the posterior vagina, and the peritoneum over the posterior wall is incised and dissected off of the vaginal tissue for several centimeters on either side. The mesh is trimmed to fit the anterior and posterior vaginal walls and transfixed using three to six stitches of nonabsorbable suture. Sutures are placed full thickness through the fibromuscular layer of the vagina, but not through the vaginal epithelium. The mesh is placed such that it reaches approximately two-thirds of the way down the

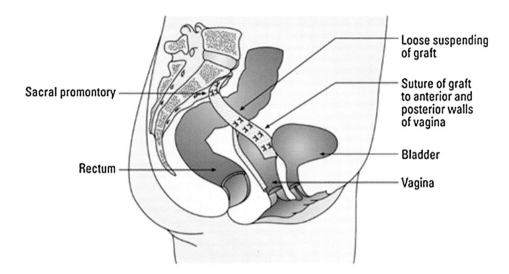

Fig. 17 Abdominal sacral colpopexy. The vaginal cuff is fixed to the anterior longitudinal ligament over the sacral promontory, using a piece of mesh or graft (Originally published in Cvach K, Dwyer P. Surgical management of pelvic organ prolapse: abdominal and vaginal approaches. World J Urol 2011;30(4):471–7; with kind permission of Springer Science+Business Media. All Rights Reserved)

anterior vagina, and a separate piece is placed at least halfway down the posterior vaginal wall. The two meshes are then sutured together above the cuff. The cul-de-sac is then obliterated using a Halban or Moschcowitz procedure.

Attention is then turned to the sacral promontory. The sigmoid colon, right ureter, aortic bifurcation, and common iliac vessels should be identified. The peritoneum over the sacral promontory is incised longitudinally and the underlying fatty tissue dissected off of the promontory. The middle sacral artery and vein should be identified at this step. The mesh is then transfixed to the anterior longitudinal ligament using two to three stitches of nonabsorbable suture. The mesh should be tensioned to avoid undue traction on the vagina. The peritoneum is then closed over the mesh.

Additional procedures at the time of sacral colpopexy may be indicated. A large randomized controlled trial showed that the addition of Burch urethropexy at the time of open sacral colpopexy reduced the rate of postoperative stress incontinence at 2 years from 57% to 37% in women who did not have stress incontinence preoperatively (Brubaker et al. 2008). As apical prolapse rarely occurs in isolation, repair of posterior prolapse may also be indicated at the time of colpopexy.

Outcomes and Complications

The success rate of abdominal sacral colpopexy for apical suspension ranges from 78% to 100% (Barber and Maher 2013). Over time, anatomic and subjective success rates tend to decrease, as prolapse tends to recur between 2 and 7 years (Nygaard et al. 2013). Severe intraoperative complications specific to colpopexy are rare and include hemorrhage from the sacral vascular plexus; complications from laparotomy may include enterotomy, ureteral damage, cystotomy, and wound infections.

The most common long-term complications after sacral colpopexy include recurrent prolapse, de novo stress incontinence, and mesh exposure. The median reoperation rates are 4.4% for recurrent prolapse, 4.9% for postoperative stress incontinence, and 3.4–5.1% for mesh exposure (Nygaard et al. 2004, 2013).

Abdominal Uterosacral Ligament Suspension

The abdominal approach to the uterosacral ligament suspension involves the same principles as the vaginal approach as described previously. The remnants of the uterosacral ligament are identified and tagged at the level of the ischial spines. The ureters are identified, and the uterosacral ligaments are fixed to the vaginal cuff using permanent or delayed absorbable sutures.

17.2 Obliterative Procedures

All of the above procedures focus on reconstructing the vagina. An alternative approach is to obliterate the vagina. This approach may be considered in women who are no longer sexually active and do not have plans to have vaginal intercourse in the future. Obliterative procedures may be performed for post-hysterectomy vault prolapse or for uterovaginal prolapse (colpectomy/colpocleisis). The uterus may be left in situ (LeFort colpocleisis) or removed. Even with removal of the uterus, these procedures offer a relatively quick operative time, low risk of morbidity, and high rate of success.

17.3 Technique/Considerations

As these procedures are generally performed on older women with multiple comorbidities, the focus of the preoperative evaluation should be on optimization of their functional status and control of their comorbidities. These patients should be carefully counseled on the procedure and the permanent loss of access to the vagina for sexual function. When the uterus is to be left in situ, these patients should be carefully screened for risk factors for endometrial and cervical pathology. They should be screened for postmenopausal vaginal bleeding and consider a pelvic ultrasound to evaluate the endometrium. Cervical cytologic screening should be up to date and negative.

17.4 Total Colpectomy/Colpocleisis

Total colpocleisis refers to the removal of the vaginal epithelium (Fig. 18) within the hymenal ring posteriorly to within 0.5–2 cm of the external

urethral meatus anteriorly (FitzGerald et al. 2006). Generally, the vaginal tissue is grasped and everted. The vaginal epithelium is excised in strips from the underlying vaginal muscularis. The muscularis is then inverted using a series of purse-string stitches. Once the prolapse is reduced, an aggressive perineorrhaphy and/or levator plication is performed. The anterior and posterior epithelia are sutured together with closure of the vagina.

17.5 Partial/LeFort Colpocleisis

A partial colpocleisis refers to when portions of the vaginal epithelium are left in place (Fig. 19). The LeFort modification is when the uterus is left in situ, and the epithelium is reconstructed in a manner to leave channels, through which vaginal discharge or blood can escape. The procedure is started by grasping the cervix and applying gentle traction. Rectangle sections are marked on the anterior and posterior vaginal walls; these are the areas to be denuded. The uterus is then reduced, and the cut edges of the remaining epithelium above and below the cervix are sewn together using interrupted sutures, such that the epithelium is inverted and it creates a tunnel in front of the cervix. A urinary catheter may be placed in this tunnel to ensure it is adequate and patent. The plication sutures are then continued laterally on either side to create lateral channels. As these sutures are placed, the prolapse is gradually reduced until it is entirely within the body. The final sutures may be placed at the level of the hymenal ring. The anterior and posterior epithelia are then reapproximated, using care to leave the lateral channels open. As above, an aggressive perineorrhaphy and levator plication are often performed to augment this repair (Evans et al. 2015).

Multiple studies have shown low rates of prolapse recurrence, high rates of patient satisfaction, and low rates of regret in appropriately counseled patients. Major complications of these procedures tend to be related to the performance of procedures on the elderly (cardiac, pulmonary, and cerebrovascular complications) and occur at a rate of

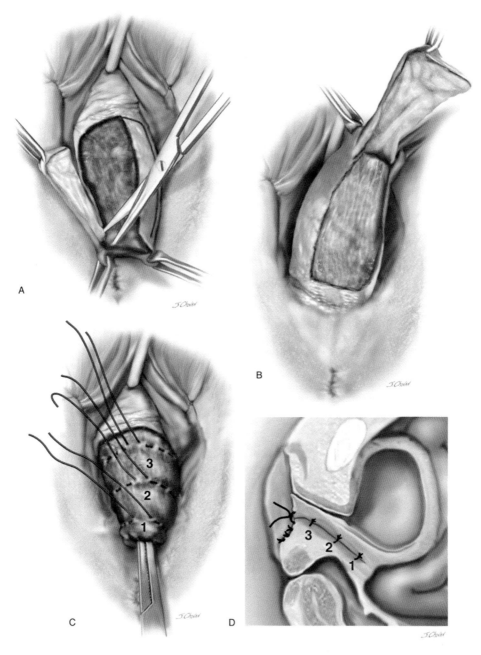

Fig. 18 Total colpectomy/colpocleisis. (**a, b**) The vagina is circumscribed and marked into quadrants. Each quadrant is removed by sharp dissection. (**c**) Purse-string sutures are placed; the leading edge is inverted by the tip of the forceps. Purse-string sutures are tied 1 before 2 and 2 before 3, with progressive inversion of the tissue. (**d**) The final relationship is shown in cross section (Reprinted from Urogynecology and reconstructive pelvic surgery, 4th Edition, Evans J, Silva WA, Karram MM. Obliterative procedures for pelvic organ prolapse, p400–410 (2015); with kind permission from Elsevier)

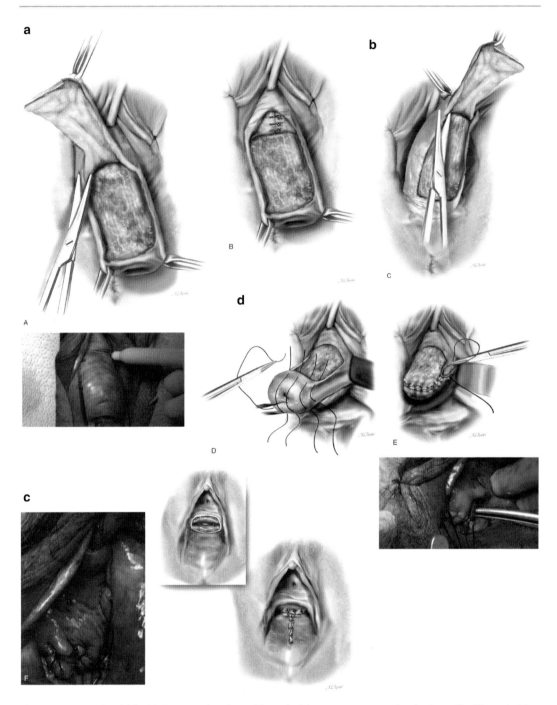

Fig. 19 LeFort colpocleisis. (**a**) A rectangular piece of the vagina has been removed. (**b**) A similar rectangular piece of the posterior vagina has been removed. (**c**) The cut edge of the interior incision is sewn to the distal cut edge of the posterior incision. Once the cervix is inverted, the sutures are continued up the lateral edges of the incisions on either side. (**d**) The entire vagina is inverted and the proximal incisions are sewn together horizontally. Note: draining channels are left in the lateral portions of the vagina to allow drainage of cervical discharge or uterine bleeding (Reprinted from Urogynecology and reconstructive pelvic surgery, 4th Edition, Evans J, Silva WA, Karram MM. Obliterative procedures for pelvic organ prolapse, p400–410 (2015); with kind permission from Elsevier)

approximately 2% (FitzGerald et al. 2006). Specific complications of the procedure include hemorrhage and pyelonephritis and appear at a rate of about 4%.

18 Posterior Prolapse

Women with symptomatic pelvic organ prolapse often have defects of the posterior vaginal wall. One study found that in women undergoing surgery for prolapse, 40% had posterior vaginal wall defects (Olsen et al. 1997). The posterior vaginal wall must usually be addressed separately from an anterior or apical suspension.

18.1 Technique

The traditional repair for posterior vaginal wall defects is the posterior colporrhaphy (Fig. 20). Two Allis clamps are placed on the perineum, which is then incised in a transverse fashion. If a perineorrhaphy is to be included, an inverted triangle of the skin is removed from the perineal body. The posterior vaginal wall is placed on gentle tension, and the vaginal epithelium is undermined using the Metzenbaum scissors up to the apex of the rectocele. The edges of the incision are grasped, and the epithelium is dissected off the underlying rectovaginal fascia bilaterally to expose the lateral attachments to the levator ani muscles. At this point, a traditional midline plication or a site-specific repair may be performed.

18.1.1 Midline Plication
The rectovaginal fascia is plicated in the midline with interrupted sutures, starting proximally and progressing toward the hymenal ring. Placement of these sutures should incorporate good purchase of the fibromuscularis and should be placed close to the junction with the epithelium to avoid injury to the rectum. The redundant vaginal epithelium is trimmed and the incision closed in a running, locked fashion. The caliber of the vagina at the end of the procedure should allow three fingerbreadths to fit comfortably.

18.1.2 Site-Specific Repair
The operator finger is placed in the rectum, and specific, palpable, or visual defects are repaired using interrupted, delayed, absorbable sutures (Fig. 21). If diffuse attenuation of the fascia is identified, a site-specific repair may not be technically feasible, and a midline plication is preferred. The redundant vaginal epithelium is trimmed and the incision closed in a running, locked fashion.

18.1.3 Graft or Mesh Augmentation
A posterior colporrhaphy may be augmented using graft or mesh. The material is cut to fit the space and sewn with permanent suture to the rectovaginal fascia at the level of the attachment to the levator ani muscles on either side. If the patient is undergoing a concomitant apical suspension, the graft may be fixed to the apical support sutures. The distal end is sutured to the perineum using absorbable sutures. The epithelium is then closed over the graft or mesh.

18.2 Outcomes and Complications

Traditional midline plication has success rates ranging from 76% to 97%. The most common complication of posterior colporrhaphy is dyspareunia. Postoperative dyspareunia is found in 11–27% after traditional posterior colporrhaphy, with de novo dyspareunia reported in 4–16% (Arnold et al. 1990; Lopez et al. 2001; Mellgren et al. 1995; Maher 2004). A three-way randomized controlled trial comparing traditional colporrhaphy to site-specific repair to porcine-derived graft showed that traditional colporrhaphy and site-specific repair had similar anatomic and functional outcomes. Porcine-derived graft augmentation resulted in improvement in symptoms similar to the other methods, but graft augmentation had significantly greater anatomic failures than the other two techniques (Paraiso et al. 2006). Graft augmentation may be considered in selected patients who have failed primary native tissue repair, with adequate preoperative counseling.

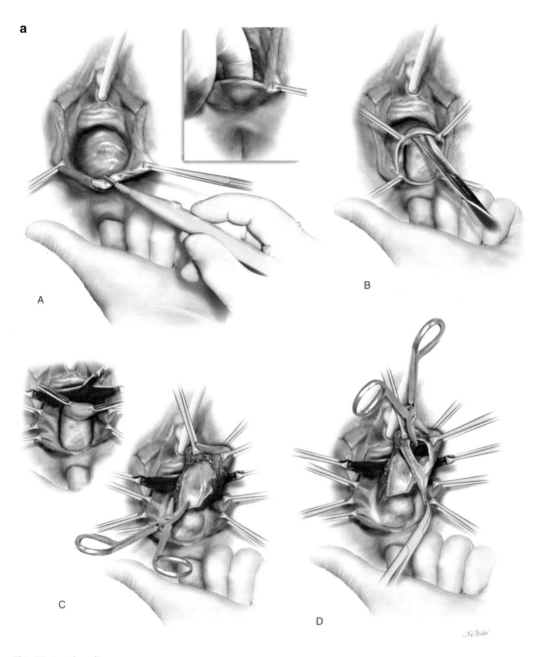

Fig. 20 (continued)

b

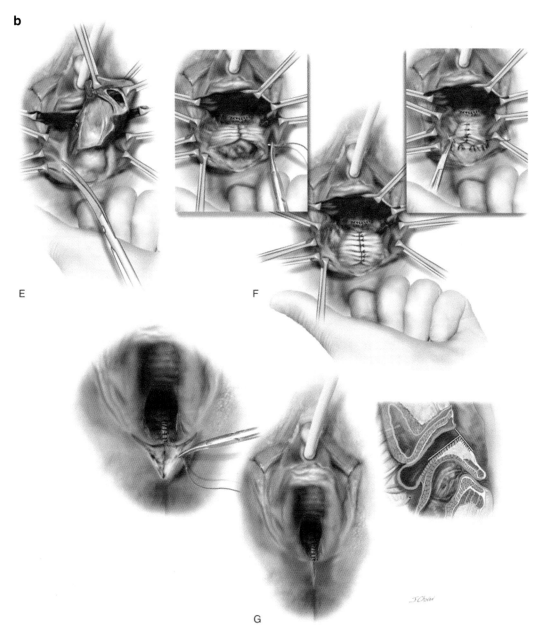

E

F

G

Fig. 20 Traditional posterior colporrhaphy. (**a**) The perineal skin is incised in the midline. (**b**) The posterior vaginal epithelium is mobilized off the rectum. (**c, d**) The enterocele sac is mobilized and entered. (**e**) The enterocele sac is excised or reduced, and the fibromuscular layer of the vagina is plicated in the midline. (**f**) A second layer may be plicated across the midline. (**g**) Perineorrhaphy is performed (Reprinted from Surgical Management of Pelvic Organ Prolapse, 1st Edition, Karram M. Surgical Correction of posterior pelvic floor defects, p139–164; with kind permission from Elsevier)

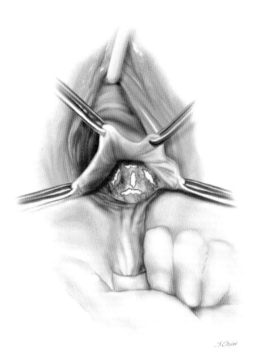

Fig. 21 Site-specific posterior defect repair. With finger in the rectum, discrete defects in the fibromuscular layer are identified. These defects are subsequently repaired using interrupted sutures (Reprinted from Surgical Management of Pelvic Organ Prolapse, 1st Edition, Karram M. Surgical Correction of posterior pelvic floor defects, p139–164; with kind permission from Elsevier)

19   Conclusion

Pelvic organ prolapse is a common problem that affects the daily activities for millions of women. The sensation of bulge in the vagina can be easily assessed and characterized by pelvic examination. Many patients may elect for expectant management or conservative management with a pessary. Radiologic testing is rarely indicated, and ancillary urodynamic testing may be indicated if the patient desires surgical intervention. Surgical treatment of prolapse is highly varied and depends greatly on the location of the prolapse, the degree of prolapse, and the patients' comorbidities and preferences. Surgical procedures are generally safe and well tolerated. Procedural success rates are hard to interpret, as success is generally considered anatomic success, symptomatic success, and absence of reoperation.

References

Abdool Z, Thakar A, Sultan AH, Oliver RS. Prospective evaluation of outcome of vaginal pessaries versus surgery in women with symptomatic pelvic organ prolapse. Int Urogynecol J. 2011;22(3):273–8.

Alnaif B, Drutz HP. Bacterial vaginosis increases in pessary users. Int Urogynecol J. 2000;11(4):219–23.

Arias BE, Ridgeway B, Barber MD. Complications of neglected vaginal pessaries: case presentation and literature review. Int Urogynecol J. 2008;19(8):1173–8.

Arnold MW, Stewart WR, Aguilar PS. Rectocele repair. Four years' experience. Dis Colon Rectum. 1990; 33(8):684–7.

Baden WF, Walker T. Fundamentals, symptoms and classification. In: Baden WF, Walker T, editors. Surgical repair of vaginal defects. Philadelphia: J.B. Lippincott; 1992. p. p14.

Barber MD, Maher C. Apical prolapse. Int Urogynecol J. 2013;24:1815–33.

Barber MD, Brubaker L, Burgio KL, Richter HE, Nygaard I, Weidner AC, Menefee SA, Lukacz ES, Norton P, Schaffer J, Nguyen JN, Borello-France D, Goode PS, Jakus-Waldman S, Spino C, Warren LK, Gantz MG, Meikle SF. Comparison of 2 transvaginal surgical approaches and perioperative behavioral therapy for apical vaginal prolapse: the OPTIMAL randomized trial. JAMA. 2014;311(10):1023–34.

Bø K. Can pelvic floor muscle training prevent and treat pelvic organ prolapse? Acta Obstet Gynecol Scand. 2006;85(3):263–8.

Braekken IH, Majida M, Engh ME, Bø K. Can pelvic floor muscle training reverse pelvic organ prolapse and reduce prolapse symptoms? An assessor-blinded, randomized, controlled trial. Am J Obstet Gynecol. 2010;203(2):170e1–7.

Brubaker L, Nygaard I, Richter HE, Visco A, Weber AM, Cundiff GW, Fine P, Chetti C, Brown MB. Two-year outcomes after sacrocolpopexy with and without Burch to prevent stress urinary incontinence. Obstet Gynecol. 2008;112(1):49–55.

Bump RC, Mattiasson A, Bø K, Brubaker LP, DeLancey JOL, Klarskov P, Shull BL, Smith ARB. The standardization of terminology of female pelvic organ prolapse and pelvic floor dysfunction. Am J Obstet Gynecol. 1996;175:10–7.

Clemons JL, Aguilar VC, Tillinghast TA, Jackson ND, Myers DL. Patient satisfaction and changes in prolapse and urinary symptoms in women who were fitted successfully with a pessary for pelvic organ prolapse. Am J Obstet Gynecol. 2004;190(4):1025–9.

Cormio L, Mancini V, Liuzzi G, Lucarelli G, Carrieri G. Cystocele repair by autologous rectus fascia graft: the pubovaginal cystocele sling. J Urol. 2015;194(3): 721–7.

Culligan PJ. Nonsurgical management of pelvic organ prolapse. Obstet Gynecol. 2012;119(4):852–60.

Cundiff GW, Weidner AC, Visco AG, Bump RC, Addison WA. A survey of pessary use by members of the

American Urogynecologic Society. Obstet Gynecol. 2000;95(6):931–5.

Cundiff GW, Amundsent CL, Bent AE, Coates KW, Schaffer JI, Strohbehn K, et al. The PESSRI study: symptom relief outcomes of a randomized crossover trial of the ring and Gellhorn pessaries. Am J Obstet Gynecol. 2007;196(4):405–8.

Dancz C, Walker D, Thomas D, Özel B. Prevalence of hydronephrosis in women with advanced pelvic organ prolapse. Urology. 2015;86(2):250–4.

DeLancey JO. Anatomic aspects of vaginal eversion after hysterectomy. Am J Obstet Gynecol. 1992;166(6 Pt 1): 1717–24. discussion 1724-28

Drake R, Vogl AW, Mitchell AWM, Ribbits R, Richardson P. Gray's Atlas of anatomy. Philadelphia: Elsevier Health Sciences; 2008. p. 229.

Evans J, Silva WA, Karram MM. Obliterative procedures for pelvic organ prolapse. In: Walters MD, Karram MM, editors. Urogynecology and reconstructive pelvic surgery. 4th ed. Philadelphia: Saunders; 2015.

FitzGerald MP, Richter HE, Siddique S, Thompson P, Zyczynski H. Colpocleisis: a review. Int Urogynecol J Pelvic Floor Dysfunct. 2006;17(3):261–71.

Francis W, Jeffcoate T. Dyspareunia following vaginal operations. J Obstet Gynaecol Br Commonw. 1961;68:1–10.

Hagen S, Stark D, Glazener C, Sinclair L, Ramsay I. A randomized controlled trial of pelvic floor muscle training for stages I and II pelvic organ prolapse. Int Urogynecol J. 2009;20(1):45–51.

Hanson LA, Schulz JA, Flood CG, Cooley B, Tam F. Vaginal pessaries in managing women with pelvic organ prolapse. Obstet Gynecol. 2006;108(1):93–9.

Haylen BT, de Ridder D, Freeman RM, Swift SE, Berghmans B, Lee J, Monga A, Petri E, Rizk DE, Sand PK, Schaer GN. An International Urogynecological Association (IUGA)/International Continence Society (ICS) Joint Report on the Terminology for Female Pelvic Floor Dysfunction. NeurourolUrodyn. 2010;29:4–20.

Hsu Y, Chen L, Summers A, Ashton-Miller JA, DeLancey JO. Anterior vaginal wall length and degree of anterior compartment prolapse seen on dynamic MRI. Int Urogynecol J Pelvic Floor Dysfunct. 2008; 19(1):137–42.

Hui SY, Chan SC, Lam SY, Lau TK, Chung KH. A prospective study on the prevalence of hydronephrosis in women with pelvic organ prolapse and their outcomes after treatment. Int Urogynecol J. 2011 Dec;22(12): 1529–34.

Inmon WB. Pelvic relaxation and repair including prolapse of vagina following hysterectomy. South Med J 1963;56:577–82.

Karram MM, Ridgeway BM, Walters MD. Surgical treatment of vaginal apex prolapse. In: Walters MD, Karram MM, editors. Urogynecology and reconstructive pelvic surgery. 4th ed. Philadelphia: Elsevier; 2015.

Koelbl H, Igawa T, Salvatore S, Laterza RM, Lowry A, Sievert KD, Sultan A. Pathophysiology of urinary

incontinence, faecal incontinence and pelvic organ prolapse. In: Abrams P, Cardozo L, Khoury S, Wein A, editors. Incontinence. 5th ed. Paris: European Association of Urology; 2013.

Lone F, Thakar R, Sultan AH, Karamalis G. A 5-year prospective study of vaginal pessary use for pelvic organ prolapse. Int J Gynecol Obstet. 2011;114(1): 56–9.

Lopez A, Anzen B, Bremmer S, Mellgren A, Nilsson BY, Zetterstrom J, et al. Durability of success after rectocele repair. Int Urogynecol J Pelvic Floor Dysfunct. 2001;12:97–103.

Maher C. Midline rectovaginal fascial plication for repair of rectocele and obstructed defecation. Obstet Gynecol. 2004;104(4):685–9.

Maher C, Karram M. Surgical management of anterior vaginal wall prolapse. In: Maher C, Karram M, editors. Surgical management of pelvic organ prolapse. 1st ed. Philadelphia: Saunders, an imprint of Elsevier; 2013.

Maher C, Feiner B, Baessler K, Schmid C. Surgical management of pelvic organ prolapse in women. Cochrane Database Syst Rev. 2013;(4).

Margulies RU, Rogers MA, Morgan DM. Outcomes of transvaginal uterosacral ligament suspension: systematic review and meta-analysis. Am J Obstet Gynecol. 2010;202(2):124–34.

Meeks GR, Washburne JF, McGehee RP, Wiser WL. Repair of vaginal vault prolapse by suspension of the vagina to iliococcygeus (prespinous) fascia. Am J Obstet Gynecol. 1994;171(6):1444–52;discussion 52–4.

Mellgren A, Anzen B, Nilsson BY, Johansson D, Dolk A, Gillgren P, et al. Results of rectocele repair. A prospective study. Dis Colon Rectum. 1995;38(1):7–13.

Menefee A, Dyer Y, Lukacz S, Simsiman J, Luber M, Nguyen N. Colporrhaphy compared with mesh or graft-reinforced vaginal paravaginal repair for anterior vaginal wall prolapse: a randomized controlled trial. Obstet Gynecol. 2011;118(6):1337–44.

Natale F, La Penna C, Padoa A, Agostini M, Panei M, Cervigni M. High levator myorrhaphy versus uterosacral ligament suspension for vaginal vault fixation: a prospective, randomized study. Int Urogynecol J Pelvic Floor Dysfunct. 2010;21(5):515–22.

Nguyen N, Burchette J. Outcome after anterior vaginal prolapse repair: a randomized controlled trial. Obstet Gynecol. 2008;111(4):891–8.

Nygaard IE, McCreery R, Brubaker L, Connolly A, Cundiff G, Weber A, Zycynski H. Abdominal sacrocolpopexy: a comprehensive review. Obstet Gynecol. 2004;104(4):805–23.

Nygaard I, Brubaker L, Zyczynski H, Cundiff G, Richter H, Gantz M, Fine P, Menefee S, Ridgeway B, Visco A, Warren LK, Zhang M, Meikle S. Long-term outcomes following abdominal sacrocolpopexy for pelvic organ prolapse. JAMA. 2013;309(19):2016–24.

Olsen AL, Smith VJ, Bergstrom JO, Colling JC, Clark AL. Epidemiology of surgically managed pelvic organ prolapse and urinary incontinence. Obstet Gynecol. 1997;89(4):501–6.

Paraiso MFR, Barber MD, Muir TW, Walters MD. Rectocele repair: a randomized trial of three techniques including graft augmentation. Am J Obstet Gynecol. 2006;195:1762–71.

Roberge RJ, Keller C, Garfinkel M. Vaginal pessary-induced mechanical bowel obstruction. J Emerg Med. 2001;20(4):367–70.

Rogo-Gupta L, Le NB, Raz S. Foreign body in the bladder 11 years after intravaginal pessary. Int Urogynecol J. 2012;23:1311–3.

Romanzi L, Chaikin D, Blaivas J. The effect of genital prolapse on voiding. J Urol. 1999;161(2):581–6.

Rooney K, Kenton K, Mueller ER, FitzGerald MP, Brubaker L. Advanced anterior vaginal wall prolapse is highly correlated with apical prolapse. Am J Obstet Gynecol. 2006;195(6):1837–40.

Shull BL, Capen CV, Riggs MW, Kuehl TJ. Bilateral attachment of the vaginal cuff to iliococcygeus fascia: an effective method of cuff suspension. Am J Obstet Gynecol. 1993;168(6 Pt 1):1669–74.

Stüpp L, Resende APM, Oliveira E, Castro RA, Girão MJBC, Sartori MGF. Pelvic floor muscle training for treatment of pelvic organ prolapse: an assessor-blinded randomized controlled trial. Int Urogynecol J. 2011; 22(10):1233–9.

Sudhakar A, Reddi V, Schein M, Gerst P. Bilateral hydroureter and hydronephrosis causing renal failure due to a procidentia uteri: a case report. Int Surg. 2001;86:173–5.

Sze EH, Karram MM. Transvaginal repair of vault prolapse: a review. Obstet Gynecol. 1997;89(3):466–75.

Thubert T, Deffieux X. Inside out: on rare occasions, ring pessaries can cause genital incarceration. Am J Obstet Gynecol. 2014;210(3):278.e1.

Trowbridge ER, Fenner DE. Practicalities and pitfalls of pessaries in older women. Clin Obstet Gynecol. 2007;50(3):709–19.

Weber A, Walters M, Piedmonte M, Ballard L. Anterior colporrhaphy: A randomized trial of three surgical techniques. Am J Obstet Gynecol. 2001;185:1299–306.

Wheeler LD, Lazarus R, Torkington J, O'Mahony MS, Woodhouse KW. Lesson of the week: perils of pessaries. Age Ageing. 2004;33(5):510–1.

Wu JM, Hundley AF, Fulton RG, Myers ER. Forecasting the prevalence of pelvic floor disorders in U.S. Women: 2010 to 2050. Obstet Gynecol. 2009;114(6):1278–83.

Wu JM, Kawasaki A, Hundley AF, Dieter AA, Myers ER, Sung VW. Predicting the number of women who will undergo incontinence and prolapse surgery, 2010 to 2050. Am J Obstet Gynecol. 2011;205(3): 230.e1–5.

Urinary Incontinence: Diagnosis, Treatment, and Avoiding Complications

Renee Rolston and Begüm Özel

Abstract

Urinary incontinence is defined as the complaint of involuntary leakage of urine. Urinary incontinence impacts physical, psychological, and social well-being. In order to achieve an accurate diagnosis, a detailed history and physical exam are important. An initial evaluation should include a detailed history, urinalysis, cough stress test, evaluation of post-void residual, focused neurologic assessment, and examination for urethral hypermobility and pelvic organ prolapse. Urodynamic testing and cystoscopy may be indicated in some patients. Treatment varies based on the type of urinary incontinence and symptom severity. First-line therapy should always consist of less invasive and more conservative treatment options as they have been shown to be highly effective with minimal risk. These therapies include pelvic floor exercises, biofeedback, bladder training, weight loss, modification in fluid and caffeine intake, urethral inserts, and incontinence pessaries. Depending on the type of incontinence characterized, more invasive treatment options can be implemented if no improvement with conservative management. Typically, women with stress incontinence who have failed conservative therapies are offered surgical intervention, whereas women with urgency incontinence may be treated with pharmacologic management, intradetrusor onabotulinum toxin A, or neuromodulation. Most incontinence can be made better with available therapies.

Keywords

Stress urinary incontinence • Urgency urinary incontinence • Mixed urinary incontinence • Sling

Contents

R. Rolston (✉) • B. Özel
Division of Female Pelvic Medicine and Reconstructive Surgery, Department of Obstetrics and Gynecology, Keck School of Medicine, University of Southern California, Los Angeles, CA, USA
e-mail: Renee.Rolston@med.usc.edu; Begum.Ozel@med.usc.edu

© Springer International Publishing AG 2017
D. Shoupe (ed.), *Handbook of Gynecology*,
DOI 10.1007/978-3-319-17798-4_71

1   Introduction

Urinary incontinence is defined as the complaint of involuntary leakage of urine (Haylen et al. 2010). The prevalence of urinary incontinence is estimated to range from 12% to 55% depending on the population studied (Castro et al. 2015). Urinary incontinence has been reported to affect up to 75% of older women (ACOG 2015). Urinary incontinence is associated with both depression and anxiety in women who are affected (Felde et al. 2016) and can lead to decrease in quality of life and negative impact on sexual function (Lim et al. 2016).

2   Diagnosis and Evaluation

2.1   History

History is a key part of the evaluation of urinary incontinence, and careful attention should be made to understanding the patient's complaints (Komesu et al. 2016). History should include duration of incontinence, precipitating events, severity, frequency of occurrence, the presence or absence of nocturia, daytime urinary frequency, hesitancy or dysuria, fluid intake, daily pad use, and interference with activities of daily living (Haylen et al. 2010). The history obtained can be used to characterize and classify the type of incontinence or to identify underlying conditions that may cause incontinence. Tools that can be utilized to aide in obtaining a detailed history include a bladder diary and validated questionnaires such as the urogenital distress inventory, incontinence impact questionnaire, questionnaire

for urinary incontinence diagnosis, incontinence quality for life questionnaire, and incontinence severity index (Staskin et al. 2005). When completing a bladder diary, patients are asked to record the timing and amount of fluid intake, voids and voided volumes, leakage episodes, and activity during leakage for 24–72-h period. As part of the history, medications should be reviewed to determine whether any of them might be contributing to urinary symptoms, such as diuretics, caffeine, alcohol, narcotic analgesics, anticholinergic drugs, antihistamines, psychotropic drugs, alpha-adrenergic blockers, alpha-adrenergic agonists, and calcium channel blockers (ACOG 2015).

2.2   Physical

Physical exam should include a pelvic exam, including evaluating for prolapse and an assessment of urethral mobility. When performing the pelvic exam, it is important to evaluate for pelvic organ prolapse and to exclude the presence of a urethral and/or pelvic mass. A urethral mass such as a diverticulum or pelvic masses such as fibroids may cause symptoms of urinary incontinence. As part of the pelvic exam, a speculum exam should be performed to evaluate for extraurethral urinary leakage which can occur if a fistula is present. A cough stress test during the pelvic exam, when positive, may confirm stress incontinence. The Q-tip or cotton-tipped swab test is a simple test to evaluate urethral hypermobility. Urethral hypermobility does not have an official definition from the International Continence Society/International Urogynecologic Association, but it can be defined as a resting angle or displacement angle of the urethra–bladder neck with maximum Valsalva of at least 30 degrees from the horizontal (Zyczynski et al. 2007). In the absence of prior anti-incontinence surgery, when point Aa is −1 or greater on the Pelvic Organ Prolapse Quantification Scale, nearly all patients demonstrate urethral hypermobility, and a Q-tip test may be deferred in these patients (Cogan et al. 2002).

During the initial evaluation of all women with incontinence, a focused neurologic examination is indicated, including assessment of gait, sensation over the perineum and perianal skin, and evaluation for sacral reflexes. A detailed neurologic examination is not necessary unless there is presence of sudden onset incontinence or new onset of neurologic symptoms. A simple test for the sacral reflexes is the anal wink in which the skin near the anus is stroked lightly with a soft cotton-tipped swab. A reflex contraction of the anus should be seen. However, the reflex can be absent in some neurologically intact women.

2.3 Additional Testing

Before initiating further therapy, it is recommended to check a urinalysis to evaluate for urinary tract infection and hematuria; a urine culture may be performed if indicated. It may be necessary to check a post-void residual (PVR) via straight catheterization or bladder ultrasound to rule out retention and overflow incontinence in women with symptoms of incomplete bladder emptying or difficulty voiding, or in women with risk factors such as neurologic disease or diabetes mellitus. A PVR volume less than 50 mL is considered indicative of adequate bladder emptying (Haylen et al. 2010), and a PVR volume greater than 200 mL is considered indicative of inadequate emptying (Gehrich et al. 2007). An isolated finding of a raised PVR requires confirmation before being considered significant.

2.4 Urodynamics

Cystometry is a graphic depiction of bladder and abdominal pressure relative to fluid volume during filling, storage, and voiding. The information obtained during cystometry can be used to assess bladder sensation, capacity, and compliance and to determine the presence and magnitude of voluntary and involuntary detrusor contractions. Uroflowmetry and pressure-flow studies measure the rate of urine flow and the mechanism of bladder emptying (Walters and Karram 2015). Urethral pressure profiles and Valsalva leak point pressures can also be measured to make the

diagnosis of urodynamic intrinsic sphincter deficiency. Studies have suggested that low urethral pressure measurements may be associated with poorer continence outcomes; a reliable cutoff measure to accurately predict surgical failure has not been found (Lim et al. 2016). Although Valsalva leak point pressures have been found to be weakly associated with subjective measures of incontinence severity, they have not been able to reliably predict surgical outcomes. Neuromuscular activity of the pelvic muscles and urethral sphincter during voiding can also be assessed during cystometry by using electromyography. The main role of electromyography is detecting coordination between detrusor muscle contraction and simultaneous urethral sphincter relaxation (Haylen et al. 2010).

Urodynamic testing should be used to evaluate patients with complicated urinary symptoms and inability to elicit evidence of stress urinary incontinence of cough stress test or to evaluate for occult stress incontinence in patients with pelvic organ prolapse. A multicenter randomized controlled study has demonstrated that for women with uncomplicated, demonstrable stress urinary incontinence, preoperative office evaluation alone was not inferior to evaluation with urodynamic testing for outcomes at 1 year; uncomplicated stress incontinence was defined as women with predominantly stress incontinence symptoms, negative urinalysis, PVR < 150 ml, the presence of urethral hypermobility, no history of pelvic irradiation, recent pelvic surgery, or significant prolapse (Nager et al. 2012).

When evaluating for urinary incontinence, cystourethroscopy is not routinely indicated. It should be considered in the setting of hematuria, acute-onset or refractory urgency incontinence, recurrent urinary tract infections, and suspicion for fistula or foreign body after gynecologic surgery.

3 Stress Incontinence

Stress urinary incontinence (SUI) is the complaint of involuntary leakage of urine on effort or exertion or on sneezing or coughing (Haylen et al.

2010). Stress incontinence is the most common type of incontinence in younger women.

> Risk factors are not well known but are believed to be attributable to age, obesity, menopause and the loss of circulating estrogen, straining when evacuating the bowels, childbirth including the number of pregnancies, vaginal delivery, and operative vaginal delivery (McIntosh et al. 2015).

A basic office evaluation as described above has been shown to be a sufficient preoperative workup for a patient with uncomplicated SUI (Nager et al. 2012).

3.1 Pathophysiology/Anatomy

The proposed mechanisms of stress urinary incontinence are urethral hypermobility and intrinsic sphincter deficiency. It is theorized that urethral hypermobility is caused by insufficient support of the pelvic floor musculature and vaginal connective tissue to the urethra and bladder neck. This causes the urethra and bladder neck to lose the ability to completely close against the anterior vaginal wall with increases in intra-abdominal pressure leading to incontinence. Treatments for hypermobility stress incontinence are aimed at providing a backboard of support for the urethra.

Intrinsic sphincter deficiency (ISD) is attributed to a loss of urethral tone that normally keeps the urethra closed. This can occur in the presence or absence of urethral hypermobility and typically results in severe urinary leakage even with minimal increases in abdominal pressure. Urodynamic ISD is defined as a maximum urethral closure pressure of ≤ 20 cm H2O and/or abdominal/Valsalva leak point pressure ≤ 60 cm H2O (Lim et al. 2016). In general, ISD results from neuromuscular damage and can be seen in women who have had multiple pelvic or incontinence surgeries. Patients with ISD can be challenging to treat and tend to have worse surgical outcomes (Lukacz 2016).

3.2 Treatment

3.2.1 Conservative

Behavioral Modifications

First-line treatment for stress incontinence includes behavioral and lifestyle modifications. Depending on symptom severity, treatment with these conservative therapies should be tried for at least 6 weeks before considering subsequent therapies (Lukacz 2016). Implementation of dietary changes in which the consumption of beverages that exacerbate incontinence such as alcohol, as well as caffeinated and carbonated beverages, is reduced may be helpful. It is also advisable for women to normalize fluid intake if they are drinking >64 oz. of fluid/day. Another behavioral modification is the management of constipation; constipation can exacerbate urinary incontinence and increase risk of urinary retention. Obesity is a known risk factor for urinary incontinence, and weight loss in obese women has been shown to reduce urinary incontinence in multiple well-designed studies (Vissers et al. 2014; Wing et al. 2010).

3.3 Pelvic Floor Muscle Training (PFMT)

In addition to behavioral and lifestyle modifications, pelvic floor muscle training is also grouped with conservative first-line treatment for SUI and has been shown to be very effective in treating stress incontinence. The Cochrane Review found that in 18 studies, there was high-quality evidence that PFMT is associated with cure of stress incontinence (RR, 8.38; 95% CI, 3.68–19.07) and moderate-quality evidence of cure or improvement of stress incontinence (RR, 17.33; 95% CI, 4.31–69.64) (Dumoulin et al. 2015).

Pelvic muscle exercises, also called Kegel exercises, aim to strengthen the pelvic floor musculature to provide a backboard for the urethra and reflexively inhibit detrusor contractions. When performing pelvic muscle exercises, different regimens have been prescribed. One simple instruction is to tell the patient to contract her pelvic floor using the same muscles they would use to stop urine flow or gas. The basic regimen consists of three sets of 8–12 contractions sustained for 8–10 s each, performed three times a day.

3.4 Incontinence Pessary

Incontinence pessary restores continence by stabilizing the proximal urethra and urethrovesical junction. Incontinence pessaries are thought to improve urinary incontinence in some women by increasing urethral functional length, urethral closure pressures, and cough profiles (McIntosh et al. 2015). The knob of the incontinence pessary should be placed at or below the bladder neck in order to stabilize the posterior urethra (McIntosh et al. 2015). A randomized controlled trial comparing the use of behavioral therapy alone (including pelvic floor muscle training), pessary alone, and combined behavioral therapy and pessary found that at 3 months pessaries were not as effective as behavioral therapy based in patient satisfaction. Therefore, although incontinence pessaries are a treatment option, they are not first line given the effectiveness of pelvic muscle exercise (Richter et al. 2010).

3.5 Urethral Inserts

A urethral insert is an occlusive device that acts as a mechanical barrier to prevent urinary leakage by sealing the urethral lumen (Sirls et al. 2002). They are self-inserted and designed for single use. The only urethral insert currently available for use is the FemSoft (Rochester Medical, Stewartville, MN). The most common side effects are urethral discomfort, hematuria, urinary tract infections, and bladder irritation. Contraindications for the use of urethral inserts include pregnancy, significant urge incontinence and unstable bladder contractions, neuropathic bladder, a history of recurrent bladder infections, the use of anticoagulants, and inflammatory or malignant lesions of the lower urinary tract.

3.6 Surgery

Stress urinary incontinence should be demonstrated objectively before any surgery is performed. This can be done with a cough stress test or with simple or multichannel urodynamic testing. A positive cough stress test is the visualization of fluid loss from the urethra simultaneously with a cough. This test should be performed with a full bladder in the supine and/or standing position. If the cough stress test is negative and patient reports symptoms of SUI, it is appropriate to perform urodynamic testing as next step. Once stress incontinence is objectively identified, surgical options include mid-urethral sling, pubovaginal sling, and Burch colposuspension. The most common surgical intervention for SUI is the mid-urethral sling procedure (Lim and Swyer 2009).

3.7 Mid-urethral Sling (MUS)

The first commercially available mid-urethral sling (MUS) was the tension-free vaginal tape (TVT) (Gynecare, Ethicon Women's Health and Urology, Somerville, New Jersey, USA), first described by Ulmsten in 1996 (Ulmsten et al. 1996) and introduced into the US market in 1998. According to the American Urogynecologic Society (AUGS) and the Society of Urodynamics, Female Pelvic Medicine and Urogenital Reconstruction (SUFU), the polypropylene mesh is considered the standard of care in the surgical treatment of SUI. There are two types of mid-urethral slings the retropubic sling and the transobturator (TOT) sling. Mid-urethral slings function by providing a backboard for the urethra, facilitating compression of the mid-urethra when intra-abdominal pressure increases.

When performing a retropubic MUS, a segment of synthetic material is inserted via the vagina and passed on each side of the urethra through the retropubic space through two exit incisions on the anterior abdominal wall. Once the sling is placed, position is assessed and confirmed to be tension-free. Absolute contraindications to the retropubic MUS include pregnancy, active oral anticoagulation, and the presence of important structures in the path of the trocars or sling, which may include a pelvic kidney, vascular graft, and low ventral hernias. A retrospective study comparing retropubic MUS, transobturator tape (TOT), and pubovaginal sling in women with ISD showed that retropubic MUS and pubovaginal slings had similar cure rates – retropubic MUS (86.9%) versus pubovaginal sling (87.3%) (Jeon et al. 2008). Potential complications of retropubic slings include bladder perforation, pelvic visceral injuries, vascular injuries and hemorrhage, mesh exposure, de novo development of urgency and urge incontinence, bladder outlet obstruction, pelvic pain, and urinary tract infection.

3.8   Transobturator

In 2001, Delorme described the transobturator technique for mid-urethral sling placement which avoided going in the retropubic space and is associated with less bladder perforation and visceral and vascular injury (Delorme 2001). The TOT can be performed via inside out or outside in technique in which the entry/exit point is the medial border of the obturator foramen at the level of the clitoris. The needle passage avoids any significant passage through the space of Retzius and nearly eliminates the possibility of intraperitoneal passage. As a result, the risk of bladder injury is lower after the TOT compared to the retropubic sling (0.6 vs. 4.5%; RR 0.13, 95% CI 0.08–0.20). Major vascular or visceral injury and operative blood loss is also lower with the TOT sling (Ford et al. 2015).

Another important complication is voiding dysfunction, which is less common after the TOT sling compared to the retropubic sling (RR 0.53, 95% CI 0.43–0.65) (Ford 2015). Groin pain appears more frequently after the TOT sling (6.4 vs. 1.3%; RR 4.12, 95% CI 2.71–6.27), whereas suprapubic pain is less common after the TOT (0.8 vs. 2.9%; RR 0.29, 95% CI 0.11–0.78). There is no difference in rates of mesh exposure or extrusion (Ford et al. 2015).

One important study that compared the TOT sling with the retropubic sling was the trial of mid-urethral slings (TOMUS); this was a multicenter, randomized equivalence trial comparing outcomes with retropubic and TOT mid-urethral slings in women with stress incontinence (Richter et al. 2010). Objective and subjective outcomes at 12 months were similar between the two approaches, with objective outcome of about 80% for both groups. Clinically important complications included voiding dysfunction requiring surgery, the use of catheter, or both, which was seen in 2.7% in women who had the retropubic sling versus none of the women who had a TOT sling ($p = 0.004$) and neurologic symptoms, seen in 9.4% of women in the TOT sling versus 4% in the retropubic sling ($p = 0.01$). Overall, the lower risk of most complications seen with the TOT sling makes it an excellent option in appropriately selected patients; however, there is a higher rate groin pain and neurologic complications, which must be considered.

Indications for TOT sling placement are the same as for retropubic MUS with the exception of intrinsic sphincter deficiency. In women with either a maximum urethral closure pressure of 20 cm H_2O or less or a pressure rise from baseline required to cause incontinence (Δ Valsalva or cough leak point pressure) of 60 cm H_2O or less, the retropubic sling appears to be more effective. Of the 138 women randomized in one study, objective failure as defined as urodynamic stress incontinence at 6 months follow-up, 45% of women who had the TOT sling and 21% of women who had the retropubic sling had USI, and 13% of women in the TOT sling group went on to have another anti-incontinence procedure (Schierlitz et al. 2008).

3.9   Pubovaginal (Autologous Sling)

Autologous slings work by supporting the proximal urethra and bladder neck achieving continence by providing a direct compressive force on the urethra/bladder outlet. Long-term success is based on the healing and fibrosis of the sling which passes through the endopelvic fascia. Autologous slings are placed at the bladder neck and are mainly reserved for women with severe stress urinary incontinence (SUI) and a non-mobile, fixed urethra, declining to have synthetic mesh implanted, recurrent SUI after a synthetic sling or history of a complication after a synthetic sling such as vaginal exposure or extrusion (Blaivas et al. 2013). It is also preferred to use an autologous sling in patients who have been irradiated, have had urethral injuries, and those who are undergoing either simultaneous or prior urethrovaginal fistula or diverticulum repair (Swierzewski and McGuire 1993). Compared to the mid-urethral sling, the pubovaginal sling is more invasive because it requires an abdominal incision to harvest fascia for the sling.

Complications of the pubovaginal sling include injury to the bladder and urethra, pelvic visceral injury, voiding dysfunction, superficial wound infection, seromas, and fascial hernias (Walters and Karram 2015).

In a meta-analysis, when compared to mid-urethral slings, the autologous sling is equally efficacious (RR 0.97 for incontinence at 12 months; 95% CI 0.78–1.20) but had longer operating time (mean difference 60 min; 5% CI 57–63 min), greater perioperative complications (RR, 1.59; 95% CI, 1.03–2.44), and greater de novo detrusor overactivity (RR, 3.21; 95% CI, 1.29–8.03) (Rehman et al. 2011). When compared to the Burch urethropexy, in a well-designed multicenter randomized trial, at 24 months of follow-up, success rates were found to be higher for women who had an autologous sling compared to the Burch urethropexy, but there were more urinary tract infections, difficulty voiding, and postoperative urgency incontinence after the autologous sling (Albo et al. 2007).

the use of permanent suture to secure the paravaginal tissue to periosteum of pubic symphysis; a known complication is osteitis pubis, a painful, noninfectious inflammation of the pubic symphysis. The Burch colposuspension involves the use of suture to secure paravaginal tissue to Cooper's ligament. The Burch colposuspension requires a low transverse incision to assess the space of Retzius. Two delayed absorbable or non-absorbable sutures are placed through the pubocervical fascia; one is placed 2 cm lateral to the mid-urethra, and the other is 2 cm lateral to bladder wall at the level of the urethrovesical junction bilaterally. The suture is then passed through Cooper's ligament. With a hand in the vagina to elevate the pubocervical fascia, the sutures are tied down; a suture bridge is created. Healing occurs by fibrosis in the space of Retzius, and support for the urethra is created.

The Burch colposuspension can be utilized in patients with SUI undergoing a concomitant abdominal procedure or in women who decline the use of mesh. Studies comparing the Burch colposuspension to slings (both mid-urethral and autologous) show similar effectiveness at 12 months (RR, 1.24; 95% CI, 0.93–1.67) (Lapitan and Cody 2016). There is a lower risk of voiding dysfunction with the Burch colposuspension compared to slings (RR, 0.41; 95% CI, 0.26–0.67). There is no difference in overall risk of perioperative complications between the Burch urethropexy and the mid-urethral slings (RR, 1.11; 95% CI, 0.66–1.87). However, women undergoing open retropubic colposuspension were nearly twice at risk of developing new or recurrent prolapse compared to those undergoing sling procedures (33.9 vs. 20.1%; RR, 1.85; 95% CI, 1.25–2.75) (Lapitan and Cody 2016).

3.10 Retropubic Urethropexy

Retropubic procedures include the Burch colposuspension and the Marshall-Marchetti-Krantz (MMK) procedure. The MMK procedure is generally no longer performed but involved in

3.11 Urethral Bulking Agents

Urethral bulking agents consist of non-biodegradable and nonimmunologic material which is injected transurethral or periurethral into the periurethral tissue around the bladder neck and proximal urethra to increase urethral resistance. Durasphere EXP (Carbon Medical Technologies, St. Paul, Minnesota, USA), Coaptite (Boston Scientific, Franksville, Wisconsin, USA), and Macroplastique (Cogentix Medical, Minnetonka, Minnesota, USA) are the bulking agents that are currently available.

The most common indications for urethral bulking agents include intrinsic sphincter deficiency with or without urethral hypermobility, persistent SUI after sling or urethropexy, and in women who cannot tolerate the risk of general anesthesia; other indications include women who cannot discontinue anticoagulation, are young and desire future fertility, and have SUI and poor bladder emptying (Cespedes and Serkin 2009). Urethral bulking agents have been shown to be less effective than surgery and usually require the need for repeat injections. Meta-analysis for the efficacy of Macroplastique found improvement rate of 75% (95% CI 69–81%) and cure/dry rates of 43% (95% CI 33–54%) at short-term follow-up (Ghoniem and Miller 2013). This is similar to success rates with other products (Reynolds and Dmochowski 2012). Managing patient expectations of outcome is important. Relative contraindications to the use of urethral bulking injections include active urinary tract infection, high post-void residual urine (>100 mL), urinary stricture/obstruction, severe detrusor overactivity, and fragile urethral mucosa. If no relief after two or three injections, further injections should not be attempted (Walters and Karram 2015).

4 Urgency Incontinence

Urgency urinary incontinence (UUI) is the complaint of involuntary urine leakage associated with urgency defined as the complaint of sudden compelling desire to pass urine that is difficult to defer, and overactive bladder (OAB) is defined as urinary urgency, usually accompanied by frequency and nocturia, with or without urgency urinary incontinence, in the absence of urinary tract infection (UTI) or other obvious pathologies

(Haylen et al. 2010). UUI is more common in older women and may be associated with comorbid conditions that occur with age. It is believed to result from detrusor overactivity, leading to involuntary detrusor muscle contractions during bladder filling (Lukacz 2016).

> The American Urological Association has identified behavioral therapy as the first-line treatment option and pharmacologic treatment as the second-line treatment option for nonneurogenic OAB in adults.

In patients with UUI refractory to behavioral and pharmacologic management, sacral nerve stimulation and intradetrusor injection of onabotulinum toxin A may be recommended (Singh et al. 2015).

4.1 Conservative

Pelvic floor exercises have been demonstrated to be effective in the treatment of UUI. They are more effective when combined with biofeedback or verbal feedback. Weight loss with diet and exercise, caffeine reduction, and 25–50% reduction in fluid intake gave all been demonstrated to be efficacious and should comprise the initial management (Olivera et al. 2016).

Bladder training has been shown to be effective for women with urgency incontinence. Bladder training starts with timed voiding. Patients should keep a voiding diary to identify their shortest voiding interval. Patients are instructed to void by the clock at regular intervals based on the shortest time interval identified between voids in voiding diary. Urgency between voiding is controlled with either distraction or relaxation techniques. When the patient can go two days without leakage, the time between scheduled voids is increased. The intervals are gradually increased until the patient is voiding every 3–4 h without urinary incontinence or frequent urgency. Successful bladder training can take up to 6 weeks (Lukacz 2016).

4.2 Pharmacologic Management

If behavioral treatments fail, the next step is a trial of antimuscarinics. Antimuscarinics block the basal release of acetylcholine during bladder filling resulting in increasing bladder capacity and decreased urgency (Lukacz 2016). The currently available antimuscarinic drugs for the treatment of UUI and OAB are listed in Table 1. Treatment should be started at the lowest dose and titrated up if there is insufficient response in treatment and minimal side effects. Improvement in symptoms may take up to 4 weeks. A systematic review, including 23 studies, concluded that improvement with anticholinergics, either alone or combined with bladder training, is significantly greater than improvement with bladder training alone (Castro et al. 2015). Despite the effectiveness of antimuscarinics therapy, it has a low adherence rate secondary to their side effect profile including dry mouth, constipation, blurred vision for near objects, tachycardia, drowsiness, and decreased cognitive function.

Antimuscarinics are contraindicated in patients with gastric retention and untreated angle-closure glaucoma.

In patients that have contraindications to antimuscarinic or cannot tolerate antimuscarinics, β3-adrenergic agonist may be an option. The current β3 agonist on the market is mirabegron, and it has been shown to be effective in the management urgency. Mirabegron acts by promoting relaxation of the detrusor muscle and increasing the bladder capacity without increasing the residual volume (Castro et al. 2015). Patients with severe or uncontrolled hypertension should not be prescribed mirabegron.

Vaginal estrogen therapy is another medication used for treatment of either stress or urgency incontinence. Vaginal atrophy can lead to symptoms of urinary frequency and dysuria and can contribute to incontinence, and correction of vaginal atrophy with topical estrogen may improve urinary symptoms. Vaginal estrogen therapy can be in the form of a cream, ring, or tablet (Cody et al. 2012). Evidence suggests that vaginal estrogen therapy may improve continence (RR, 0.74;

95% CI, 0.64–0.86). There are 1–2 fewer voids in 24 h among women treated with vaginal estrogen, and there is less urgency and frequency (Cody et al. 2012).

4.3 Percutaneous Tibial Nerve Stimulation

Percutaneous tibial nerve stimulation (PTNS) delivers neuromodulation to the pelvic floor through the S2–4 junction of the sacral nerve plexus via the posterior tibial nerve. A 34-gauge needle electrode is inserted above the ankle, and the tibial nerve is accessed. This area has projections to the sacral nerve plexus, creating a feedback loop that modulates bladder innervation. Initial therapy consists of 12-weekly 30-min treatments (Gaziev et al. 2013). In a randomized trial of 220 adults, the 13-week subject global response assessment for overall bladder symptoms demonstrated statistically significant improvement in bladder symptoms from baseline with PTNS over sham therapy; 54.5% reported being moderately or markedly improved with PTNS compared to 20.9% of participants who received the sham therapy ($p < 0.001$) (Peters et al. 2010).

4.4 Intradetrusor Onabotulinum Toxin A

Onabotulinum toxin A blocks neuromuscular transmission by binding to receptor sites on nerve terminals and inhibiting the release of acetylcholine. This inhibition occurs as the neurotoxin cleaves SNAP-25, a protein integral to the successful docking and release of acetylcholine from vesicles situated within nerve endings (Balchandra and Rogerso 2014). The most commonly recommended dose for nonneurogenic UUI/DO is BoNT-A 100 units. It is administered under cystoscopic visualization by evenly distributed intradetrusor injections across 20 sites approximately 1 cm apart, sparing the trigone of the bladder (Liao and Kuo 2015). Onabotulinum toxin A is indicated in urgency refractory to medical

Table 1 Antimuscarinic medications for treatment of women with urgency urinary incontinence or overactive bladder

Medication	Available formulations
Darifenacin	Extended release
Fesoterodine	Extended release
Oxybutynin	Immediate release Extended release Transdermal patch Transdermal gel
Solifenacin	Extended release
Tolterodine	Immediate release Extended release
Trospium	Immediate release Extended release

treatment. Contraindications include active infection, acute urinary retention, unwillingness or inability to self-catheterize, and known hypersensitivity to the toxin (Liao and Kuo 2015). In a large, randomized controlled trial of onabotulinum toxin A compared to placebo, at 12 weeks, onabotulinum toxin A significantly decreased urinary incontinence episodes per day (-2.95 vs. -1.03, $p < 0.001$), and reduction in all OAB symptoms as assessed by validated quality of life questionnaires was significantly greater with onabotulinum toxin A compared to placebo (Chapple et al. 2013). The need to self-catheterize occurred in 6.9% of participants, and urinary tract infections were seen in 20.4%, which was the most common complication seen (Chapple et al. 2013).

4.5   Sacral Neuromodulation

Sacral neuromodulation consists of the surgical implantation of electrodes in the S3 sacral nerve root and of an electric impulse generator, which is implanted in the subcutaneous tissue. It is reserved for severe cases of urgency refractory to conventional treatments. The mechanism of action is not fully understood, but electrical impulses are believed to act in both afferent and efferent fibers. The electrode implantation is performed in two stages in order to reduce complications and false-negative rates (Balchandra and Rogerso 2014). The first stage is the testing phase in which the electrode is implanted and positioned using radioscopy.

The definitive implant is offered to patients who exhibit a positive response at least a 50% symptom improvement in the first stage after 1–4 weeks. Cure and improvement rates are 30–50% and 60–90%, respectively (Castro et al. 2015; Yamanishi et al. 2015). Complication rates are low and include adverse change in bowel habits, electrically induced discomfort, pain at the implantable pulse generator site, and infection (Olivera et al. 2016).

4.6   Mixed Urinary Incontinence

Mixed urinary incontinence is defined as the complaint of involuntary loss of urine associated with urgency and also with effort or physical exertion or on sneezing or coughing. The pathophysiology is poorly understood. Initial treatment is conservative and should aim at treating both the SUI and UUI components. Subsequent therapy needs to be individualized to the patient's primary complaint and degree of bother from the SUI and UUI. Typically, outcomes with anti-incontinence surgery for women with MUI are poorer than women with SUI alone. Persistent DO after anti-incontinence surgeries is seen in up to 74% of women, typically leading to lower satisfaction with outcome of surgery (Bandukwala and Gousse 2015). Preoperative counseling on persistent UUI and DO after surgery is important when offering these women surgical treatment (Komesu et al. 2016).

5   Conclusion

Urinary incontinence is a treatable medical condition that significantly affects quality of life. A variety of conservative, pharmacologic, and interventional therapies exist to treat this condition.

6   Cross-References

▶ Minimally Invasive Procedures for Incontinence and Lower Urinary Tract Disorders: Indications and Avoiding Complications
▶ Pelvic Organ Prolapse: Diagnosis, Treatment, and Avoiding Complications

References

Albo M, Richter H, Brubaker L, Norton P, et al. Burch colposuspension versus fascial sling to reduce urinary stress incontinence. N Engl J Med. 2007;356 (21):2143–55.

American College of Obstetricians and Gynecologists (ACOG). Urinary incontinence in women. Practice Bulletin No. 155. American College of Obstetricians and Gynecologists. 2015.

Balchandra P, Rogerso L. Women's perspective: intra-detrusor botox versus sacral neuromodulation for over-active bladder symptoms after unsuccessful anticholinergic treatment. Int Urogynecol J. 2014;25(8):1059–64.

Bandukwala NQ, Gousse AE. Mixed urinary incontinence: what is first? Curr Urol Rep. 2015;16(3):9.

Blaivas J, Purohit R, Weinberger J, Tsui J, et al. Surgery after failed treatment of synthetic mesh sling complications. J Urol. 2013;190(4):1281–6.

Castro R, Arruda R, Bortolini M. Female urinary incontinence: effective treatment strategies. Climacteric. 2015;18(2):135–41.

Cespedes RD, Serkin FB. Is injection therapy for stress urinary incontinence dead? No Urology. 2009;73(1): 11–3.

Chapple C, Sievert K, MacDiarmid S, Khullar V, et al. Onabotulinum toxin A 100 U significantly improves all idiopathic overactive bladder symptoms and quality of life in patients with overactive bladder and urinary incontinence: a randomised, double-blind, placebo-controlled trial. Eur Urol. 2013;64(2):249–56.

Cody J, Jacobs M, Richardson K, Moehrer B, Hextall A. Oestrogen therapy for urinary incontinence in post-menopausal women. Cochrane Database Syst Rev. 2012;10:CD001405. doi:10.1002/14651858.cd001405.pub3.

Cogan SL, Weber AM, Hammel JP. Is urethral mobility really being assessed by the pelvic organ prolapse quantification (POP-Q) system? Obstet Gynecol. 2002;99(3):473–6.

Delorme E. Transobturator urethral suspension: mini-invasive procedure in the treatment of stress urinary incontinence in women. Prog Urol. 2001;11(6): 1306–13.

Dumoulin C, Hay-Smith J, Habée-Séguin GM, Mercier J. Pelvic floor muscle training versus no treatment, or inactive control treatments, for urinary incontinence in women: a short version Cochrane systematic review with meta-analysis. Neurourol Urodyn. 2015;34(4): 300–8.

Felde G, Ebbesen MH, Hunskaar S. Anxiety and depression associated with urinary incontinence. A 10-year follow-up study from the Norwegian HUNT study (EPINCONT). Neurourol Urodynam. 2016; doi:10.1002/nau.22921.

Ford A, Rogerson L, Cody JD, Ogah J. Mid-urethral sling operations for stress urinary incontinence in women. Cochrane Database Syst Rev. 2015;7:CD006375. doi:10.1002/14651858.cd006375.pub3.

Gaziev G, Topazio L, Lacovelli V, Asimakopoulos A, et al. Percutaneous Tibial Nerve Stimulation (PTNS) efficacy in the treatment of lower urinary tract dysfunctions: a systematic review. BMC Urol. 2013; doi:10.1186/1471-2490-13-61.

Gehrich A, Stany M, Fischer J, Buller J, Zahn C. Establishing a mean postvoid residual volume in asymptomatic perimenopausal and postmenopausal women. Obstet Gynecol. 2007;110(4):827–32.

Ghoniem G, Miller C. A systematic review and meta-analysis of Macroplastique for treating female stress urinary incontinence. Int Urogynecol J. 2013;24(1):27–36.

Haylen B, De Ridder D, Freeman R, Swift S, et al. An International Urogynecological Association (IUGA)/ International Continence Society (ICS) joint report on the terminology for female pelvic floor dysfunction. Neurourol Urodyn. 2010;29:4–20.

Jeon M, Jung H, Chung S, Sei-Kwang K, et al. Comparison of the treatment outcome of pubovaginal sling, tension-free vaginal tape, and transobturator tape for stress urinary incontinence intrinsic sphincter deficiency. Am J Obstet Gynceol. 2008;199(1):76.e1–4.

Komesu Y, Schrader R, Ketai L, Rogers R, Dunivan C. Epidemiology of mixed, stress, and urgency urinary incontinence in middle-aged/older women: the importance of incontinence history. Int Urogynecol J. 2016;27(5):763–72.

Lapitan M, Cody J. Open retropubic colposuspension for urinary incontinence in women. Cochrane Database Syst Rev. 2016;6:CD002912. doi:10.1002/14651858.CD002912.pub5.

Liao C, Kuo H. Practical aspects of Botulinum Toxin-A treatment in patients with overactive bladder syndrome. Int Neurourol J. 2015;19(4):213–9.

Lim Y, Swyer P. Effectiveness of midurethral slings in intrinsic sphincteric-related stress urinary incontinence. Curr Opin Obstet Gynecol. 2009;21(5):428–33.

Lim R, Liong M, Leong W, Khan N, Yuen K. Effect of stress urinary incontinence on the sexual function of couples and the quality of life of patients. J Urol. 2016; doi:10.1016/j.juro.2016.01.090.

Lukacz E. Treatment of urinary incontinence in women[Internet]; 2016. Available from: http://www.uptodate.com/contents/treatment-of-urinary-incontinence-in-women

McIntosh L, Andersen E, Reekie M. Conservative treatment of stress urinary incontinence in women: a 10-year (2004-2013) scoping review of the literature. Urologic Nursing. 2015;35(4):179–86.

Nager C, Brubaker L, Litman H, Zyczynski H, et al. A randomized trial of urodynamic testing before stress-incontinence surgery. Urinary Incontinence Treatment Network. N Engl J Med. 2012;366(21):1987–97.

Olivera C, Meriwether K, El-Nashar S, et al. Systematic review group for the society of gynecological surgeons. Nonantimuscarinic treatment for overactive bladder: a systematic review. Am J Obstet Gynecol. 2016; doi:10.1016/j.ajog.2016.01.156.

Peters K, Carrico D, Perez-Marrero R, et al. Randomized trial of percutaneous tibial nerve stimulation versus sham efficacy in the treatment of overactive bladder syndrome: results from the SUMIT trial. J Urol. 2010;183(4):1438–43.

Rehman H, Berzerra C, Bruschini H, Cody J. Traditional suburethral sling operations for urinary incontinence in women. Cochrane Database Syst Rev. 2011;1: CD001754. doi:10.1002/14651858.CD001754.pub3.

Reynolds W, Dmochowski R. Urethral bulking: a urology perspective. Urol Clin North Am. 2012;39(3):279–87.

Richter H, Albo M, Zyczynski H, Kenton K, et al. Urinary incontinence treatment network. Retropubic versus transobturator midurethral slings for stress incontinence. N Engl J Med. 2010;362(22):2066–76.

Schierlitz L, Dwyer P, Rosamilia A, Murray C, et al. Effectiveness of tension-free vaginal tape compared with transobturator tape in women with stress urinary incontinence and intrinsic sphincter deficiency: a randomized controlled trial. Obstet Gynecol. 2008;112(6): 1253–61.

Singh E, El Nashar A, Trabuco E, et al. Comparison of short term outcomes of sacral nerve stimulation and intradetrusor injection of Onabotulinum toxin A (Botox) in women with refractory overactive bladder. Female Pelvic Med Reconstr Surg. 2015; 21(6):369–73.

Sirls L, Foote J, Kaufman J, Lightner D, et al. Long-term results of the FemSoft urethral insert for the management of female stress urinary incontinence. Int Urogynecol J Pelvic Floor Dysfunct. 2002;13(2): 88–95.

Staskin D, Hilton P, Emmanuel A, et al. Initial assessment of incontinence. In: Abrams P, Cardozo L, Khoury S, Wein A, editors. Incontinence: 3rd international consultation on incontinence. Paris: Health Publications Ltd; 2005. p. 485.

Swierzewski S, McGuire E. Pubovaginal sling for treatment of female stress urinary incontinence complicated by urethral diverticulum. J Urol. 1993;149(5): 1012–4.

Ulmsten U, Henriksson L, Johnson P, Varhos G. An ambulatory surgical procedure under local anesthesia for treatment of female urinary incontinence. Int Urogynecol J Pelvic Floor Dysfunct. 1996;7(2):81–5.

Vissers D, Neels H, Vermandel A, De Wachter S, et al. The effect of non-surgical weight loss interventions on urinary incontinence in overweight women: a systematic review and meta-analysis. Obes Rev. 2014;15 (7):610–7.

Walters M, Karram M. Urogynecology and reconstructive pelvic surgery. 4th ed. Philadelphia: Saunders Elsevier; 2015.

Wing R, West D, Grady D, Creasman J, et al. Effect of weight loss on urinary incontinence in overweight and obese women: results at 12 and 18 months. Program to reduce incontinence by diet and exercise group. J Urol. 2010;184(3):1005–10.

Yamanishi T, Kaga K, Fuse M, Shibata C, Uchiyama T. Neuromodulation for the treatment of lower urinary tract symptoms. Low Urin Tract Symptoms. 2015;7(3): 121–32.

Zyczynski H, Lloyd L, Kenton K, Menefee S, et al. Correlation of Q-tip values and point Aa in stress-incontinent women. Urinary Incontinence Treatment Network (UITN). Obstet Gynecol. 2007;110(1):39–43.

Diagnosis and Management of Delayed Postoperative Complications in Gynecology: Neuropathy, Wound Complications, Fistulae, Thromboembolism, Pelvic Organ Prolapse, and Cuff Complications

Christina Dancz and Anastasiya Shabalova

Abstract

Surgical complications are an inevitable occurrence for any surgeon. Such complications may be a source of significant morbidity and even mortality. Delayed surgical complications typically present after the patient is discharged from the hospital. This chapter describes the presentation, evaluation, and management of the most common delayed postoperative complications. Delayed complications may be broadly categorized into those found in the early postoperative period and those in the later postoperative period. The first 2 weeks after surgery is a key time to evaluate and diagnose nerve injuries and wound complications, including infectious complications. Genital tract fistulae and thromboembolism may also present in this time period, but are also commonly seen in the first 3 months after surgery. Pelvic organ prolapse and cuff complications may present months to years after surgical intervention. The surgeon must be vigilant in the postoperative period for any sign of a delayed surgical complication, as prompt diagnosis and management is critical to minimize the effect upon the patient.

Keywords

Coagulation • Cuff complications • Fistula • Nerve injury • Postoperative • Prolapse • Thromboembolism • Wound

Contents

C. Dancz (✉) • A. Shabalova
University of Southern California, Los Angeles, CA, USA
e-mail: christina.dancz@med.usc.edu; anastasiya.
shabalova@med.usc.edu

© Springer International Publishing AG 2017
D. Shoupe (ed.), *Handbook of Gynecology*,
DOI 10.1007/978-3-319-17798-4_73

1   Introduction

Some of the most commonly performed surgical procedures are performed by obstetrician/gynecologists. Cesarean section and hysterectomies are among the most commonly performed major surgeries in the United States, accounting for 1.8 million procedures in 2010 alone (National Center for Health Statistics (NCHS) 2010). These procedures are generally safe; however, occasionally complications may occur. Surgical complications range in both severity and acuity. When injuries occur during surgery, they may be immediately repaired, often with minimal impact on the patient. Intraoperative injuries that are not recognized until the postoperative period generally have worse outcomes than those repaired at the time of surgery. In order to minimize the impact on patients, it is critical for any surgeon to promptly identify and appropriately manage any complications of these common surgical procedures.

2   Delayed Complications Presenting in the Immediate Postoperative Period (Within 2 Weeks)

2.1   Neurologic Injury

Neurologic injury complicates approximately 1–2% of gynecological surgery. Many injuries are due to improper positioning or self-retaining retractors; however, direct surgical trauma, suture entrapment, or hematoma formation can also be involved (Bohrer et al. 2009; Warner et al. 2000). Symptoms almost always present soon after

surgery, and, although most resolve completely with appropriate treatment, some patients continue to have long-term neurologic consequences. Therefore, prevention, early recognition, and treatment initiation are paramount.

Nerves that may be injured after pelvic surgery include: femoral, lateral femoral cutaneous, ilioinguinal, iliohypogastric, genitofemoral, common perineal, sciatic, and obturator.

2.2   Femoral Nerve

Femoral nerve (L2-L4) is the largest branch of the lumbar plexus that courses between the psoas and the iliacus muscles in the abdomen, then passes under the inguinal ligament, and enters the thigh. Gynecologic surgery and particularly the abdominal hysterectomy are the most frequent causes of iatrogenic injury to the femoral nerve.

Injury to the femoral nerve can occur throughout its course due to variable mechanisms. The most frequent cause is related to the use of self-retaining retractors. Retractor blades placed on the psoas muscle cause injury by compressing the nerve, particularly with the use of longer retractor blades. The retractor can also compress the nerve where it traverses the abdominal wall by lateral displacement of the psoas muscle.

To avoid such injury, the shortest retractor blades should be used, particularly in thin patients. Folded laparotomy sponges or towels can be placed between the retractor and the abdominal wall. Disposable retractors that don't use blades and therefore distribute the pressure evenly can be considered. The risk of injury is directly related to length of surgery.

Another mechanism of injury of the femoral nerve is patient positioning. In dorsal lithotomy position excessive hip flexion, external rotation or abduction can compress the nerve against the inguinal ligament. Close attention to proper positioning is imperative to decrease the risk of compression injury. Thighs should not be excessively abducted or externally rotated and hip flexion should not exceed 80–90°.

Although less common, injury can also occur due to direct transection, incorporation into a suture, or a hematoma causing nerve compression.

The classic presentation of postoperative femoral nerve injury is a patient who cannot climb stairs or falls when trying to get out of bed. The motor deficits include inability to flex the hip or extend the knee as well as an absent patellar reflex.

Sensory deficits usually involve paresthesia over the anterior-medial thigh and leg.

If a neurological injury is suspected after surgery, a thorough neurological examination may provide the diagnosis. Electromyography and nerve conduction studies may narrow down the location of injury. Imaging studies such as MRI, CT scan, or ultrasound can be used to detect formation of a hematoma or other fluid collections causing nerve compression.

After diagnosis, treatment should be initiated immediately. In cases of suspected transection or suturing, surgical reexploration and repair may be needed. Nerve compression from a hematoma can be relieved with drainage. Physical therapy should be initiated as soon as possible to prevent muscle atrophy. Knee stabilizers may be used to counteract thigh muscle weakness during standing.

Most patients will achieve full recovery, although time till recovery varies and may take up to several months (Bradshaw and Advincula 2010; Chan and Manetta 2002; Craig 2013; Irvin et al. 2004).

2.3 Lateral Femoral Cutaneous Nerve

Lateral femoral cutaneous nerve (L2-L3) courses over the iliacus muscle and passes under the inguinal ligament near the anterior superior iliac spine. Similarly to the femoral nerve, it is at risk of compression from excessive hip flexion in dorsal lithotomy position as well as with inappropriate placement of lateral retractor blades. Neurologic deficits associated with this nerve are loss of sensation, paresthesia, and pain over the anterior lateral thigh from the inguinal ligament to the knee, a condition sometimes referred to as **meralgia paresthetica** (Bradshaw and Advincula 2010; Craig 2013; Irvin et al. 2004).

2.4 Ilioinguinal and Iliohypogastric

Ilioinguinal (T12-L1) and iliohypogastric (T12-L1) nerves are frequently grouped together due to difficulty in distinguishing individual effects. The nerves run laterally through the head of the psoas muscle, pass diagonally along the anterior surface of quadratus lumborum, penetrate transversus abdominis, and enter the anterior abdominal wall. The nerves are susceptible to injury if a transverse abdominal incision is extended laterally, particularly beyond the edge of the rectus muscle at which point the edge of the fascia is close to the nerve branches. Injury from trocar placement in laparoscopic surgery has also been reported.

The nerve damage typically occurs from direct surgical injury or nerve incorporation during fascial closure as well as scar formation after surgery. To decrease the risk of injury, the width of a transverse incision should be kept within the width of the rectus muscle. Neuropathy typically manifests with burning or pain at the incision site that radiates to the groin as well as paresthesia over mons pubis, labia, and inner thigh. The symptoms typically improve after infiltration with local anesthetic.

Treatment typically includes pharmacologic agents such as tricyclic antidepressants or gabapentin; however, nerves blocks, trigger point injection, or surgical nerve resection may also be necessary. Resecting the nerve requires extending the prior transverse incision to the anterior superior iliac spine and exposing the interface between the external oblique and the internal oblique muscle. The two nerves course between these two muscles and can be identified and sectioned close to the lateral sidewall.

Complete relief of pain can occur after nerve resection in more than 70% of patients. Ilioinguinal and iliohypogastric nerve entrapment is typically under recognized and should be considered in cases of chronic pelvic pain associated with history of abdominal surgery (Bradshaw and Advincula 2010; Irvin et al. 2004).

2.5   Genitofemoral

The genitofemoral nerve (L1-L2) runs along the ventral surface of the psoas muscle, lies lateral to the external iliac artery, and branches near the inguinal ligament. Similarly to the femoral nerve, it is at risk of compression during laparotomy with the use of self-retaining retractors. In addition it can be directly damaged during retroperitoneal dissection, removal of pelvic masses adherent to the side wall, or with removal of external iliac lymph nodes. During such dissections the nerve should be isolated and preserved if possible. Neural deficits include groin pain and paresthesia over the ipsilateral mons, labia, and anterior thigh below the inguinal ligament (Bradshaw and Advincula 2010; Irvin et al. 2004).

2.6   Common Peroneal

Common peroneal nerve (L4-S2) courses laterally across the knee in close proximity to bone with little superficial protection. It can be injured due to poor positioning of the knee and lower leg by pressing against the hard surface of stirrups. The nerve may be pressed against the fibular head; therefore, careful positioning, avoiding pressure on the lateral knee, and use of padding may decrease the chance of injury. Neurological deficits include paresthesia over the lateral lower leg and dorsum of the foot, weakness of ankle extension, or foot dorsiflexion. The patients typically present with foot drop (Bradshaw and Advincula 2010; Craig 2013; Irvin et al. 2004).

2.7   Sciatic Nerve

Sciatic nerve (L4-S3) courses beneath the piriformis muscle and through the greater sciatic foramen as it exits the pelvis to travel down the posterior thigh to the popliteal fossa. Injury during open surgery is rare but may result in an event of a sudden hemorrhage requiring placement of sutures deep within lateral pelvis to control bleeding. The injury has also been reported with pelvic exenteration surgery.

Symptoms of injury typically involve pain as well as weakness affecting most of the lower leg musculature and hamstrings while sparing hip flexion, extension, abduction, adduction, and knee extension. Sensory loss involves the lower leg. The ankle reflex is absent, while the knee reflex is normal (Craig 2013; Irvin et al. 2004).

2.8   Obturator Nerve

Obturator nerve (L2-L4) courses through psoas muscle, passes behind the common iliac arteries and laterally to the internal iliac artery and ureter, then runs along the lateral wall of pelvis anterior to the obturator vessels to the obturator foramen, and enters the thigh through the obturator canal. In gynecologic surgery it is most frequently injured during retroperitoneal dissection for malignancies or endometriosis resection (Cardosi et al. 2002). The nerve can be exposed with gentle medial or lateral traction on the external iliac artery and vein.

If perioperative injury is diagnosed, the damage should be immediately repaired with microsurgical technique. Nerve injury can also occur during mid-urethral sling operations, particularly the transobturator tape (TOT) procedure (Aydogmus et al. 2014). Nerve injury presents postoperatively with loss of sensation over the inner thighs and motor loss in the hip adductors. Postoperative physical therapy should be initiated promptly including neuromuscular electrical stimulation, electromyographic biofeedback, exercise, and home-treatment regimen. Complete motor recovery is common after physiotherapy (Craig 2013; Irvin et al. 2004).

3   Wound Complications

Wound complications are one of the most common causes of postoperative morbidity. Wound complications (separation, hematoma, seroma, and infection) are estimated to affect 2–5% of abdominal incisions (Sherertz et al. 1992). Poor wound healing or collections of fluid/blood under the skin may cause the incision to separate and predispose the wound to infection.

Wound complications usually present as swelling, pain, and/or drainage of fluid from the incision, most often within 3–10 days after surgery. When infected, the wound is often erythematous, indurated, and tender. Wound infections may be accompanied by fever and/or leukocytosis.

Patients presenting in the postoperative period with any of these symptoms should be carefully evaluated with a thorough history and physical exam. Most of these complications may be managed without imaging or surgical intervention.

Wound separation: Wound separation is defined as separation of the superficial layers of the wound (subcutaneous fat and skin). The underlying fascia is intact. Wound separation in the absence of a fluid collection or infection is uncommon, and if identified within 7–10 days of the initial surgery, delayed surgical re-approximation of the wound may be considered.

Seroma/hematoma: A seroma is a collection of serum under the skin, while a hematoma is a similar collection of blood. A seroma or hematoma separates the superficial layers under the skin and prevents adequate wound healing. These wound complications are commonly related to obesity, immunocompromised and inadequate hemostasis. The fluid collects under the skin and gradually leaks out the incision line. Small hematomas and seromas (<2 cm) may be managed expectantly, while most need to be opened up and drained. During drainage of the fluid collection, it is important to evaluate whether the fascia is intact (see below on wound dehiscence). After drainage of a hematoma or seroma, the wound is generally packed with clean gauze and the wound is allowed to heal by secondary intention. This gauze packing should be removed and replaced one to two times per day to promote healing and decrease the risk of infection. When there is healthy granulation tissue present and no evidence of infection, delayed surgical re-approximation of the wound may be considered.

Abscess/superficial surgical site infection: Fluid collections under the skin are prone to infection. Infection of a fluid collection is by definition an abscess. Clinical suspicion for abscess is high when the wound appears erythematous, indurated,

or warm and when the patient has fevers or leukocytosis. Superficial wound infection in the absence of abscess may be treated with antibiotics alone and close follow-up. Any wound abscess must be opened up and drained. If there is suspicion for a deep surgical site infection (infection of the fascia) or fascial disruption, then the wound exploration should be conducted in the operating room (Figs. 1 and 2). The infected wound should be irrigated, debrided down to the healthy-appearing tissue, and packed open with clean gauze. Once the infection has resolved and granulation tissue is visible, the wound may be closed secondarily. Systemic antibiotics should be considered based on the severity/extent of the infection, presence of systemic symptoms, and medical comorbidities.

A severe form of surgical site infection is necrotizing fasciitis. Necrotizing fasciitis is usually caused by Group A *Streptococcus*, but may be polymicrobial. Necrotizing fasciitis should be considered when patients appear acutely ill, have pain out of proportion to the examination, and demonstrate significant tissue disruption or where the fluid and tissue appear gray and dusky. The skin and more superficial layers may appear relatively unaffected, while the infection involves the fascia and deep muscle layers. Necrotizing fasciitis is an acute infection with significant morbidity and mortality. It is a surgical emergency and should be aggressively treated with surgical debridement with experienced surgeons. Surgical exploration is the only way to accurately diagnose necrotizing fasciitis.

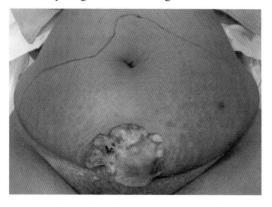

Fig. 1 Abdominal incision surgical site wound infection showing erythema, induration, exudate, and necrosis

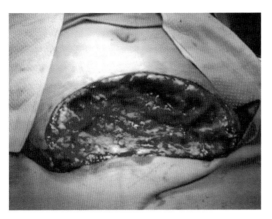

Fig. 2 Wound infection after extensive debridement showing healthy granulation tissue

Wound (fascial) dehiscence: Wound dehiscence occurs when there is separation of the fascial layers, which provide the majority of support for the abdominal wall. Fascial dehiscence is estimated to affect 0.4–3.5% of abdominal surgeries (van Ramshorst et al. 2010). With early fascial dehiscence, the skin may be intact. The patient may report a "popping" sensation upon sitting up or coughing, or the wound may start to leak copious amounts of serosanguinous fluid. The wound should be evaluated for fascial integrity, and any suspicion for fascial dehiscence is a surgical emergency, as the patient is at risk for evisceration.

Evisceration: Evisceration is fascial dehiscence with extrusion of abdominal contents into the incision or onto the abdomen. Evisceration is a surgical emergency, as the exposed bowel may undergo swelling and necrosis. Patients with evisceration should be covered with sterile towels and taken immediately for surgical repair.

4   Cuff Infection

Deep surgical site infections are an uncommon complication after hysterectomy. The rate of infection generally ranges from 1% to 3% (Mahdi et al. 2014). Deep surgical site infections after gynecologic surgery are usually polymicrobial and often represent the endogenous flora of the patient's skin or vagina (Duff and Park 1980; ACOG 2009).

Patients generally present with pain, fever, tachycardia, and tachypnea. Cuff infections are usually identified in the first few days to weeks after hysterectomy. On pelvic exam, the vaginal cuff is diffusely tender and a fluctuant mass may be palpable. Laboratory findings are consistent with systemic infection and include leukocytosis with left shift, elevated erythrocyte sedimentation rate, and an elevated C-reactive protein (Jaiyeoba 2012). Cuff tenderness and evidence of infection are indicative of cuff cellulitis, while such evidence of infection in the setting of a complex fluid collection is suggestive of pelvic abscess.

Any patient with a suspecte pelvic abscess should undergo imaging, usually via computed tomography (CT). CT allows for delineation of the abscess, as well as evaluation of the surrounding organs, which can help rule out bowel or bladder injury as the etiology of the infection.

Postoperative cuff cellulitis may be treated empirically with antibiotics and close monitoring. Broad spectrum antibiotics covering aerobic and anaerobic bacteria are usually effective for cellulitis and for abscesses less than 2 cm (Greenstein et al. 2013). For larger abscesses, percutaneous or surgical drainage should be considered. Percutaneous drainage can be accomplished using ultrasound or CT guidance and may be approached transabdominally,   transgluteally,   or transvaginally.

In patients with abscesses that fail to respond to percutaneous drainage and antibiotics, surgical drainage should be considered. Surgical drainage can be accomplished via laparotomy or laparoscopy, depending on the stability of the patient. Surgical evaluation can confirm the diagnosis, obtain cultures to guide postoperative antibiotic treatment, and remove the abscess/necrotic tissue. Copious irrigation is used and a drain is usually left in situ.

5   Cuff Evisceration

Vaginal cuff evisceration is the dehiscence of the vaginal tissue with associated prolapse of small bowel through the vagina (Fig. 8). Vaginal cuff evisceration is extremely rare, and estimates range from 0.032% to 1.2% (Ceccaroni et al. 2011; Croak et al. 2004; Kho et al. 2009). Patients with cuff evisceration most commonly present with pelvic/abdominal pain and vaginal bleeding or watery discharge (Cronin et al. 2012). However, they may be asymptomatic. These patients typically present in the first 6 weeks after surgery, but may present up to 30 years later (Cronin et al. 2012). Some cases are precipitated by intercourse, defecation, or Valsalva (such as cough or sneeze); however, the majority of cases are spontaneous (Croak et al. 2004; Nick et al. 2011).

Asymptomatic cuff separation without evisceration may be managed expectantly and left to close by secondary intention. Once the bowel has eviscerated, surgical management is necessary. Surgical closure of the cuff may be accomplished vaginally, laparoscopically, or via laparotomy. There is not enough data to recommend one approach over another. If the bowel is compromised, then laparoscopic or open technique should be undertaken with resection of non-viable bowel. If the prolapsed bowel is viable, then the approach may be laparoscopic, open, or vaginal (Gandhi and Jha 2011). Laparoscopic and open techniques allow the surgeon to fully evaluate the bowel for any injuries. The vaginal approach has lower morbidity and allows recovery without any abdominal incisions (Cronin et al. 2012).

6   Delayed Complications Presenting in the Early Postoperative Period (Within 3 Months)

6.1   Urinary Tract Fistulae

The most common operative complication during hysterectomy or cesarean section is urinary tract injury. The exact prevalence of bladder and ureteral injury during obstetric/gynecologic surgery is unknown, though estimates range from 0.3% to 4.3% (Teeluckdharry et al. 2015).

The bladder is most commonly injured during (1) entry into the peritoneal cavity, (2) development of the bladder flap at the time of cesarean section or hysterectomy, or (3) closure of the vaginal cuff at the time of hysterectomy. The ureters are less commonly injured, but are most vulnerable at the time of ligation of the ovarian vessels and ligation of the uterine vessels or during transection of the vaginal cuff.

Many urinary tract injuries are recognized and repaired intraoperatively and usually heal well. Sometimes injuries may be detected in the immediate postoperative period (within 1–4 days). These usually present as fever, unilateral or bilateral flank pain, and/or the inability to urinate. Damage to the ureter or bladder may result in leakage of urine into the peritoneal cavity, which then is reabsorbed, causing an elevation in creatinine. This collection of fluid may be detected on ultrasound or computed tomography (CT) scan, and any postoperative patient with these symptoms should be evaluated with a high index of suspicion for ureteral or bladder injury. The typical workup includes: careful physical examination, measurement of serum creatinine, pelvic/abdominal ultrasound, or CT scan. If a collection of urine (urinoma) is found, then prompt consultation by a urologic surgeon is needed to determine if immediate surgical repair may be indicated to reduce further postoperative complications, such as genitourinary fistula (Tables 1 and 2).

6.1.1   Postoperative Recognition

It is impossible to know how many unrecognized injuries heal spontaneously. However, it is clear that some unrecognized injuries may result in serious sequelae. The most common sequela of a bladder or ureteral injury is an abnormal communication between two organs called a fistula. The incidence of genitourinary fistulae after

Table 1 Examples of common fistulae and their nomenclature

Organ 1	Organ 2	Fistula
Bladder	Vagina	Vesico-vaginal
Bladder	Uterus	Vesico-uterine
Ureter	Vagina	Ureterovaginal
Ureter	Uterus	Uretero-uterine
Rectum	Vagina	Rectovaginal
Small bowel	Vagina	Enterovaginal
Small bowel	Skin	Entero-cutaneous

Table 2 Nerves commonly injured in gynecologic surgery

Nerve	Nerve roots	Motor function	Sensory function	Presenting symptom	Mode of injury
Ilioinguinal, iliohypogastric	T12-L1	None	Mons pubis, labia, and inner thigh	Pain at the incision site that radiates to the groin. Paresthesia over mons pubis, labia, and inner thigh	Direct surgical injury or nerve incorporation during fascial closure
Genitofemoral	L1-L2	None	Mons, labia, and anterior thigh below the inguinal ligament	Groin pain and paresthesia over the ipsilateral mons, labia, and anterior thigh below the inguinal ligament	Compression from retractors. Retroperitoneal dissection
Femoral	L2-L4	Hip flexion, adduction, knee extension	Anterior thigh, medial leg	Weakness of hip flexion, knee extension. Unstable knee, unable to climb stairs, absent patellar reflex	Compression from retractors. Improper positioning in lithotomy
Lateral femoral cutaneous	L2-L3	None	Anterior lateral thigh	Numbness, paresthesia, and pain over the anterior lateral thigh from the inguinal ligament to the knee	Compression from retractors. Improper positioning in lithotomy
Obturator	L2-L4	Thigh adduction	Inner thigh	Weakness of thigh adduction. Paresthesias/ numbness over inner thigh	Retroperitoneal dissection. Transobturator mid-urethral sling
Sciatic	L4-S3	Lower leg musculature and hamstrings	Lower leg	Weakness of most of the lower leg musculature and hamstrings, spared hip flexion, extension, abduction, adduction, and knee extension. Paresthesia/ numbness of the lower leg. Absent ankle reflex, but normal knee reflex	Placement of sutures deep within lateral pelvis to control bleeding. Pelvic exenteration surgery
Common peroneal	L4-S2	Ankle extension and foot dorsiflexion	Lateral lower leg and dorsum of the foot	Foot drop (poor foot dorsiflexion). Paresthesia over lateral lower leg and dorsum of foot	Poor positioning of the knee and lower leg against the hard surface of stirrups

gynecologic surgery is estimated to range between 0.13% and 2% (Meeks and Roth 2011; Adelman et al. 2014).

Fistulae classically present within 7–30 days after surgery. Patients usually complain of painless leakage of urine or fluid from the vagina. Anyone with leakage of fluid from the vagina should undergo a careful physical exam to determine the source and consistency of the leakage. The fluid may be examined by wet mount and culture to evaluate for infection and by urinalysis to confirm a urinary source. Often it may be difficult to identify the source of the leakage of the fluid, and the bladder may be evaluated by one of several techniques:

1. Filling the bladder with blue fluid (usually normal saline with a few drops of methylene blue) and looking for leakage of blue fluid in the vagina.
2. Cystoscopy: A cystoscope is inserted through the urethra to directly visualize the inside surface of the bladder. A fistula may be directly identified using this technique.
3. Cystogram: Radio-opaque dye is instilled into the bladder and leakage is identified by X-ray.

Care must be taken to exclude urinary incontinence (leakage from the urethra) that may mimic a fistula on X-ray (Fig. 3).

4. CT Urogram: Computerized tomography is used to evaluate the integrity of the bladder and upper urinary tract.

It is important to remember that multiple injuries may coexist. Injury to the bladder may signify additional injury to the distal ureter, and ureterovaginal fistula must be ruled out, even if a vesico-vaginal fistula has been diagnosed. The ureter is usually evaluated using a CT urogram or an intravenous pyelogram.

When identified, the first treatment for a genitourinary fistula is continuous bladder drainage while the injury heals. With continuous drainage via transurethral catheter, small fistulas may heal without surgical intervention. Continuous catheterization is usually recommended for 6 weeks to 3 months after the initial injury. Once the inflammatory stage of wound healing is completed, if the connection is still present, then surgery is necessary to treat the fistula.

Surgical repair may be attempted vaginally, laparoscopically, or via open abdominal surgery. Surgical approach depends on surgeon preference, health of the surrounding tissue, the size and location of the fistula, and whether it has been repaired before. Generally the first repair of most fistulas is attempted vaginally, especially for small fistulas just above the trigone of the bladder. Abdominal/laparoscopic procedures are reserved for complicated repairs, repeat procedures, and patients who have been irradiated or those with extremely large injuries or ureteral involvement.

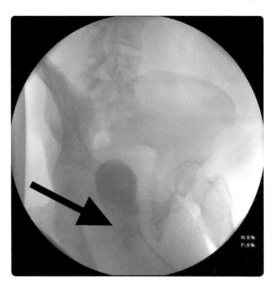

Fig. 3 Cystogram showing large defect in the bladder with extravasation of dye into the vagina (Originally published in: Wild et al. 2012; with kind permission of Elsevier. All rights reserved)

within the first few days of surgery and is discussed elsewhere. Chronic injury may result in a fistulous tract.

Any leakage of fecal contents from the vagina should be evaluated promptly. Rectal injuries are common after vaginal deliveries, particularly after instrumented deliveries using vacuum or forceps. These injuries are usually repaired at the time of delivery, but may break down or be inadequately repaired.

Leakage of gas or liquid stool from the vagina is the presenting complaint of women with a rectovaginal fistula. Leakage of solid stool is usually indicative of a large fistula or a defect in the anal sphincter. These distal connections can often be found on careful physical exam with a finger in the rectum. Any defect can be gently probed with a cotton-tipped swab or a small instrument. The connection can usually be identified in this manner (Fig. 4).

Similar to urinary tract fistulae, rectovaginal fistulae are generally allowed to heal until all inflammatory and granulation tissue is resolved. The tract is then surgically excised and the intervening tissue repaired in layers. Postoperatively, the patient is encouraged to have bulky, soft bowel

7 Rectovaginal and Enterovaginal Fistulae

Injury to the large or small intestines is one of the most dreaded intraoperative complications from ob/gyn surgery. Acute injury, when repaired intraoperatively, generally has little consequence. However, unrecognized bowel injury is one of the most significant causes of postoperative morbidity and mortality. Acute injury may be identified

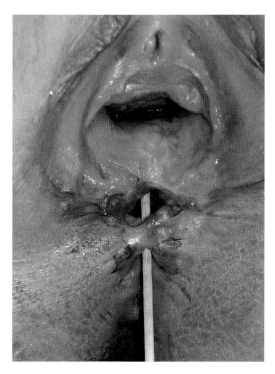

Fig. 4 Rectovaginal fistula

movements for 3 months, through aggressive dietary and bowel management.

Connections higher up in the rectum or involving the large bowel may be identified on colonoscopy or using X-ray in conjunction with a radio-opaque enema. Connections involving the small intestines are difficult to diagnose and may require computed tomography. Fistulas involving the small or large bowel should be managed in cooperation with a colorectal surgeon.

8   Thromboembolism

Venous thromboembolism is the leading cause of postoperative mortality. Deep vein thrombosis (DVT) is usually occult and may resolve without complication, and death from DVT-associated pulmonary embolism (PE) is responsible for up to 300,000 deaths annually in the United States alone (Tapson 2008).

Venous thrombosis is caused by activation of the clotting mechanism within the venous circulation. These blood clots may become dislodged and migrate to the right heart and pulmonary artery, where they may result in occlusion and cardiac strain.

The postoperative period is a time of increased risk for venous thromboembolism due to: (1) venous stasis due to paralysis during surgery, (2) perioperative release of coagulation factors, and (3) the relative immobility of the postoperative period. Many studies have shown that perioperative treatment with sequential compression devices, chemoprophylaxis, and early/aggressive ambulation are all effective at decreasing the risk of perioperative thromboembolism.

The most common presentation of DVT is (often unilateral) edema, leg pain, leg tenderness, and warmth or erythema of the skin over the thrombosis. Pulmonary embolism may manifest as acute shortness of breath or chest pain and may be the presenting symptom of DVT.

Physical exam findings are nonspecific. Patients may demonstrate calf pain upon dorsiflexion of the foot (Homans' sign). They may demonstrate a palpable cordlike section of vein along the posterior of the calf. This "cord" may or may not be tender to palpation.

Further evaluation is necessary when considering a diagnosis of DVT. The American Academy of Family Physicians (AAFP) and the American College of Physicians (ACP) recommend a complete workup including the following (Qaseem et al. 2007; Snow et al. 2007):

Clinical parameter to predict DVT (Wells et al. 1997)	Score
Active cancer	+1
Paralysis or recent plaster immobilization of lower extremities	+1
Recently bedridden for more than 3 days or major surgery within 12 weeks	+1
Local tenderness in the distribution of the deep venous system	+1
Entire leg swollen	+1
Calf swelling 3 cm larger than asymptomatic side (measured 10 cm below tibial tuberosity)	+1
Pitting edema confined to the symptomatic leg	+1

(*continued*)

Clinical parameter to predict DVT (Wells et al. 1997)	Score
Collateral superficial veins (non-varicose)	+1
Alternative diagnosis at least as likely as DVT	−2

Pretest assessment of clinical factors uses validated criteria, such as the Wells criteria. The Wells criteria to predict DVT include nine different clinical factors, which are scored as a clinical probability. A score of $< = 0$ is low, 1–2 is intermediate, and $> = 3$ is high.

In patients with a low pretest probability based on clinical criteria, a high-sensitivity D-dimer assay may be used to rule out DVT. If the D-dimer assay is positive, or if the patient is older/has significant comorbidities, then further testing is indicated.

Doppler ultrasound testing of the venous system is recommended for anyone with intermediate or high scoring of clinical criteria. Doppler ultrasound of the calf may be negative; therefore, if suspicious of DVT confined to the calf, repeat ultrasound testing or contrast venography may be indicated.

If suspicious for pulmonary embolism, pretest assessment of clinical factors should similarly be performed. Wells criteria to predict PE include six different clinical factors, and similar to the Wells score for DVT, the Wells score for PE is scored as low, intermediate, or high probability; a score of 0–1 is low risk, 2–6 is intermediate risk, and $>= 7$ is high risk.

Clinical parameter to predict PE (van Belle et al. 2006)	Score
Previous PE or DVT	+1.5
Heart rate >100 beats per minute	+1.5
Recent surgery or immobilization	+1.5
Clinical signs of deep venous thrombosis	+3
Alternative diagnosis less likely than pulmonary embolism	+3
Hemoptysis	+1
Cancer	+1

If the clinical suspicion for DVT or PE is high, it is reasonable to begin treatment while the workup is confirming the diagnosis. The risks of untreated DVT or PE are high and may outweigh the risks of a brief treatment of anticoagulation, even if such treatment is ultimately unnecessary.

Once diagnosed, the mainstay of treatment for DVT or PE is anticoagulation. Low-molecular-weight heparin (LMWH) should be used for initial inpatient treatment of DVT. LMWH is superior to unfractionated heparin for the treatment of DVT for ease of dosing and maintenance, as well as an overall reduction in mortality and major bleeding. Treatment is generally administered for 3–6 months for DVT due to transient risk factors such as surgery. Outpatient treatment is reasonable and may consist of daily injections with LMWH or transition to an oral treatment, such as a vitamin K antagonist. Compression stockings should be used to prevent post-thrombotic syndrome, a chronic syndrome of leg pain, swelling, and ulceration that occurs in up to half of patients with DVT. The stockings should be worn staring within 1 month of DVT diagnosis and continued for at least a year (Vazquez and Kahn 2010).

9 Delayed Complications Presenting in the Late Postoperative Period (Months to Years)

9.1 Pelvic Organ Prolapse

Pelvic organ prolapse is the descent of any of the pelvic organs. Hysterectomy is a known risk factor for the development of pelvic organ prolapse. A large study of community dwelling women found that women with prolapse were 1.68× more likely to have undergone a prior hysterectomy (Lawrence et al. 2008). The incidence of prolapse after hysterectomy is higher for women who had a hysterectomy for prolapse (1.6–11.6%) compared to women who had a hysterectomy for other indications (0.3–1.8%) (Mant et al. 1997; Marchionni et al. 1999).

The main symptom of pelvic organ prolapse is the sensation of pressure or bulge in the vagina (Fig. 5). Severe complications of prolapse are rare. Prolapse diagnosis is usually based on physical exam, though several formal staging systems exist. Asymptomatic or minimally symptomatic prolapse may not require any intervention.

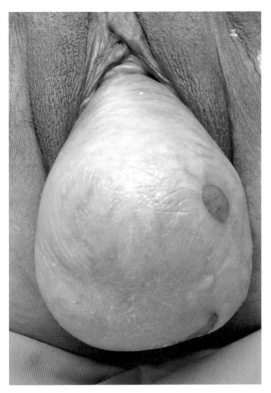

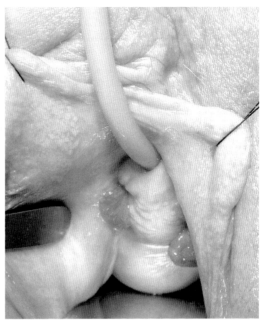

Fig. 6 Granulation tissue at cuff (Originally published in: Stember et al. 2003; with kind permission of Springer Science + Business Media. All rights reserved)

Fig. 5 Pelvic organ prolapse after hysterectomy

Patients with significant bother may elect to use a plastic device (pessary) to hold their prolapsed organs in place, or they may elect for surgery. There are a variety of surgical procedures for prolapse, depending on the patient's health, preferences, degree, and location of prolapse.

9.1.1 Cuff Complications

Granulation Tissue

The most common abnormal postoperative finding at the vaginal cuff is granulation tissue. Granulation tissue is an over-proliferation of healing tissue that may be found on any wound. Granulation tissue is usually described as beefy red and friable (see Fig. 6).

Most cases of vaginal granulation tissue are asymptomatic, but may also cause vaginal bleeding, particularly after intercourse. Granulation tissue at the cuff is benign and may be treated with topical cautery using (Saropola and Ingsirorat 1998) sticks or may be excised. Excision may be preferred when the tissue is large and symptomatic or if the diagnosis is in question. Other conditions may occasionally be mistaken for granulation tissue, including malignancy or fallopian tube prolapse (Song et al. 2005).

Fallopian Tube Prolapse

Fallopian tube prolapse is a rare complication of hysterectomy, whereby the fallopian tube is either incorporated into the vaginal cuff or prolapses through an open cuff. This complication usually presents with severe low abdominal pain or a pulling sensation and tenderness to palpation of the cuff. The tube may be visible at the apex of the vagina, and biopsy or excisional biopsy can confirm the diagnosis (Figs. 7 and 8).

If the diagnosis is confirmed, revision of the cuff is usually necessary to relieve symptoms. This revision may be performed vaginally, and the cuff is opened up, the damaged tube is often excised, and the remaining cuff is closed. Laparoscopic/open approach may also allow confirmation of diagnosis and evaluation for additional etiologies of the pain.

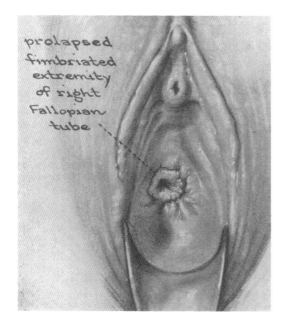

prolapsed fimbriated extremity of right Fallopian tube

Fig. 7 Fallopian tube prolapse (Originally published in: Bower et al. 1940; with kind permission of Elsevier. All rights reserved)

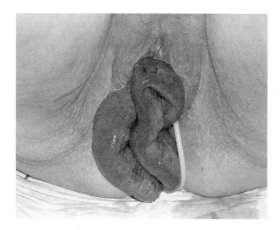

Fig. 8 Vaginal evisceration of small bowel through vaginal cuff (Originally published in: Partsinevelos et al. 2008; with kind permission of Springer Science + Business Media. All rights reserved)

10   Conclusion

All surgical procedures have the risks of postoperative complications. These complications may be immediate or delayed. Delayed postoperative complications can have serious effects for patients, and prompt diagnosis and management is critical. This chapter discusses a variety of complications that can be managed clinically or operatively. A thorough understanding of the mechanism of neurologic injury allows for insight into prevention and recognition, which can reduce the effect on the patient. Wound complications can generally be managed conservatively, and only the most severe infections or fascial dehiscences need surgical management. Fistulae are among the most dreaded complications by surgeons, as they generally represent unrecognized surgical injury; however, with prompt recognition and surgical treatment, most fistulae can be completely cured. Thromboembolism is probably the most dangerous of the postoperative complications, though studies have shown improvement of morbidity and mortality with aggressive prevention and early diagnosis. Finally, pelvic organ prolapse and cuff complications are varied and require clinical insight into diagnosis and management. There is no such thing as a surgeon with no complications, but with enough understanding, preparation, and care, a surgeon can minimize their complications and mitigate the impact upon their patients.

References

ACOG practice bulletin #104: antibiotic prophylaxis for gynecologic procedures. Obstet Gynecol. 2009; 113 (5):1180–9.

Adelman MR, Bardsley TR, Sharp HT. Urinary tract injuries in laparoscopic hysterectomy: a systematic review. J Minim Invasive Gynecol. 2014;21(4):558–66.

Aydogmus S, Kelekci S, Aydogmus H, Ekmekci E, Secil Y, Ture S. Obturator nerve injury: an infrequent complications of TOT procedure. Case Rep Obstet Gynecol. 2014; 1–3.

Bohrer JC, Walters MD, Park A, Polston D, Barber MD. Pelvic nerve injury following gynecologic surgery: a prospective cohort study. Am J Obstet Gynecol. 2009;209:1–7.

Bower JO, Pearce AE, Conway EW. Prolapse and torsion of the right fallopian tube with vaginal bleeding, following vaginal hysterectomy. Am J Obstet Gynecol. 1940;40(6):1047–50.

Bradshaw A, Advincula A. Postoperative neuropathy in gynecologic surgery. Obstet Gynecol Clin North Am. 2010;37:451–9.

Cardosi RJ, Cox CS, Hoffman MS. Postoperative neuropathies after major pelvic surgery. Obstet Gynecol. 2002;100(2):240–4.

Ceccaroni M, Berretta R, Malzoni M, Scioscia M, Roviglione G, Spagnolo E, Rolla M, Farina A, Malzoni C, De Iaco P, Minelli L, Bovicelli L. Vaginal cuff dehiscence after hysterectomy: a multicenter retrospective study. Eur J obstet Gynecol Repro Bio. 2011;158:308–13.

Chan JK, Manetta A. Prevention of femoral nerve injuries in gynecologic surgery. Am J Obstet Gynecol. 2002;186:1–7.

Craig A. Entrapment neuropathies of the lower extremity. Phys Med Rehabil. 2013;5:31–40.

Croak AJ, Gebhart JB, Klingele CJ, Schroeder G, Lee RA, Podratz KC. Characteristics of patients with vaginal rupture and evisceration. Obstet Gynecol. 2004;103:572–6.

Cronin B, Sung VW, Matteson KA. Vaginal cuff dehiscence: risk factors and management. Am J Obstet Gynecol. 2012;206:284–8.

Duff P, Park RC. Antibiotic prophylaxis in vaginal hysterectomy: a review. Obstet Gynecol. 1980;55(5):193s.

Gandhi P, Jha S. Review: vaginal vault evisceration. Obstetrician Gynecologist. 2011;13:231–7.

Greenstein Y, Shah AJ, Vragovic O, Cabral H, Soto-Wright V, Borgatta L, Kuching W. Tuboovarian abscess. Factors associated with operative intervention after failed antibiotic therapy. J Reprod Med. 2013;58(3–4):101–6.

Irvin W, Anderson W, Taylor P, Rice L. Minimizing the risk of neurologic injury in gynecologic surgery. Obstet Gynecol. 2004;103:374–82.

Jaiyeoba O. Postoperative infections in obstetrics and gynecology. Clin Obstet Gyencol. 2012;55(4):904–13.

Kho RM, Akl MN, Cornella JL, Magtibay PM, Wechter ME, Magrina JF. Incidence and characteristics of patients with vaginal cuff dehiscence after robotic procedures. Obstet Gynecol. 2009;114:231–5.

Lawrence JM, Lukacz ES, Nager CW, Hsu JY, Luber KM. Prevalence and co-occurrence of pelvic floor disorders in community-dwelling women. Obstet Gynecol. 2008;111:670–85.

Mahdi H, Goodrich S, Lockhart D, DeBernardo R, Moslemi-Kebria M. Predictors for surgical site infection in women undergoing hysterectomy for benign gynecologic disease: a multicenter analysis using the national surgical quality improvement program data. J Minim Invasive Gynecol. 2014;21(5):901–9.

Mant J, Painter R, Vessey M. Epidemiology of genital prolapse observations from the Oxford Family Planning Association study. Br J Obstet Gynaecol. 1997;104:579–85.

Marchionni M, Bracco GL, Checcucci V, Carabaneanu A, Coccia EM, Mecacci F, Scarselli G. True incidence of vaginal vault prolapse: thirteen years experience. J Reprod Med. 1999;44:679–84.

Meeks GR, Roth TM. Vesicovaginal fistula and urethrovaginal fistula. In: Rock JA, Jones III HW, editors. Te Linde's operative gynecology. 10th ed. Philadelphia: J.B. Lippincott; 2011. p. 973–93.

National Center for Health Statistics. National Hospital Discharge Survey, 2010. [Internet] Number of all-listed procedures for discharges for short-stay hospitals, by procedure category and age: United States, 2010. [Cited 2016 Mar 15]. Available from: http://www.cdc.gov/nchs/data/ndsp/4procedures/2010pro4_numberprocedureage.pdf

Nick AM, Lange J, Frumovitz M, Soliman PT, Schmeler KM, Schlumbrecht MP, dos Reis R, Ramirez PT. Rate of vaginal cuff separation following laparoscopic or robotic hysterectomy. Gynecol Oncol. 2011;120:47–51.

Partsinevelos GA, Rodolakis A, Athanasiou S, Antsaklis A. Vaginal evisceration after hysterectomy: a rare condition a gynecologist should be familiar with. Arch Gynecol Obstet. 2008;279(2):267.

Qaseem A, Snow V, Barry P, Hornbake ER, Rodnick JE, Tobolic T, Ireland B, Segal JB, Bass EB, Weiss KB, Green L, Owens DK. Current diagnosis of venous thromboembolism in primary care: a clinical practice guideline from the American Academy of Family Physicians and the American College of Physicians. Ann Fam Med. 2007;5:57–62.

Saropola N, Ingsirorat C. Conservative treatment of vaginal vault granulation tissue following total abdominal hysterectomy. Int J Gynecol Obstet. 1998;62:55–8.

Sherertz RJ, Garibaldi RA, Marosok RD, Mayhall CG, Scheckler WE, Berg R, Gaynes RP, Jarvis WR, Martone WJ, Lee JT. Consensus paper on the surveillance of surgical wound infections. Infect Control Hosp Epidemiol. 1992;13(10):599.

Snow V, Qaseem A, Barry P, Hornbake ER, Rodnick JE, Tobolic T, Ireland B, Segal J, Bass E, Weiss KB, Green L, Owens DK. Management of venous thromboembolism: a clinical practice guideline from the American College of Physicians and the American Academy of Family Physicians. Ann Intern Med. 2007;146(3):204–10.

Song YS, Kang JS, Park MH. Fallopian tube prolapse misdiagnosed as vault granulation tissue: a report of three cases. Pathol Res Pract. 2005;201(12):819–22.

Stember DS, Scarpero HM, Nitti VW. Vaginal granulation tissue secondary to bone anchors: experience in two patients. J Urol. 2003;169(6):2300–1.

Tapson VF. Acute pulmonary embolism. N Engl J Med. 2008;358(10):1037–52.

Teeluckdharry B, Gilmour D, Flowerdew G. Urinary tract injury at benign gynecologic surgery and the role of cystoscopy: a systematic review and meta-analysis. Obstet Gynecol. 2015;126(6):1161.

van Belle A, Buller HR, Huisman MV, Huisman P, Kaasjager K, Kamphuisen PW, Kramer MHH, Kruip MJHA, Kwakkel-vanErp JM, Leebeek FWG, Nijkeuter M, Prins MH, Sohn M, Tick LW. Effectiveness of managing suspected pulmonary embolism using an algorithm combining clinical probability, d-dimer testing and computed tomography. JAMA. 2006;295:172.

van Ramshorst GH, Nieuwenhuizen J, Hob WCJ, Arends P, Boom J, Jeekel J, Lange JF. Abdominal wound dehiscence in adults: development and validation of a risk model. World J Surg. 2010;34(1):20–7.

Vazquez SR, Kahn SR. Postthrombotic syndrome. Circulation. 2010;121:e217–9.

Warner MA, Warner DO, Harper CM, Schroeder DR, Maxson PM. Lower extremity neuropathies associated with lithotomy positions. Anesthesiology. 2000;93:938–42.

Wells PS, Anderson DR, Bormanis J, Guy F, Mitchell M, Gray L, et al. Value of assessment of pretest probability of deep-vein thrombosis in clinical management. Lancet. 1997;350:1795–8.

Wild TT, Bradley CS, Erickson BA. Successful conservative management of a large iatrogenic vesicovaginal fistula after loop electrosurgical excision procedure. Am J Obstet Gynecol. 2012;207(3):e4–6.

Part IX

Management of Gynecologic Neoplasms and Cancers (Koji Matsuo)

Diagnosis and Management of Gestational Trophoblastic Disease

Jocelyn Garcia-Sayre, Antonio V. Castaneda, Lynda D. Roman, and Koji Matsuo

Abstract

Gestational trophoblastic disease (GTD) refers to all tumors that arise from the maternal placenta. Gestational trophoblastic neoplasm (GTN) is a subset of GTD and refers to choriocarcinoma, placental site trophoblastic tumor, and epithelioid trophoblastic tumor. Persistent GTD may develop after treatment of a molar pregnancy and is also referred to as GTN. The treatment of GTN is stratified based on whether the patient is low risk or high risk as determined by the World Health Organization (WHO) score and International Federation of Gynecology and Obstetrics (FIGO) staging system. Low-risk GTN is treated with single-agent chemotherapy, whereas high-risk GTN should be treated with combination regimens. GTN that does not respond to first-line treatment is said to be resistant or refractory. Resistance to a particular chemotherapeutic regimen is evidenced by a plateau or rise in beta-hCG levels. The overall prognosis for GTN is excellent, even in the setting of refractory disease. GTN affects women of reproductive age, and comprehensive counseling must be performed prior to initiation of gonadotoxic treatment. This chapter also discusses the management of GTN with special considerations such as brain and vaginal metastasis, role of secondary curettage, and post-molar prophylactic chemotherapy.

Keywords

Gestational trophoblastic neoplasm • Persistent gestational trophoblastic disease • Invasive mole • Choriocarcinoma • Placental site trophoblastic tumor • Epithelioid trophoblastic tumor • High-risk gestational trophoblastic neoplasm • Low-risk gestational trophoblastic neoplasm

Contents

J. Garcia-Sayre • L.D. Roman • K. Matsuo (✉)
Division of Gynecologic Oncology, Department of Obstetrics and Gynecology, University of Southern California, Los Angeles, CA, USA
e-mail: Jocelyn.Garcia@med.usc.edu; lroman@med.usc.edu; koji.matsuo@med.usc.edu

A.V. Castaneda
Department of Obstetrics and Gynecology, University of Southern California, Los Angeles, CA, USA
e-mail: Antonio.Castaneda@med.usc.edu

© Springer International Publishing AG (outside the USA) 2017
D. Shoupe (ed.), *Handbook of Gynecology*,
DOI 10.1007/978-3-319-17798-4_11

1   Introduction

Gestational trophoblastic disease (GTD) is the general term used to describe growth disturbances of the placental trophoblast. GTD encompasses the complete mole, partial mole, invasive mole, choriocarcinoma, placental site trophoblastic tumor (PSTT), and epithelioid trophoblastic tumor (ETT). Gestational trophoblastic neoplasia (GTN) is a subset of GTD and refers to the latter four. The term persistent GTD is often used interchangeably with GTN when referring to the diagnosis of post-hydatidiform mole trophoblastic neoplasia. Typically, GTN will arise after a molar pregnancy but can occur in the setting of a normal pregnancy and in rare cases may not be associated with pregnancy. With the advent of various chemotherapeutic regimens, the prognosis for GTN is excellent.

1.1   Epidemiology

The overall incidence of GTD and GTN is low within the general population. The incidence varies widely based on geographical location and race. Southeast Asia and Japan have the highest incidence of GTD. It is unknown at this time why various ethnicities have a higher incidence of GTD and GTN. Currently, the incidence of GTD is documented at 1–3 per 1000 pregnancies (Froeling and Seckl 2014). Given that GTN typically arises from GTD, the incidence of GTN is much lower. In North America the incidence is quoted to be 1 in 40,000 and at 9 per 40,000 in Southeast Asia and Japan (Lurain 2010).

1.2   Presentation

The presentation of GTN is diverse and dependent on the type of neoplasm. Benign moles such as the complete hydatidiform mole present most often with vaginal bleeding and significantly elevated beta-hCG. The elevation in beta-hCG often correlates to the burden of trophoblastic disease (Froeling and Seckl 2014). A single elevated beta-hCG should not be used to make the diagnosis of GTD or GTN. When an ultrasound is performed, hydropic villi are observed, and this is often referred to as a snowstorm appearance (Froeling and Seckl 2014).

Following evacuation of GTD, beta-hCG levels should steadily decline. The majority of patients will have normal beta-hCG levels around 12–14 weeks after evacuation. A plateauing or increase of the beta-hCG is concerning for the development of GTN or persistent GTD. Regression curves have been developed to help identify patients at risk (Schlaerth et al. 1981). Persistent GTD develops when molar tissue invades into the myometrium. Typically, this is seen with the invasive mole but can also be seen in choriocarcinoma, PSTT, and ETT. Table 1 describes the criteria for the diagnosis of post-hydatidiform mole trophoblastic neoplasia or GTN (Committee 2002). GTN can be diagnosed if any one of the criteria is established.

Histologically, the invasive mole appears as excessive growth of the trophoblastic tissue which invades into the myometrium of the uterus. Invasive

Table 1 Criteria for the diagnosis of post-hydatidiform mole trophoblastic neoplasia

GTN may be diagnosed when the plateau of beta-hCG lasts for four measurements over a period of 3 weeks or longer, that is, days 1, 7, 14, and 21[a]
GTN may be diagnosed when there is a rise of beta-hCG of three weekly consecutive measurements or longer, over at least a period of 2 weeks or more, days 1, 7, and 14[a]
GTN is diagnosed when the beta-hCG level remains elevated for 6 months or more

Adopted and modified from FIGO committee report on FIGO staging for gestational trophoblastic neoplasia 2000 (Committee 2002)
[a]A difference of 10% or less between measurements is considered stable and should not be interpreted as a change

Table 2 Summary of clinical presentation and histopathologic findings

GTN type	Presentation /behavior	Histopathology	Management
Invasive mole	• Presents with irregular bleeding after dilation and curettage • Associated with localized invasion; however 15% metastasize to the lung or vagina • High levels of beta-hCG	• Molar tissue which invades the myometrium. • Growth of trophoblastic tissue with the presence of chorionic villi invading myometrium	Chemotherapy
Choriocarcinoma	• Associated with irregular bleeding after dilation and curettage • 50% arise from hydatidiform moles • Increased risk of hemorrhage and vaginal bleeding • Highly malignant tumor with propensity for widespread metastasis via vascular channels- spreading to the lung, liver, and brain • High levels of beta-hCG	• Sheets of anaplastic cytotrophoblasts and syncytiotrophoblasts with absence of chorionic villi	Chemotherapy
Placental Site Trophoblastic Tumor (PSTT)	• Rare • Presents with non-specific vaginal bleeding • Chemoresistant, persistent low levels beta-hCG • Presence of human placental lactogen (hPL) • Metastasizes via lymphatics	• Intermediate trophoblastic tissue without chorionic villi seen invading into the myometrium	Hysterectomy +/− Chemotherapy
Epithelioid Trophoblastic Tumor (ETT)	• Rare • Majority occur after term pregnancy • Presents with non-specific vaginal bleeding • Chemoresistant • Elevated beta-hCG but usually less than 2500	• Mononucleate trophoblastic cells arranged in cords associated with eosinophilic, fibrillary and necrotic debris	Hysterectomy +/− Chemotherapy

Adopted and modified from Lurain (2010)

moles often have local invasion and are less often associated with metastasis. Choriocarcinoma is a highly malignant tumor associated with hemorrhage, widespread metastasis, and sheets of anaplastic cytotrophoblasts and syncytiotrophoblasts. Choriocarcinomas are typically very chemosensitive. Placental site trophoblastic tumor is a rare form of GTN that arises after a term pregnancy and histologically consists of intermediate trophoblasts. PSTT has slow growth within the uterus and only metastasizes late in its course. Patients with PSTT usually present with low levels of beta-hCG and irregular vaginal bleeding. Surgery of the primary tumor and multi-agent chemotherapy are the mainstays of treatment for PSTT (Lurain 1990); (Abrão et al. 2008; Papadopoulos et al. 2002). Epithelioid trophoblastic tumor is an extremely rare type of GTN

with little documentation in the literature. ETT can arise from either a previously gestation or without a previously documented gestation. ETT is chemoresistant; therefore, surgery is the mainstay of treatment when confined to the uterus. Histologically, ETT develops from the chorionic-type intermediate trophoblast (Allison et al. 2006; Lurain 1990) (Table 2).

1.3 Treatment Overview

The treatment for GTN is determined by whether the patient is found to be low risk or high risk. There are two classification systems for GTN: International Federation of Gynecology and Obstetrics (FIGO) and the World Health Organization (WHO). The FIGO staging criteria defines stage based on extent of disease (Table 3). The World Health Organization (WHO) proposed a classification system that divides patients into low-risk and high-risk categories with the purpose of defining the best course of treatment (Table 4). It uses independent prognostic factors to risk stratify patients based on the likelihood of being successfully treated with single-agent versus multi-agent chemotherapy. Low-risk patients are likely to achieve 90% response to single-agent chemotherapy, whereas high-risk patient will need multi-agent chemotherapy (Lurain et al. 1991).

After successful treatment for GTD, it is imperative to follow the patient with serial beta-hCG levels weekly until undetectable levels are noted for 3 weeks. Monthly beta-hCG measurements should then be drawn for

6–12 months. Six months follow-up may be sufficient if the decline in beta-hCG follows the normal regression curve as detailed by Morrow et al. (1977). However, 12 months follow-up is recommended if regression is irregular. During the monitoring for declining serial beta-hCG, it is necessary for the patient to be on effective contraception. A concomitant pregnancy at the time of beta-hCG evaluation will lead to an inability to monitor for disease recurrence. The intrauterine device, however, is not recommended as birth control for patients with GTD given the risk for uterine perforation. Oral contraceptive pills and implantable devices are both safe for use (Berkowitz and Goldstein 2009).

2 Management of Primary GTN

Primary GTN is highly curable with chemotherapy. Primary treatment is dictated by the WHO and FIGO score as above. A WHO score of 6 or less with FIGO stages I–III is considered to be low-risk disease and can be treated with a single chemotherapeutic agent. A score of 7 or greater with FIGO stages I–III or FIGO stage IV is considered to be high-risk disease and calls for treatment with a combination of agents.

Table 3 FIGO staging system

Stage	Extent of disease
I	Limited to the uterus
II	Extension beyond uterus to adnexa, broad ligament, or the vagina
III	Extension to the lungs with or without extension to genital tract
IV	Other metastatic sites

Adopted and modified from FIGO Committee on Gynecologic Oncology (Oncology 2009)

Table 4 WHO prognostic scoring system

Score assigned	0	1	2	4
Age at diagnosis	Less than 40	40 or greater	-	-
Prior pregnancy	Mole	Abortion	Term	-
Interval between index pregnancy (months)	Less than 4	4–6	7–12	More than 1 year
Pretreatment beta-hCG	Less than 1000	1000–10,000	10,000–100,000	Greater than 100,000
Tumor size (cm); including uterine mass size	Less than 3	Greater than 3 but less than 5	5 or greater	-
Metastatic location	Lung*	Kidney/spleen	GI	Brain or liver
Number of metastases	0	1–4	5–8	9 or more
Failed chemotherapy	-	-	Single agent	Multi-agent

*Lung metastases should only be included in the WHO score if seen on Chest X-Ray (CXR). Lung CT-Scan may be used but should not influence the score because of the likely presence of lung micro-metastases. If counted, they would increase the score without adding any clinical benefit. While a lung metastasis receives a score of 0, it may be included when counting the total number of metastatic lesions if visualized on CXR
Adopted and modified from FIGO Committee on Gynecologic Oncology (Abrão et al. 2008; Oncology 2009)

Table 5 Response rate for chemotherapy regimens for low-risk GTN

Regimen	Primary Remission Rate (%)
(a) MTX 0.4 mg/kg IM for 5 days, repeated q2 weeks	87–93
(b) MTX 50 mg IM or 1 mg/kg QOD for four doses with leucovorin 15 mg or 0.1 mg/kg administered 24–30 h after each MTX dose	74–90
(c) MTX 30 mg/m^2 or 50 mg/m2 IM given weekly	49–74
(d) Act-D 1.25 mg/m^2 IV q2 weeks (pulsed regimen)	69–90
(e) Act-D 12 µg/kg for 5 days, repeated q2 weeks	77–94
(f) (i) MTX 20 mg IM on D1–D5 with 500ug Act-D IV on D1–D5 q2 weeks (ii) Act-D 0.6 mg/m^2 on D1 and D2 with MTX 100 mg/m^2 IV push and then infusion of 300 mg/m^2 on D1–D2 followed by leucovorin for 2 weeks	100

Adopted and modified from Lurain (2011)
Abbreviations: *MTX*, methotrexate; *Act-D*, actinomycin D; *QOD*, every other day; *q2 week*, every 2 weeks

2.1 Low-risk GTN: Chemotherapy

As mentioned above, low-risk GTN is usually treated with single-agent chemotherapy. Two agents are typically used for treatment of low-risk disease, methotrexate and actinomycin D with cure rates of approximately 100%. Etoposide was historically used for low-risk disease, but this has fallen out of favor due to the slightly increased risk of secondary malignant tumors, especially leukemia (Rustin et al. 1996). Several different dosing regimens have been studied for methotrexate and actinomycin D; these are discussed below. Table 5 summarizes the regimens and includes their primary remission rates.

(a) Methotrexate 0.4 mg/kg intramuscularly (IM) for 5 days, repeated every 2 weeks. The primary failure rate is approximately 11% for non-metastatic disease (Lurain and Elfstrand 1995). The response rate in women with metastatic disease has been quoted to be 60% (Soper et al. 1994).

(b) Methotrexate with folinic acid (leucovorin) rescue: Methotrexate 50 mg IM or 1 mg/kg every other day for four doses with leucovorin 15 mg or 0.1 mg/kg administered 24–30 h after each methotrexate dose. In patients with nonmetastatic disease, only 7.7% of those treated with methotrexate alone developed resistant disease requiring a change in chemotherapy for induction of remission, while 27.5% of patients initially treated with the leucovorin rescue required a change in regimen to achieve remission. Thus, the frequency of drug resistance is significantly higher in those treated with the leucovorin rescue (Matsui et al. 2005). However, the use of methotrexate alone has been shown to be more toxic than the methotrexate-folinic acid combination.

(c) Methotrexate 30 mg/m^2 or 50 mg/m^2 IM given weekly. This regimen was used in GOG-174 to compare response rates to those of actinomycin D 1.25 mg/m^2 IV every 2 weeks (Osborne et al. 2011). Actinomycin D was found to be more effective with a response rate of 70% compared to 53% for weekly methotrexate.

(d) Actinomycin D 1.25 mg/m^2 IV every 2 weeks (pulsed regimen). Actinomycin D is associated with alopecia and is therefore less favored by patients.

(e) Actinomycin D 12 µg/kg for 5 days. This is an alternative to the 5-day methotrexate regimen. This regimen has shown to be effective in patients who failed to respond to the 1.25 mg/m^2 pulse actinomycin D regimen with an 80% response rate (Kohorn 2002).

(f) Combined methotrexate and actinomycin D: The following dosing regimens have been used for this combination regimen:
  (i) Methotrexate 20 mg IM on D1–D5 with 500 µg actinomycin D IV on D1–D5 every 14 days (Abrão et al. 2008).

(ii) Actinomycin D 0.6 mg/m^2 on D1 and D2 with methotrexate 100 mg/m^2 IV push and then infusion of 300 mg/m^2 on D1–D2 followed by leucovorin for 14 days (Eiriksson et al. 2012). Higher remission rates have been reported when the combination is used as compared to each drug alone. It is has also proven to lead to a cure faster, requiring a fewer number of cycles (Eiriksson et al. 2012). The combination regimens ultimately yielded a greater number of grades 3 and 4 toxicities as defined by the Common Terminology Criteria of Adverse Events (CTCAE). Therefore, taking into consideration the frequency of toxic effects and a modest increase in remission rate, a combined regimen may be better suited for second-line therapy (Abrão et al. 2008).

GOG-275 is an ongoing multicenter phase III randomized control trial that compares the use of multiday methotrexate versus actinomycin D in treating patients with low-risk GTN. At present, the question of whether methotrexate versus actinomycin D should be used as first-line treatment for GTN remains unanswered (Alazzam et al. 2012a). While GOG-174 attempted to answer this question, it used the weekly methotrexate regimen which has been shown to be inferior to the multiday regimen. A Cochrane review meta-analysis concluded that actinomycin D is much more likely to achieve a primary cure when compared to methotrexate (82% in the actinomycin D group compared to 53% in the methotrexate group); however, the review included data from different dosing regimens making it difficult to draw a clear conclusion. The results from GOG-275 will help determine whether actinomycin D or methotrexate should be first-line choice for treatment of low-risk GTN (Alazzam et al. 2012a).

In general, treatment should be continued beyond the first negative beta-hCG titer; this is known as consolidation therapy (Lybol et al. 2012). Usually 2–3 cycles of chemotherapy are recommended, especially if the decrease in beta-hCG is slow or if there is extensive disease.

2.2   Low-risk GTN: Adjuvant Surgery

2.2.1   Second Curettage

Attempts have been made to curtail chemotherapy in the setting of low-risk GTN. The theory behind a second curettage is that debulking the tumor will lead to a decreased need for chemotherapy. Single institution retrospective studies have reported varying outcomes. The Dutch published a retrospective cohort study evaluating the effect of a second curettage on low-risk GTN (van Trommel et al. 2005). Their primary outcome measures were the need for chemotherapy and the number of chemotherapy courses required. Unfortunately, only 9.4% of patients were cured after curettage and required no further chemotherapy. However, those patients who received a second curettage required a fewer number of chemotherapy cycles, and the authors concluded that the second curettage offers a "debulking" effect. A second curettage is not without complications; 4.8% of patients in this study had a major complication such as uterine perforation and hemorrhage. Another retrospective study from the United Kingdom concluded that 60% of their patients did not require chemotherapy after a second evacuation (Pezeshki et al. 2004).

Until recently there was only one published prospective study from Iran evaluating the clinical response to a second curettage, with a small sample size of 12 (Yarandi et al. 2014): 83% of patients did not require chemotherapy and were cured by a second curettage. Eight percent of patients experienced a complication such as uterine perforation.

A second curettage has not been considered standard practice. Most practitioners believe that a second curettage should be reserved for patients who experience significant vaginal bleeding and anemia after the first curettage. The GOG recently published a multicenter prospective phase II study evaluating the efficacy and safety of a second curettage in lieu of chemotherapy for patients with low-risk GTN (persistent GTD). The study population included women with non-metastatic low-risk GTN. Patients whose first curettage revealed choriocarcinoma, PSTT, or ETT were excluded. Patients with previously treated low-risk GTN were excluded. The method of

Table 6 Efficacy of second curettage for persistent GTD/low-risk GTN

Author	Year	Study type	No.[a]	Response rate (%)	Complication rate
van Trommel et al. 2005	2005	Retrospective, multicenter	85	9.4	4.8 %
Pezeshki et al. 2004	2004	Retrospective, multicenter	282	60	n.a.
Yarandi et al. 2014	2014	Prospective, single institution	12	83	8 %
Osborne et al. 2016	2016	Prospective, multicenter	60	40	10 %

[a]Patients who underwent second curettage for persistent GTD

evacuation was not specified by the study but could include intraoperative ultrasound localization of the residual trophoblast or directed hysteroscopic resection. Forty percent of the patients were cured after the second curettage with only 10% of patients experiencing a complication. 1.6% of patients experienced uterine perforation that was managed by observation, 6.7% grade 1, and 1.6% grade 3 incidents of uterine hemorrhage as defined by the CTCAE 3.0. They concluded that a second curettage as initial treatment for low-risk GTN cures 40% of patients without significant morbidity (Osborne et al. 2016).

Table 6 provides a summary of the above-referenced studies evaluating the use of second curettage in the setting of low-risk GTN. Generally, the decision for second curettage should not be taken lightly, and patients must be counseled regarding the risks including hysterectomy if profuse bleeding and/or uterine perforation are encountered. Whether or not to perform a second curettage should be determined on a case-by-case basis given that methotrexate and actinomycin D are generally well tolerated and have excellent response rates.

2.2.2 Adjuvant Hysterectomy

Historically, the accepted indications for hysterectomy in women with GTN were removal of chemoresistant disease and to control hemorrhage or infection in emergency cases. However, a hysterectomy can be employed to help decrease the amount of chemotherapy required for treatment of low-risk GTN. The Japanese published a prospective trial evaluating the efficacy of adjuvant hysterectomy in women with and without metastatic disease (Suzuka et al. 2001). They treated 115 women with single-agent

chemotherapy (the majority treated with etoposide) and then performed interval hysterectomy. Adjuvant hysterectomy decreased the total dose of etoposide given to achieve primary remission in women with nonmetastatic disease. There was no difference in the number of chemotherapy cycles required for remission in patients with metastatic disease. Thus, the authors concluded that adjuvant hysterectomy is a viable option for women who have completed childbearing and whose disease is confined to the uterus. Another study also concluded that adjuvant hysterectomy significantly reduced the amount of chemotherapy used to achieve remission (Hammond et al. 1980).

2.3 High-Risk GTN: Chemotherapy

Unlike treatment of low-risk GTN, high-risk GTN should be treated with combination regimens, as opposed to single-agent therapy. High-risk GTN patients are at risk of developing drug resistance to methotrexate when it is used as a single agent. Below are the most widely studied combination regimens and associated toxicities:

(a) Cyclophosphamide, hydroxyurea, actinomycin D, methotrexate, doxorubicin, melphalan, and vincristine (CHAMOMA). In 1981 the GOG instituted a prospective randomized protocol comparing CHAMOMA and methotrexate, actinomycin D, and chlorambucil (MAC) (Curry et al. 1989). At that time, MAC was the standard of care for patients with high-risk disease, and their goal was to find a less toxic and more effective regimen. The study, however, concluded the opposite; the CHAMOMA regimen was more toxic and

Table 7 EMA-CO regimen

Day	Agents	Dosing
1	Etoposide	100 mg/m^2 IV over 30 min
	Actinomycin D	0.5 mg IV push
	Methotrexate	100 mg/m^2 IV and 200 mg/m^2 IV in 1000 mL of D5W over 12 h
2	Etoposide	100 mg/m^2 IV over 30 min
	Actinomycin D	0.5 mg IV bolus
	Folinic acid	15 mg IM or PO every 12 h for four doses starting 24 h after initiation of methotrexate
8	Cyclophosphamide	600 mg/m^2 IV
	Vincristine	1.0 mg/m^2 IV push

Adopted and modified from Escobar et al. (2003)
Repeat cycle on days 15, 16, and 22 (every 2 weeks)

possibly less effect. It closed prematurely because of a 30% death rate in the CHAMOMA arm, compared to a 4% death rate in the MAC arm.

(b) MAC: This regimen has a response rate of approximately 77% and was routinely used up until the 1990s when the combination regimen of EMA-CO was found to be well tolerated and has a response rate of approximately 83% (Curry et al. 1989) (Bower et al. 1997). EMA-CO has now become the preferred first-line combination regimen in the United States and Europe.

(c) MEA: This regimen, like EMA-CO, uses etoposide, methotrexate, and actinomycin D but omits the use of etoposide and Oncovin (vincristine); it has a 74.4% response rate (Matsui et al. 2000). It has been favored by some European centers because of its tolerability.

(d) 5-Flurouracil, methotrexate, etoposide (5-FUME): This regimen is mostly used in China and has an 80.8% remission rate in high-risk patients, which appears to be comparable to the published results seen with EMA-CO. It also appears that the toxicity profile of this regimen may be slightly better than that of EMA-CO. However, this regimen is far less studied, and further investigation is warranted (Wang et al. 2006).

(e) EMA-CO: In the late 1970s, it was discovered that etoposide was a very effective chemotherapeutic agent for GTD. EMA-CO was subsequently formulated by Newlands et al. (1986). Table 7 outlines the treatment regimen. As mentioned above, complete response rates and long-term survival rates of well over 80% have been reported with this regimen (Newlands et al. 1991). The toxicities of this regimen are manageable with the most common being anemia and neutropenia which may require a treatment delay of about a week (Schink et al. 1992; Escobar et al. 2003). Colony-stimulating factors (G-CSF 300 μg subcutaneous) can be administered on days 9–14 of the cycle if any neutropenia-related treatment delays are experienced. Treatment delays should be minimized as resistance can develop if interruption is experienced. This regimen is now the preferred first-line regimen for high-risk GTN.

3 Management of Refractory/Persistent Disease

GTN that does not respond to first-line treatment is said to be resistant or refractory. Resistance to a particular chemotherapeutic regimen is evidenced by a plateau or rise in beta-hCG levels. Approximately 5% of low-risk patients and 25% of high-risk patients will have an incomplete response or experience a recurrence following the first-line therapy (Lurain and Nejad 2005). In this setting, salvage chemotherapy and surgical resection, when appropriate, are employed. A new WHO score must be assigned, and treatment is once again determined based on low- versus high-risk WHO score.

3.1 Low-Risk Refractory GTN

In treating low-risk GTN, if resistance to methotrexate is noted, it is common practice to use the sequential 5-day actinomycin D, followed

Table 8 EMA-EP schedule

Day	Agents	Dosing
EP		
1	Etoposide	150 mg/m² IV in 250 mL NS over 30 min
	Cisplatin	25 mg/m² IV in 1 L NS + 20 mmol KCL 4 h
EMA		
1	Etoposide	100 mg/m² IV in 250 mL NS over 30 min
	Methotrexate	300 mg/m² IV in 1 L NS over 12 h
	Actinomycin D	0.5 mg IV bolus
2	Folinic acid	15 mg PO or IM[a] BID for four doses 24 h after start of methotrexate

Adopted and modified from Newlands et al. (2000)
EP and EMA are alternated at weekly intervals
[a]The decision as to route of administration depends on development of nausea and ability to tolerate oral intake

by MAC or EMA-CO if further salvage treatment is required (Alazzam et al. 2012b).

3.2 High-Risk Refractory/ Recurrent GTN

Patients with persistent or recurrent high-risk GTN who develop resistance to methotrexate-containing regimens should be treated with platinum-containing combination regimens.

EMA-EP substitutes etoposide and cisplatin for cyclophosphamide and Oncovin in the EMA-CO protocol and is commonly the initial approach employed for patients who responded to EMA-CO and have plateauing beta-hCG levels or experience a recurrence (Table 8) (Lurain and Nejad 2005). Response rates can be as high as 75% in patients who previously failed EMA-CO. This regimen is moderately toxic; in particular it can be nephrotoxic and myelosuppressive, thus renal function must be closely monitored (Newlands et al. 2000).

Other regimens have also been described for use in this setting: BEP (bleomycin, etoposide, and cisplatin), VIP (vinblastine, ifosfamide, and cisplatin), ICE (ifosfamide, cisplatin, and

etoposide), and TP/TE (paclitaxel, cisplatin/ paclitaxel, etoposide) (Lurain and Nejad 2005); (Wang et al. 2008). At the Brewer Trophoblastic Disease Center, BEP is the first choice for treating high-risk patients who are resistant to EMA-CO/ EMA-EP (Lurain and Nejad 2005). Charing Cross Hospital in London has presented TP/TE as an effective, relatively well-tolerated salvage regimen for patients with heavily pretreated high-risk GTN (Wang et al. 2008).

Figure 1 provides a proposed chemotherapy treatment algorithm for both low-risk/high-risk GTN and refractory disease as described above. It is important to note that refractory cases should be referred to a trophoblastic disease center for consultation.

3.3 Non-gestational Trophoblastic Tumors (Non-GTT)

In the setting of high-risk refractory GTN, one must also think of and evaluate for non-gestational trophoblastic tumors (Alifrangis et al. 2013). These are choriocarcinomas that are not associated with pregnancy. Oftentimes, the distinction can be made on histopathology by finding the absence of syncytiotrophoblasts. However, some non-GTTs can exhibit trophoblastic differentiation making the distinction difficult. Genetic testing of the tumor with microsatellite genotyping can be employed to examine the genetic origin of these tumors (Fisher et al. 2007). Non-GTTs do not respond to chemotherapy and have a very poor prognosis; being able to distinguish between GTT and non-GTT helps optimize patient care.

4 Special Considerations

4.1 Vaginal Metastases

The incidence of vaginal metastasis in choriocarcinoma is 8.6% (Yingna et al. 2002). The vagina is the second most common metastatic site in GTN, with the lung being the most common. These patients present with friable, vascular lesions located in the anterior wall of

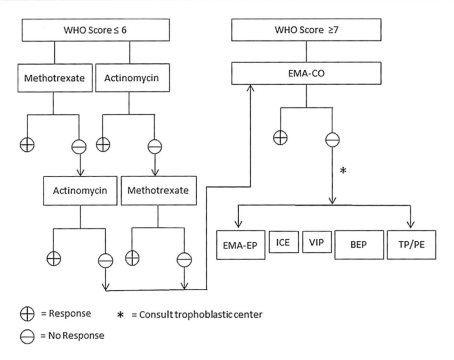

Fig. 1 Proposed chemotherapy treatment algorithm. Abbreviations: *WHO*, World Health Organization; *EMA-CO*, etoposide, methotrexate, actinomycin D, cyclophosphamide, and Oncovin; *EMA-EP*, etoposide, methotrexate, actinomycin D, etoposide, and cisplatin; *BEP*, bleomycin, etoposide, and cisplatin; *ICE*, ifosfamide, cisplatin, and etoposide; and *TP/TE*, paclitaxel, cisplatin/paclitaxel, etoposide

the lower vagina. Though performing a biopsy for diagnostic conformation may be tempting, it puts the patient at great risk for hemorrhage and is therefore discouraged when metastatic GTN is suspected. If patients present with spontaneous hemorrhage, vaginal packing with the use of hemostatic agents should be employed. Selective angiographic embolization by interventional radiology is another viable option in the setting of acute hemorrhage. Treatment for vaginal metastasis includes systemic treatment with chemotherapy as well as local injection with 5-FU (Yingna et al. 2002).

4.2 Brain Metastases

Metastases to the brain and central nervous system (CNS) are observed in up to 10–15% of patients with GTN. CNS involvement is frequent enough that it is one of the criteria used to assign patients to the high-risk category. Treatment of CNS

metastasis has evolved to include whole brain radiation (WBRT). It has shown to have significant therapeutic benefit in the treatment of GTN with improved overall survival. The survival of patients with metastatic GTN to the brain is excellent if extracranial disease is controlled (Schechter et al. 1998). It is recommended that WBRT be initiated simultaneously with the start of multi-agent systemic chemotherapy (Yordan et al. 1987). Should chemotherapy be initiated before WBXRT there is increased risk of intracranial hemorrhage. Treatment initiation with WBRT can reduce the incidence of hemorrhage and resultant sequela in the first 2 weeks of chemotherapy administration (Schechter et al. 1998).

When treating patients with brain metastases, the systemic dose of methotrexate administered IV must be increased because the concentrations of methotrexate in the cerebrospinal fluid have been found to be less than 5% of plasma concentrations. The use of high-dose methotrexate regimens without concomitant

WBRT has achieved remission rates as high as 69%; the addition of WBRT can increase remission rates to 78% (Schechter et al. 1998).

Intrathecal chemotherapy in conjunction with systemic chemotherapy has also been evaluated in the setting of CNS metastasis and has yielded excellent survival rates (Small et al. 1996). A direct comparison between intrathecal chemo administration and WBRT has yet to be made. However, it appears that treatment with WBRT is more commonly employed.

WBRT is not without toxicity. It can lead to long-term sequelae including impaired cognitive function, dementia, behavioral changes, and ataxia. For this reason, in the setting of a solitary brain lesion, craniotomy with surgical resection should be employed in efforts to avoid WBRT. More recently, the use of stereotactic radiosurgery has been employed and reported by Charing Cross to treat multiple brain metastases or solitary lesions in locations that are inaccessible with surgery (Soper et al. 2007).

If a CNS recurrence is suspected during surveillance and no lesion is noted on imaging, a plasma to spinal fluid ratio can be obtained. In the absence of brain metastases, the spinal fluid beta-hCG level is proportional to that of plasma. A plasma to spinal fluid ratio less than 60 is confirmatory of CNS recurrence (Bagshawe and Harland 1976). Overall patients with brain metastases have a good prognosis; however, those who develop brain metastases during treatment with systemic therapy or recur to brain after WBRT have the poorest prognosis (Evans et al. 1995).

4.3 Reproductive Outcomes After Treatment for GTN

GTN affects women of reproductive age; thus, fertility and reproductive outcomes following treatment are of utmost importance. Studies evaluating the reproductive outcome of patients treated for both low- and high-risk GTN have concluded that reproductive outcomes do not differ from the general population. In addition the chemotherapy regimen does not affect reproductive performance when comparing single-agent methotrexate to multi-agent therapy (Woolas et al. 1998). However, data regarding the risk of congenital malformation appears to be conflicting; while some studies conclude that the risk is similar to that of the general population in both frequency and type for both single and multi-agent therapy, another concluded that the risk of congenital heart abnormalities (particularly ventricular septal defects) is higher in the group receiving multi-agent treatment (Goto et al. 2004). The overall risk of congenital anomalies is relatively low but should be discussed with patients receiving multi-agent therapy for GTN. The American Society of Clinical Oncology stresses the importance of discussing the potential for infertility with all patients undergoing treatment for cancer. While treatment for GTN appears to have minimal effect on reproductive outcomes, the possibility of infertility should be addressed and documented.

4.4 Post-molar Prophylactic Chemotherapy

To date, the use of chemotherapy for primary prevention of post-molar GTN remains controversial as there is conflicting data regarding efficacy (Ayhan et al. 1990). Patients with high-risk hydatidiform moles, as defined in Table 9, have up to a 50% chance of developing post-molar GTN (Uberti et al. 2009). It has been argued that chemotherapy administered at the time of uterine evacuation in this patient population can prevent the development of GTN; however, studies have shown that prophylactic chemotherapy is not without risk. Those who receive chemoprophylaxis are known to have prolonged hospital stays and chemotherapy-related toxicities and require more courses of chemotherapy to cure subsequent GTN, all of which may seem too risky for a disease with an excellent cure rate. Nevertheless, it does not affect reproductive outcomes and has also been shown to reduce psychological angst, medical visits, and operational costs associated with management of post-molar GTN/persistent GTD (Uberti et al.

Table 9 Risk scoring system for the prediction of developing GTN in women with a molar pregnancy

Score	0	1	2	3
Ultrasound diagnosis of HM in current pregnancy	Partial	Complete	Recurrent	-
Uterine size for gestational age at diagnosis of molar pregnancy	Size = or < dates	Size 4 weeks greater than corresponding gestational age	Size 8 weeks greater than corresponding gestational age	Size 12 weeks greater than corresponding gestational age
Beta-hCG levels (mU/mL)	<50,000	50,000–100,000	100,000–1,000,000	>1,000,000
Diameter of theca lutein cyst (cm)	-	<6	6–10	>10
Patient's age (years)	-	<20	≥40	>
Associated medical complications[a]	-	≥1	-	-

Adopted and modified from Uberti et al. (2006)

Final score of <4 is low risk; ≥4 is high risk

HM, hydatidiform mole

[a]Hyperthyroidism, hyperemesis, preeclampsia, trophoblastic embolization, disseminated intravascular coagulation

2009). Though the use of chemoprophylaxis is not widely accepted, most agree that its use is most appropriate for patients with high-risk moles in settings where serial beta-hCG levels cannot be followed and in those with poor compliance, such as in the adolescent population (Uberti et al. 2006). Table 9 offers a scoring system for the prediction of developing GTN in women with a molar pregnancy. Women with a score of greater than or equal to 4 are deemed to be high-risk of developing GTN and may benefit from post-molar prophylactic chemotherapy. Table 10 provides a summary of the published studies evaluating the efficacy of post-molar chemoprophylaxis. Methotrexate administered at 0.4 mg/kg IM for 5 days did not prove effective for post-molar prophylaxis. However, actinomycin D at 1.25 mg/m^2 IV X 1 dose has shown to reduce the rate of post-molar GTN in high-risk molar pregnancies.

4.5 Phantom Beta-hCG, Quiescent GTD, and Physiologic Beta-hCG

After treatment for GTN is complete, it is recommended that quantitative serum beta-hCG levels be followed monthly for 6–12 months after normalization as the risk of relapse is about 3%

Table 10 Summary of prophylactic chemotherapeutic regimens and response

Chemotherapy	Schedule	Rate of post-molar GTN in high-risk mole Control versus Prophylactic Chemotherapy
Methotrexate (Ayhan et al. 1990)	0.4 mg/kg IM, 5 days	26.2% vs 25%
Actinomycin D (Uberti et al. 2009)	1.25 mg/m^2 IV, one dose	34.3% vs 18.4%
Actinomycin D (Uberti et al. 2006)	1.25 mg/m^2 IV, one dose	29% vs 6.9%

during the first year and significantly decreases thereafter (Lurain 2011). Women with persistent mildly elevated beta-hCG levels can exhibit false-positive results caused by non-specific heterophilic antibodies. This can lead to unnecessary workup and treatment intervention for presumed persistent or recurrent disease. Two criteria have been developed to identify false-positive beta-hCG levels: (1) elevated serum beta-hCG levels in the setting of a negative urine pregnancy test and (2) finding of more than a fourfold difference between commercially available immunoassays employed in the common clinical setting and those used by reference laboratories (Rotmensch and Cole 2000).

False-positive beta-hCG must be differentiated from quiescent GTD. Quiescent GTD is defined by persistent low levels of beta-hCG present for at least 3 months with no changed in beta-hCG trend. It is caused by a small focus of persistent slow-growing syncytiotrophoblasts that produce low levels of beta-hCG but do not typically progress to invasive disease (Cole 2010). Testing for hyperglycosylated hCG (h-hCG) can be employed to discriminate quiescent GTD from active trophoblastic malignancy. Quiescent GTD does not respond to chemotherapy. H-hCG is produced by invasive cytotrophoblasts and therefore a marker of invasive cells. It can be used by clinicians to decide when treatment is not indicated but also help detect active disease at its inception so that appropriate treatment can be initiated (Cole et al. 2006).

Low levels of physiologic beta-hCG are secreted from the pituitary alongside luteinizing hormone (LH) during the LH surge of the ovulatory cycle. Pituitary beta-hCG production increases with age and is frequently detected in perimenopausal or postmenopausal women. Physiologic expression of beta-hCG has led to unnecessary treatment for GTN. Pituitary expression of beta-hCG can be suppressed with a short course of combined oral contraceptives and can help rule out GTN (Cole et al. 2008).

References

Abrão RA, de Andrade JM, Tiezzi DG, Marana HR, Candido dos Reis FJ, Clagnan WS. Treatment for low-risk gestational trophoblastic disease: comparison of single-agent methotrexate, dactinomycin and combination regimens. Gynecol Oncol. 2008;108:149–53.

Alazzam M, Tidy J, Hancock BW, Osborne R, Lawrie TA. First-line chemotherapy in low-risk gestational trophoblastic neoplasia. Cochrane Database Syst Rev. 2012a: p. CD007102.

Alazzam M, Tidy J, Osborne R, Coleman R, Hancock BW, Lawrie TA. Chemotherapy for resistant or recurrent gestational trophoblastic neoplasia. Cochrane Database Syst Rev. 2012b;12:CD008891.

Alifrangis C, Agarwal R, Short D, Fisher RA, Sebire NJ, Harvey R, Savage PM, Seckl MJ. EMA/CO for high-risk gestational trophoblastic neoplasia: good outcomes with induction low-dose etoposide-cisplatin and genetic analysis. J Clin Oncol. 2013;31:280–6.

Allison KH, Love JE, Garcia RL. Epithelioid trophoblastic tumor: review of a rare neoplasm of the chorionic-type intermediate trophoblast. Arch Pathol Lab Med. 2006;130:1875–7.

Ayhan A, Ergeneli MH, Yüce K, Yapar EG, Kisnisci AH. Effects of prophylactic chemotherapy for postmolar trophoblastic disease in patients with complete hydatidiform mole. Int J Gynaecol Obstet. 1990;32:39–41.

Bagshawe KD, Harland S. Immunodiagnosis and monitoring of gonadotrophin-producing metastases in the central nervous system. Cancer. 1976;38:112–8.

Berkowitz RS, Goldstein DP. Current management of gestational trophoblastic diseases. Gynecol Oncol. 2009;112:654–62.

Bower M, Newlands ES, Holden L, Short D, Brock C, Rustin GJ, Begent RH, Bagshawe KD. EMA/CO for high-risk gestational trophoblastic tumors: results from a cohort of 272 patients. J Clin Oncol. 1997;15:2636–43.

Cole LA. Hyperglycosylated hCG, a review. Placenta. 2010;31:653–64.

Cole LA, Butler SA, Khanlian SA, Giddings A, Muller CY, Seckl MJ, Kohorn EI. Gestational trophoblastic diseases: 2 hyperglycosylated hCG as a reliable marker of active neoplasia. Gynecol Oncol. 2006;102:151–9.

Cole LA, Khanlian SA, Muller CY. Detection of perimenopause or postmenopause human chorionic gonadotropin: an unnecessary source of alarm. Am J Obstet Gynecol. 2008;198:275.e1–7.

Committee, F. O. FIGO staging for gestational trophoblastic neoplasia 2000. Int J Gynaecol Obstet. 2002;77:285–7.

Curry SL, Blessing JA, DiSaia PJ, Soper JT, Twiggs LB. A prospective randomized comparison of methotrexate, dactinomycin, and chlorambucil versus methotrexate, dactinomycin, cyclophosphamide, doxorubicin, melphalan, hydroxyurea, and vincristine in "poor prognosis" metastatic gestational trophoblastic disease: a gynecologic oncology group study. Obstet Gynecol. 1989;73:357–62.

Eiriksson L, Wells T, Steed H, Schepansky A, Capstick V, Hoskins P, Pike J, Swenerton K. Combined methotrexate-dactinomycin: an effective therapy for low-risk gestational trophoblastic neoplasia. Gynecol Oncol. 2012;124:553–7.

Escobar PF, Lurain JR, Singh DK, Bozorgi K, Fishman DA. Treatment of high-risk gestational trophoblastic neoplasia with etoposide, methotrexate, actinomycin D, cyclophosphamide, and vincristine chemotherapy. Gynecol Oncol. 2003;91:552–7.

Evans AC, Soper JT, Clarke-Pearson DL, Berchuck A, Rodriguez GC, Hammond CB. Gestational trophoblastic disease metastatic to the central nervous system. Gynecol Oncol. 1995;59:226–30.

Fisher RA, Savage PM, MacDermott C, Hook J, Sebire NJ, Lindsay I, Seckl MJ. The impact of molecular genetic diagnosis on the management of women with hCG-producing malignancies. Gynecol Oncol. 2007;107:413–9.

Froeling FE, Seckl MJ. Gestational trophoblastic tumours: an update for 2014. Curr Oncol Rep. 2014;16:408.

Goto S, Ino K, Mitsui T, Kikkawa F, Suzuki T, Nomura S, Mizutani S. Survival rates of patients with choriocarcinoma treated with chemotherapy without hysterectomy: effects of anticancer agents on subsequent births. Gynecol Oncol. 2004;93:529–35.

Hammond CB, Weed JC, Currie JL. The role of operation in the current therapy of gestational trophoblastic disease. Am J Obstet Gynecol. 1980;136:844–58.

Kohorn EI. Is lack of response to single-agent chemotherapy in gestational trophoblastic disease associated with dose scheduling or chemotherapy resistance? Gynecol Oncol. 2002;85:36–9.

Lurain JR. Gestational trophoblastic tumors. Semin Surg Oncol. 1990;6:347–53.

Lurain JR. Gestational trophoblastic disease I: epidemiology, pathology, clinical presentation and diagnosis of gestational trophoblastic disease, and management of hydatidiform mole. Am J Obstet Gynecol. 2010;203:531–9.

Lurain JR. Gestational trophoblastic disease II: classification and management of gestational trophoblastic neoplasia. Am J Obstet Gynecol. 2011;204:11–8.

Lurain JR, Casanova LA, Miller DS, Rademaker AW. Prognostic factors in gestational trophoblastic tumors: a proposed new scoring system based on multivariate analysis. Am J Obstet Gynecol. 1991;164:611–6.

Lurain JR, Elfstrand EP. Single-agent methotrexate chemotherapy for the treatment of nonmetastatic gestational trophoblastic tumors. Am J Obstet Gynecol. 1995;172:574–9.

Lurain JR, Nejad B. Secondary chemotherapy for high-risk gestational trophoblastic neoplasia. Gynecol Oncol. 2005;97:618–23.

Lybol C, Sweep FC, Harvey R, Mitchell H, Short D, Thomas CM, Ottevanger PB, Savage PM, Massuger LF, Seckl MJ. Relapse rates after two versus three consolidation courses of methotrexate in the treatment of low-risk gestational trophoblastic neoplasia. Gynecol Oncol. 2012;125:576–9.

Matsui H, Suzuka K, Iitsuka Y, Seki K, Sekiya S. Combination chemotherapy with methotrexate, etoposide, and actinomycin D for high-risk gestational trophoblastic tumors. Gynecol Oncol. 2000;78:28–31.

Matsui H, Suzuka K, Yamazawa K, Tanaka N, Mitsuhashi A, Seki K, Sekiya S. Relapse rate of patients with low-risk gestational trophoblastic tumor initially treated with single-agent chemotherapy. Gynecol Oncol. 2005;96:616–20.

Morrow CP, Kletzky OA, Disaia PJ, Townsend DE, Mishell DR, Nakamura RM. Clinical and laboratory correlates of molar pregnancy and trophoblastic disease. Am J Obstet Gynecol. 1977;128:424–30.

Newlands ES, Bagshawe KD, Begent RH, Rustin GJ, Holden L. Results with the EMA/CO (etoposide, methotrexate, actinomycin D, cyclophosphamide, vincristine) regimen in high risk gestational trophoblastic tumours, 1979 to 1989. Br J Obstet Gynaecol. 1991;98:550–7.

Newlands ES, Bagshawe KD, Begent RH, Rustin GJ, Holden L, Dent J. Developments in chemotherapy for medium- and high-risk patients with gestational trophoblastic tumours (1979-1984). Br J Obstet Gynaecol. 1986;93:63–9.

Newlands ES, Mulholland PJ, Holden L, Seckl MJ, Rustin GJ. Etoposide and cisplatin/etoposide, methotrexate, and actinomycin D (EMA) chemotherapy for patients with high-risk gestational trophoblastic tumors refractory to EMA/cyclophosphamide and vincristine chemotherapy and patients presenting with metastatic placental site trophoblastic tumors. J Clin Oncol. 2000;18:854–9.

Oncology, F. C. o. G. Current FIGO staging for cancer of the vagina, fallopian tube, ovary, and gestational trophoblastic neoplasia. Int J Gynaecol Obstet. 2009;105:3–4.

Osborne RJ, Filiaci V, Schink JC, Mannel RS, Alvarez Secord A, Kelley JL, Provencher D, Scott Miller D, Covens AL, Lage JM. Phase III trial of weekly methotrexate or pulsed dactinomycin for low-risk gestational trophoblastic neoplasia: a gynecologic oncology group study. J Clin Oncol. 2011;29:825–31.

Osborne RJ, Filiaci VL, Schink JC, Mannel RS, Behbakht K, Hoffman JS, Spirtos NM, Chan JK, Tidy JA, Miller DS. Second curettage for low-risk nonmetastatic gestational trophoblastic neoplasia. Obstet Gynecol. 2016;128:535–42.

Papadopoulos AJ, Foskett M, Seckl MJ, McNeish I, Paradinas FJ, Rees H, Newlands ES. Twenty-five years' clinical experience with placental site trophoblastic tumors. J Reprod Med. 2002;47:460–4.

Pezeshki M, Hancock BW, Silcocks P, Everard JE, Coleman J, Gillespie AM, Tidy J, Coleman RE. The role of repeat uterine evacuation in the management of persistent gestational trophoblastic disease. Gynecol Oncol. 2004;95:423–9.

Rotmensch S, Cole LA. False diagnosis and needless therapy of presumed malignant disease in women with false-positive human chorionic gonadotropin concentrations. Lancet. 2000;355:712–5.

Rustin GJ, Newlands ES, Lutz JM, Holden L, Bagshawe KD, Hiscox JG, Foskett M, Fuller S, Short D. Combination but not single-agent methotrexate chemotherapy for gestational trophoblastic tumors increases the incidence of second tumors. J Clin Oncol. 1996;14:2769–73.

Schechter NR, Mychalczak B, Jones W, Spriggs D. Prognosis of patients treated with whole-brain radiation therapy for metastatic gestational trophoblastic disease. Gynecol Oncol. 1998;68:183–92.

Schink JC, Singh DK, Rademaker AW, Miller DS, Lurain JR. Etoposide, methotrexate, actinomycin D, cyclophosphamide, and vincristine for the treatment of metastatic, high-risk gestational trophoblastic disease. Obstet Gynecol. 1992;80:817–20.

Schlaerth JB, Morrow CP, Kletzky OA, Nalick RH, D'Ablaing GA. Prognostic characteristics of serum human chorionic gonadotropin titer regression following molar pregnancy. Obstet Gynecol. 1981;58:478–82.

Small W, Lurain JR, Shetty RM, Huang CF, Applegate GL, Brand WN. Gestational trophoblastic disease metastatic to the brain. Radiology. 1996;200:277–80.

Soper JT, Clarke-Pearson DL, Berchuck A, Rodriguez G, Hammond CB. 5-day methotrexate for women with metastatic gestational trophoblastic disease. Gynecol Oncol. 1994;54:76–9.

Soper JT, Spillman M, Sampson JH, Kirkpatrick JP, Wolf JK, Clarke-Pearson DL. High-risk gestational trophoblastic neoplasia with brain metastases: individualized multidisciplinary therapy in the management of four patients. Gynecol Oncol. 2007;104:691–4.

Suzuka K, Matsui H, Iitsuka Y, Yamazawa K, Seki K, Sekiya S. Adjuvant hysterectomy in low-risk gestational trophoblastic disease. Obstet Gynecol. 2001;97:431–4.

Uberti EM, Diestel MC, Guimarães FE, De Nápoli G, Schmid H. Single-dose actinomycin D: efficacy in the prophylaxis of post-molar gestational trophoblastic neoplasia in adolescents with high-risk hydatidiform mole. Gynecol Oncol. 2006;102:325–32.

Uberti EM, Fajardo MC, da Cunha AG, Rosa MW, Ayub AC, Graudenz MS, Schmid H. Prevention of postmolar gestational trophoblastic neoplasia using prophylactic single bolus dose of actinomycin D in high-risk hydatidiform mole: a simple, effective, secure and low-cost approach without adverse effects on compliance to general follow-up or subsequent treatment. Gynecol Oncol. 2009;114:299–305.

van Trommel NE, Massuger LF, Verheijen RH, Sweep FC, Thomas CM. The curative effect of a second curettage in persistent trophoblastic disease: a retrospective cohort survey. Gynecol Oncol. 2005;99:6–13.

Wang J, Short D, Sebire NJ, Lindsay I, Newlands ES, Schmid P, Savage PM, Seckl MJ. Salvage chemotherapy of relapsed or high-risk gestational trophoblastic neoplasia (GTN) with paclitaxel/cisplatin alternating with paclitaxel/etoposide (TP/TE). Ann Oncol. 2008;19:1578–83.

Wang S, An R, Han X, Zhu K, Xue Y. Combination chemotherapy with 5-fluorouracil, methotrexate and etoposide for patients with high-risk gestational trophoblastic tumors: a report based on our 11-year clinical experiences. Gynecol Oncol. 2006;103:1105–8.

Woolas RP, Bower M, Newlands ES, Seckl M, Short D, Holden L. Influence of chemotherapy for gestational trophoblastic disease on subsequent pregnancy outcome. Br J Obstet Gynaecol. 1998;105:1032–5.

Yarandi F, Jafari F, Shojaei H, Izadi-Mood N. Clinical response to a second uterine curettage in patients with low-risk gestational trophoblastic disease: a pilot study. J Reprod Med. 2014;59:566–70.

Yingna S, Yang X, Xiuyu Y, Hongzhao S. Clinical characteristics and treatment of gestational trophoblastic tumor with vaginal metastasis. Gynecol Oncol. 2002;84:416–9.

Yordan EL, Schlaerth J, Gaddis O, Morrow CP. Radiation therapy in the management of gestational choriocarcinoma metastatic to the central nervous system. Obstet Gynecol. 1987;69:627–30.

Diagnosis and Management of Vulvar Cancer

Mariko Shindo, Yutaka Ueda, Tadashi Kimura, and Koji Matsuo

Abstract

Vulvar cancer is rare, comprising only 5% of all gynecologic malignancies. However, the incidence of invasive vulvar carcinoma has been increasing moderately over the past two decades, and the incidence of in situ vulvar carcinoma has increased more than fourfold in the same period. Vulvar squamous cell carcinoma, the most common form of this cancer, is commonly divided into two basic types: HPV-associated and HPV-independent. To improve vulvar cancer survival, early detection by careful screening is important. FIGO surgical staging system for vulvar cancer was updated in 2009, incorporating prognostic factors such as inguinal lymph node metastasis. The number and morphology including the size, extracapsular spread of the involved nodes have been taken into account. The presence of fixed or ulcerated inguino-femoral nodes is also included to a staging system. The standard treatment for vulvar cancer has been primarily surgery; however, to decrease morbidity and improve survival outcome, more conservative and individualized treatment practices have recently been explored. The benefit of postoperative adjuvant therapy has been shown in the past decades; although an indication for adjuvant therapy needs further discussion. In advanced vulvar cancer, multimodality therapy including neoadjuvant chemoradiotherapy followed by surgical resection and definitive chemoradiotherapy has been investigated to avoid exenterative surgery or stoma formation. For patients with clinical positive inguino-femoral lymph nodes, node dissection or neoadjuvant chemoradiation therapy are now recommended.

Keywords

Vulvar cancer • Squamous cell carcinoma • HPV • Conservative therapy • Management

Contents

M. Shindo • Y. Ueda • T. Kimura
Department of Obstetrics and Gynecology, Osaka University Graduate School of Medicine, Suita, Osaka, Japan
e-mail: s.mariko0206@gmail.com; zvf03563@nifty.ne.jp; tadashi@gyne.med.osaka-u.ac.jp

K. Matsuo (✉)
Division of Gynecologic Oncology, Department of Obstetrics and Gynecology, University of Southern California, Los Angeles, CA, USA
e-mail: koji.matsuo@med.usc.edu

© Springer International Publishing AG 2017
D. Shoupe (ed.), *Handbook of Gynecology*,
DOI 10.1007/978-3-319-17798-4_9

1   Introduction

Vulvar cancer is a relatively rare disease of the female genital tract, accounting for roughly only 5% of all gynecologic cancers. In 2015, the estimated number of expected new cases of vulvar cancer in the United States alone will be 5,150, with 1,080 accompanying deaths (Siegel et al. 2015). One large retrospective study found that, from the years 1973 to 2000, the incidence of invasive vulvar cancer in women had increased by approximately 20%, from 1.8 cases per 100,000 to 2.2 cases per 100,000 (Judson et al. 2006), whereas the incidence of in situ carcinoma rose by an alarming 411%, from 0.56 cases per 100,000 women to 2.86 per 100,000, during the same period. The same study observed that the incidence of invasive vulvar cancer begins to increase quickly after age 50 and that it peaks between the ages of 65–70. Conversely, the incidence of the noninvasive in situ form increases only until roughly the age of 40–49, whereupon it declines

Histologically, vulvar squamous cell carcinoma (SCC) is the most common histologic subtype of vulvar cancer, accounting for 80–90% of such malignancies (Beller et al. 2006), with vulvar melanoma being the second most common type. Other significant histological types include vulvar basal cell carcinoma, Paget's disease of the vulva, vulvar adenocarcinoma, and Bartholin's gland carcinoma. Vulvar Paget's disease is discussed in the separate chapter.

There are at least three main histological types of vulvar SCC: warty, basaloid, and keratinizing.

Rarer histological variants of SCC are verrucous carcinoma, keratoacanthoma-like SCC, sarcomatoid carcinoma, and SCC with giant tumor cells. The warty and basaloid patterns affect younger women, having risk factors similar to cervical cancer, and both are highly associated with high-grade vulvar dysplasia. The keratinizing pattern, which is a dominant pattern consisting 65–80% of invasive vulvar SCC, affects older women and often accompanies lichen sclerosis or squamous hyperplasia.

In the large study which reports over 1,700 cases of vulvar SCC, 25.1% were human papilloma virus (HPV) positive. Of all invasive vulvar SCC, 72.2% was the keratinizing pattern and 19.1% was the warty and basaloid patterns. The warty and basaloid patterns were more likely to be HPV positive (69.5%) compared to the keratinizing pattern (11.5%). HPV type16 was the most common type in invasive vulvar SCC (de Sanjosé et al. 2013).

Two distinct pathways, HPV-associated and non-HPV-associated, were proposed for development of vulvar SCC. In the HPV-associated vulvar SCC, the virus-encoded E6 and E7 oncoproteins cause inactivation of at least two important tumor suppressor proteins, p53 and Rb. In the non-HPV-associated type, it is the direct inactivation of *p53* by missense and deletion mutations that is most frequently identified, although a number of other somatic mutational events are usually present as well.

Because of the rarity of vulvar cancer, most studies have been retrospective clinicopathological reviews. Such studies have shown that the management of vulvar cancer has been making steady progress towards more conservative and individualized treatment plans. The standard treatment for early stage vulvar cancer remains surgery; however, more advanced disease cases are now treated with additional radiation and/or chemotherapy. Unfortunately, the choices of which treatments to use, and when, are still based mostly on case by case.

2   Diagnosis and Staging

The vulva consists of several distinct anatomical structures, the labia majora and minora, clitoris, mons pubis, vaginal vestibule, urinary meatus, and perineum. Over 70% of vulvar cancers arise in the labia majora and minora. The overt symptoms of vulvar cancer can include pruritus, a palpable mass, a localized pain, vaginal discharge, dysuria, bleeding, or ulceration. However, a significant diagnostic delay for patients with vulvar cancer frequently occurs because the lesion is so often asymptomatic or lacks many of the more alarming symptoms, like unexpected bleeding, associated with other gynecological cancers. This lack of early warning symptoms means that, unfortunately, almost 40% of patients with vulvar cancer are at advanced stage when first diagnosed (Homesley et al. 1991). Lack of suspicion for vulvar cancer is another reason for delay in diagnosis.

At exam presentation, neoplastic vulvar lesions are usually visible and palpable (Fig. 1). Careful visual evaluation by a physician is important so as not to miss frequently occurring multiple skip lesions. To detect and treat these neoplasms at the earliest possible stages, all suspicious vulvar lesions need to be carefully biopsied. The biopsy will include the surface epithelial lesion and stroma to evaluate depth of lesion invasion, and each lesion needs to be fully histologically assessed. Clinically viable tumor sites but not necrotic areas are recommended for the biopsy site. Along with assessment of the vulva, the groin lymph nodes need to be evaluated carefully. Colposcopy of the cervix and vagina can be performed to detect other squamous intraepithelial neoplasms.

Invasive vulvar cancer usually spreads in two distinct ways: (i) by lymphatic spread to the regional lymph nodes or (ii) by direct expansion into any adjacent structures, such as the vagina, urethra, bladder, rectum, or anal sphincter. Distal hematogenous spread of vulvar cancer is relatively rare.

During lymphatic spread, the first nodal metastasis usually involves the superficial inguino-femoral nodes, and moves subsequently into the deep inguino-femoral and pelvic nodes. Deep inguinal lymph node involvement occurs only in patients with superficial inguinal node metastasis (Andrews et al. 1994). The presence of pelvic lymph node metastasis with an absence of groin nodal metastasis is very rare. Lateral lesions generally drain to the ipsilateral groin nodes. Midline lesions and lesions within 1 cm of the midline can drain to bilateral nodes.

In 1988, the International Federation of Gynecology and Obstetrics (FIGO) committee adopted a surgical staging system for vulvar cancer in which the pathological evaluation of the primary tumor and regional nodes was emphasized, based on the fact that, at the time, metastasis to regional nodes was the most important known prognostic factor and that clinical palpation evaluation of the lymph nodes was known to be unreliable. For example, in one study of 477 patients assessed with vulvar lesions, but having palpably normal groin lymph nodes, 24% were later found at surgery to have positive nodes (Hoffman et al. 1985; Homesley et al. 1991).

In 1991, problems with the 1988 FIGO surgical staging system for vulvar cancer became more apparent when the Gynecologic Oncology Group (GOG) reported on an analysis of survival outcome of 588 patients. When the patient had both a primary tumor <8 cm in diameter and no nodal metastasis, the 5-year survival was found to be 87%. This means that lesions up to 8 cm in size are low risk of disease relapse as long as there is no nodal metastasis. Secondly, patients with stage III tumors represented a wide range of survival rates, from 34% to 100%. Thirdly, the study found a 5-year survival of 90.9% for patients with surgically negative nodes, 75.2% for patients with 1–2

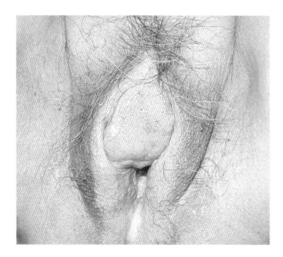

Fig. 1 Squamous cell carcinoma of vulva

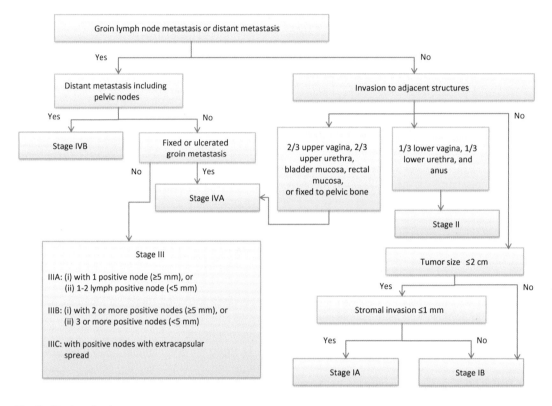

Fig. 2 Staging of vulvar cancer

positive nodes, 36.1% for patients with 3–4 positive nodes, 24.0% for patients with 5–6 positive nodes, and 0% for patients with ≥7 positive nodes.

In 2009, after consideration of these problems, FIGO revised the staging for vulvar cancers: Stages I and II in the 1988 classification were combined, and the number and morphology of the involved nodes were now to be taken into account (Pecorelli et al. 2009). Stage IA, the group considered to be at negligible risk of lymph node metastasis, remained unchanged (Fig. 2).

3   Tumor Imaging

There is currently only limited data available on the efficacy of various imaging modalities for the diagnosis and treatment of primary vulvar cancer, although imaging techniques, such as MRI, CT, and PET/CT, currently play important roles in the diagnosis of local, regional, and distal metastasis

for treatment planning. This is especially true in advanced vulvar carcinoma, since these patients need more individualized treatment planning, including surgery and chemoradiation, to minimize morbidity.

Kim et al. reported that imaging with MRI was the most accurate modality for evaluation of the primary lesions. To detect lymph nodal metastasis, combined ultrasound imaging and ultrasound-guided aspiration biopsy was found to be the most reliable method, with its high specificity (82–100%) and sensitivity (80–93%). The sensitivity of MRI for detecting nodal metastasis was moderate (50–89%), but the specificity was high (89–100%).

CT may be an important staging tool for nodal and distant metastasis and for surveillance monitoring after treatment, although CT is less sensitive for detecting a nodal metastasis with size <1 cm because of CT's size criteria (Kim et al. 2013). Cohn et al. showed that the sensitivity of PET/CT is 80% and the specificity is 90% for assessment of nodal metastasis (Cohn et al. 2002).

However, PET/CT has a limited value in evaluation of lymph nodes with size <0.5 cm. MRI appears to be the better method for determining the extent and degree of invasion of local lesions, and for detection of small inguino-femoral nodal metastasis, while CT and PET/CT can help detect distant metastasis. PET/CT also plays an important role in the assessment of nodal and distant metastasis, when the clinical diagnosis is difficult.

4 Prognostic Factors

Many studies have retrospectively assessed the prognostic factors that are in play for vulvar cancer. Collectively, they have found that the most significant factor is nodal status. FIGO staging, tumor size, patient age, tumor grade, depth of stromal invasion, and lymphatic capillary space invasion are also predictive for survival probability. In the 26th FIGO Annual Report, involving 1,600 patients with vulvar cancer, the respective 5-year overall survival (OS) rate for each stage was: stage I 78.5%, stage II 58.8%, stage III 43.2%, and stage IV 13.0%, respectively (Beller et al. 2006).

The previously mentioned GOG study of 588 patients reported that, of all the pathologic findings based on surgery, the status of the inguino-femoral lymph nodes and the tumor diameter were the only significant independent factors for prognosis. In their study, there were 34% of patients with nodal metastasis. The 5-year survival rate was 91% in the negative-node patients but only 57% in the positive-node patients. Histological nodal metastasis was significantly related to clinical node status, lymphatic capillary space involvement, tumor differentiation, patient age, and tumor thickness (Homesley et al. 1993).

5 Treatment of Early Stage Disease

5.1 Surgical Therapy

Historically, the surgery for vulvar cancer was a "classic radical vulvectomy". It required en bloc removal of the entire vulva, including the complete vulvar skin and subcutaneous tissue and the bilateral groin nodes through a butterfly-shaped incision. This procedure achieved an overall survival of around 70%; however, it could also cause severe complications, including postoperative wound breakdown. Additionally, infection occurred in 50–80% of these vulvectomy cases, and lymphedema of the lower extremities and psychosexual disturbances were also prevalent. In the past few decades, to decrease surgical morbidities and improve the quality of life of the patient without compromising survival outcome, surgeons have made several modifications to their surgical treatment plans. Contemporarily, the treatment of vulvar cancer is far more individualized. Some of the more important modifications are as follows: an en bloc dissection has been replaced by three separate groin incisions, a unilateral lymphadenectomy is now used for selected lesions, the radical vulvectomy has been replaced by a more localized radical excision, and the pelvic lymphadenectomy has been replaced by radiation therapy of the pelvic nodes (Ansink and van der Velden 2000; Burke et al. 1995; Hacker et al. 1981; Hacker and Van der Velden 1993).

As a result of these modifications, especially the separate groin incisions and the localized radical excision, groin complications such as wound infection and breakdown have decreased dramatically, to as low as 17–22% compared to previously reported rates. However, significant chronic complications, including lymphedema, still occur in about 30% of cases.

5.2 Surgical Management of the Primary Tumor

A stage IA vulvar carcinoma is defined as one being ≤2 cm in size and having ≤1 mm of stromal invasion. These microinvasive carcinomas can be treated with a wide local excision, which is a removal of the lesion with a 1–2 cm lateral margin and at least a 1 cm deep surgical margin. It is generally felt that a groin lymphadenectomy is not necessary for stage IA because local recurrence and lymph node metastasis are rare for this type of lesion (Hacker et al. 1984b).

Table 1 Terminology and definition of vulvectomy

Wide local resection	A lesion is excised with 1 cm margin. The depth of excision needs at least 1 cm including the skin and superficial subcutaneous tissues
Simple vulvectomy	Removal of the entire vulva, including the skin and superficial subcutaneous tissues. Usually, performed for benign or premalignant lesion of the vulva that are extensive or multifocal
Radical local excision	Radical excision of the portion of the vulva. The surgical margins should be at least 1 cm. The depth of the dissection is from the skin to the urogenital diaphragm. This terminology is sometimes included in modified radical vulvectomy in the broad sense
Modified radical vulvectomy	Radical excision of the portion of the vulva containing the tumor with approximately a 2 cm margin. This usually implies an intermediate resection between a radical vulvectomy and a radical local excision, where most of vulva is removed. This terminology include radical hemivulvectomy, anterior or posterior radical vulvectomy
Radical hemivulvectomy	Radical excision of unilateral of the vulva. This would not remove midline structures like clitoris, urethra, vagina, perineal body, or anus
Radical vulvectomy	Radical removal of the entire vulva down to the level of the urogenital diaphragm. At least 2 cm margins are needed. When the radical vulvectomy is performed through a separate incision, elliptical outer skin incision is used. The anterior border is on the mons pubis. The lateral incision is made along labiocrural folds. The posterior border is the perineal body. The inner vulvar incision is created circumscribing the urethra and vaginal introitus. The traditional or classic radical vulvectomy mean en bloc removal of bilateral groin nodes and the entire vulva, and intervening skin bridge through butterfly skin incision or longhorn skin incision

For more invasive tumors, but that are still confined to the vulva and have clinically negative nodes, a radical local excision or a modified radical vulvectomy, rather than radical vulvectomy, is indicated to reduce surgical morbidity. A radical local excision includes 1–2 cm of tumor-free margin and the deep surgical margin will be carried down to the inferior fascia of the urogenital diaphragm, which is coplanar with the fascia lata and the fascia over the pubic symphysis. The surgical defect is usually closed without tension. A modified radical vulvectomy is an intermediate resection between a radical vulvectomy and a radical local excision, including a radical hemivulvectomy. A modified vulvectomy is more appropriate for patients with multifocal lesions. Definition of terminology for vulvar surgery is shown in Table 1 (Burke et al. 1995; Heaps et al. 1990; De Hullu et al. 2002; Tantipalakorn et al. 2009).

In a report by Heaps et al., 135 patients with vulvar SCC were treated by primary radical resection. The majority had stage I disease (45.9%). Approximately one sixth of patients (15.6%) developed a local vulvar recurrence after the primary radical resection. On examination of formalin-fixed tissue specimens, 67.4% of the patients had a tumor-free histopathologic margin of ≥8 mm, and none of these cases had a local vulvar recurrence. Of the 44 patients that had a margin of <8 mm, nearly a half of the patients (48%) recurred. Taking the 25% shrinkage of tissue that occurs in formalin fixative into consideration, Heaps et al. have suggested that 10 mm of actual tumor-free surgical margin is needed (Heaps et al. 1990).

De Hullu et al. (2002) reported on a series of 253 patients with T1 and T2 disease, in which 168 patients (66.4%) underwent classical radical vulvectomy with an en bloc inguino-femoral lymphadenectomy and 85 patients (33.6%) underwent a revised, less radical, wide local excision with inguino-femoral lymphadenectomy through separate incisions. The overall recurrence rate within 4 years was increased in the less radical treatment group (33.3%) compared with radical treatment group (19.9%). In the less radical group, 6.3% of patients developed fatal recurrences, compared with 1.3% of patients in the radical group. In the less radical group, approximately a half of patients had histologic tumor-free margins ≤8 mm, resulting in 11.3% of local recurrence rate; whereas in the other half patients, with margins measuring >8 mm, there were no

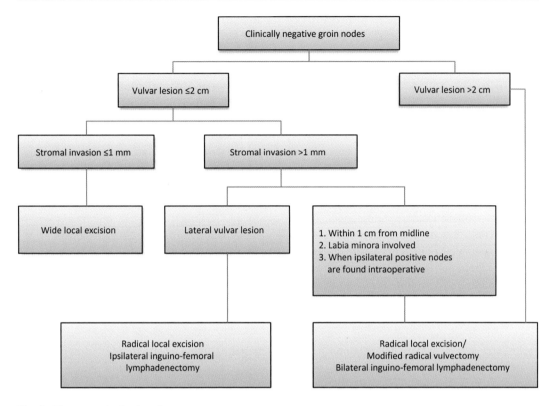

Fig. 3 Management of early vulvar cancer

recurrences. In their study, 50% of patients had histologic tumor-free margins measuring <8 mm, despite the intended surgical margins of 10 mm. Therefore, the authors recommended obtaining surgical margins of at least 20 mm for the localized surgical treatment of patients with vulvar carcinoma.

A surgical management of early vulvar cancer is shown in Fig. 3.

If a reexcision cannot be performed for patients with a close margin (<8 mm) or a tumor-involved margin, adjuvant radiation therapy may be considered. If the tumor is close to the urethra, the distal 10 mm of the urethra can usually be resected without affecting urinary continence.

5.3 Management of Lymph Nodes

In patients with early stage vulvar disease, with nodes negative by palpation and imaging,

metastases to the inguino-femoral lymph nodes are present at surgery in approximately 20–35% of the cases. Therefore, an appropriate evaluation of nodal status is the most important to decrease vulvar cancer mortality.

The standard procedure for nodal evaluation is a bilateral inguino-femoral lymphadenectomy, which is defined as removal of all the lymph nodes contained in the adipose tissue between the inguinal ligament, the sartorius muscle, and the adductor longus muscle and dissection of the femoral lymph nodes located in the fossa ovalis medial to the femoral vein. To reduce morbidity, a separate groin incision is performed for the vast majority of patients. For selected patients with clinically normal lymph nodes, a more conservative lymph node resection has been suggested. As previously mentioned, the physician can safely omit lymph nodes dissection for stage IA disease. To determine the indication for lymphadenectomy, an excisional biopsy of the primary lesion at the vulva needs to be performed under local anesthesia to evaluate the stromal invasion.

Ipsilateral groin dissection can be offered to stage IB patients with a unilateral lesion. Some studies have reported that patients diagnosed as having stage I and II vulvar cancer (using the 1988 FIGO standards) can be treated more effectively by ipsilateral inguinal lymphadenectomy. Burke et al. studied 76 patients with T1 and T2 lesions and clinically uninvolved groin nodes, who were treated with radical wide excision and selected inguinal lymphadenectomy. Groin node failure was seen in 5.3% of the patients; three of the failures were in cases of prior negative dissected ipsilateral groin nodes, only one failure occurred in the undissected contralateral groin nodes (Burke et al. 1995). In a study by Andrews et al., of 84 patients with a lateral T1 and T2 vulvar lesion, 56.7% of the patients were treated with radical vulvectomy with bilateral inguino-femoral lymphadenectomy, and 33.3% of the patients were treated with radical hemivulvectomy and superficial ipsilateral inguinal lymphadenectomy. No contralateral metastases or recurrences were observed, whereas 10.7% of patients developed ipsilateral recurrences. The frequency of recurrence was independent of the type of radical surgery performed (Andrews et al. 1994).

The incidence of contralateral node metastasis is <1% in patients with a unilateral lesion measuring ≤2 cm, if the ipsilateral nodes are free of disease (Hacker and Van der Velden 1993). A unilateral lesion is defined as one having the closest tumor margin being >1 cm from the midline structure. Patients with a unilateral tumor measuring >2 cm confined to the vulva (T2 by 1988 FIGO staging) had metastasis to contralateral nodes in 2.4% (Homesley et al. 1991, 1993).

Under the newer 2009 FIGO classification, the definition of stage II was changed to include a part of the previous stage III. Before determining ipsilateral groin lymphadenectomy to patients diagnosed with stage II disease under the present 2009 FIGO system, it is suggested that a large number of cases need to be further examined. Other risk factors, such as lymphatic capillary space invasion, depth of stromal tumor invasion, and tumor size also need to be considered to better identify a subgroup of patients with lateral T2 tumors who have a low risk of contralateral groin metastasis. Bilateral inguino-femoral node dissection needs to be performed for midline or bilateral tumors, or for those tumors involving the anterior labia minora, and for tumors presenting with any ipsilateral positive nodes.

Conducting only a superficial inguinal lymphadenectomy is correlated with a relatively high rate of groin recurrence, even though the lymphadenectomy-associated morbidity is reduced. Although the groin recurrence rate in patients with no groin nodal involvement at primary surgery is historically <1%, recent reports indicate that about 4–8% of patients with negative superficial lymphadenectomy had a recurrence (Burke et al. 1995; Gordinier et al. 2003; Stehman et al. 1992). Because most patients with a groin recurrence of vulvar cancer die, both inguinal and femoral lymphadenectomy are highly recommended. Role of sentinel lymph node in vulvar cancer surgery is discussed in the separate chapter.

5.4   Adjuvant Radiotherapy

Adjuvant postoperative therapy for the primary tumor site can be used when adverse pathologic features are found in the surgical specimen. This includes patients with a positive or close margin (<8 mm), lymphatic capillary space invasion, or a depth of stromal invasion >5 mm, as these characteristics are associated with a higher risk of local recurrence (Heaps et al. 1990).

While it may be a possible approach to include the vulvar tumor site within the radiation field if the tumor express any high-risk factor, current available data remain insufficient to adequately support this concept, especially adjuvant radiotherapy except for close and positive margin and further studies are warranted.

For cases with surgically positive groin nodes, adjuvant irradiation is generally adopted. Pelvic lymphadenectomy alone is no longer preformed for patients with vulvar cancer. One GOG study (Kunos et al. 2009) compared the outcome for pelvic and groin irradiation after groin dissection with the outcome from solely using pelvic lymphadenectomy. For patients randomized to receive pelvic radiation, the radiation treatment fields encompassed both groins, obturator, and external and internal iliac nodal areas. After a median survival follow-up of 74 months, the relative risk of progression was significantly reduced in the radiation treatment patients (hazard ratio 0.61 $p = 0.02$). At 6 years, overall survival in the radiation patients was 36%, compared with 13% for those who received only lymph node dissection. Their data showed a clear benefit for radiation in patients having clinically suspected or fixed ulcerated groin nodes and ≥ 2 positive nodes. Subsequent studies have emphasized further factors. Patients with one macroscopic metastasis (≥ 5 mm diameter), extracapsular spread, or ≥ 2 lymph nodes with micrometastasis (<5 mm) should receive bilateral pelvic and groin irradiation (Hacker et al. 2012).

Recently, in a retrospective multicenter study analyzing over 1,600 patients, the efficacy of adjuvant radiotherapy for node-positive patients was examined. Of all 447 patients (27.9%) who have groin nodal metastasis, 244 patients (51.1%) received adjuvant therapy. The majority (84%) received adjuvant radiotherapy, while 14% received chemoradiation therapy. Three-year progression-free survival (PFS) rates in these patients were better compared with node-positive patients without adjuvant radiotherapy (40% vs. 26%, hazard ratio 0.67, $p = 0.004$), whereas the difference in 3-year overall survival rate was statistically not significant. This study suggest that adjuvant radiotherapy is associated with better outcome in patients with ≥ 2 positive lymph nodes, although the effects of adjuvant radiotherapy on patients with single lymph node metastasis remains unclear (Mahner et al. 2015).

A medium- or high-energy photon beam (6–18 MV), with anterior-posterior and posterior-anterior fields, is recommended for the standard radiotherapy modality. CT-based planning is essential to determine the depth of the inguinal nodes to be treated. The treatment field should include the inguino-femoral nodes, the obturator

Table 2 Suggested radiation field based on tumor factor

Tumor site		Radiation field		
Vulva	Groin node metastasis	Pelvis	Groin	Vulva
High-risk (−)	Negative	No	No	No
High-risk (+)	Negative	No	No	RT if positive margin[a,b]
High-risk (−)	Positive[c]	Yes[d]	Yes[e]	No
High-risk (+)	Positive[c]	Yes[d]	Yes[e]	RT if positive margin[a,b]

Vulvar high-risk factor: close <8 mm or positive margin, large tumor >4 cm, lymphovascular space invasion, stromal invasion >5 mm
[a]Re-resection is another option
[b]Controversy to give RT for other high-risk factors such as close margin, large tumor, LVSI+, and deep stromal invasion
[c]Groin and pelvic radiation is indicated for following factor: one macroscopic micrometastasis (≥5 mm diameter), extracapsular spread, or ≥2 or more lymph nodes with micrometastasis (<5 mm)
[d]Radiate whole pelvis if bilaterally positive or unknown contralateral side in unilaterally positive case; radiate ipsilateral pelvis if unilateral positive after bilateral dissection (Morrow and Curtin 1998)
[e]Bilateral groin radiotherapy is recommended

nodes, and the external and internal iliac nodes. The cephalad border of the pelvic field needs to extend to the mid sacroiliac or L5/S1 joints. If the patient has suspected or proven internal or external iliac involvement, the cephalad border can be extended to the L3/4 or L4/5 level, so as to include the common iliac nodes. The caudal border needs to cover the vulva or the inferior margin of the tumor; the lateral border extends 2 cm laterally, to the widest point of the pelvic inlet. The suggested treatment fields for adjuvant radiation therapy, where vulvar adverse factors and groin nodal metastasis are integrated, are shown in Table 2 based on our best practice.

For treatment of microscopic groin metastases or the primary site, a dose of 50 Gy is recommended. If there are multiple metastases, or an extracapsular extension, the dose is 50–60 Gy. For gross residual disease, the dose needs to be brought to 60–70 Gy (Halperin et al. 2013).

A midline radiation block can be used to protect the radiosensitive vulvar tissues from the radiation, if there is no indication to treat the vulva itself. However, because of the reported high local recurrence rate found with use of a midline block, its routine use should be avoided (Dursenbey et al. 1994).

The effectiveness of chemoradiation treatments in an adjuvant setting in patients with groin nodal metastasis has not been systematically studied. A few studies, each evaluating fewer than ten patients, have treated patients with a combination of 5-fluorouracil (5-FU) and CDDP or mitomycin C with radiation therapy. The role of adjuvant chemotherapy alone has also not been adequately investigated. Bellati et al. enrolled 14 patients with inguinal node metastases after primary surgery. Cisplatin (100 mg/m^2) was administered at 21 day intervals for four cycles. Four of 14 patients (29%) had recurrence, including 14% recurrence rate in the groin, during a median of 57 months of follow-up. The 3-year OS and PFS were 86% and 71%, respectively. The author concluded that adjuvant chemotherapy is feasible, with an acceptable complication rate (Bellati et al. 2005). Further studies are necessary to compare these strategies in patients affected by high-risk disease.

The most significant acute complication of radiation alone or chemoradiation therapy is mucocutaneous reactions such as erythema and moist desquamation in the vulva, perineum, and inguinal lesion, which are expected early during the course of the treatment. This skin reactions may require a treatment break depending on degree of reactions, so that skin care is important. Acute hematologic toxicity is common under the setting of chemoradiation therapy. For severe leukocytopenia, colony-stimulating factors may be needed, and severe anemia can be treated with blood transfusions. The late complications include vulvar skin atrophy, telangestasis, dryness of the vaginal mucosa, and vaginal stenosis. When the pelvis is included in the radiation field, acute enteritis may occur during the treatment, and late complications may occur several months to years after the completion of radiotherapy including proctitis and cystitis.

6 Management of Advanced Stage Tumors

6.1 Surgery Advanced Disease

For patients with stage III or IV vulvar cancer, combinations of multimodal treatments are needed. A primary surgical resection is the best option, if the tumor can be resected without a need for a stoma by conducting modified radical vulvectomy or radical vulvectomy. For some patients, with tumors involving the distal urethra, anus, anal sphincter, rectovaginal septum, or rectum, exenterative operations, combined with radical vulvectomy, have been used to achieve an adequate surgical margin. For larger vulvar tumors, plastic reconstruction procedures are considered following an exenterative surgery or radical vulvectomy. However, because an exenterative procedure compromises the quality of life, with significant amounts of physical and psychological morbidity, alternative therapies, such as chemoradiation followed by radical vulvectomy and lymphadenectomy, have been explored to reduce the tumor burden and to allow for a more conservative surgery. If the primary surgical treatment would compromise sphincter function, such that a bowel or urinary stoma would be needed, preoperative chemoradiation is more desirable.

6.2 Management of Groin Lymph Nodal Metastasis

A thorough evaluation of the status of groin nodes needs to be initially performed to plan the overall treatment. When the primary tumor is advanced and needs a stoma formation if proceeds upfront surgical treatment, groin nodal biopsy or node resection, and inguino-femoral lymphadenectomy can be performed first, based on the groin nodal status. So that postoperative groin radiotherapy can be delivered with the radiation for primary tumor at the same time.

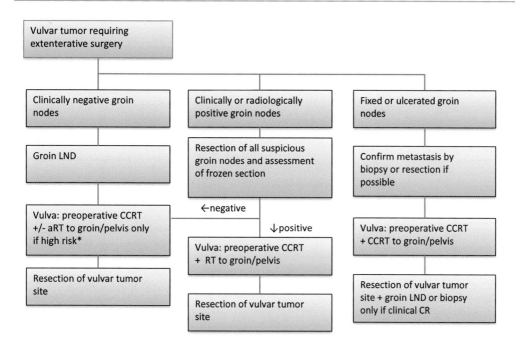

*one macrometastasis (≥5 mm diameter), extracapsular spread, or ≥2 lymph nodes with micrometastasis (<5 mm).
LND: lymphadenectomy, RT: radiation thearapy, aRT: adjuvant radiation therapy, CCRT: concurrent chemoradiotherapy, CR: complete response

Fig. 4 Proposed management of advanced vulvar tumor requiring extenterative surgery

If there is a clinically determined high suspicion of inguino-femoral lymph node metastasis, node resection is recommended and a complete inguino-femoral lymphadenectomy is suggested to avoid because a complete groin dissection, together with postoperative groin irradiation, may result in severe lymphedema. Only the palpably enlarged nodes from the groin and pelvis are to be removed. If nodal metastasis is confirmed, the patient should be given postoperative groin and pelvic radiation.

If there are pathologically positive unresectable nodes, as in ulcerative or fixed nodes, after confirming the presence of the pathologically positive nodes by biopsies, preoperative combined chemotherapy and radiation therapy are recommended prior to the groin lymphadenectomy. In one GOG study of patients with vulvar cancer, with what was considered to be unresectable N2/N3 lymph nodes, the patients were first treated with radiotherapy (total 57.6 Gy, 1.7 Gy fraction) and cisplatin combined with 5-FU. Following the chemoradiation, the residual disease in the lymph nodes became resectable in 95% of the patients, which was combined with surgical resection of the residual tumor. Of those patients who completed the chemoradiation, 88.1% of the patients received both vulvectomy and lymphadenectomy. In the patients who were treated with chemoradiotherapy, the resulting resected lymph nodes were histologically negative in 41% of the cases (Montana et al. 2000). By integrating primary tumor and groin nodal metastasis, a suggested management of advanced tumors which otherwise require exenterative surgery including stoma formation if proceeds upfront surgical treatment is shown in Fig. 4, and a management of advanced tumors resectable without stoma formation is shown in Fig. 5.

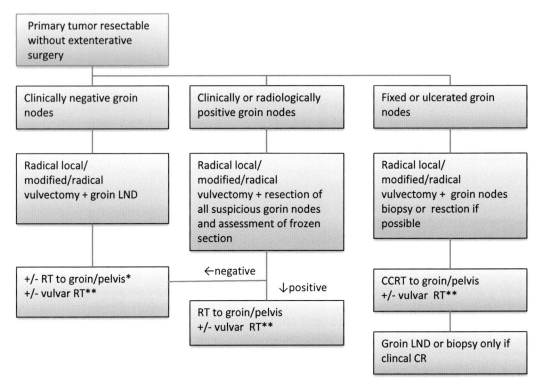

*one macrometastasis (≥5 mm diameter), extracapsular spread, or ≥2 lymph nodes with micrometastasis (<5 mm)
** if there is positive margin , re-excision or vulvar RT are recommended.
LND: lymphadenectomy, RT: radiation thearapy , aRT: adjuvant radiation therapy, CCRT: concurrent chemoradiotherapy,
CR: complete response

Fig. 5 Proposed management of advanced vulvar tumor resectable without extenterative surgery

6.3 Role of Chemoradiation Therapy

The GOG101 trial has studied the effectiveness of cisplatin and 5-fluorouracil (5-FU) as part of the chemoradiation therapy used as a neoadjuvant therapy for patients with locally advanced vulvar cancer, who otherwise would require exenteration to achieve negative surgical margins. Seventy-three patients received 47.6 Gy (1.7 Gy fraction). After chemoradiation, 46.5% of the patients had no evidence of residual tumor at the time of the planned surgery. Only 2.8% of these patients still had residual unresectable disease (Moore et al. 1998).

The existing series of retrospective studies regarding the efficacy of chemoradiation have shown a range of complete clinical responses,

from 47% to 90% (Cunningham et al. 1997; Moore et al. 1998; Tans et al. 2011). To allow better organ preservation, some of these studies describe encouraging evidence for the efficacy of replacing exenterative surgery with primary chemoradiation, forgoing subsequent surgery (Cunningham et al. 1997; Landoni et al. 1996; Moore et al. 1998). In a prospective study by Landoni et al., 58 patients with locally advanced or recurrent vulvar cancer received preoperative radiotherapy (54 Gy) with 5-FU and mitomycin C. The majority (89%) completed the chemoradiotherapy. Objective responses were observed in 80% of the vulvar tumors and in 79% of the cases with groin metastases. Approximately one-fourth (27%) had a complete clinical response confirmed by vulvar biopsy.

A radiation dose of 45–55 Gy is recommended (Hacker et al. 1984a; Halperin et al. 2013).

Following chemoradiation, to reduce complications when a complete response is achieved, instead of conducting a radical vulvectomy, a surgical biopsy of the vulva can be alternatively performed (Moore et al. 2012). A lymphadenectomy is recommended regardless of whether or not there has been a clinical complete response, because residual disease is often found in the lymph nodes (Montana et al. 2000). For patients unable to tolerate radical vulvectomy, or for those who are deemed unsuitable for surgery because of the site or the extent of the disease, definitive chemoradiation therapy is a treatment choice. A total radiation dose of 60–70 Gy is recommended.

Combined chemotherapeutic agents, such as 5-FU/cisplatin and 5-FU/mitomycin C, are often used for chemoradiation treatment for vulvar cancer. For the treatment of locally advanced vulvar cancer, a recent phase II trial conducted by GOG examined the effectiveness of a radiotherapy (total 57.6 Gy, 1.8 cGy fraction) with weekly cisplatin (40 mg/m^2) followed by surgical resection of the residual tumor (or biopsy to confirm complete clinical response) for the treatment of locally advanced vulvar cancer. Among 58 evaluable patients, there were 69% of the patients who completed treatment. High rates of complete clinical response (64%) and histological response (78%) were demonstrated. In the GOG101 study, the total radiation dose was 47.6 Gy. In this latter study, a 20% higher dose of radiation, 57.6 Gy, was delivered, in hopes of achieving better results. The treatment-related toxicity of this approach was found to be acceptable. Common adverse effects included leukopenia, pain, radiation dermatitis, pain, or metabolic change. There were four patients who experienced anemia (grade 3–4) and one of these patients received a blood transfusion (Moore et al. 2012).

Recently, intensity-modulated radiation therapy (IMRT) has been suggested be highly beneficial for lowering the incidence of severe toxicity, by reducing the radiation dose to normal tissue. Beriwal et al. presented results from 42 patients treated with IMRT and 5-FU/cisplatin; they showed a high rate of complete pathologic response (48.5%) (Beriwal et al. 2013). The treatment in this series was well tolerated, with only 2.5% of the patients requiring hospitalization for intravenous hydration after developing severe diarrhea.

6.4 Role of Chemotherapy

Although attempts have been made to decrease the risks of surgical morbidities and to palliate the symptoms of locally advanced disease, the role of neoadjuvant chemotherapy is still limited in vulvar cancer. There have been only a few studies with single- or combination-agent chemotherapies. The most studied single agent chemotherapy regimen is bleomycin, which has been shown to induce a response rate of between 45% and 80% (Aragona et al. 2012; Deppe et al. 1979; Domingues et al. 2010; Tropé et al. 1980). Additional single agents that have been tested in vulvar cancer are cisplatin, paclitaxel, and adriamycin. Table 3 shows a list of examples of combination chemotherapies that have been studied in vulvar cancer (Aragona et al. 2012; Domingues et al. 2010; Durrant et al. 1990; Geisler et al. 2006; Tropé et al. 1980; Wagenaar et al. 2001).

The Gynecological Cancer Cooperative Group of EORTC conducted two different phase II trials with bleomycin, methotrexate, and the alkylating agent lomustine/CCNU (BMC). The overall response rate in the two studies was 56% and 64%, and the complete response rate was 8% and 11%, respectively. In the latter study, the median progression-free survival was 4.8 months and the median survival was 7.8 months. The 1-year overall survival rate was 32%. Unfortunately, severe and life-threatening toxicities were documented in both studies. Severe mucositis was observed in 21% of the patients, and 14% had a severe infection. Severe pulmonary toxicity was seen in up to 7% of cases, and there was one death in each of the studies. Hematologic toxicity and nausea/vomiting were also common. These toxicities suggested that the BMC schedule was not well tolerated in the group, consisting of elderly women (Durrant et al. 1990; Wagenaar et al. 2001). Geisler et al. reported using a

Table 3 Combination chemotherapy for advanced/recurrent vulvar cancer (Based on Wagenaar et al. 2001)

Author	Date	Chemotherapy regimen	No. of patients	Complete response (%)	Partial response (%)	Response rate (%)	Postchemotherapy operability rate (%)
Mosher et al.	1973	BM	1	100		100	
Morrow et al.	1973	AP	1				
Vogl et al.	1976	MHO	2				
Guthrie et al.	1978	MOB + VB	3		100	100	
Hakes et al.	1979	MO	2				
Trope et al.	1980	BMc	9	11	44	55	
Belinson et al.	1985	BOMcP	3				
Chambers et al.	1989	BOMcP	2		50	50	
Durrant et al.	1990	BMC	28	10	54	64	29
Shimizu et al.	1990	BOMcP	1	100			
Benedetti-Panici et al.	1993	PBM	21		10	10	90
Behbakht et al.	1996	BIP	1				
Wagenaar et al.	2001	BMC	25	8	48	56	40
Geisler et al.	2006	P + 5-FU	10	10	90	100	90
Domingues et al.	2010	P + 5-FU	10		20	20	20
Aragona et al.	2012	VBPx	6		100	100	83
Aragona et al.	2012	PPx	6		83	83	83
Aragona et al.	2012	PPx + 5-FU	6		83	83	83
Aragona et al.	2012	P + 5-FU	12		83	83	58

Abbreviations used: *A* adriamycin (doxorubicin), *B* bleomycin, *C* CCNU (lomustine), *Cb* carboplatin, *H* hydroxyurea, *I* ifosfamide, *M* methotrexate, *Mc* mitomycin C, *O* vincristine (oncovin), *P* cisplatin, *Px* paclitaxel, *V* vinblastine

combination of cisplatin and 5-FU on ten patients with locally advanced vulvar cancer and showed a 100% response rate. Interestingly, three patients treated with cisplatin alone in the same study had no response (Geisler et al. 2006). Assessing the efficacy of these single and combination drugs is challenging because these series are based only on small cohorts of cases. Although no particular drug regimen can be recommended at this time, it should be noted that bleomycin, cisplatin, and 5-FU have been shown to have significant activity as key drugs. However, bleomycin has also been associated with severe pulmonary toxicity.

The epidermal growth factor receptor (EGFR) is overexpressed on the cell membrane of invasive vulvar SCC cases, and higher EGFR expression is significantly associated with the depth of stromal tumor invasion and with disease recurrence. The anti-EGFR monoclonal cetuximab has been used successfully to treat some vulvar cancers. Erlotinib, a small-molecule inhibitor of EGFR,

has also been evaluated as a targeted therapy for vulvar cancer. Of 41 patients treated with erlotinib in one study, the overall rate of clinical benefit was 67.5%, with 27.5% having a partial response and 40.0% having a stable disease response (Horowitz et al. 2012).

6.5   Recurrence and Prognosis

Groin recurrences occur in 1–10% of early stage vulvar cancers (Hacker et al. 1981; Homesley et al. 1991; De Hullu et al. 2002; Stehman et al. 1992). Nodal metastasis has been the most important factor in recurrent diseases. Metastasis to groin nodes is diagnosed in approximately 25–35% of patients undergoing surgery.

The site of vulvar cancer recurrence varies. One multicenter study evaluating cases of primary invasive vulvar SCC focused on the patterns of recurrence and clinical outcomes. Of 502 patients,

37.3% of the patients developed a recurrence; these were: perineum, 53.4%; inguinal nodes, 18.7%; and pelvis, 5.7%. Recurrence at distant or multiple sites occurred in 7.9% and 14.2% of cases, respectively. Isolated perineal recurrences were more common; they developed in 70% of the stage I patients. Perineal recurrences appeared during the first year after treatment in 39% of cases; 72% of inguinal recurrences also appeared during the first year (Maggino et al. 2000).

The site of recurrence further weighs heavily against patient survival. Groin recurrence occurs earlier and is more likely to be fatal. In one GOG study, of 143 patients who received one or more modifications of therapy, approximately one-fourth (25.9%) of the patients with vulvar cancer had recurrence, and 54.0% of these patients died of the disease (Stehman et al. 1996). The median interval to recurrence was 35.9 months, and the median survival time after recurrence was 52.4 months. The median time to recurrence in the groin was 7.0 months, and the median survival time after recurrence was only 9.4 months. Most significantly, 91% of those with a groin recurrence died of the disease.

6.6 Follow-up

As in other cancers, most authors recommend regular follow-up for patients after treatment. Most centers adopt a follow-up schedule of every 3 months for 2 year, every 6 months for 5 years, and every 12 months thereafter. Because the majority of vulvar cancer is HPV-related, all the areas with possible HPV-related cancer also need a careful examination during follow-up period (cervix, vagina, and anus).

6.7 Melanoma of the Vulva

Melanoma is the second most frequent type of vulvar cancer, representing 5–10% of such cases. Vulvar melanoma arises from melanocytic cells and is usually pigmented. The mean age of the patients is approximately 60 years. For a primary melanoma without metastasis, the most important prognostic factors are tumor thickness, ulcerations, mitotic rate, and depth of invasion. Symptoms are similar to those of vulvar SCC. The most common melanoma symptom is a vulvar mass. Pain, bleeding, and pruritus are also frequent. Most vulvar melanomas will involve either the labia majora or minora, and multiple sites often occur.

In most cases the clinical appearance of the melanoma varies by subtype. There are four basic histologic types: (i) the superficial spreading melanoma, (ii) the mucosal lentiginous melanoma, (iii) the nodular melanoma, and (iv) acral lentiginous melanoma. Dermoscopy should be used for the differential diagnosis of pigmented lesions. Not only pigmented lesions but also nonpigmented lesions should be examined carefully because there is a unique and rare variant of melanoma which is called amelanotic melanoma. Amelanotic melanoma is difficult to differentiate from other epithelial and nonepithelial malignant tumor due to absence of melanin pigmentation. Adding to the clinical diagnosis, a histopathologic diagnosis for any suspicious lesions is also needed, and the specimen must be examined by dermatopathologists experienced in melanoma. If an excisional biopsy is possible, an incisional biopsy is usually avoided as the latter may lead to misdiagnosis. Immunohistochemical stains, such as S-100, HMB45, or Melan-A, can be helpful, if the histologic diagnosis is unclear.

Melanoma staging is defined by the American Joint Commission on Cancer (AJCC) TNM classification system. Historically, some microstaging systems have been used, including the Clark system (based on the depth of invasion) and Breslow system (tumor thickness) for staging cutaneous melanomas. Currently, Breslow's depth is included as a major prognostic factor in the AJCC staging guidelines for melanoma.

The primary treatment of vulvar melanoma is surgical excision. A wide local excision of the primary lesion, with a negative safety margin, is recommended. Radical vulvectomy is not necessary for most cases. The recommended minimal margin for melanoma is 1 cm for a lesion with ≤ 2 mm thickness, and 2 cm margins are needed for a lesion with >2 mm thickness. Although limited, there is data to suggest that a more radical excision results in lower local recurrence and better survival. As for cutaneous melanomas with clinically negative nodes, elective node dissection has not been shown to have any therapeutic advantage, and sentinel lymph node mapping is now considered the standard approach. Most studies do not indicate a survival advantage for adjuvant therapy for vulvar melanoma. In advanced cases, an individualized treatment plan should be considered (Garbe et al. 2010; Leitao et al. 2014). Melanoma often metastasizes systematically resulting in poor prognosis in such metastatic disease. Recently, targeting programmed death-1 pathway is found to be effective in melanoma. In a large phase III trial presented at European Society for Medical Oncology in 2014, nivolumab showed a higher rate of objective response than chemotherapy (32% vs. 11%) in patients with ipilumamab-refractory melanoma (Gunturi and McDermott 2015). Further development is expected in vulvar melanoma.

6.8   Vulvar Cancer in Pregnancy

Vulvar cancer diagnosed during pregnancy is extremely rare. Matsuo et al. conducted a systematic review of the literature to evaluate managements and feto-maternal outcomes of vulvar cancer during pregnancy (Matsuo et al. 2014). In their study, 32 cases were analyzed. The mean age was 30.7; the most common presenting symptom was vulvar mass/swelling (75.0%). Vulvectomy and inguino-femoral lymphadenectomy were performed in 97.1% and 63.9% of the cases, respectively. Cesarean delivery was performed in 46.2% of the cases. Live birth and full-term delivery rates were 96.3% and 74.0%, respectively. Vulvectomy, with the fetus in situ, was performed in 42.4% cases, and it did not increase the risk of preterm delivery or stillbirth.

The authors pointed out a frequent significant delay of diagnosis in these cases, leading to decreasing both the disease-free survival and overall survival rates. A biopsy of the vulvar lesion, observed at the time of initial presentation for pregnancy care, was conducted in only 46.7%

of the cases. Among the 53% of biopsy-delayed cases, the mean duration of the delay was 12.8 weeks and the majority (62.5%) had a delay for more than 8 weeks. Sixty percent of patients who had a delay that exceeded 8 weeks were initially staged at a more advanced stage, compared to 15% of the patients who had less than 8 weeks of delay. The 5-year disease-free rate was 0% for the cases with >8 weeks delay in diagnosis compared to 69.1% for the cases with ≤8 weeks delay in diagnosis. The majority (70%) of delays in biopsy were due to the observed lesions having a low suspicion for malignancy, mainly because vulvar cancer is predominantly considered a disease of postmenopausal women.

Similarly, in the general population there is also often described a delay in the diagnosis of vulvar cancer, which is usually attributed to both the patient and the physician. Patients often hesitate to tell their physician about their vulvar symptoms, and, because it is so rare, physicians may not always recognize the risk for vulvar malignancy. For early diagnosis, an active approach, including a biopsy for suspicious lesions, even during pregnancy, is strongly recommended.

7   Conclusion

For decades we have been making advances in the treatment of vulvar cancer. Investigators and clinicians are now exploring more individualized treatments and multimodal approaches for it. However, we are greatly hampered in developing new clinical trials because of the relative rarity of this disease. Further studies will help us better understand how to integrate chemoradiation, neoadjuvant chemotherapy, sentinel lymph node sampling, and newer approaches, including IMRT and gene-targeted therapy, into our management of vulvar cancer, helping us to decrease its morbidities and improve its treatment outcome for our patients.

Disclosure The authors have declared that no conflicts of interest exist.

References

Andrews SJ, Williams BT, DePriest PD, Gallion HH, Hunter JE, Buckley SL, et al. Therapeutic implications of lymph nodal spread in lateral T1 and T2 squamous cell carcinoma of the vulva. Gynecol Oncol. 1994; 55(1):41–6.

Ansink A, van der Velden J. Surgical interventions for early squamous cell carcinoma of the vulva. Cochrane Database Syst Rev. 2000;(2):CD002036.

Aragona AM, Cuneo N, Soderini AH, Alcoba E, Greco A, Reyes C, et al. Tailoring the treatment of locally advanced squamous cell carcinoma of the vulva: neoadjuvant chemotherapy followed by radical surgery: results from a multicenter study. Int J Gynecol Cancer. 2012;22(7):1258–63.

Bellati F, Angioli R, Manci N, Angelo Zullo M, Muzii L, Plotti F, et al. Single agent cisplatin chemotherapy in surgically resected vulvar cancer patients with multiple inguinal lymph node metastasis. Gynecol Oncol. 2005;96(1):227–31.

Beller U, Quinn MA, Benedet JL, Creasman WT, Ngan HYS, Maisonneuve P, et al. Carcinoma of the vulva. FIGO 26th Annual Report on the results of treatment in gynecological cancer. Int J Gynaecol Obstet. 2006; 95 Suppl 1:S7–27.

Beriwal S, Shukla G, Shinde A, Heron DE, Kelley JL, Edwards RP, et al. Preoperative intensity modulated radiation therapy and chemotherapy for locally advanced vulvar carcinoma: analysis of pattern of relapse. Int J Radiat Oncol Biol Phys. 2013;85 (5):1269–74.

Burke TW, Levenback C, Coleman RL, Morris M, Silva EG, Gershenson DM. Surgical therapy of T1 and T2 vulvar carcinoma: further experience with radical wide excision and selective inguinal lymphadenectomy. Gynecol Oncol. 1995;57(2):215–20.

Cohn DE, Dehdashti F, Gibb RK, Mutch DG, Rader JS, Siegel BA, et al. Prospective evaluation of positron emission tomography for the detection of groin node metastases from vulvar cancer. Gynecol Oncol. 2002;85(1):179–84.

Cunningham MJ, Goyer RP, Gibbons SK, Kredentser DC, Malfetano JH, Keys H. Primary radiation, cisplatin, and 5-fluorouracil for advanced squamous carcinoma of the vulva. Gynecol Oncol. 1997;66(2):258–61.

Deppe G, Cohen CJ, Bruckner HW. Chemotherapy of squamous cell carcinoma of the vulva: a review. Gynecol Oncol. 1979;7(3):345–8.

Domingues AP, Mota F, Durão M, Frutuoso C, Amaral N, de Oliveira CF. Neoadjuvant chemotherapy in advanced vulvar cancer. Int J Gynecol Cancer. 2010;20(2):294–8.

Durrant KR, Mangioni C, Lacave AJ, George M, van der Burg ME, Guthrie D, et al. Bleomycin, methotrexate, and CCNU in advanced inoperable squamous cell carcinoma of the vulva: a phase II study of the EORTC Gynaecological Cancer Cooperative Group (GCCG). Gynecol Oncol. 1990;37(3):359–62.

Dursenbey KE, Carlson JW, LaPorte RM, Unger JA, Goswitz JJ, Roback DM, et al. Radical vulvectomy with postoperative irradiation for vulvar cancer: therapeutic implications of a central block. Int J Radiat Oncol Biol Phys. 1994;29(5):989–98.

Garbe C, Peris K, Hauschild A, Saiag P, Middleton M, Spatz A, et al. Diagnosis and treatment of melanoma: European consensus-based interdisciplinary guideline. Eur J Cancer. 2010;46(2):270–83.

Geisler JP, Manahan KJ, Buller RE. Neoadjuvant chemotherapy in vulvar cancer: avoiding primary exenteration. Gynecol Oncol. 2006;100(1):53–7.

Gordinier ME, Malpica A, Burke TW, Bodurka DC, Wolf JK, Jhingran A, et al. Groin recurrence in patients with vulvar cancer with negative nodes on superficial inguinal lymphadenectomy. Gynecol Oncol. 2003;90 (3):625–8.

Gunturi A, McDermott DF. Nivolumab for the treatment of cancer. Expert Opin Investig Drugs. 2015; 24(2):253–60.

Hacker NF, Van der Velden J. Conservative management of early vulvar cancer. Cancer. 1993;71(4 Suppl):1673–7.

Hacker NF, Leuchter RS, Berek JS, Castaldo TW, Lagasse LD. Radical vulvectomy and bilateral inguinal lymphadenectomy through separate groin incisions. Obstet Gynecol. 1981;58(5):574–9.

Hacker NF, Berek JS, Juillard GJ, Lagasse LD. Preoperative radiation therapy for locally advanced vulvar cancer. Cancer. 1984a; 54(10):2056–61.

Hacker NF, Berek JS, Lagasse LD, Nieberg RK, Leuchter RS. Individualization of treatment for stage I squamous cell vulvar carcinoma. Obstet Gynecol. 1984b; 63(2):155–62.

Hacker NF, Eifel PJ, van der Velden J. Cancer of the vulva. Int J Gynecol Obstet. 2012;119:S90–6.

Halperin EC, Brady LW, Perez CA, Wazer DE. Perez & Brady's principles and practice of radiation oncology. 6th ed. Philadelphia. Lippincott Williams & Wilkins; 2013.

Heaps JM, Fu YS, Montz FJ, Hacker NF, Berek JS. Surgical-pathologic variables predictive of local recurrence in squamous cell carcinoma of the vulva. Gynecol Oncol. 1990;38(3):309–14.

Hoffman JS, Kumar NB, Morley GW. Prognostic significance of groin lymph node metastases in squamous carcinoma of the vulva. Obstet Gynecol. 1985; 66(3):402–5.

Homesley HD, Bundy BN, Sedlis A, Yordan E, Berek JS, Jahshan A, et al. Assessment of current International Federation of Gynecology and Obstetrics staging of vulvar carcinoma relative to prognostic factors for survival (a Gynecologic Oncology Group study). Am J Obstet Gynecol. 1991;164(4):997–1003.

Homesley HD, Bundy BN, Sedlis A, Yordan E, Berek JS, Jahshan A, et al. Prognostic factors for groin node metastasis in squamous cell carcinoma of the vulva (a Gynecologic Oncology Group study). Gynecol Oncol. 1993;49(3):279–83.

Horowitz NS, Olawaiye AB, Borger DR, Growdon WB, Krasner CN, Matulonis UA, et al. Phase II trial of erlotinib in women with squamous cell carcinoma of the vulva. Gynecol Oncol. 2012;127(1):141–6.

De Hullu JA, Hollema H, Lolkema S, Boezen M, Boonstra H, Burger MPM, et al. Vulvar carcinoma: the price of less radical surgery. Cancer. 2002; 95(11):2331–8.

Judson PL, Habermann EB, Baxter NN, Durham SB, Virnig BA. Trends in the incidence of invasive and in situ vulvar carcinoma. Obstet Gynecol. 2006;107 (5):1018–22.

Kim KW, Shinagare AB, Krajewski KM, Howard SA, Jagannathan JP, Zukotynski K, et al. Update on imaging of vulvar squamous cell carcinoma. Am J Roentgenol. 2013;201(1):147–57.

Kunos C, Simpkins F, Gibbons H, Tian C, Homesley H. Radiation therapy compared with pelvic node resection for node-positive vulvar cancer: a randomized controlled trial. Obstet Gynecol. 2009;114(3):537–46.

Landoni F, Maneo A, Zanetta G, Colombo A, Nava S, Placa F, et al. Concurrent preoperative chemotherapy with 5-fluorouracil and mitomycin C and radiotherapy (FUMIR) followed by limited surgery in locally advanced and recurrent vulvar carcinoma. Gynecol Oncol. 1996;61(3):321–7.

Leitao MM, Cheng X, Hamilton AL, Siddiqui NA, Jurgenliemk-Schulz I, Mahner S, et al. Gynecologic Cancer InterGroup (GCIG) consensus review for vulvovaginal melanomas. Int J Gynecol Cancer. 2014;24(9 Suppl 3):S117–22.

Maggino T, Landoni F, Sartori E, Zola P, Gadducci A, Alessi C, et al. Patterns of recurrence in patients with squamous cell carcinoma of the vulva. A multicenter CTF Study. Cancer. 2000;89(1):116–22.

Mahner S, Jueckstock J, Hilpert F, Neuser P, Harter P, de Gregorio N, et al. Adjuvant therapy in lymph node-positive vulvar cancer: the AGO-CaRE-1 study. J Natl Cancer Inst. 2015;107(3):dju426.

Matsuo K, Whitman SA, Blake EA, Conturie CL, Ciccone MA, Jung CE, et al. Feto-maternal outcome of pregnancy complicated by vulvar cancer: a systematic review of literature. Eur J Obstet Gynecol Reprod Biol. 2014;179:216–23.

Montana GS, Thomas GM, Moore DH, Saxer A, Mangan CE, Lentz SS, et al. Preoperative chemo-radiation for carcinoma of the vulva with N2/N3 nodes: a Gynecologic Oncology Group study. Int J Radiat Oncol Biol Phys. 2000;48(4):1007–13.

Moore DH, Thomas GM, Montana GS, Saxer A, Gallup DG, Olt G. Preoperative chemoradiation for advanced vulvar cancer: a phase II study of the Gynecologic Oncology Group. Int J Radiat Oncol Biol Phys. 1998;42(1):79–85.

Moore DH, Ali S, Koh W-J, Michael H, Barnes MN, McCourt CK, et al. A phase II trial of radiation therapy and weekly cisplatin chemotherapy for the treatment of locally-advanced squamous cell carcinoma of the vulva: a Gynecologic Oncology Group study. Gynecol Oncol. 2012;124(3):529–33.

Morrow CP, Curtin JP. Tumors of the vulva. In: Synopsis of gynecologic oncology. 5th ed. New York: Churchill Livingstone; 1998. p. 61–87.

Pecorelli S, Zigliani L, Odicino F. Revised FIGO staging for carcinoma of the vulva, cervix, and endometrium. Int J Gynecol Obstet. 2009;105(2):107–8. Elsevier B.V.

de Sanjosé S, Alemany L, Ordi J, Tous S, Alejo M, Bigby SM, et al. Worldwide human papillomavirus genotype attribution in over 2000 cases of intraepithelial and invasive lesions of the vulva. Eur J Cancer. 2013;49 (16):3450–61.

Siegel RL, Miller KD, Jemal A. Cancer statistics. CA Cancer J Clin. 2015;65(1):5–29.

Stehman FB, Bundy BN, Dvoretsky PM, Creasman WT. Early stage I carcinoma of the vulva treated with ipsilateral superficial inguinal lymphadenectomy and modified radical hemivulvectomy: a prospective study of the Gynecologic Oncology Group. Obstet Gynecol. 1992;79(4):490–7.

Stehman FB, Bundy BN, Ball H, Clarke-Pearson DL. Sites of failure and times to failure in carcinoma of the vulva treated conservatively: a Gynecologic Oncology Group study. Am J Obstet Gynecol. 1996;174(4):1128–32.

Tans L, Ansink AC, van Rooij PH, Kleijnen C, Mens JW. The role of chemo-radiotherapy in the management of locally advanced carcinoma of the vulva: single institutional experience and review of literature. Am J Clin Oncol. 2011;34(1):22–6.

Tantipalakorn C, Robertson G, Marsden DE, Gebski V, Hacker NF. Outcome and patterns of recurrence for International Federation of Gynecology and Obstetrics (FIGO) stages I and II squamous cell vulvar cancer. Obstet Gynecol. 2009;113(4):895–901.

Tropé C, Johnsson JE, Larsson G, Simonsen E. Bleomycin alone or combined with mitomycin C in treatment of advanced or recurrent squamous cell carcinoma of the vulva. Cancer Treat Rep. 1980;64(4–5):639–42.

Wagenaar HC, Colombo N, Vergote I, Hoctin-Boes G, Zanetta G, Pecorelli S, et al. Bleomycin, methotrexate, and CCNU in locally advanced or recurrent, inoperable, squamous-cell carcinoma of the vulva: an EORTC Gynaecological Cancer Cooperative Group Study. European Organization for Research and Treatment of Cancer. Gynecol Oncol. 2001;81(3):348–54.

Diagnosis and Management of Vaginal Cancer

E. Clair McClung, Ardeshir Hakam, and Mian M. K. Shahzad

Abstract

Primary malignancies of the vagina are rare, comprising only about 1–4% of all gynecologic malignancies. The majority of vaginal cancers are metastases from other sites. Among primary vaginal tumors, squamous cell carcinoma (SCC) is the most common, followed by adenocarcinoma, melanoma, and other rare histologies. Squamous cell carcinomas are frequently associated with chronic human papillomavirus (HPV) infection, whereas adenocarcinomas are associated with in utero diethylstilbestrol (DES) exposure. Vaginal intraepithelial neoplasia (VAIN) is a premalignant condition thought to progress to invasive squamous cell carcinoma if untreated. Vaginal intraepithelial neoplasia is generally asymptomatic and diagnosed by abnormal vaginal cytology followed by vaginal colposcopy and biopsies. Most vaginal cancers present with abnormal vaginal bleeding or a vaginal mass. Diagnosis is made by physical exam and confirmatory biopsy. Treatment of vaginal cancer depends on the primary histology, stage at diagnosis, and patient characteristics. Treatment options include surgical excision, radiation therapy, and chemotherapy. The majority of vaginal cancers are treated with radiation, frequently in combination with chemotherapy. Prognosis varies depending on underlying histology and stage at presentation; however, with advances in radiation techniques, survival rates are similar to those seen in cervical cancer.

Keywords

Vaginal intraepithelial neoplasia (VAIN) • Vaginal squamous cell carcinoma • Vaginal adenocarcinoma • Vaginal melanoma • Vaginal rhabdomyosarcoma

Contents

E.C. McClung • M.M.K. Shahzad (✉)
Department of Gynecologic Oncology, University of South Florida/H. Lee Moffitt Cancer Center, Tampa, FL, USA
e-mail: Emily.mcclung@moffitt.org;
Mian.Shahzad@moffitt.org

A. Hakam
Department of Pathology, University of South Florida/H. Lee Moffitt Cancer Center, Tampa, FL, USA
e-mail: Ardeshir.Hakam@moffitt.org

© Springer International Publishing AG 2017
D. Shoupe (ed.), *Handbook of Gynecology*,
DOI 10.1007/978-3-319-17798-4_8

1 Introduction

Primary malignancies of the vagina are quite rare, comprising only about 1–4% of all gynecologic malignancies (Siegel et al. 2015). In the USA, approximately 4000 women are diagnosed with vaginal cancer each year, and approximately 900 women die of the disease (Siegel et al. 2015). The majority of cancers involving the vagina are actually secondary metastases or direct extensions from other primary sites. In a series of 355 invasive carcinomas involving the vagina, only 58 (16%) represented primary vaginal lesions. Among secondary sites metastatic to the vagina, the cervix was most common (32%), followed by the endometrium (18%), colon and rectum (9%), ovary (6%), vulva (6%), bladder and urethra (4%) (Fu and Reagan 1989).

In this chapter, we will focus on the diagnosis and management of primary vaginal malignant neoplasms and premalignant conditions. Due to the rarity of the disease, most treatment strategies are derived from small retrospective case series and extrapolated from prospective studies for the treatment of cervical and anal cancers. Squamous cell carcinoma is the most common and well-studied histology, representing 65–79% of vaginal cancers in two large cancer registry studies (Creasman et al. 1998; Shah et al. 2009). Adenocarcinoma is the second most common histology representing 9–14% of tumors, followed by melanoma (3–6%) and other rare histologies including mesenchymal, germ cell, neuroendocrine, and hematologic cell types collectively accounting for the remaining 4–15% (Creasman et al. 1998; Shah et al. 2009). The majority of vaginal cancers are treated with radiation, frequently in combination with chemotherapy. Prognosis varies depending on underlying histology and stage at presentation;

however, with advances in radiation techniques, survival rates are similar to those seen in cervical cancer.

2 Vaginal Anatomy

The vagina is a fibro-muscular, distensible tube extending from the uterine cervix superiorly to the vestibule of the vagina, vulva, and perineum inferiorly. Embryologically, the vagina is formed by fusion of the urogenital sinus epithelium inferiorly with the mullerian ducts superiorly. Structural support for the vagina includes the cardinal and uterosacral ligaments superiorly and the muscular supports of the pelvic floor including the levator ani, the bulbospongiosus muscle, and urogenital diaphragm. The vagina shares fascial support anteriorly with the bladder and posteriorly with the rectum. Between these attachments, the lateral vaginal wall opens into the paravaginal space. The vaginal fornix describes the recesses around the uterine cervix and can be divided into anterior, posterior, and lateral regions. The posterior fornix is the largest and is separated from the rectum by a fold of peritoneum, forming the pouch of Douglas.

The vaginal wall consists of three layers: the mucosa, the muscularis, and the adventitia. The mucosa is lined by the nonkeratinized stratified squamous epithelium, rich in glycogen and estrogen. There are no glands or crypts in the vagina, and the mucosa is primarily lubricated by cervical glands. Vaginal atrophy, characterized by mucosal thinning and blunting of the vaginal rugae, is common in low estrogen states such as prior to onset of puberty and after menopause. Underlying the epithelial basement membrane is the submucosal layer, highly vascular and rich in lymphatics. The muscularis layer consists of smooth muscle fibers, and adventitia is a thin layer of connective tissue continuous with the adventitia layer of other surrounding organs.

The arterial supply of the upper vagina comes from the internal iliac artery frequently off a trunk shared with the uterine artery, called vaginal artery, while the middle and lower portions of the vagina are supplied by branches of the middle rectal and internal pudendal arteries. Venous drainage is facilitated by vaginal venous plexuses in the lateral vagina which drain into the internal iliac vein. The vagina is innervated by nerves derived from the inferior hypogastric plexus.

Classically, lymphatic vessels from the upper 2/3 of the vagina drain into the internal iliac and external iliac lymph nodes, while vessels from the lower 1/3 drain into the superficial inguinal lymph nodes via lymphatic channels in the lateral vagina (Plentl and Friedman 1971). Posterior vaginal lesions may also drain into para-rectal nodes (Plentl and Friedman 1971).

3 Natural History

Most data about the natural history of vaginal carcinoma emanates from early case reports where few treatment modalities were available, and many patients presented with advanced disease. In a compilation of early case series, Plentl and Friedman report that of 1204 vaginal cancer cases, 57.2% were located on the posterior wall, 26.9% on the anterior wall, and 15.9% on the lateral wall (Plentl and Friedman 1971). Among 743 cases with data available, 50.7% of tumors were located in the upper 1/3 of the vagina, 18.8% in the middle 1/3, and 30.4% in the lower 1/3. VAIN also has a predilection for the upper vagina, which is thought to be due to an HPV-related field effect in patients with cervical HPV infections.

Vaginal cancers may spread by contiguous growth and local invasion, lymphatic drainage, and hematogenously. Because of closely approximated structures including the urethra, bladder, rectum, and pelvic bones, locally advanced disease is generally symptomatic and carries a high rate of morbidity. Due to the rich lymphatic drainage of the vagina, lymph node metastases occur relatively early in the disease. By contrast, hematogenous dissemination to distant sites, such as the liver, lung, or bone, occurs late in the disease process.

4 Epidemiology

Vaginal squamous cell carcinoma is primarily a disease of older women, with peak incidence between ages 60 and 80 (Creasman et al. 1998; Shah et al. 2009). Vaginal squamous cell carcinoma is considered to be an HPV-related disease and shares many risk factors with other HPV-related squamous cell carcinomas, including prior documented HPV infection (particularly HPV 16), history of cervical or vulvar dysplasia (CIN or VIN), immunosuppression, five or more sexual partners or sexual debut prior to age 17, smoking, and low socioeconomic status (Daling et al. 2002). VAIN and squamous cell carcinomas are strongly associated with a prior history of cervical cancer. Prior radiation therapy (Hellman et al. 2004) and chronic vaginal irritation related to pelvic organ prolapse and pessary use have also been proposed as possible risk factors (Wang et al. 2014).

Vaginal adenocarcinoma is associated with precursor lesions including vaginal adenosis, endometriosis, and mesonephric rests. Vaginal clear cell carcinoma, associated with in utero diethylstilbestrol (DES) exposure is the most commonly described form in the literature. DES is a nonsteroidal estrogen that has been implicated in congenital reproductive tract abnormalities including persistence of vaginal glandular tissue in a condition called vaginal adenosis. In review of registry cases, Herbst reported that among women exposed to DES in utero, the risk of clear cell carcinoma of the vagina or cervix was approximately 1/1000, with age at diagnosis ranged from 7 to 34 years, with peak incidence at age 14–22 (Herbst and Andersond 1990). Vaginal adenosis occurred in 45%, and structural genital tract anomalies in 25%. The incidence of vaginal clear cell carcinoma has declined significantly since the 1990s. Non-DES-related vaginal adenocarcinomas occur in older women, with a median age at diagnosis of 54 (Frank et al. 2007).

A small subset of vaginal cancer has a predilection for the pediatric population. Vaginal rhabdomyosarcoma, also known as sarcoma botryoides, accounts for approximately 4% of rhabdomyosarcomas, which are the most common tumors in childhood. The median age at presentation is 16.3 months (Magné et al. 2008). Vaginal and cervical yolk sac tumors, also known as endodermal sinus tumors, are another rare vaginal tumor of childhood. Only about 100 cases have been reported in the literature, all diagnosed prior to age 3.

5   Signs and Symptoms

Approximately 15–17% of vaginal cancers are asymptomatic and identified by abnormal cytology or incidental mass on routine pelvic examination (Eddy et al. 1991; Hellman et al. 2004). Abnormal vaginal bleeding is the most commonly reported symptom of invasive carcinoma; however, abnormal vaginal discharge and dysuria are also frequently reported. In the case of more advanced disease, patients may present with pain, the sensation of a mass, or symptoms related to the involvement of adjacent pelvic organs. Tumors involving the bladder may present with urinary incontinence or retention, hematuria, urgency, or frequency. Tumors involving the rectum may present with constipation, tenesmus, or rectal bleeding. Sarcoma botryoides presents with a characteristic edematous, grape-like mass protruding from the vagina.

Vaginal intraepithelial neoplasia (VAIN) is generally asymptomatic, but may present with abnormal vaginal discharge which is often the result of a coincidental vaginitis. Most cases of VAIN are diagnosed after abnormal vaginal cytology in women who have a history of cervical dysplasia

6   Diagnosis

Vaginal cancer should be diagnosed after a thorough focused history and physical exam, careful inspection of the vagina, confirmatory biopsies, and exclusion of more common gynecologic malignancies which may have metastasized to the vaginal mucosa. According to the International Federation of Gynecology and Obstetrics

(FIGO) definitions, any vaginal lesion also involving the cervix or the vulva should be classified as a cervical or vulvar primary cancer, respectively (Hacker et al. 2015). Similarly, in women with a prior history of cervical carcinoma, a vaginal carcinoma lesion should not be considered a second primary unless the patient has been without evidence of disease for at least 5 years (Hacker et al. 2015).

Inquiry of clinical history should include symptoms and risk factors associated with vaginal carcinoma and a complete past medical and gynecological history. Physical examination should focus on evaluation of potential metastatic sites, with particular care to palpate the inguinal and supraclavicular lymph nodes, which may be enlarged in advanced disease.

During pelvic examination, the vulva and anus should be carefully inspected for HPV-related lesions, with care to visualize folds of the labia and the vaginal vestibule prior to speculum insertion. The entire vaginal surface should be visualized, which may require an exam under anesthesia in women with locally advanced disease or vaginal stenosis secondary to severe vaginal atrophy or prior radiation. Most vaginal cancers are located in the upper vagina, frequently on the posterior wall. A speculum examination should be performed with care to inspect the anterior and posterior fornix as well as the distal vagina. Lesions in the distal anterior and posterior vagina may be obscured by the blades of the speculum unless the speculum is gently rotated to expose the circumferential surface of the vagina. Small lesions may be difficult to identify in parous or obese women with redundant vaginal folds. In women who have had a prior hysterectomy, lesions also may be concealed by folds of mucosa buried within the vaginal cuff closure. Partial upper vaginectomy may be required to adequately evaluate these patients.

Vaginal cancers are frequently exophytic, papillary appearing tumors, but infiltrating, ulcerative and flat spreading forms are also seen (Morrow and Curtin 1998). Carcinomas arising in the setting of extensive VAIN may be multifocal. Any visible lesions should be evaluated with full-thickness mucosal biopsies. Vaginal cytology may also be useful to identify cellular atypia, but should not be used alone to evaluate for VAIN or vaginal malignancies. Any woman with a suspicious vaginal lesion who has not had a total hysterectomy should also have consideration of cervical biopsies and endocervical sampling to evaluate for an occult cervical malignancy. Similarly, women with abnormal bleeding and an intact uterus should have an endometrial biopsy or dilation and curettage to evaluate for endometrial cancer. A bimanual exam should be performed to palpate the size and extent of an intravaginal mass and assess for any pelvic masses. This exam should be followed by a rectovaginal exam to identify gross invasion through the rectal mucosa, tumor infiltration of the rectovaginal septum, and parametrial or pelvic sidewall involvement. When locally advanced disease is suspected based on the size and location of the primary tumor, cystourethroscopy and/or proctoscopy are indicated. Biopsies should be obtained if there is any question of mucosal bowel or bladder involvement. Sigmoidoscopy may also be considered for women with large tumors in the posterior vaginal fornix that are suspected to extend into the pelvis.

All patients with abnormal cytology but no grossly visible lesion should be further evaluated with vaginal colposcopy. Some providers advocate colposcopy for all cases of vaginal carcinoma in order to visualize any areas of occult mucosal involvement or associated dysplasia. Colposcopy can be performed in the office during initial examination and may be repeated in the operating room as needed to guide biopsies or excision of lesions identified. Acetic acid solution should be liberally applied to the vagina, and the mucosa should be inspected under magnification using a colposcope. Lugol's iodine solution may be a useful adjunct to identify nonstaining mucosa. Colposcopically abnormal mucosa should be biopsied for diagnosis. When there is a question of high-grade dysplasia versus invasive carcinoma, lesions should be excised, as a large superficial lesion may contain a small focus of deeper invasion that could be missed on biopsy alone. A complete upper vaginectomy may be necessary in order to adequately rule out invasive carcinoma in

the setting of multifocal or extensive high-grade VAIN. In a series of sequential upper vaginectomies for VAIN2 or VAIN3 from 1985 to 2004, Indermaur et al. reported that 12/105 (12%) had a previously unsuspected invasive carcinoma (Indermaur et al. 2005).

7 Evaluation and Staging

Similar to cervical cancer, vaginal cancer staging is clinical. Two commonly used staging systems are defined by the International Federation of Gynecology and Obstetrics (FIGO) and American Joint Committee on Cancer (AJCC) TNM staging system (Edge et al. 2010; Hacker et al. 2015). In both systems stage I/T1 describes tumors confined to the vaginal wall; stage II/T2 tumors invade the paravaginal tissues; stage III/T3 involves the pelvic sidewall; stage IV/T4 invades the bladder or rectal mucosa; and distant metastases (M) are labeled stage IVB (Table 1).

Table 1 FIGO stage and 5-year overall survival rates for vaginal cancer

FIGO stage[a]	Definition	Creasman et al. 1998[b] (NCDB data, $n = 4885$)	Shah et al. 2009[c] (SEER data, $n = 2149$)
I	Limited to the vaginal wall	73%	84%
II	Involving subvaginal tissue	58%	75%
III	Pelvic sidewall involvement	36% (stages III and IV)	57% (stages III and IV)
IVA	Bladder or rectum invasion or extension beyond the pelvis		
IVB	Distant metastases		

Compiled from:
[a]Hacker et al. (2015)
[b]Creasman et al. (1998)
[c]Shah et al. (2009)

Lymph node involvement is not directly addressed in the FIGO system, whereas in the AJCC system it is designated by N, and all patients with positive pelvic or inguinal lymph nodes are assigned to N1 (clinical stage III). Metastatic sites (AJCC designation M1) include, but are not limited to, aortic lymph nodes, lungs, liver, bone, and others outside the pelvis. Currently FIGO staging is used more commonly in the treatment of vaginal cancer.

In the FIGO system, studies officially recommended for clinical staging of a tumor are limited in order to preserve consistent labeling across historical data and low resource settings. These studies include pelvic examination, cystoscopy, proctoscopy, chest radiograph, and intravenous pyelogram. Where advanced imaging techniques such as computed tomographic (CT) scans and magnetic resonance imaging (MRI) are available, many providers extrapolate results from these studies into the clinical staging model. Because of its high resolution and ability to discriminate soft tissue plains, MRI of the pelvis can be a particularly useful adjunct to physical exam for determining the extent of tumor invasion into the bladder, rectum, or parametrial tissues. Taylor et al. correlated MRI findings with clinical outcomes in 25 vaginal cancer patients and concluded that MRI could identify 95% of primary lesions and accurately predicted clinical stage (Taylor et al. 2007). Primary vaginal lesions appear with low-intermediate intensity on T1- and hyperintensity on T2-weighted images (Taylor et al. 2007) and may be better visualized if the vagina is instilled with gel during the study to separate and distend the vaginal walls. Positron emission tomography (PET) scans have become a standard tool for evaluating local, nodal, and metastatic disease for initial evaluation and surveillance of cervical cancer. Not surprisingly, PET has also been widely adopted for evaluation of vaginal cancers and has been shown to have superior sensitivity compared with standard CT for detecting both primary vaginal tumors (100% with PET vs. 43% for CT) and nodal metastasis (Lamoreaux et al. 2005).

8   Screening and Prevention

Similar to other rare cancers, screening for vaginal cancer among low-risk populations is not recommended. The American Cancer Society and American Society for Colposcopy and Cervical Pathology (ASCCP) recommend routine vaginal cytology in women who have had a hysterectomy *only* if there is a history of high-grade cervical dysplasia (CIN2/CIN3) (Saslow et al. 2012). Because VAIN and squamous cell carcinomas are closely associated with HPV infection, HPV vaccination campaigns are likely to be the most important strategy to prevent these diseases.

9   Histologic Subtypes and Management

9.1   Vaginal Intraepithelial Neoplasia (VAIN)

Vaginal intraepithelial neoplasia (VAIN), also known as vaginal carcinoma in situ, is a form of squamous cell atypia that is confined to the squamous epithelium of the vagina, without any evidence of invasion. The characteristics of VAIN include nuclear atypia, loss of squamous cell maturation, and the presence of suprabasilar mitoses. Similar to cervical intraepithelial neoplasia (CIN), VAIN1 involves the deepest 1/3 of the epithelium, VAIN2 the deepest 2/3, and VAIN3 the full thickness of the epithelial layer (Fig. 1). VAIN is almost always associated with HPV infection in more than 90% of cases, with HPV 16 being the most common subtype, found in up to 65% of cases of VAIN2/VAIN3 (Smith et al. 2009). The true natural history of VAIN is not known; however, it is considered premalignant because of its association with high-risk HPV types. Invasive squamous cell carcinoma has been identified in up to 12% of vaginectomies performed for VAIN2/VAIN3 (Indermaur et al. 2005).

Treatment strategies for VAIN include observation, local excision, partial or total vaginectomy, ablation with laser vaporization or

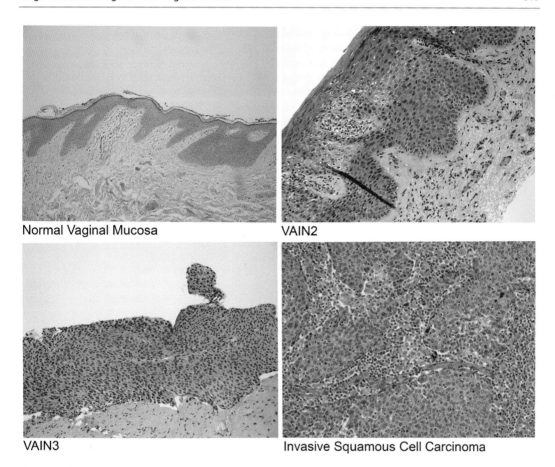

Normal Vaginal Mucosa   VAIN2

VAIN3   Invasive Squamous Cell Carcinoma

Fig. 1 Vaginal mucosa, high-grade dysplasia, and invasive carcinoma (Ardeshir Hakam 2015)

electrocoagulation, topical 5% fluorouracil, or intracavitary radiation therapy. Observation is limited to the treatment of VAIN1, which is more likely to regress spontaneously. For VAIN2/VAIN3, published disease control rates are similar for all approaches. Most studies consist of small, single institutional case series, and modalities have not been directly compared for efficacy. The choice of therapy should be individualized based on the size, location, and severity of VAIN lesions, as well as the patient's age, general health and life expectancy, desire for sexual function, and prior history of treatment failures. In a significant subset of women, VAIN is chronically persistent and recurrent and may require repeated treatment with multiple modalities. Risk factors for recurrence include multifocal disease, VAIN3, and older age (Dodge et al. 2001). In all cases,

invasive carcinoma should be ruled out with adequate sampling biopsies prior to initiating treatment. Treatment strategies are summarized in Table 2.

Surgical excision is the most appropriate management when invasive carcinoma cannot be ruled out, as this is the only approach that will provide tissue for diagnosis. For patients with a focal, well-circumscribed lesion, local excisional colpectomy is the best choice. In more extensive disease, an upper or total vaginectomy may be necessary to obtain adequate margins. These procedures are usually performed vaginally; however upper vaginectomy may require an abdominal approach in some cases, ideally using minimally invasive technique. Vaginectomy can lead to shortening or stenosis of the vagina and loss of sexual function. Reconstructive procedures and

Table 2 Treatment modalities for vaginal intraepithelial neoplasia

Method of treatment	Applications/advantages	Risks and side effects
Surgical excision	Pathologic diagnosis Evaluate for invasive cancer Total vaginectomy provides definitive treatment	Vaginal shortening or stenosis (large excision) Loss of sexual function (vaginectomy) Possible laparotomy or other surgical complications Generally requires anesthesia
Ablation (CO_2 laser or electrocautery)	Preservation of vaginal length Treatment of multifocal or extensive disease Lower rates of sexual dysfunction	Vaginal stenosis may occur Diagnosis of invasive cancer can be delayed Generally requires anesthesia
5-Fluorouracil	Coverage of diffuse or multifocal disease Does not require anesthesia	Vaginal burning Vaginal ulceration Diagnosis of invasive cancer can be delayed May cause vaginal adenosis in rare cases after CO_2 ablation
Imiquimod	Coverage of diffuse or multifocal disease Does not require anesthesia	Vaginal burning Vaginal ulceration Diagnosis of invasive cancer can be delayed
Vaginal estrogen	May augment other treatment modalities	Unproven as monotherapy
Radiation therapy	Usually definitive Effective when other modalities have failed	Vaginal shortening or stenosis Vaginal fibrosis Sexual dysfunction or loss of function Impaired wound healing Radiation cystitis/proctitis Premature menopause/ovarian ablation

skin grafts may be necessary after total vaginectomy. Women with a prior history of radiation therapy are also at increased risk of surgical complications and fistula formation following colpectomy and vaginectomy procedures.

CO₂ laser vaporization is proposed as relatively noninvasive approach that may be useful for large VAIN lesions and multifocal disease in women who want to retain sexual function. The procedure is generally well tolerated, and patients report minimal sexual dysfunction. Ablation procedures should only be performed if an underlying invasive carcinoma can be adequately ruled out and if the entire lesion can be visualized. Lesions that are partially obscured should be excised.

Topical therapies may be useful for women with low-grade persistent VAIN or diffuse, multifocal disease in women who are poor surgical candidates, after invasive carcinoma has been ruled out. The advantage of these modalities is that the entire vaginal surface can be treated, including difficult to access crevices at the vaginal apex. Proposed topical agents include 5-fluorouracil (5FU), imiquimod, and vaginal estrogen. Of these, **5FU** is the best studied. Several 5FU dose regimens have been proposed, but none have been directly compared, and the most commonly used dose is 2 g once weekly for 10–12 weeks (Gurumurthy and Cruickshank 2012). Side effects of vaginal 5FU include burning and vaginal ulceration. Zinc and other barrier creams may be used to protect unaffected areas, and vaginal estrogen may reduce vaginal discomfort. Vaginal columnar metaplasia (adenosis) has been reported when 5FU is administered after prior CO_2 laser ablation, but the significance of this finding is unknown (Paczos et al. 2010; Gurumurthy and Cruickshank 2012). **Imiquimod**, a topical immune modulator, has also been shown to have activity against VAIN in a few small studies. As with 5FU, dosing regimens vary from series to series. Buck et al. reported that 86% of a 42-patient series experience regression of VAIN after a 3-week course of once weekly application of 0.25 g 5%

Table 3 Histologic subtypes of vaginal cancer and their characteristics

	Squamous cell carcinoma	Adenocarcinoma	Melanoma	Rhabdomyosarcoma (sarcoma botryoides)
Epidemiology	Age >60 HPV (HPV 16) History of cervical dysplasia Chronic irritation	Age 14–22 or >60 DES exposure (clear cell) Vaginal adenosis, endometriosis, or mesonephric rests	Age ~60 White, non-Hispanic	Early childhood
Signs/ symptoms	Abnormal pap (ASCUS-HSIL) Vaginal bleeding Vaginal mass	Abnormal pap (AGUS) Vaginal bleeding Vaginal mass	Pigmented lesion Vaginal bleeding Discharge	Grape-like vaginal mass
Treatment modalities	Chemoradiation (EBRT + brachytherapy) Vaginectomy (localized stage I in upper vagina) Pelvic exenteration (central disease)	Conservative surgery Fertility sparing (young patients) Chemoradiation	Surgery Targeted therapies Immunotherapy	Chemotherapy Conservative surgery Radiation

Other histologies: **leiomyosarcoma, carcinosarcoma, endometrial stromal sarcoma, yolk sac tumors, neuroendocrine tumor, glassy cell carcinoma, verrucous carcinoma, Wilms tumor, Ewing sarcoma, lymphoma**

HPV human *papillomavirus*, *ASCUS* atypical squamous cells of undetermined significance, *HSIL* high-grade squamous intraepithelial lesion, *AGUS* atypical glandular cells of undetermined significance, *EBRT* external beam radiation therapy

imiquimod cream (Buck and Guth 2003). Side effects of Imiquimod include vaginal burning and irritation. In the Buck et al. series, these side effects were well tolerated, and there were no reports of vaginal ulceration. **Topical estrogen cream** has been advocated as a useful adjunct to all VAIN treatment modalities. Particularly in postmenopausal women with significant vaginal atrophy, topical estrogen therapy may improve detection of VAIN by normalizing adjacent epithelium. Estrogen may also play a role in promoting regression of VAIN (Rhodes et al. 2014).

Radiation therapy is one of the most effective therapies for VAIN, but is less commonly used because of toxicities associated with radiation including vaginal shortening, stenosis, and fibrosis which may interfere with both sexual function and future examinations. Other toxicities include impaired wound healing, risk of inducing premature menopause through ovarian ablation, and radiation cystitis or proctitis. Vaginal intracavitary brachytherapy is most frequently used for definitive treatment of persistent and recurrent VAIN that has failed other modalities, with disease control rates of 86–100% (Gurumurthy and Cruickshank 2012).

Posttreatment surveillance should be similar to follow up schedules in women with cervical dysplasia: every 6 months for 1–2 years and then annually, with vaginal cytology at each visit. HPV testing has not yet been established in the follow-up of VAIN, but may improve the sensitivity of surveillance exams and allow for improved risk stratification and less frequent follow-up.

9.2 Invasive Squamous Cell Carcinoma

(*Summarized in* Table 3)

Invasive squamous cell carcinoma (SCC) shares cytologic features with VAIN, along with evidence of invasion beyond the epithelial basement membrane. Approximately 65% of vaginal SCC is HPV positive (Smith et al. 2009). Similar to VAIN, HPV 16 is the most common HPV type found in vaginal cancer, and p16 staining is highly sensitive and specific for HPV infection in vaginal tumors. SCC may be divided into keratinizing and nonkeratinizing subtypes, and other variants including basaloid, warty, and papillary squamotransitional have also been described.

Vaginal SCC is graded by the degree of differentiation. Grade 1 tumors are keratinizing and generally very similar in appearance to squamous epithelium, with abundant cytoplasm. Grade 2 tumors have less cytoplasm, but are easily recognized as squamous cells, whereas grade 3 tumors are both nonkeratinizing and poorly differentiated. Verrucous carcinoma is a distinct type of SCC also found on the cervix and vulva which presents with a large exophytic mass and is generally very well differentiated and cytologically bland appearing. Verrucous carcinoma spreads locally and is generally treated surgical resection.

Treatment strategies for vaginal SCC may include surgery, radiation, or chemotherapy – alone or in combination. Chemoradiation including a combination of external beam and brachytherapy is currently the most recommended treatment modality for vaginal cancer of all stages. Because of the rare incidence of the disease, there are no phase III clinical trials to guide management. Overall, management strategies are based on the results of small case series; extrapolation of treatment strategies for cervical, vulvar, and anal cancers; and expert opinion. Therapy should be individualized for each patient based on the stage of disease, size and location of the tumor, and personal goals for vaginal function. Whenever possible, patients should be referred to tertiary centers to receive care from providers experienced in treating vaginal cancers.

Surgery has limited utility in the treatment of vaginal cancer because of the close proximity of other organs including the bladder and rectum making it nearly impossible to obtain adequate margins with organ-sparing approach, especially when the tumor has invaded beyond the vaginal mucosa. In the 2015 FIGO Cancer Report, Hacker et al. recommend only four situations in which surgery may be useful (Hacker et al. 2015):

1. Patients with stage I disease located in the upper posterior vagina: When a negative tumor margin of at least 1 cm can be obtained, and an adequate pelvic lymph node dissection performed, patients with small stage I tumors

may benefit from radical upper vaginectomy (and hysterectomy if the uterus is in situ).

2. Ovarian transposition prior to radiation therapy for young patients. The authors note that debulking of large primary tumors and/or pelvic nodes larger than 2 cm in diameter may be performed at the time of this procedure.

3. Patients with locally advanced, stage IVA tumors may benefit from primary pelvic exenteration, but should also have a pelvic lymphadenectomy and consideration of bilateral groin dissection. This approach may also be combined with preoperative radiation therapy.

4. Patients with a central recurrence following primary radiation therapy should be offered pelvic exenteration if there is no evidence of distant metastases.

Surgical case series report 5-year overall survival rates of 56–90% for patients with stage I disease treated with partial or total vaginectomy (Davis et al. 1991; Creasman et al. 1998; Ling et al. 2008; Di Donato et al. 2012). Laparoscopic radical vaginectomy with neovagina construction has also been described with excellent overall survival and patient satisfaction. Cancer registry-based studies suggest a survival advantage for patients who are treated surgically when compared with radiation therapy (Ling et al. 2008). Creasman et al. report a 5-year survival rate of 90% for women with stage I disease in the National Cancer Data Base treated with surgery, compared with 63% for women who received radiation therapy alone and 79% for women who received combined surgery and radiation therapy (Creasman et al. 1998). Similarly, Shah et al. also reported a trend toward improved survival in the SEER database for women with stage I disease treated by primary surgery; however, differences in the hazard ratios were only statistically significant when surgery was compared with no treatment for stage I disease (Shah et al. 2009). Trends toward improved survival with surgical management have also been reported for women with stage II disease, but these are not statistically significant, and survival rates are lower overall when compared to women with stage I disease.

In general, improved survival among women treated with primary surgery likely reflects careful selection criteria biased toward women with small, superficial tumors and little comorbidity. The true advantage of primary surgery for patients with early-stage vaginal cancer is preservation of ovarian and sexual function and avoidance of other radiation-related toxicities.

For women with locally advanced disease, anterior, posterior, or total pelvic exenteration is necessary in order to achieve adequate margins around the tumor. Eddy et al. reported 50% 5-year survival among six patients with stage IVA disease who underwent pelvic exenteration following preoperative radiation (Eddy et al. 1991). In general, exenteration should only be offered to patients who have a reasonable chance of long-term survival after the procedure. Preoperative evaluation should include efforts to rule out pelvic sidewall involvement or nodal and distant metastases. Most surgeons advocate beginning the procedure with exploratory laparotomy and pelvic lymphadenectomy to evaluate for peritoneal or nodal disease prior to beginning the exenteration.

Radiation therapy techniques may include intracavitary or interstitial brachytherapy, external beam radiation therapy (EBRT), or intensity-modulated radiation therapy (IMRT). Practical considerations in the selection of radiation modality, dosing, and technique are summarized in the American Brachytherapy Society consensus guidelines and American College of Radiology Appropriateness Criteria for the management of vaginal cancer (Beriwal et al. 2012; Lee et al. 2013). Because of the high rate of local recurrence and lymph node involvement, most vaginal cancers should be treated with a combination of EBRT and brachytherapy.

Most vaginal cancers are treated with pelvic EBRT to a dose of 45–50.4Gy in 25–28 fractions, followed by a boost to a cumulative dose of approximately 70Gy to the primary tumor site. The clinical target volume includes the gross tumor volume with a 1–2 cm margin, the entire vagina and paravaginal/parametrial tissues out to the pelvic sidewalls, and the bilateral pelvic lymph nodes, which generally correspond to the L5/S1 interspace. For tumors involving the middle or distal 1/3 of the vagina, inguinal nodes should also be included (Yeh et al. 2001). When pelvic lymph nodes are known to be involved, or bulky para-aortic nodes are present on pretreatment imaging studies, extended field coverage of the para-aortic region may be necessary.

The boost to the primary tumor site may be accomplished through brachytherapy or IMRT or a combination. Selection of brachytherapy technique depends on the residual tumor thickness following EBRT. Vaginal cylinder brachytherapy is appropriate for residual disease mainly confined to the mucosa. Tandem and ovoids are typically used for women who have an intact uterus. When the depth of tumor involvement is greater than 5 mm, interstitial implants are required to adequately provide a definitive dose to the entire tumor. Interstitial applicator placement is usually done with epidural anesthesia in order to provide adequate pain control during the procedure and therapy. Laparoscopy or laparotomy may be necessary for appropriate interstitial catheter placement in large tumors in order to prevent inadvertent injury to the bowel. Marker seeds of fiducial gold, platinum, or carbon fiber can be used to define the extent of gross disease. Both low and high dose rate (LDR and HDR) protocols have been reported for the treatment of vaginal cancer, and neither has been definitively shown to be superior. There are fewer studies describing HDR; however, the advantage of this dose schedule is fewer fractions, and rather than continuous radiation dosing requiring radiation precautions, HDR protocols allow for visits and nursing care in between treatments (Beriwal et al. 2012).

Among radiation therapy series of more than ten patients, 5-year disease-specific survival ranges from 36 to 100% for stage I disease, 31 to 80% for stage II disease, 8 to 80% for stage III disease, and 0 to 40% for stage IV disease (Di Donato et al. 2012). The range of survival rates likely reflects differences in radiation protocol as well as differences in the characteristics of each tumor.

Concurrent chemoradiation therapy has become the standard of care for locally advanced cervical cancer and has been increasingly adopted as the primary treatment strategy for most vaginal cancers (Lee et al. 2013). In small series, chemotherapeutics including 5FU, mitomycin C, and cisplatin with concurrent radiation therapy resulted in 5-year survival rates of approximately 65% (Di Donato et al. 2012). Some authors report locoregional recurrence rates as high as 61% following chemoradiation (Roberts et al. 1991), but these reports are difficult to interpret due to variations in stage and tumor size among studies. In the largest single institution report, Miyamoto et al. present a significantly lower recurrence rate (15% vs. 45%, $p = 0.027$) for 20 patients with stage I–IV disease who received chemoradiation (mainly weekly cisplatin) compared with 51 patients who received radiation therapy alone (Miyamoto and Viswanathan 2013). Recently, a large National Cancer Data Base study by Rajagopalan et al. found that 48.6% of 8086 patients who received radiation also received concurrent chemotherapy. Concurrent chemoradiation therapy was significantly associated with improved 5-year overall survival in all stages and for the entire cohort (48.8% for chemoradiation vs. 41.9% for radiation alone). Median overall survival was also significantly increased for all stages of disease when compared with patients who received radiation alone (109 vs. 85 months for stage I, 85.8 vs. 41.7 months for stage II, 43 vs. 19.9 months for stage III, and 18.5 vs. 9 months for stage IV) (Rajagopalan et al. 2014).

Neoadjuvant chemotherapy prior to radical surgery has also been advocated in patients with stage II disease. Panici et al. describe 11 patients who received 3 cycles of cisplatin and paclitaxel followed by radical surgery. In this series, 27% had a complete response and 64% had a partial response prior to surgery, and 73% were disease-free at a median follow-up of 75 months (Panici et al. 2008).

Posttreatment surveillance for vaginal cancer should follow Society of Gynecologic Oncology guidelines (Salani et al. 2011). For high-risk patients (those who were treated with chemotherapy, radiation, or surgery followed by adjuvant therapy or who had advanced disease), a focused history and careful exam should be performed every 3 months for the first 2 years after completing therapy and then every 6 months until 5 years without evidence of disease, after which visits can be repeated annually. Low-risk patients who have stage I disease and were treated by surgery alone may follow up every 6 months for the first 2 years and then annually. Vaginal cytology should be obtained annually to screen for microscopic recurrence, and any cytologic abnormalities should be evaluated with colposcopy. Symptoms such as vaginal bleeding or discharge, pelvic or abdominal pain, new palpable mass, or change in bowel or bladder habits should prompt a CT abdomen pelvis or PET CT to assess for recurrence. There is no evidence to support routine imaging in the absence of symptoms.

Treatment complications affecting vaginal function and the lower urinary and GI tracts are the most common due to the close proximity of vaginal cancers to these pelvic structures. Radiation-related toxicity to the pelvic organs may include radiation cystitis or proctitis and vesicovaginal or rectovaginal fistula. Vesicovaginal and rectovaginal fistulas have also been reported as a complication of radical surgery. Vaginal radiation toxicity includes acute vaginitis, vaginal stricture, vaginal stenosis, or, rarely, vaginal necrosis. In series reporting rates of toxicity, the incidence of grade 2 complications has been reported to be 15–25% (Gadducci et al. 2015). Factors that increase risk of complications include older age, smoking, medical comorbidities affecting vascular profusion and healing such as diabetes and hypertension, and prior pelvic surgery.

Vaginal stricture and stenosis can be reduced with a combination of topical estrogen cream and dilator use. Women who are sexually active should continue to have intercourse on a regular basis if tolerated. Sexual dysfunction following treatment for vaginal cancer is likely multifactorial, and alterations in body image are common.

Loss of fertility and premature menopause are important considerations in the treatment of young women. We recommend that women of reproductive age be offered consultation with reproductive endocrinology regarding fertility preservation options such as oocyte or embryo cryopreservation prior to initiating therapy for vaginal cancer. Ovarian transposition to the anterior abdominal wall may reduce the likelihood of radiation-induced menopause and should be considered for some young patients.

Patterns and rates of recurrence vary with initial stage at diagnosis. For stage I disease, the recurrence risk is approximately 10–20%, compared with 30–40% for stage II, and 50–70% for stage III and IV (Davis et al. 1991; Chyle et al. 1996; Perez et al. 1999; Tabata et al. 2002). Among patients with stage I disease, locoregional recurrence is far more common, whereas patients with advanced locoregional disease at the time of diagnosis also have higher rates of both persistent disease and new distant metastases, which may occur in up to 47% of patient (Perez et al. 1999; Tabata et al. 2002). Recurrent disease portends a very poor prognosis, with a 5-year survival rate of only 12% (Chyle et al. 1996).

As in the primary setting, salvage treatment strategies include surgical resection, radiation, and chemotherapy. Patients with stage I disease who did not receive radiation initially may be may receive radiation therapy with curative intent. Radiation protocols in this setting are similar to those used at the time of diagnosis and should include EBRT for empiric coverage of pelvic lymph nodes. Recurrences in the distal 1/3 of the vagina should also be treated with empiric sterilization of the bilateral groins. Similarly, in patients with a prior history of radiation, radiation may still be a reasonable option for disease outside the previously radiated field. Patients who have previously received chemoradiation present a therapeutic challenge because bone marrow reserves have been depleted. Women with local recurrence limited to the central pelvis should be offered pelvic exenteration, which offers the only path to long-term disease-free survival, particularly among patients who have failed definitive radiation.

Distant metastases are best treated with systemic chemotherapy, palliative radiation if focal in nature, or best supportive care. Few studies evaluating chemotherapy for recurrent vaginal cancer exist, and most report a poor response to therapy. In a phase II trial presented by Thigpen et al. of the Gynecologic Oncology Group (GOG 26C), only 1/22 women experienced a complete response to cisplatin 50 mg/m^2 given every 3 weeks. Combination therapy appears to be similarly ineffective. In a study of combination of bleomycin, vincristine (Oncovin), mitomycin C, and cisplatin (BOMP), only 1/15 women treated for recurrent disease experienced a response, compared with 5/6 treated in the primary setting (Belinson et al. 1985). For this reason, many patients who are not candidates for exenteration pursue palliative care.

Prognosis has improved with advances in radiation and chemotherapy and particularly with adoption of chemoradiation (Rajagopalan et al. 2014). In a SEER database study by Shah et al. in 2009, stage is the most important predictor of prognosis. A summary of survival rates by stage at diagnosis is provided in Table 1. Other factors linked to shorter overall survival in large cancer registry studies include larger tumor size (>4 cm), lymph node involvement, and older age (Creasman et al. 1998; Shah et al. 2009; Rajagopalan et al. 2014; Gadducci et al. 2015).

9.3 Adenocarcinomas

(*Summarized in* Table 3)

As discussed earlier in this chapter, most vaginal adenocarcinomas reported in the literature are DES-related clear cell carcinomas occurring in adolescents and young women. The prognosis of vaginal clear cell carcinoma is better than for squamous cell carcinoma, with 5-year survival rates of 92% for stage I and 83% for stage II disease (Senekjian et al. 1987, 1988). In contrast, non-DES-related vaginal adenocarcinomas carry a relatively poor prognosis. In a series from MD Anderson, the median age at diagnosis was 54 and 5-year survival of only 34%, compared with 58% among squamous cell carcinoma patients at the same institution (Frank et al. 2007). Both DES-related and non-DES-related adenocarcinomas are treated similarly to vaginal squamous cell carcinoma. The management of adolescent and young women should include efforts to preserve fertility and sexual function when possible. When a tumor is too large for local excision and radiation is planned, laparoscopic ovarian transposition should be considered to reduce risk of premature menopause.

9.4 Melanoma

(*Summarized in* Table 3)

Primary vaginal melanoma is the third most common primary malignancy of the vagina, representing 3–6% of all vaginal cancers (Creasman et al. 1998; Shah et al. 2009) and only approximately 1% of all melanomas. Vaginal melanomas most often present as a pigmented or ulcerated lesion in the distal 1/3 of the vagina. Amelanotic lesions have also been described and can be mistaken for squamous cell carcinoma. Immunohistochemistry staining for S-100, HMB45, or Melan-A may be helpful in confirming the diagnosis. The average age at diagnosis is approximately 60, and the majority of patients are white non-Hispanic (Leitao et al. 2014).

The prognosis of vaginal melanoma is very poor, with 5-year overall survival of 5–20% (Creasman et al. 1998; Leitao et al. 2014). Survival for vaginal melanoma is also poor compared to melanomas arising in other sites, likely due to diagnosis at later stages of disease. Melanomas are classically thought to be resistant to radiation, and few traditional systemic chemotherapies have been shown to be active. As a result, surgical resection is the mainstay of therapy for vaginal melanoma, with clear surgical margins being the most important determinant of disease control. Acceptable clinical margins for melanoma are 0.5 cm for melanoma in situ, 1 cm for Breslow thickness less than or equal to 2 mm (AJCC T1 or T2 tumors), and 2 cm for Breslow thickness greater than 2 mm (Garbe et al. 2010). Breslow thickness has not been evaluated for vaginal melanoma, and FIGO staging of vaginal cancer is frequently used. Pelvic exenteration has not demonstrated superior survival compared with wide local excision. Even though sentinel lymph node dissection (SLND) is associated with improved survival in cutaneous melanoma, it has not been widely adopted or evaluated in vaginal melanoma cases. Adjuvant radiation using a similar approach to that used for vaginal squamous cell carcinoma has also been reported, with the possibility of cure. Preoperative radiation can also be considered as a way to improve the chance of complete resection for larger tumors.

Treatment should be approached with consultation with a melanoma specialist at a tertiary center whenever possible. Traditional chemotherapeutics have not been demonstrated to improve overall survival, but there is promising data supporting combination of chemotherapy with targeted agents and immunotherapies. While targeted therapies have not been formally evaluated for primary vaginal melanoma, the BRAF inhibitor vemurafenib and immune modulator ipilimumab have yielded promising results in the melanoma field. In light of recent developments and rapidly improving outcomes using novel agents, women with vaginal melanoma should be encouraged to consider clinical trial participation when such opportunities are available.

9.5 Mesenchymal Tumors

Vaginal leiomyosarcoma, a bulky, rapidly growing smooth muscle tumor with a high mitotic index, is the most common mesenchymal tumor of the vagina in adults, but is extremely rare in general. Radical surgical resection offers the best chance of cure, but 5-year overall survival is only 36% (Peters et al. 1985). **Vaginal carcinosarcoma and primary vaginal endometrial stromal sarcoma** have also been reported. Treatment of these tumors is generally extrapolated from strategies employed for the corresponding uterine primaries.

Embryonal rhabdomyosarcoma (sarcoma botryoides, summarized in Table 3**)** is characterized by the presence of cross-striated rhabdomyoblasts. This rare tumor has been treated with radical surgery including pelvic exenteration in the past, but is now more commonly treated with chemotherapy in combination with more conservative surgery and radiation. The Intergroup Rhabdomyosarcoma Study Group (IRSG) has conducted four clinical trials from 1972 to 1997, including all tumor sites that are used to guide therapy and is now in the process of a fifth study (Raney et al. 2001). The IRSG classifies tumors into four groups: (I) localized disease that is completely excised with no microscopic residual tumor; (II) complete gross resection of disease with microscopic residual disease, including regional disease with positive lymph nodes; (III) incomplete resection with gross residual disease; and (IV) distant metastases. In the IRS-I through IRS-IV studies, patients in groups I–III received a combination of vincristine, actinomycin D, and cyclophosphamide (VAC) for 12 months sometimes in combinations with ifosfamide, or etoposide, and patients in group IV were randomized to receive vincristine and melphalan (VM) or ifosfamide and doxorubicin (ID) followed by VAC and radiation therapy.

9.6   Other Histologies

Rare variants of vaginal cancer have been reported including primary vaginal lymphoma, Wilms tumor, and Ewing sarcoma, as well as germ cell tumors including childhood vaginal endodermal sinus tumors and variants of epithelial carcinomas such as glassy cell and small cell neuroendocrine carcinomas. Treatment of such variants should be individualized and may include elements of management for vaginal cancer combined with therapies adapted for similar histologies at more common disease sites.

10   Summary

Primary vaginal cancer is a rare entity. Squamous cell carcinoma is the most commonly seen histology affecting women in their sixth and seventh decade of life. Most, but not all, squamous cell carcinomas of the vagina are related to HPV infection. Majority of women are asymptomatic or present with vaginal bleeding or a vaginal mass. The diagnosis and staging are accomplished primarily through physical exam, with confirmatory biopsies, although PET and MRI studies are likely to have an increasing role in predicting prognosis and determining optimal treatment. Radiation is the mainstay of therapy except in select cases of focal, early-stage disease or central recurrences. With the introduction of chemoradiation, overall survival approaches rates seen in cervical cancer. Because of the rarity of this disease, there is no recommended screening; however HPV vaccination efforts hold promise for reducing the incidence of this disease in the future.

References

Belinson JL, Stewart JA, Richards AL, McClure M. Bleomycin, vincristine, mitomycin-C, and cisplatin in the management of gynecological squamous cell carcinomas. Gynecol Oncol. 1985;20(3):387–93.

Beriwal S, Demanes DJ, Erickson B, Jones E, Jennifer F, Cormack RA, Yashar C, Rownd JJ, Viswanathan AN. American Brachytherapy Society consensus guidelines for interstitial brachytherapy for vaginal cancer. Brachytherapy. 2012;11(1):68–75.

Buck HW, Guth KJ. Treatment of vaginal intraepithelial neoplasia (primarily low grade) with imiquimod 5% cream. J Low Genit Tract Dis. 2003;7(4):290–3.

Chyle V, Zagars GK, Wheeler JA, Wharton JT, Delclos L. Definitive radiotherapy for carcinoma of the vagina: outcome and prognostic factors. Int J Radiat Oncol Biol Phys. 1996;35(5):891–905.

Creasman WT, Phillips JL, Menck HR. The National Cancer Data Base report on cancer of the vagina. Cancer. 1998;83(5):1033–40.

Daling JR, Madeleine MM, Schwartz SM, Shera KA, Carter JJ, McKnight B, Porter PL, Galloway DA, McDougall JK, Tamimi H. A population-based study of squamous cell vaginal cancer: HPV and cofactors. Gynecol Oncol. 2002;84(2):263–70.

Davis KP, Stanhope CR, Garton GR, Atkinson EJ, O'Brien PC. Invasive vaginal carcinoma: analysis of early-stage disease. Gynecol Oncol. 1991;42(2):131–6.

Di Donato V, Bellati F, Fischetti M, Plotti F, Perniola G, Panici PB. Vaginal cancer. Crit Rev Oncol Hematol. 2012;81(3):286–95.

Dodge JA, Eltabbakh GH, Mount SL, Walker RP, Morgan A. Clinical features and risk of recurrence among patients with vaginal intraepithelial neoplasia. Gynecol Oncol. 2001;83(2):363–9.

Eddy GL, Marks Jr RD, Miller MC, Underwood Jr PB. Primary invasive vaginal carcinoma. Am J Obstet Gynecol. 1991;165(2):292–8.

Edge SB, Byrd DR, Compton CC, Fritz AG, Greene FL, Trotti A. AJCC cancer staging manual. New York: Springer; 2010.

Frank SJ, Deavers MT, Jhingran A, Bodurka DC, Eifel PJ. Primary adenocarcinoma of the vagina not associated with diethylstilbestrol (DES) exposure. Gynecol Oncol. 2007;105(2):470–4.

Fu YS, Reagan JW. Pathology of the uterine cervix, vagina, and vulva. Philadelphia: WB Saunders; 1989.

Gadducci A, Fabrini MG, Lanfredini N, Sergiampietri C. Squamous cell carcinoma of the vagina: natural history, treatment modalities and prognostic factors. Crit Rev Oncol Hematol. 2015; 93(3):211–24.

Garbe C, Peris K, Hauschild A, Saiag P, Middleton M, Spatz A, Grob J-J, Malvehy J, Newton-Bishop J, Stratigos A. Diagnosis and treatment of melanoma: European consensus-based interdisciplinary guideline. Eur J Cancer. 2010;46(2):270–83.

Gurumurthy M, Cruickshank ME. Management of vaginal intraepithelial neoplasia. J Low Genit Tract Dis. 2012;16(3):306–12.

Hacker NF, Eifel PJ, van der Velden J. Cancer of the vagina. Int J Gynaecol Obstet. 2015;131 Suppl 2:S84–7. PubMed PMID: 26433679. Epub 2015/10/05. eng.

Hellman K, Silfverswärd C, Nilsson B, Hellström A, Frankendal B, Pettersson F. Primary carcinoma of the vagina: factors influencing the age at diagnosis. The Radiumhemmet series 1956–96. Int J Gynecol Cancer. 2004;14(3):491–501.

Herbst AL, Andersond D. Clear cell adenocarcinoma of the vagina and cervix secondary to intrauterine exposure to diethylstilbestrol. Semin Surg Oncol. 1990;6(6):343–346. Wiley Online Library.

Indermaur MD, Martino MA, Fiorica JV, Roberts WS, Hoffman MS. Upper vaginectomy for the treatment of vaginal intraepithelial neoplasia. Am J Obstet Gynecol. 2005;193(2):577–81.

Lamoreaux WT, Grigsby PW, Dehdashti F, Zoberi I, Powell MA, Gibb RK, Rader JS, Mutch DG, Siegel BA. FDG-PET evaluation of vaginal carcinoma. Int J Radiat Oncol Biol Phys. 2005;62(3):733–7.

Lee LJ, Jhingran A, Kidd E, Cardenes HR, Elshaikh MA, Erickson B, Mayr NA, Moore D, Puthawala AA, Rao GG. Acr appropriateness criteria management of vaginal cancer. Oncology (Williston Park). 2013;27(11):1166–73.

Leitao Jr MM, Cheng X, Hamilton AL, Siddiqui NA, Jurgenliemk-Schulz I, Mahner S, Avall-Lundqvist E, Kim K, Freyer G. Gynecologic Cancer InterGroup (GCIG) consensus review for vulvovaginal melanomas. Int J Gynecol Cancer. 2014;24(9 Suppl 3): S117–22.

Ling B, Gao Z, Sun M, Sun F, Zhang A, Zhao W, Hu W. Laparoscopic radical hysterectomy with vaginectomy and reconstruction of vagina in patients with stage I of primary vaginal carcinoma. Gynecol Oncol. 2008;109(1):92–6.

Magné N, Oberlin O, Martelli H, Gerbaulet A, Chassagne D, Haie-Meder C. Vulval and vaginal rhabdomyosarcoma in children: update and reappraisal of Institut Gustave Roussy brachytherapy experience. Int J Radiat Oncol Biol Phys. 2008;72(3):878–83.

Miyamoto DT, Viswanathan AN. Concurrent chemoradiation for vaginal cancer. PLoS One. 2013; 8(6):e65048.

Morrow CP, Curtin JP. Synopsis of gynecologic oncology. Newyork: Churchill Livingstone; 1998.

Paczos TA, Ackers S, Odunsi K, Lele S, Mhawech-Fauceglia P. Primary vaginal adenocarcinoma arising in vaginal adenosis after CO_2 laser vaporization and 5-fluorouracil therapy. Int J Gynecol Pathol. 2010; 29(2):193–6.

Panici PB, Bellati F, Plotti F, Di Donato V, Antonilli M, Perniola G, Manci N, Muzii L, Angioli R. Neoadjuvant chemotherapy followed by radical surgery in patients affected by vaginal carcinoma. Gynecol Oncol. 2008;111(2):307–11.

Perez CA, Grigsby PW, Garipagaoglu M, Mutch DG, Lockett MA. Factors affecting long-term outcome of irradiation in carcinoma of the vagina. Int J Radiat Oncol Biol Phys. 1999;44(1):37–45.

Peters III WA, Kumar NB, Andersen WA, Morley GW. Primary sarcoma of the adult vagina: a clinico-pathologic study. Obstet Gynecol. 1985; 65(5):699–704.

Plentl AA, Friedman EA. Lymphatic system of the female genitalia. Philadelphia: WB Saunders; 1971.

Rajagopalan MS, Xu KM, Lin JF, Sukumvanich P, Krivak TC, Beriwal S. Adoption and impact of concurrent chemoradiation therapy for vaginal cancer: a National Cancer Data Base (NCDB) study. Gynecol Oncol. 2014;135(3):495–502.

Raney RB, Maurer HM, Anderson JR, Andrassy RJ, Donaldson SS, Qualman SJ, Wharam MD, Wiener ES, Crist WM. The Intergroup Rhabdomyosarcoma Study Group (IRSG): major lessons from the IRS-I through IRS-IV studies as background for the current IRS-V treatment protocols. Sarcoma. 2001;5(1):9–15.

Rhodes HE, Chenevert L, Munsell M. Vaginal intraepithelial neoplasia (VaIN 2/3): comparing clinical outcomes of treatment with intravaginal estrogen. J Low Genit Tract Dis. 2014;18(2):115–21.

Roberts WS, Hoffman MS, Kavanagh JJ, Fiorica JV, Greenberg H, Finan MA, Cavanagh D. Further experience with radiation therapy and concomitant intravenous chemotherapy in advanced carcinoma of the lower female genital tract. Gynecol Oncol. 1991; 43(3):233–6.

Salani R, Backes FJ, Fung MFK, Holschneider CH, Parker LP, Bristow RE, Goff BA. Posttreatment surveillance and diagnosis of recurrence in women with gynecologic malignancies: Society of Gynecologic Oncologists recommendations. Am J Obstet Gynecol. 2011;204(6):466–78.

Saslow D, Solomon D, Lawson HW, Killackey M, Kulasingam SL, Cain JM, Garcia FAR, Moriarty AT, Waxman AG, Wilbur DC, Wentzensen N, Downs LSJ, Spitzer M, Moscicki A-B, Franco EL, Stoler MH, Schiffman M, Castle PE, Myers ER. American Cancer

Society, American Society for Colposcopy and Cervical Pathology, and American Society for Clinical Pathology screening guidelines for the prevention and early detection of cervical cancer. J Low Genit Tract Dis. 2012;16(3):175–204.

Senekjian EK, Frey KW, Anderson D, Herbst AL. Local therapy in stage I clear cell adenocarcinoma of the vagina. Cancer. 1987;60(6):1319–24.

Senekjian EK, Frey KW, Stone C, Herbst AL. An evaluation of stage II vaginal clear cell adenocarcinoma according to substages. Gynecol Oncol. 1988;31(1):56–64.

Shah CA, Goff BA, Lowe K, Peters III WA, Li CI. Factors affecting risk of mortality in women with vaginal cancer. Obstet Gynecol. 2009;113(5):1038.

Siegel RL, Miller KD, Jemal A. Cancer statistics, 2015. CA Cancer J Clin. 2015;65(1):5–29.

Smith JS, Backes DM, Hoots BE, Kurman RJ, Pimenta JM. Human papillomavirus type-distribution in vulvar and vaginal cancers and their associated precursors. Obstet Gynecol. 2009;113(4):917–24.

Tabata T, Takeshima N, Nishida H, Hirai Y, Hasumi K. Treatment failure in vaginal cancer. Gynecol Oncol. 2002;84(2):309–14.

Taylor MB, Dugar N, Davidson SE, Carrington BM. Magnetic resonance imaging of primary vaginal carcinoma. Clin Radiol. 2007;62(6):549–55.

Wang Y, Li Q, Du H, Lv S, Liu H. Uterine prolapse complicated by vaginal cancer: a case report and literature review. Gynecol Obstet Invest. 2014;77(2):141–4.

Yeh AM, Marcus Jr RB, Amdur RJ, Morgan LS, Million RR. Patterns of failure in squamous cell carcinoma of the vagina treated with definitive radiotherapy alone: what is the appropriate treatment volume? Int J Cancer. 2001;96(S1):109–16.

Cervical Cancer: General Overview

Seiji Mabuchi, Mahiru Kawano, Yuri Matsumoto, and
Tadashi Kimura

Abstract

Cervical cancer is the most common cancer
affecting women in developing countries and
the fourth most common type of malignancy
affecting women worldwide, with almost half a
million cases diagnosed each year. The median
age at diagnosis of cervical cancer patients is
49 years. Persistent human papilloma virus
(HPV) infection is the most important factor
influencing the development of cervical cancer. According to previous research, the prevalence rate of HPV is >99%. Cervical cancer
progresses slowly from cervical intraepithelial
neoplasia to invasive cancer. Thus, screening
asymptomatic women with Papanicolaou cytological smears allows preinvasive disease to be
diagnosed. Although widespread screening has
significantly reduced the impact of cervical
cancer on women in industrialized countries,
such screening is not performed routinely in
less developed countries, where most patients
present with advanced disease and cervical
cancer remains a leading cause of cancer
death in women. This chapter outlines some
general information that clinicians need to
know in order to understand and manage uterine cervical cancer.

Keywords

Cervical cancer • HPV • Diagnosis • Clinical
stage • Treatment

Contents

S. Mabuchi (✉) • M. Kawano • Y. Matsumoto • T. Kimura
Department of Obstetrics and Gynecology, Osaka
University Graduate School of Medicine, Suita, Osaka,
Japan
e-mail: smabuchi@gyne.med.osaka-u.ac.jp;
tsukue1205@yahoo.co.jp; yuriri49@gmail.com;
tadashi@gyne.med.osaka-u.ac.jp

© Springer International Publishing AG 2017
D. Shoupe (ed.), *Handbook of Gynecology*,
DOI 10.1007/978-3-319-17798-4_36

1   Introduction

Cervical cancer is the most common form of cancer affecting women in developing countries and the fourth most common type of malignancy affecting women worldwide, with almost half a million cases diagnosed each year. This section outlines some general information that clinicians need to know in order to understand and manage uterine cervical cancer.

2   Epidemiology

2.1   Prevalence

Worldwide, cervical cancer is the fourth most common form of cancer affecting women, with approximately 530,000 new cases arising in 2012 and accounts for 7.5% of all female cancer deaths. It is estimated that cervical cancer causes >270,000 deaths each year worldwide, with >85% of them occurring in less developed regions (Torre et al. 2015).

2.2   The Role of Human Papilloma Virus and Vaccines Against It

Virtually all cases of cervical cancer are caused by specific types of human papillomavirus (HPV). There are more than 100 types of HPV, of which more than 40 can be sexually transmitted. Among these, at least 13 are considered to be high-risk cancer-causing types (Bouvard et al. 2009). Two of these high-risk types, HPV-16 and HPV-18, cause about 70% of cervical cancers worldwide (Wheeler et al. 2009). HPV is mainly transmitted through sexual contact, and most people are infected with HPV shortly after their first sexual encounter. Despite the high prevalence of HPV, the majority of HPV infections clear up, and only a minority persist and progress to cervical intraepithelial neoplasia (CIN) or invasive cancer. The 2-year clearance rate of HPV infections is as high as 90% (Ho et al. 1998). As our understanding of the role played by HPV infections in cervical cancer has improved, vaccines against HPV

have emerged as an important cancer prevention tool. Currently, vaccines against HPV-16 and −18 have been approved for use in many countries. Such vaccines were found to be highly effective at preventing CIN as well as adenocarcinoma in situ due to HPV-16 and −18 in previously unexposed women (Ault and Group FIS 2007).

2.3   Risk Factors

The risk factors for cervical cancer are mostly associated with an increased risk of acquiring an HPV infection. They include first having sexual intercourse at a young age, having multiple sexual partners, delivering your first child at a young age, experiencing an increased number of full-term pregnancies (Berrington de González et al. 2007; Muñoz et al. 2002), and having a history of sexually-transmitted infections (Anttila et al. 2001). Oral contraceptive use appears to be associated with an increased risk of cervical cancer, especially adenocarcinoma (Appleby et al. 2007), and cigarette smoking seems to be associated with an increased risk of squamous cell carcinoma but not adenocarcinoma (Berrington de González et al. 2007). As people living with HIV/AIDS are susceptible to infection by oncogenic viruses including HPV, cervical cancer is considered to be an AIDS-defining cancer together with Kaposi's sarcoma and some types of lymphoma (Rubinstein et al. 2014).

3   Diagnosis

3.1   Clinical Manifestations

Early cervical cancer patients are frequently asymptomatic; therefore, cancer screening is important for identifying such patients. The first symptom of early cervical cancer is usually a watery or mucinous vaginal discharge, but this often goes unnoticed by the patient. The most common presenting symptom is irregular, intermenstrual, or abnormal vaginal bleeding after sexual intercourse (vaginal bleeding, after sexual intercourse). As the cervical tumor enlarges, the bleeding episodes become heavier and more frequent. Indicators of more advanced disease include pain that seems to arise from the flank or leg (such pain is usually a secondary symptom of pelvic wall or sciatic nerve involvement); dysuria, hematuria, or rectal bleeding resulting from bladder or rectal invasion; fatigue; weight loss; loss of appetite; or a single swollen leg caused by lymphatic or venous blockade.

3.2 Diagnosis

During physical examinations, the cervix and entire vagina should be inspected and palpated to identify overt tumors or subepithelial vaginal extension. The lesion can manifest as an exophytic tumor in the exocervix, an infiltrating tumor of the endocervix, or an ulcerative tumor. Tumors that arise in the endocervical canal can result in an enlarged, indurated cervix with a smooth surface (referred to as a "barrel-shaped cervix"). Tumor size and parametrial involvement are best assessed using a rectovaginal examination. Palpation of the liver, supraclavicular lymph nodes, and groin should be used to diagnose distant metastasis. In women with visible lesions, a suspected diagnosis of cancer must be confirmed by a biopsy of the lesion. Symptomatic women without visible lesions and those who only present with abnormal cervical cytological findings should undergo a colposcopy-directed biopsy (followed by endocervical curettage) and, if necessary, diagnostic conization. Conization can also be used to determine whether conservative or radical surgery is required in cases of microinvasive cancer.

4 Staging

4.1 Clinical Staging

The most widely accepted staging system for cervical cancer is the four-stage system developed by the International Federation of Gynecologists and Obstetricians (FIGO) (Table 1) (Pecorelli 2009). The FIGO classification of cervical cancer was originally based on the results of clinical examinations. Cervical tumors are staged using the FIGO system at the time of the initial diagnosis. Thus, it is of critical importance that pelvic examinations are performed by experienced examiners. Since the revised FIGO staging system for uterine cervix was published in 2009, the FIGO Committee on Gynecologic Oncology has encouraged the use of imaging techniques for evaluating lesion size and growth. Other investigations (i.e., examinations performed under anesthesia, cystoscopy, sigmoidoscopy, or intravenous pyelography) are considered optional (Pecorelli et al. 2009).

4.2 Diagnostic Studies

4.2.1 Tumor Size and Local Spread

It remains unclear whether imaging studies can assess tumor size and local spread more accurately than clinical examinations in cervical cancer patients. However, a prospective multi-institutional study involving 208 women with early-stage cervical cancer showed that magnetic resonance imaging (MRI) is superior to computed tomography (CT) and clinical examinations for evaluating tumor size (Mitchell et al. 2006). Moreover, in a meta-analysis of 57 studies, it was suggested that MRI is superior to CT for evaluating parametrial involvement (Bipat et al. 2003).

4.2.2 Lymph Node and Distant Metastases

The FIGO staging system does not take lymph node involvement into account, but the information regarding the lymphatic spread of cervical cancer is important in determining its prognosis and the most appropriate treatment. Historically, surgery with lymphadenectomy was required to evaluate for lymph node metastasis. Currently, the options for evaluating for lymph node metastasis include lymph node dissection, imaging studies, or both. The initial evaluation of the lymph nodes is usually performed with CT to minimize costs, but positron emission tomography (PET) and PET/CT might be able to evaluate patients' lymph node status more accurately. According to a meta-analysis of 72 studies involving 5042

Table 1 2009 modification of FIGO staging for carcinoma of the cervix uteri[a]

Stage			Descriptions
Stage I			The carcinoma confined to the cervix[b]
	IA		Invasive carcinoma which can be diagnosed only by microscopy, with deepest invasion ≤5 mm and largest extension ≥7 mm[b]
		IA1	Measured stromal invasion of ≤3.0 mm in depth and extension of ≤7.0 mm
		IA2	Measured stromal invasion of >3.0 mm and not >5.0 mm with an extension of not >7.0 mm
	IB		Macroscopically visible lesions limited to the cervix uteri or preclinical cancers greater than stage IA[c]
		IB1	Lesion ≤4.0 cm in greatest dimension
		IB2	Lesion >4.0 cm in greatest dimension
Stage II			Clinically visible cervical carcinoma invades beyond the uterus but not to the pelvic wall or to the lower third of the vagina
	IIA		Lesion without parametrial invasion
		IIA1	Lesion ≤4.0 cm in greatest dimension
		IIA2	Lesion >4 cm in greatest dimension
	IIB		Lesion with obvious parametrial invasion
Stage III			The tumor extends to the pelvic wall and/or involves lower third of the vagina and/or causes hydronephrosis or nonfunctioning kidney
	IIIA		Tumor involves lower third of the vagina, with no extension to the pelvic wall
	IIIB		Extension to the pelvic wall and/or hydronephrosis or nonfunctioning kidney
Stage IV			The carcinoma has extended beyond the true pelvis or has involved (biopsy proven) the mucosa of the bladder or rectum. A bullous edema, as such, does not permit a case to be allotted to Stage IV
	IVA		Spread of the growth to adjacent organs
	IVB		Spread to distant organs

[a]Adopted and modified from the original source
[b]Extension to the corpus would be disregarded
[c]The involvement of vascular/lymphatic spaces should not change the stage allotment

women (Selman et al. 2008), the sensitivity and specificity of the abovementioned imaging modalities for detecting lymph node metastases are as follows: PET: 75% and 98%, respectively; MRI: 56% and 93%, respectively; CT: 58% and 92%, respectively.

5 Histology

The World Health Organization recognizes three general categories of invasive carcinoma of the cervix: squamous cell carcinoma, adenocarcinoma, and other epithelial tumors (IARC. WHO histological classification of tumors of the uterine cervix) (Table 2). Squamous cell carcinoma is the most common histological subtype, accounting for 60–70% of invasive carcinomas. Adenocarcinoma and adenosquamous carcinoma comprise 20–25% of all cases, and the other types account

for 10–15% of cases. However, the proportion of cervical adenocarcinoma has recently been increasing (Smith et al. 2000).

6 Spread and Metastasis

6.1 Direct Invasion

Cervical cancer principally spreads via direct local invasion of the adjacent tissues and lymphatic system and, less commonly, through blood vessels. Initially, the malignant cells penetrate the basement membrane, and then progressively infiltrate into the underlying stroma. Cervical tumors grow laterally into the paracervical and parametrial areas and can also invade the uterine cavity and vagina, before progressing into the urinary bladder and rectum.

Table 2 WHO histological classification of invasive carcinomas of the uterine cervix[a]

Histological classification			
Squamous cell carcinoma	Microinvasive squamous cell carcinoma		
	Invasive squamous cell carcinoma	Keratinizing	
		Nonkeratinizing	
		Basaloid	
		Verrucous	
		Warty	
		Papillary	
		Lymphoepithelioma-like	
		Squamotransitional	
Adenocarcinoma	Early invasive adenocarcinoma		
	Invasive adenocarcinoma	Mucinous adenocarcinoma	Endocervical
			Intestinal
			Signet-ring cell
			Minimal deviation
			Villoglandular
		Endometrioid adenocarcinoma	
		Clear cell adenocarcinoma	
		Serous adenocarcinoma	
		Mesonephric adenocarcinoma	
Other epithelial tumors		Adenosquamous carcinoma	
		Glassy cell carcinoma variant	
		Adenoid cystic carcinoma	
		Adenoid basal carcinoma	
		Neuroendocrine tumors	Carcinoid
			Atypical carcinoid
			Small cell carcinoma
			Large cell neuroendocrine carcinoma
		Undifferentiated carcinoma	

[a]Adopted and modified from the original source

6.2 Lymphatic Spread

The lymphatic spread of cervical cancer occurs relatively early, and the risk of lymph node metastasis increases with the depth of invasion. The reported incidence of lymph metastasis in each FIGO stage of cervical cancer is as follows: stage IA1: 0–0.8%; stage IA2: 0–7.4%; stage IB: 11.7–23.2%; stage IIA: 10.0–26.8%; stage IIB: 35.2–48.6% (Buckley et al. 1996; Cosin et al. 1998; Creasman et al. 1998; Elliott et al. 2000; Hirai et al. 2003; Kasamatsu et al. 2002; Lee et al. 1989, 2006; Östör and Rome 1994; Poynor et al. 2006; van Meurs et al. 2009).

The lymphatic spread of cervical cancer usually occurs in an orderly fashion from the pelvic lymph nodes, most commonly the obturator or external iliac lymph nodes, to the common iliac lymph nodes, and then the para-aortic lymph nodes (PALN). However, cervical cancer can directly metastasize to the PALN, although this is very rare. According to a retrospective study involving 61 patients with invasive cervical cancer who displayed solitary positive lymph nodes after radical hysterectomy (RH) plus systematic lymphadenectomy, metastasis to each nodal site occurred at the following frequencies: external iliac lymph nodes: 43%, obturator lymph nodes: 26%, parametrial lymph nodes: 21%, common iliac lymph nodes: 7%, presacral lymph nodes: 1%, and PALN: 1% (Bader et al. 2007).

Ovarian involvement due to direct invasion is rare. Instead, it usually occurs via lymphatic spread. In a study of patients with stage IB cervical cancer, the Gynecologic Oncology Group reported that ovarian involvement was detected in 4 of 770 patients (0.5%) with squamous cell carcinoma and 2 of 121 patients (1.7%) with adenocarcinoma (Sutton et al. 1992).

6.3 Hematogenous Metastasis

Hematogenous metastasis can also occur in cervical cancer patients. The most common sites of hematogenous spread are the lungs, liver, and bone.

6.4 Surgical Staging of the PALN

PALN metastases are seen in 9–24% of stage II cases, 12–38% of stage III cases, and 13–50% of stage IVA cases (Heller et al. 1990; Michel et al. 1998). Failure to detect metastases to the PALN can lead to suboptimal treatment and lower survival.

Pretreatment surgical staging might be beneficial as it allows adequate histological evaluations of the retrieved PALN and can lead to treatment modification in certain cases. In addition, debulking enlarged positive lymph nodes during surgical staging might be of therapeutic benefit. However, the role of surgical staging of the PALN in cervical cancer has never been investigated in a randomized study, and thus, its clinical value remains unclear.

Pretreatment surgical staging is associated with an increased postoperative morbidity rate and treatment delays. According to a previous report, the mean complications rate of surgical PALN staging procedures is 9% (range: 4–24%) (Fine et al. 1995; Hughes et al. 1980). Retrospective studies have suggested that a retroperitoneal approach, laparoscopic surgery, and robotic surgery are all associated with lower rates of postoperative complications compared with an intraperitoneal approach (Smits et al. 2014). Thus, these less invasive approaches might be recommended for surgical PALN staging procedures.

It has been suggested that PET (with or without CT) is the most accurate imaging modality for assessing extrapelvic disease in cervical cancer (PET, extrapelvic disease in cervical cancer). It was reported that PET produces a high true-positive rate (50–100%), indicating that surgical staging might not be necessary if uptake is detected in the para-aortic region. Nevertheless, false-negative results in the para-aortic region have been recorded in 12–22% of patients, indicating the weakness of PET for detecting small metastases (Gouy et al. 2012). The comparative advantages of the surgical staging of the PALN over clinical assessments based on imaging technologies, such as PET, in terms of the complications rate and survival need to be investigated in large randomized controlled trials.

7 Treatment

The treatment of invasive cervical cancer involves the management of both the primary lesion and any metastatic disease. For early-stage cervical

Table 3 Classification of radical hysterectomy according to Piver, Rutledge, and Smith[a]

Class	Description
Class I: Extrafascial hysterectomy	
	Deflection and retraction of the ureters without dissection of the ureteral bed
	Uterine artery is laterouterine sectioned and ligated
	Uterosacral ligament and cardinal ligament are not removed
	No vaginal portion is excised
Class II: Modified radical hysterectomy (Wertheim)	
	Ureters are freed from the paracervical position but are not resected from the pubovesical ligament
	Uterine arteries are ligated just medial to the ureter
	Uterosacral ligaments are resected midway between the uterus and their sacral attachments
	Medial half of the cardinal ligaments are removed
	Upper one-third of the vagina is removed
	Elective pelvic lymphadenectomy
Class III: Classical radical hysterectomy (Meigs')	
	Complete dissection of the ureter from the pubovesical ligament to entry into the bladder except for a small lateral part of the pubovesical ligament
	Uterine vessels are ligated at the origin of the internal iliac artery
	Uterosacral ligaments are resected at their sacral attachments
	Cardinal ligaments resected as close to the pelvic wall
	Upper half of the vagina is removed
	Routine pelvic lymphadenectomy
Class IV: More radical than class III in three aspects	
	(i) Complete dissection of the ureter from the pubovesical ligament
	(ii) The superior vesicle artery is sacrificed
	(iii) Upper three-fourth of the vagina is removed
Class V: More radical than class IV	
	Involved portions of the distal ureter or bladder are excised

[a]Adopted and modified from the original source

cancer, both surgery and radiotherapy can be used to treat the primary lesion. In contrast, radiotherapy is the only curative treatment for advanced disease. The choice of treatment should be based on the extent of the cervical cancer, the patient's age and general health, and the complications of the patient.

The advantages of a primary surgical approach are as follows: First, it facilitates accurate tumor staging. Second, it allows ovarian function to be preserved in premenopausal patients. Third, it makes it possible to remove bulky lymph nodes that cannot be cured with external beam radiotherapy. The main advantage of radiotherapy is that it is applicable to almost all patients, whereas radical surgery cannot be used to treat patients with medically inoperable disease.

7.1 Surgical Treatment

7.1.1 Classification of Radical Hysterectomy

The first case series in which RH was used to treat cervical cancer was reported by Ernst Wertheim in 1912 and was followed by a study by Okabayashi (Okabayashi 1921; Werheim 1912). Today, RH is commonly categorized according to the amount of the parametrium that is resected.

In 1974, Piver et al. published a classification of RH (Piver et al. 1974) (Table 3). This classification is still widely used, although two newer classifications have been proposed to overcome the ambiguities of the original one (Mota et al. 2008; Querleu and Morrow 2008).

7.1.2 Morbidities Associated with Radical Surgery for Cervical Cancer

RH is associated with various postoperative morbidities, including bladder dysfunction, sexual dysfunction, and colorectal motility disorders. Accidental damage to the pelvic autonomic nerves during surgery is considered to be a major cause of such morbidities.

According to previous studies, bladder dysfunction including incomplete bladder emptying and a need to strain to micturate occur in 16–40% of patients (Bergmark et al. 2006; Kenter et al. 1989), 9–18% of patients suffer constipation (Bergmark et al. 2006; Sood et al. 2002), fecal or flatal incontinence is seen in 33% of patients (Kenter et al. 1989), fistulas develop in 1–6.7% of patients (Kenter et al. 1989; Lee et al. 1989), lymphedema occurs in 3–19% of patients (Bergmark et al. 2006; Pieterse et al. 2006), and 19–36% of patients experience sexual dysfunction (Bergmark et al. 2006; Pieterse et al. 2006).

7.1.3 Nerve-Sparing Radical Hysterectomy

In an effort to reduce the postoperative morbidity rate, nerve-sparing RH (NSRH), which protects the pelvic nerves that can be damaged during RH, was developed by Japanese gynecologists, and the procedure has been improved over the last 20 years (Fujii et al. 2007). A recent meta-analysis suggested that although NSRH exhibited a significantly longer operating time than RH, NSRH results in greater postoperative recovery of pelvic organ function and a lower postoperative morbidity rate than RH (Long et al. 2014).

7.2 Radiotherapy

Radiotherapy is an extremely useful treatment for cervical cancer because the uterine cervix is able to tolerate high-radiation doses. Radiotherapy can be used to treat all stages of cervical cancer; however, as the volume of the primary cervical lesion increases, the likelihood of sterilizing it with radiation decreases. Thus, for patients with bulky tumors or locally advanced disease, the risk of locoregional recurrence remains significant, leading to poor survival.

Pelvic external beam radiotherapy involving a dose of 50 Gy combined with brachytherapy is the gold standard treatment for cervical cancer. During such treatment, initial external beam radiotherapy involving the delivery of 40–45 Gy to the whole pelvis is often necessary to induce tumor shrinkage and facilitate the intracavitary installation of the radiation source. In cases involving gross disease in the parametrial or pelvic lymph nodes, an external beam boost to 60–65 Gy can be administered.

8 Prognosis

The survival outcomes of cervical cancer patients according to the FIGO 26th Annual Report on the Results of Treatment in Gynecological Cancer are shown in Table 4 (Quinn et al. 2006).

9 Conclusion

Cervical cancer remains a significant health problem for women worldwide. However, the introduction of widespread screening and/or HPV vaccines would significantly reduce its impact. Moreover, the use of multidisciplinary approaches to the treatment of cervical cancer has led to marked improvements in patient outcomes.

Table 4 Prognosis of cervical cancer according to FIGO stage[a]

	Overall survival (%) at	
FIGO stage	3 year	5 year
IA1	98.3	97.5
IA2	95.2	94.8
IB1	92.6	89.1
IB2	81.7	75.7
IIA	81.5	73.4
IIB	73.0	65.8
IIIA	54.0	39.7
IIIB	51.0	41.5
IVA	28.3	22.0
IVB	16.4	9.3

[a]Adopted and modified from the original source

References

Anttila T, Saikku P, Koskela P, Bloigu A, Dillner J, Ikäheimo I, Jellum E, Lehtinen M, Lenner P, Hakulinen T, Närvänen A, Pukkala E, Thoresen S, Youngman L, Paavonen J. Serotypes of *Chlamydia trachomatis* and risk for development of cervical squamous cell carcinoma. JAMA. 2001;285(1):47–51.

Appleby P, Beral V, Berrington de González A, Colin D, Franceschi S, Goodhill A, Green J, Peto J, Plummer M, Sweetland S, Cancer ICoESoC. Cervical cancer and hormonal contraceptives: collaborative reanalysis of individual data for 16,573 women with cervical cancer and 35,509 women without cervical cancer from 24 epidemiological studies. Lancet. 2007;370 (9599):1609–21.

Ault KA, Group FIS. Effect of prophylactic human papillomavirus L1 virus-like-particle vaccine on risk of cervical intraepithelial neoplasia grade 2, grade 3, and adenocarcinoma in situ: a combined analysis of four randomised clinical trials. Lancet. 2007;369 (9576):1861–8.

Bader AA, Winter R, Haas J, Tamussino KF. Where to look for the sentinel lymph node in cervical cancer. Am J Obstet Gynecol. 2007;197(6):678.e671–677.

Berrington de González A, Green J, Cancer ICoESoC. Comparison of risk factors for invasive squamous cell carcinoma and adenocarcinoma of the cervix: collaborative reanalysis of individual data on 8,097 women with squamous cell carcinoma and 1,374 women with adenocarcinoma from 12 epidemiological studies. Int J Cancer. 2007;120(4):885–91.

Bergmark K, Avall-Lundqvist E, Dickman PW, Henningsohn L, Steineck G. Lymphedema and bladder-emptying difficulties after radical hysterectomy for early cervical cancer and among population controls. Int J Gynecol Cancer. 2006;16(3):1130–9.

Bipat S, Glas AS, van der Velden J, Zwinderman AH, Bossuyt PM, Stoker J. Computed tomography and magnetic resonance imaging in staging of uterine cervical carcinoma: a systematic review. Gynecol Oncol. 2003;91(1):59–66.

Bouvard V, Baan R, Straif K, Grosse Y, Secretan B, El Ghissassi F, Benbrahim-Tallaa L, Guha N, Freeman C, Galichet L, Cogliano V, Group WIAfRoCMW. A review of human carcinogens – part B: biological agents. Lancet Oncol. 2009;10(4):321–2.

Buckley SL, Tritz DM, Van Le L, Higgins R, Sevin BU, Ueland FR, DePriest PD, Gallion HH, Bailey CL, Kryscio RJ, Fowler W, Averette H, van Nagell JR. Lymph node metastases and prognosis in patients with stage IA2 cervical cancer. Gynecol Oncol. 1996;63(1):4–9.

Cosin JA, Fowler JM, Chen MD, Paley PJ, Carson LF, Twiggs LB. Pretreatment surgical staging of patients with cervical carcinoma: the case for lymph node debulking. Cancer. 1998;82(11):2241–8.

Creasman WT, Zaino RJ, Major FJ, DiSaia PJ, Hatch KD, Homesley HD. Early invasive carcinoma of the cervix (3 to 5 mm invasion): risk factors and prognosis. A Gynecologic Oncology Group study. Am J Obstet Gynecol. 1998;178(1 Pt 1):62–5.

Elliott P, Coppleson M, Russell P, Liouros P, Carter J, MacLeod C, Jones M. Early invasive (FIGO stage IA) carcinoma of the cervix: a clinico-pathologic study of 476 cases. Int J Gynecol Cancer. 2000;10(1):42–52.

Fine BA, Hempling RE, Piver MS, Baker TR, McAuley M, Driscoll D. Severe radiation morbidity in carcinoma of the cervix: impact of pretherapy surgical staging and previous surgery. Int J Radiat Oncol Biol Phys. 1995;31 (4):717–23.

Fujii S, Takakura K, Matsumura N, Higuchi T, Yura S, Mandai M, Baba T, Yoshioka S. Anatomic identification and functional outcomes of the nerve sparing Okabayashi radical hysterectomy. Gynecol Oncol. 2007;107(1):4–13.

Gouy S, Morice P, Narducci F, Uzan C, Gilmore J, Kolesnikov-Gauthier H, Querleu D, Haie-Meder C, Leblanc E. Nodal-staging surgery for locally advanced cervical cancer in the era of PET. Lancet Oncol. 2012;13(5):e212–20.

Heller PB, Maletano JH, Bundy BN, Barnhill DR, Okagaki T. Clinical-pathologic study of stage IIB, III, and IVA carcinoma of the cervix: extended diagnostic evaluation for paraaortic node metastasis – a Gynecologic Oncology Group study. Gynecol Oncol. 1990;38 (3):425–30.

Hirai Y, Takeshima N, Tate S, Akiyama F, Furuta R, Hasumi K. Early invasive cervical adenocarcinoma: its potential for nodal metastasis or recurrence. BJOG. 2003;110(3):241–6.

Ho GY, Bierman R, Beardsley L, Chang CJ, Burk RD. Natural history of cervicovaginal papillomavirus infection in young women. N Engl J Med. 1998;338 (7):423–8.

Hughes RR, Brewington KC, Hanjani P, Photopulos G, Dick D, Votava C, Moran M, Coleman S. Extended field irradiation for cervical cancer based on surgical staging. Gynecol Oncol. 1980;9(2):153–61.

IARC. WHO histological classification of tumours of the uterine cervix. http://screening.iarc.fr/atlasclassifwho. php?lang=1

Kasamatsu T, Okada S, Tsuda H, Shiromizu K, Yamada T, Tsunematsu R, Ohmi K. Early invasive adenocarcinoma of the uterine cervix: criteria for nonradical surgical treatment. Gynecol Oncol. 2002;85(2):327–32.

Kenter GG, Ansink AC, Heintz AP, Aartsen EJ, Delemarre JF, Hart AA. Carcinoma of the uterine cervix stage I and IIA: results of surgical treatment: complications, recurrence and survival. Eur J Surg Oncol. 1989;15 (1):55–60.

Lee KB, Lee JM, Park CY, Cho HY, Ha SY. Lymph node metastasis and lymph vascular space invasion in microinvasive squamous cell carcinoma of the uterine cervix. Int J Gynecol Cancer. 2006;16(3):1184–7.

Lee YN, Wang KL, Lin MH, Liu CH, Wang KG, Lan CC, Chuang JT, Chen AC, Wu CC. Radical hysterectomy with pelvic lymph node dissection for treatment of cervical cancer: a clinical review of 954 cases. Gynecol Oncol. 1989;32(2):135–42.

Long Y, Yao DS, Pan XW, Ou TY. Clinical efficacy and safety of nerve-sparing radical hysterectomy for cervical cancer: a systematic review and meta-analysis. PLoS One. 2014;9(4):e94116.

Mitchell DG, Snyder B, Coakley F, Reinhold C, Thomas G, Amendola M, Schwartz LH, Woodward P, Pannu H, Hricak H. Early invasive cervical cancer: tumor delineation by magnetic resonance imaging, computed tomography, and clinical examination, verified by pathologic results, in the ACRIN 6651/GOG 183 Intergroup Study. J Clin Oncol. 2006; 24(36):5687–94.

Michel G, Morice P, Castaigne D, Leblanc M, Rey A, Duvillard P. Lymphatic spread in stage Ib and II cervical carcinoma: anatomy and surgical implications. Obstet Gynecol. 1998;91(3):360–3.

Mota F, Vergote I, Trimbos JB, Amant F, Siddiqui N, Del Rio A, Verheijen R, Zola P. Classification of radical hysterectomy adopted by the Gynecological Cancer Group of the European Organization for Research and Treatment of Cancer. Int J Gynecol Cancer. 2008; 18(5):1136–8.

Muñoz N, Franceschi S, Bosetti C, Moreno V, Herrero R, Smith JS, Shah KV, Meijer CJ, Bosch FX, Group IAfRoCMCCS. Role of parity and human papillomavirus in cervical cancer: the IARC multicentric case–control study. Lancet. 2002;359 (9312):1093–101.

Okabayashi H. Radical hysterectomy for cancer of the uteri. Modification of the Takayama operation. Surg Gynecol Obstet. 1921;33:335–41.

Östör AG, Rome RM. Micro-invasive squamous cell carcinoma of the cervix: a clinico-pathologic study of 200 cases with long-term follow-up. Int J Gynecol Cancer. 1994;4(4):257–64.

Pecorelli S. Revised FIGO staging for carcinoma of the vulva, cervix, and endometrium. Int J Gynaecol Obstet. 2009;105(2):103–4.

Pecorelli S, Zigliani L, Odicino F. Revised FIGO staging for carcinoma of the cervix. Int J Gynaecol Obstet. 2009;105(2):107–8.

Pieterse QD, Maas CP, ter Kuile MM, Lowik M, van Eijkeren MA, Trimbos JB, Kenter GG. An observational longitudinal study to evaluate miction, defecation, and sexual function after radical hysterectomy with pelvic lymphadenectomy for early-stage cervical cancer. Int J Gynecol Cancer. 2006;16(3): 1119–29.

Piver MS, Rutledge F, Smith JP. Five classes of extended hysterectomy for women with cervical cancer. Obstet Gynecol. 1974;44(2):265–72.

Poynor EA, Marshall D, Sonoda Y, Slomovitz BM, Barakat RR, Soslow RA. Clinicopathologic features of early adenocarcinoma of the cervix initially managed with cervical conization. Gynecol Oncol. 2006;103(3):960–5.

Querleu D, Morrow CP. Classification of radical hysterectomy. Lancet Oncol. 2008;9(3):297–303.

Quinn MA, Benedet JL, Odicino F, Maisonneuve P, Beller U, Creasman WT, Heintz AP, Ngan HY, Pecorelli S. Carcinoma of the cervix uteri. FIGO 26th Annual Report on the Results of Treatment in Gynecological Cancer. Int J Gynaecol Obstet. 2006;95 Suppl 1: S43–103.

Rubinstein PG, Aboulafia DM, Zloza A. Malignancies in HIV/AIDS: from epidemiology to therapeutic challenges. AIDS. 2014;28(4):453–65.

Selman TJ, Mann C, Zamora J, Appleyard TL, Khan K. Diagnostic accuracy of tests for lymph node status in primary cervical cancer: a systematic review and meta-analysis. CMAJ. 2008;178(7):855–62.

Smith HO, Tiffany MF, Qualls CR, Key CR. The rising incidence of adenocarcinoma relative to squamous cell carcinoma of the uterine cervix in the United States – a 24-year population-based study. Gynecol Oncol. 2000;78(2):97–105.

Smits RM, Zusterzeel PL, Bekkers RL. Pretreatment retroperitoneal para-aortic lymph node staging in advanced cervical cancer: a review. Int J Gynecol Cancer. 2014;24(6):973–83.

Sood AK, Nygaard I, Shahin MS, Sorosky JI, Lutgendorf SK, Rao SS. Anorectal dysfunction after surgical treatment for cervical cancer. J Am Coll Surg. 2002; 195(4):513–9.

Sutton GP, Bundy BN, Delgado G, Sevin BU, Creasman WT, Major FJ, Zaino R. Ovarian metastases in stage IB carcinoma of the cervix: a Gynecologic Oncology Group study. Am J Obstet Gynecol. 1992;166(1 Pt 1):50–3.

Torre LA, Bray F, Siegel RL, Ferlay J, Lortet-Tieulent J, Jemal A. Global cancer statistics, 2012. CA Cancer J Clin. 2015;65(2):87–108.

van Meurs H, Visser O, Buist MR, Ten Kate FJ, van der Velden J. Frequency of pelvic lymph node metastases and parametrial involvement in stage IA2 cervical cancer: a population-based study and literature review. Int J Gynecol Cancer. 2009;19(1):21–6.

Werheim E. The extended abdominal operation for carcinoma uteri (based on 500 operative cases). Am J Obstet Dis Women Child. 1912;66:169–232.

Wheeler CM, Hunt WC, Joste NE, Key CR, Quint WG, Castle PE. Human papillomavirus genotype distributions: implications for vaccination and cancer screening in the United States. J Natl Cancer Inst. 2009;101 (7):475–87.

Fertility-Sparing Treatment for Early-Stage Cervical Cancer

Hiromasa Kuroda, Seiji Mabuchi, Katsumi Kozasa, and Tadashi Kimura

Abstract

Fertility preservation is of paramount importance for young women that are diagnosed with early-stage cervical cancer. Women with stage IA1 disease can be treated with conization. Radical trachelectomy has been developed as a surgical method for preserving reproductive function, and the radical trachelectomy procedure has evolved significantly over the last 25 years. The candidates for radical trachelectomy include women of reproductive age with early-stage disease (stage IA2 or IB1) who do not possess any risk factors for recurrence (i.e., a lesion size of >2 cm or lymph node metastasis). Lymphovascular space invasion within the tumor is a risk factor for lymph node recurrence, but is not a contraindication for fertility-sparing surgery in cases in which it is the only risk factor present. Recently, neoadjuvant chemotherapy followed by fertility-preserving surgery has been proposed as an option for patients with larger lesions. Pregnancy after radical trachelectomy is associated with an increased risk of obstetric complications, including preterm delivery, infection, and preterm premature rupture of membranes. However, there are no effective interventions for preventing these complications.

Keywords

Cervical cancer • Fertility-preserving surgery • Trachelectomy

Contents

H. Kuroda • S. Mabuchi (✉) • K. Kozasa • T. Kimura
Department of Obstetrics and Gynecology, Osaka University Graduate School of Medicine, Suita, Osaka, Japan
e-mail: monjirota@hotmail.com

© Springer International Publishing AG 2017
D. Shoupe (ed.), *Handbook of Gynecology*,
DOI 10.1007/978-3-319-17798-4_6

1   Introduction

In the United States, 46% of uterine cervical cancers are diagnosed in women below the age of 44 (National Cancer Institute: Browse the SEER Cancer Statistics Review (CSR) 1975–2010). Thus, information regarding fertility-sparing options is an important part of pretreatment counseling, especially for women of childbearing age that are diagnosed at an early stage. The fertility-sparing options for such patients include conization and radical trachelectomy. Observational studies have suggested that these procedures result in good oncological and obstetric outcomes in carefully selected patients with early-stage cervical cancer.

2   Patients

2.1   Stage IA1 Disease Without LVSI

A cohort study of stage IA1 squamous cell carcinoma of the uterine cervix that analyzed data from the National Cancer Institute's Surveillance, Epidemiology, and End Results (SEER) database showed that there was no difference between the 5-year survival rates of patients that were treated with conization and those that underwent hysterectomy (98% vs. 99%) (Wright et al. 2010). Thus, stage IA1 patients without lymphovascular space involvement (LVSI) are indicated for conization alone. In cases in which the margins of the excised cone are positive, repeated conization or trachelectomy is recommended. Clinicians have to recognize that the risk of preterm delivery is increased after conization if the depth of the excised cone is >10 mm (Kyrgiou et al. 2006).

2.2   Stage IA1 Disease with LVSI, Stage IA2 Disease, and Stage IB1 Disease

A previous report has shown that 8.2% of stage IA1 patients with LVSI have lymph node metastasis, compared with 0.8% of those without LVSI (Mota 2003). Thus, pelvic lymphadenectomy should be included in the fertility-sparing surgical options for stage IA1 patients with LVSI. Radical trachelectomy plus pelvic lymphadenectomy or conization plus pelvic lymphadenectomy is recommended for childbearing women with stage IA1 disease and LVSI, stage IA2 disease, or stage IB1 disease.

2.2.1   Radical Trachelectomy Plus Pelvic Lymphadenectomy

Regarding cases in which the patient wants to preserve their fertility, women with stage IA1 disease and LVSI, stage IA2 disease, or stage IB1 disease are indicated for radical trachelectomy plus pelvic lymphadenectomy. Radical trachelectomy can be performed either through a vaginal or abdominal approach and can also be carried out using laparoscopic or robotic methods.

The criteria for radical trachelectomy vary slightly among institutions, but remain essentially unchanged from the original set proposed by Roy et al. in 1998 (Table 1) (Roy and Plante 1998). Although previous studies have shown that a tumor size of >2 cm is associated with increased

Table 1 Criteria of radical trachelectomy

1. A desire for fertility
2. Histologically proven invasive cervical cancer
3. Squamous cell carcinoma, adenocarcinoma, or adenosquamous carcinoma, without high-risk histology (e.g., neuroendocrine carcinoma)
4. Stage IA1 with lymphovascular space invasion, stage IA2, or stage IB1
5. Tumor size ≤ 2 cm
6. Tumor limited to the cervix
7. No evidence of lymph node metastasis and distant metastasis

Table 2 Oncological outcomes according to surgical procedures

Surgery	Author	No. of surgeries	Follow-up	Recurrences	Deaths
	Year		Months	n (%)	n (%)
VRT	Burnett et al. 2003	21	31	2 (9.5)	0 (0)
	Mathevet et al. 2003	109	76	4 (3.7)	3 (2.8)
	Shepherd et al. 2006	123	45	5 (4.1)	4 (3.3)
	Hertel et al. 2006	108	29	4 (3.7)	2 (1.9)
	Marchiole et al. 2007	118	95	7 (5.9)	5 (4.2)
	Beiner et al. 2008	90	51	5 (5.5)	3 (3.3)
	Sonoda et al. 2008	43	21	1 (2.3)	0 (0)
	Plante et al. 2011	125	93	6 (4.8)	2 (1.6)
	Cao et al. 2013	71	34.4	7 (9.9)	2 (2.8)
	Total	765		41 (5.4)	21 (2.6)
ART	Ungár et al. 2005	30	47	0 (0)	0 (0)
	Abu-Rustum et al. 2008	22	12	0 (0)	0 (0)
	Pareja et al. 2008	15	32	0 (0)	0 (0)
	Nishio et al. 2009	61	27	6 (9.8)	NA[a]
	Cibula et al. 2009	17	21.2	1 (5.9)	0 (0)
	Yao et al. 2010	10	NA	0 (0)	0 (0)
	Saso et al. 2012	30	24	3 (10)	2 (6.7)
	Muraji et al. 2012	23	NA	0 (0)	0 (0)
	Wethington et al. 2012	93	32	4 (4.3)	0 (0)
	Cao et al. 2013	55	20.6	0 (0)	0 (0)
	Total	356		14 (3.9)	2 (0.7)[b]
VRH	Steed et al. 2004	71	17	4 (5.6)	NA
	Jackson et al. 2004	50	52	2 (4.0)	2 (4.0)
	Marchiole et al. 2007	139	113	9 (6.4)	7 (5.0)
	Beiner et al. 2008	90	58	1 (1.1)	1 (1.1)
	Total	350		16 (4.6)	10 (3.6)[c]
ARH	Roy et al. 1996	27	27	1 (3.7)	NA
	Steed et al. 2004	205	21	13 (6.3)	NA
	Jackson et al. 2004	50	49	2 (4.0)	2 (4.0)
	Malzoni et al. 2009	62	71.5	4 (6.5)	NA
	Zhang et al. 2014	90	12.5	0 (0)	0 (0)
	Total	434		20 (4.6)	2 (1.4)[d]

NA not available, *VRT* vaginal radical trachelectomy, *ART* abdominal radical trachelectomy, *VRH* vaginal radical hysterectomy, *ARH* abdominal radical hysterectomy
[a]Three of six patients were lost to follow-up as of the time of the review
[b]Estimated without the data of Nishio et al. 2009
[c]Estimated without the data of Steed et al. 2004
[d]Estimated with the data of Jackson et al. 2004 and Zhang et al. 2014

risk of recurrence after radical trachelectomy (Marchiole et al. 2007; Mathevet et al. 2003; Plante et al. 2011), tumors that measure >2 cm, are very exophytic, and exhibit minimal stromal invasion might also be considered for radical trachelectomy.

A previous study of radical trachelectomy for cervical cancer found that 28% of cervical tumors that are resected by radical trachelectomy exhibit LVSI and that LVSI is associated with an increased risk of recurrence (Beiner and Covens 2007). However, when LVSI is the only risk factor present, it is not an exclusion criterion for radical trachelectomy, as it does not justify adjuvant therapy (Beiner and Covens 2007; Plante et al. 2011).

2.2.2 Conization Plus Pelvic Lymphadenectomy

Radical trachelectomy plus pelvic lymphadenectomy is a safer approach for stage IA1–IA2 disease when LVSI is present; however, conization plus pelvic lymphadenectomy might also be a useful treatment option (Maneo et al. 2011).

3 Outcomes

3.1 Surgical Outcomes

Approximately 10% of planned radical trachelectomy procedures have to be abandoned because of the presence of lymph node metastasis on frozen sections or positive endocervical margins (Tables 3 and 4). In a previous study, the mortality rate of patients who underwent vaginal radical trachelectomy (VRT) was 3.1%, which was comparable with the 0–1.4% observed in patients that were treated with abdominal radical hysterectomy (ARH) or abdominal radical trachelectomy (ART) (Averette et al. 1993).

3.2 Oncological Outcomes

A previous study suggested that the oncological outcomes of patients who undergo ART or VRT are similar to those of patients treated with ARH. As shown in Table 2, these procedures result in recurrence and death rates of approximately 5% and 2%, respectively. According to a recent review of VRT, recurrent lesions can develop predominantly in the parametrium or pelvis (Beiner and Covens 2007).

3.3 Prognostic Factors

The risk factors for recurrence have been intensively investigated, and tumors that measure

>2 cm in diameter are consistently associated with an increased risk of recurrence. In addition, some studies have suggested that the presence of LVSI (Marchiole et al. 2007; Mathevet et al. 2003; Plante et al. 2011) and deep stromal invasion (DSI) of >10 mm (Diaz et al. 2008) are risk factors for recurrence; however, others have found that they are not associated with a higher risk of recurrence (Hertel et al. 2006; Plante et al. 2011). Although the prognostic significance of LVSI and DSI needs to be investigated further in larger studies, they are not considered to be contraindications for radical trachelectomy at this point. As neuroendocrine tumors are an aggressive subtype of cervical cancer and often recur rapidly, even if they have been completely removed and there is no lymph node or distant metastasis, radical trachelectomy cannot be recommended for women with this histological subtype of cervical cancer (Beiner and Covens 2007; Marchiole et al. 2007).

4 Surgical Procedures

The first successful trachelectomy procedure was performed via a vaginal approach by Dargent et al. in 1986, and the oncological and reproductive outcomes of patients who underwent VRT were presented at the Society of Gynecologic Oncologists meeting in 1994 (Ribeiro Cubal et al. 2012). A laparoscopic pelvic lymph node evaluation should be performed prior to VRT to rule out lymph node metastasis.

The abdominal approach was first reported by Smith et al. in 1997 (Ribeiro Cubal et al. 2012). The main advantages of ART are its greater radicality and feasibility compared with VRT.

Basically, the procedure for radical trachelectomy begins with the creation of paravesical and pararectal spaces and the dissection of the caudal bladder. Then, after the vesicouterine ligaments and cardinal ligaments have been divided, the cervix is removed. Finally, the uterine corpus and vaginal stump are reconstructed.

The endocervical margin of the specimen needs to be evaluated after the cervix has been

Table 3 Reproductive outcomes for patients who underwent vaginal radical trachelectomy

Author (year)	No. of planned trachelectomies	Trachelectomy done	Fertility preserved	Attempting to conceive	Pregnant women	Pregnancies	Miscarriages 1st trimester	Miscarriages 2nd trimester	Deliveries At term	Deliveries Preterm	Patients pregnant at the time of report
Schlaerth et al. 2003	12	10	10	NA	4	4	0	2	1	1	0
Burnett et al. 2003	21	19	18	NA	3	3	0	1	1	1	0
Mathevet et al. 2003	108	95	95	NA	33	56	14	8	29	5	0
Hertel et al. 2006	108	106	106	NA	18	18	3	0	4	8	3
Chen et al. 2008	16	16	16	NA	5	5	0	2	1	1	1
Sonoda et al. 2008	43	41	36	11	11	11	3	0	4	0	4
Pahisa et al. 2008	15	13	13	NA	3	3	0	0	1	0	2
Shepherd and Milliken 2008	158	158	138	NA	NA	88	19	12	19	25	7
Diaz et al. 2008	135	NA	118	NA	33	56	14	8	29	5	NA
Plante et al. 2011	140	125	122	NA	58	106	21	3	58	19	0
Dańska-Bidzińska et al. 2011	14	14	14	NA	2	2	1	0	1	0	0
Speiser et al. 2011	NA	212	212	76	50	60	5	3	27	18	4
Hauerberg et al. 2015	NA	120	108	72	55	77	16	2	20	33	3
Total number	770	929	1006	159	275	489	96	41	195	116	24

NA not available

Table 4 Reproductive outcomes for patients who underwent abdominal radical trachelectomy

Author (year)	No. of planned trachelectomies	Trachelectomy done	Fertility preserved	Attempting to conceive	Pregnant women	Pregnancies	Miscarriages		Deliveries		Patients pregnant at the time of report
							1st term	2nd term	At term	Preterm	
Ungár et al. 2005	33	30	NA	NA	3	3	1	0	2	0	0
Pareja et al. 2008	15	15	14	6	3	3	0	0	2	1	0
Olawaiye et al. 2009	10	10	10	3	3	3	1	0	1	1	0
Nishio et al. 2009	71	61	57	29	4	4	0	0	2	2	0
Cibula et al. 2009	24	20	17	9	6	6	1	0	2	3	0
Yao et al. 2010	10	10	10	NA	2	2	0	0	1	1	0
Li et al. 2011	64	62	59	10	2	2	0	0	1	0	1
Du et al. 2011	68	60	60	15	5	8	1[a]		3	2	2
Nick et al. 2012	25	24	21	NA	NA	3	1	1	0	1	0
Saso et al. 2012	30	30	NA	10	3	3	0	1	2	0	0
Muraji et al. 2012	23	21	20	NA	1	1	0	0	0	1	0
Wethington et al. 2012	101	81	70	38	28	31	3	6	16[b]		6
Karateke and Kabaca 2012	8	8	8	NA	3	3	0	1	1	1	0
Total	482	432	346	120	63	72	7	9	17	13	9

NA not available

[a]The timing of miscarriage was not described

[b]The timing of delivery was not described

removed to ensure that no residual disease remains. It is well known that the outcomes of post-conization pregnancies are influenced by the depth and size of the excised cervical tissue specimen (Kyrgiou et al. 2006), which also holds true for post-radical trachelectomy pregnancies. As a shorter cervix can provide an easy route for ascending infections, which increase the risk of premature delivery, most clinicians aim to preserve at least 5 mm–1 cm of the endocervix during both procedures. There is no clear consensus regarding whether cervicoisthmic cerclage should be performed during radical trachelectomy or only after a patient has become pregnant.

Radical trachelectomy can also be performed via either a laparoscopic (Marchiole et al. 2007) or robotic approach (Persson et al. 2008). A previous retrospective study involving a relatively small number of patients suggested that these approaches are feasible, less invasive, and similarly effective, i.e., achieve comparable oncological outcomes, to conventional vaginal or abdominal approaches (Marchiole et al. 2007).

5 Surgical Complications

The intraoperative complications rate of VRT seems to be higher than that of ART (5.6% vs. 0.7%) (Pareja et al. 2013; Plante et al. 2011). The most common intraoperative complication of VRT is urinary tract damage. However, in comparisons of laparoscopic-assisted VRT versus laparoscopic-assisted vaginal radical hysterectomy (Marchiole et al. 2007) or ART versus ARH (Cao et al. 2013), all of the procedures exhibited similar perioperative complication rates, indicating that radical trachelectomy can be performed safely in carefully selected cases of early-stage cervical cancer.

The immediate postoperative complications associated with radical trachelectomy include bladder dysfunction, lymphedema, and lymphocele, which are comparable to the complications associated with RH (Pareja et al. 2013). In addition, the specific long-term postoperative complications associated with radical trachelectomy include cervical stenosis, dyspareunia, dysmenorrhea, prolonged amenorrhea, and chronic discharge. Similar rates of these complications are seen after VRT and ART (Beiner and Covens 2007; Cao et al. 2013; Pareja et al. 2013).

6 Adjuvant Treatments

The recommendations for post-trachelectomy adjuvant therapy are based on the presence/absence of pathological risk factors, such as nodal metastasis, parametrial involvement, LVSI, or DSI. Clinicians have to recognize that adjuvant radiotherapy affects patients' fertility (Beiner and Covens 2007; Hertel et al. 2006; Marchiole et al. 2007). Chemotherapy is an alternative adjuvant therapy. However, the clinical efficacy of adjuvant chemotherapy remains unclear.

7 Radical Trachelectomy for Tumors Larger Than 2 cm in Diameter

As the ART is more radical than VRT (Ungár et al. 2005; Wethington et al. 2012), it might have broader indications than other types of trachelectomy. However, in patients with larger tumors, radiotherapy is often indicated postoperatively because of the patient's pathological risk factors, which usually results in a loss of fertility.

Neoadjuvant chemotherapy (NACT) is the only way to reduce the size of cervical tumors, which might allow some patients with bulky tumors to undergo radical trachelectomy. Recent retrospective studies have suggested that NACT followed by radical trachelectomy is feasible and effective (Plante 2015). However, the oncological and reproductive issues have not been fully investigated. To draw a definitive conclusion regarding the benefits of NACT, further large-scale prospective studies are needed.

8   Hysterectomy in the Post-Childbearing Period

So far, there is no evidence that hysterectomy has beneficial effects in patients that do not want any more children.

9   Reproductive Issues

9.1   Fertility Issues

There is no clear consensus about the optimal interval between radical trachelectomy and attempts to get pregnant. However, as the tissue healing process can last at least 3 months, most authors suggest that patients should wait for 6–12 months before attempting to get pregnant.

Fertility might be impaired after radical trachelectomy because of anatomical and physiological changes, such as adhesion, cervical stenosis, and a loss of cervical function. In addition, the impact of pre-radical trachelectomy NACT on fertility remains unknown; however, a retrospective study found that 50% of patients who received NACT followed by trachelectomy and retained their fertility subsequently became pregnant (Robova et al. 2014).

The pregnancy outcomes seen in previous studies are summarized in Tables 3 and 4. Among the women who attempted to get pregnant after VRT, 73.0% (116 out of 159 women) were able to conceive, which is higher than the 45% (54 out of 120 women) observed in the women who underwent ART. The reasons for the worse fertility outcomes of the ART group remain to be elucidated.

9.2   Obstetric Outcomes

Clinicians should inform patients who undergo radical trachelectomy that post-radical trachelectomy pregnancies are associated with an increased risk of obstetric complications.

As shown in Tables 3 and 4, the first-trimester miscarriage rate was 19.6% (96 of 489 pregnancies) in the VRT group and 11.0% (7 of 64 pregnancies) in the ART group, which are comparable to those of the general population. However, the second-trimester miscarriage rates of the patients in the VRT (8.4%; 41 out of 489 pregnancies) and ART groups (14.1%; 9 out of 64 pregnancies) were higher than that observed in the general population. Of the women who reached the third trimester, roughly two-thirds delivered their babies at term, and the remaining women (37.8%) delivered prematurely (Tables 3 and 4). At present, there are no effective interventions for preventing preterm labor or preterm premature rupture of membranes.

9.3   Cesarean Section for Women Who Undergo Radical Trachelectomy

Cesarean section should be selected as the mode of delivery after radical trachelectomy. However, the optimal timing of cesarean section remains unclear. Moreover, it is disputed whether a low transverse incision or a low vertical incision should be performed in such cases.

10   Oocyte Cryopreservation for Women with Advanced Disease

Oocyte cryopreservation has been proposed to be an option for patients who are at risk of infertility due to RH or gonadotoxic adjuvant treatment. However, it is recommended that patients should be counseled about the current lack of data about the efficacy, risks, and costs of oocyte cryopreservation (Oocyte cryopreservation. Committee Opinion No. 584. American College of Obstetricians and Gynecologists).

11   Conclusion

Previous studies have shown that trachelectomy is a safe and feasible procedure and produces good oncological and reproductive outcomes in patients with early-stage cervical cancer. To optimize the fertility and oncological outcomes of such patients, the strict indications for radical trachelectomy should be emphasized.

References

Abu-Rustum NR, Neubauer N, Sonoda Y, Park KJ, Gemignani M, Alektiar KM, Tew W, Leitao MM, Chi DS, Barakat RR. Surgical and pathologic outcomes of fertility-sparing radical abdominal trachelectomy for FIGO stage IB1 cervical cancer. Gynecol Oncol. 2008;111(2):261–4.

Averette HE, Nguyen HN, Donato DM, Penalver MA, Sevin BU, Estape R, Little WA. Radical hysterectomy for invasive cervical cancer. A 25-year prospective experience with the Miami technique. Cancer. 1993;71:1422–37.

Beiner ME, Covens A. Surgery insight: radical vaginal trachelectomy as a method of fertility preservation for cervical cancer. Nat Clin Pract Oncol. 2007;4(6):353–61.

Beiner ME, Hauspy J, Rosen B, Murphy J, Laframboise S, Nofech-Mozes S, Ismiil N, Rasty G, Khalifa MA, Covens A. Radical vaginal trachelectomy vs. radical hysterectomy for small early stage cervical cancer: a matched case–control study. Gynecol Oncol. 2008;110(2):168–71.

Burnett AF, Roman LD, O'Meara AT, Morrow CP. Radical vaginal trachelectomy and pelvic lymphadenectomy for preservation of fertility in early cervical carcinoma. Gynecol Oncol. 2003;88(3):419–23.

Cao DY, Yang JX, Wu XH, Chen YL, Li L, Liu KJ, Cui MH, Xie X, Wu YM, Kong BH, Zhu GH, Xiang Y, Lang JH, Shen K, China Gynecologic Oncology Group. Comparisons of vaginal and abdominal radical trachelectomy for early-stage cervical cancer: preliminary results of a multi-center research in China. Br J Cancer. 2013;109(11):2778–82.

Chen Y, Xu H, Zhang Q, Li Y, Wang D, Liang Z. A fertility-preserving option in early cervical carcinoma: laparoscopy-assisted vaginal radical trachelectomy and pelvic lymphadenectomy. Eur J Obstet Gynecol Reprod Biol. 2008;136(1):90–3.

Cibula D, Sláma J, Svárovský J, Fischerova D, Freitag P, Zikán M, Pinkavová I, Pavlista D, Dundr P, Hill M. Abdominal radical trachelectomy in fertility-sparing treatment of early-stage cervical cancer. Int J Gynecol Cancer. 2009;19(8):1407–11.

Dańska-Bidzińska A, Sobiczewski P, Bidziński M, Gujski M. Radical trachelectomy – retrospective analysis of our own case material. Ginekol Pol. 2011;82(6):436–40.

Diaz JP, Sonoda Y, Leitao MM, Zivanovic O, Brown CL, Chi DS, Barakat RR, Abu-Rustum NR. Oncologic outcome of fertility-sparing radical trachelectomy versus radical hysterectomy for stage IB1 cervical carcinoma. Gynecol Oncol. 2008;111(2):255–60.

Du XL, Sheng XG, Jiang T, Li QS, Yu H, Pan CX, Lu CH, Wang C, Song QQ. Sentinel lymph node biopsy as guidance for radical trachelectomy in young patients with early stage cervical cancer. BMC Cancer. 2011;11:157.

Hauerberg L, Høgdall C, Loft A, Ottosen C, Bjoern SF, Mosgaard BJ, Nedergaard L, Lajer H. Vaginal radical trachelectomy for early stage cervical cancer. Results of the Danish National Single Center Strategy. Gynecol Oncol. 2015;S0090-8258(15)30001-9.

Hertel H, Köhler C, Grund D, Hillemanns P, Possover M, Michels W, Schneider A, German Association of Gynecologic Oncologists (AGO). Radical vaginal trachelectomy (RVT) combined with laparoscopic pelvic lymphadenectomy: prospective multicenter study of 100 patients with early cervical cancer. Gynecol Oncol. 2006;103(2):506–11.

Jackson KS, Das N, Naik R, Lopes AD, Godfrey KA, Hatem MH, Monaghan JM. Laparoscopically assisted radical vaginal hysterectomy vs. radical abdominal hysterectomy for cervical cancer: a match controlled study. Gynecol Oncol. 2004;95(3):655–61.

Karateke A, Kabaca C. Radical abdominal trachelectomy is a safe and fertility preserving option for women with early stage cervical cancer. Eur J Gynaecol Oncol. 2012;33(2):200–3.

Kyrgiou M, Koliopoulos G, Martin-Hirsch P, Arbyn M, Prendiville W, Paraskevaidis E. Obstetric outcomes after conservative treatment for intraepithelial or early invasive cervical lesions: systematic review and meta-analysis. Lancet. 2006;367:489–98.

Li J, Li Z, Wang H, Zang R, Zhou Y, Ju X, Ke G, Wu X. Radical abdominal trachelectomy for cervical malignancies: surgical, oncological and fertility outcomes in 62 patients. Gynecol Oncol. 2011;121(3):565–70.

Malzoni M, Tinelli R, Cosentino F, Fusco A, Malzoni C. Total laparoscopic radical hysterectomy versus abdominal radical hysterectomy with lymphadenectomy in patients with early cervical cancer: our experience. Ann Surg Oncol. 2009;16(5):1316–23.

Maneo A, Sideri M, Scambia G, Boveri S, Dell'anna T, Villa M, Parma G, Fagotti A, Fanfani F, Landoni F. Simple conization and lymphadenectomy for the conservative treatment of stage IB1 cervical cancer. An Italian experience. Gynecol Oncol. 2011;123:557–60.

Marchiole P, Benchaib M, Buenerd A, Lazlo E, Dargent D, Mathevet P. Oncological safety of laparoscopic-assisted vaginal radical trachelectomy (LARVT or Dargent's operation): a comparative study with laparoscopic-assisted vaginal radical hysterectomy (LARVH). Gynecol Oncol. 2007;106(1):132–41.

Mathevet P, Laszlo de Kaszon E, Dargent D. Fertility preservation in early cervical cancer. Gynecol Obstet Fertil. 2003;31(9):706–12.

Mota F. Microinvasive squamous carcinoma of the cervix: treatment modalities. Acta Obstet Gynecol Scand. 2003;82(6):505–9.

Muraji M, Sudo T, Nakagawa E, Ueno S, Wakahashi S, Kanayama S, Yamada T, Yamaguchi S, Fujiwara K, Nishimura R. Type II versus type III fertility-sparing abdominal radical trachelectomy for early-stage cervical cancer: a comparison of feasibility of surgical outcomes. Int J Gynecol Cancer. 2012;22(3): 479–83.

National Cancer Institute: Browse the SEER Cancer Statistics Review (CSR) 1975–2010. Available from http://seer.cancer.gov/archive/csr/1975_2010/browse_csr.php?sectionSEL=5&pageSEL=sect_05_table.07.html

Nick AM, Frumovitz MM, Soliman PT, Schmeler KM, Ramirez PT. Fertility sparing surgery for treatment of early-stage cervical cancer: open vs. robotic radical trachelectomy. Gynecol Oncol. 2012;124(2):276–80.

Nishio H, Fujii T, Kameyama K, Susumu N, Nakamura M, Iwata T, Aoki D. Abdominal radical trachelectomy as a fertility-sparing procedure in women with early-stage cervical cancer in a series of 61 women. Gynecol Oncol. 2009;115(1):51–5.

Olawaiye A, Del Carmen M, Tambouret R, Goodman A, Fuller A, Duska LR. Abdominal radical trachelectomy: Success and pitfalls in a general gynecologic oncology practice. Gynecol Oncol. 2009;112(3):506–10.

Oocyte cryopreservation. Committee opinion no. 584. American College of obstetricians and gynecologists. Obstet Gynecol. 2014;123:221–2.

Pahisa J, Alonso I, Torné A. Vaginal approaches to fertility-sparing surgery in invasive cervical cancer. Gynecol Oncol. 2008;110:S29–32.

Pareja FR, Ramirez PT, Borrero FM, Angel CG. Abdominal radical trachelectomy for invasive cervical cancer: a case series and literature review. Gynecol Oncol. 2008;111(3):555–60.

Pareja R, Rendón GJ, Sanz-Lomana CM, Monzón O, Ramirez PT. Surgical, oncological, and obstetrical outcomes after abdominal radical trachelectomy – a systematic literature review. Gynecol Oncol. 2013;131 (1):77–82.

Persson J, Kannisto P, Bossmar T. Robot-assisted abdominal laparoscopic radical trachelectomy. Gynecol Oncol. 2008;111(3):564–7.

Plante M. Bulky early-stage cervical cancer (2–4 cm lesions): upfront radical trachelectomy or neoadjuvant chemotherapy followed by fertility-preserving surgery: which is the best option? Int J Gynecol Cancer. 2015;25(4):722–8.

Plante M, Gregoire J, Renaud MC, Roy M. The vaginal radical trachelectomy: an update of a series of 125 cases and 106 pregnancies. Gynecol Oncol. 2011;121 (2):290–7.

Ribeiro Cubal AF, Ferreira Carvalho JI, Costa MF, Branco AP. Fertility-sparing surgery for early-stage cervical cancer. Int J Surg Oncol. 2012;2012:936534.

Robova H, Halaska MJ, Pluta M, Skapa P, Matecha J, Lisy J, Rob L. Oncological and pregnancy outcomes after high-dose density neoadjuvant chemotherapy and fertility-sparing surgery in cervical cancer. Gynecol Oncol. 2014;135(2):213–6.

Roy M, Plante M. Pregnancies after radical vaginal trachelectomy for early-stage cervical cancer. Am J Obstet Gynecol. 1998;179:1491–6.

Roy M, Plante M, Renaud MC, Têtu B. Vaginal radical hysterectomy versus abdominal radical hysterectomy in the treatment of early-stage cervical cancer. Gynecol Oncol. 1996;62(3):336–9.

Saso S, Ghaem-Maghami S, Chatterjee J, Naji O, Farthing A, Mason P, McIndoe A, Hird V, Ungar L, Del Priore G, Smith JR. Abdominal radical trachelectomy in West London. BJOG. 2012;119(2):187–93.

Schlaerth JB, Spirtos NM, Schlaerth AC. Radical trachelectomy and pelvic lymphadenectomy with uterine preservation in the treatment of cervical cancer. Am J Obstet Gynecol. 2003;188(1):29–34.

Shepherd JH, Milliken DA. Conservative surgery for carcinoma of the cervix. Clin Oncol (R Coll Radiol). 2008;20(6):395.

Shepherd JH, Spencer C, Herod J, Ind TE. Radical vaginal trachelectomy as a fertility-sparing procedure in women with early-stage cervical cancer-cumulative pregnancy rate in a series of 123 women. BJOG. 2006;113(6):719–24.

Sonoda Y, Chi DS, Carter J, Barakat RR, Abu-Rustum NR. Initial experience with Dargent's operation: the radical vaginal trachelectomy. Gynecol Oncol. 2008;108(1):214–9.

Speiser D, Mangler M, Köhler C, Hasenbein K, Hertel H, Chiantera V, Gottschalk E, Lanowska M. Fertility outcome after radical vaginal trachelectomy: a prospective study of 212 patients. Int J Gynecol Cancer. 2011; 21(9):1635–9.

Steed H, Rosen B, Murphy J, Laframboise S, De Petrillo D, Covens A. A comparison of laparoscopic-assisted radical vaginal hysterectomy and radical abdominal hysterectomy in the treatment of cervical cancer. Gynecol Oncol. 2004;93(3):588–93.

Ungár L, Pálfalvi L, Hogg R, Siklós P, Boyle DC, Del Priore G, Smith JR. Abdominal radical trachelectomy: a fertility-preserving option for women with early cervical cancer. BJOG. 2005;112(3):366–9.

Wethington S, Cibula D, Duska LR, Garrett L, Kim CH, Chi DS, Sonoda Y, Abu-Rustum NR. An international series on abdominal radical trachelectomy: 101 patients and 28 pregnancies. Int J Gynecol Cancer. 2012; 22(7):1251–7.

Wright JD, NathavithArana R, Lewin SN, Sun X, Deutsch I, Burke WM, Herzog TJ. Fertility-conserving surgery for young women with stage IA1 cervical cancer: safety and access. Obstet Gynecol. 2010;115(3):585–90.

Yao T, Mo S, Lin Z. The functional reconstruction of fertility-sparing radical abdominal trachelectomy for early stage cervical carcinoma. Eur J Obstet Gynecol Reprod Biol. 2010;151(1):77–81.

Zhang D, Li J, Ge H, Ju X, Chen X, Tang J, Wu X. Surgical and pathological outcomes of abdominal radical trachelectomy versus hysterectomy for early-stage cervical cancer. Int J Gynecol Cancer. 2014;24(7):1312–8.

Management of Early-Stage and Locally Advanced Cervical Cancer

Seiji Mabuchi, Mahiru Kawano, Tomoyuki Sasano, and Hiromasa Kuroda

Abstract

Carcinoma of the cervix remains a significant health problem for women worldwide. However, the use of a multidisciplinary approach to the treatment of cervical cancer has led to a marked improvement in patient outcomes. It has been demonstrated that early-stage cervical cancer can be effectively treated with radical surgery or definitive radiotherapy, which achieve similar survival outcomes. To reduce the frequency of postoperative complications, less invasive surgical procedures involving laparoscopic or robotic approaches have been introduced. Moreover, for patients who wish to preserve their fertility, fertility-preserving surgery has been developed. Concurrent chemoradiotherapy with a platinum-based agent is the recommended treatment for locally advanced cervical cancer. The standard concurrent chemotherapy regimen involves the administration of single-agent cisplatin at a weekly dose of 40 mg/m^2 during external beam radiotherapy. Overall, when added to radiotherapy, cisplatin was demonstrated to reduce the risk of death from cervical cancer; i.e., it resulted in an absolute overall survival benefit of 10%. In this chapter, we summarize the current management strategies for early and locally advanced cervical carcinoma.

Keywords

Cervical cancer • Surgery • Neoadjuvant chemotherapy • Radiotherapy • Prognostic factors

Contents

1 Introduction

Currently, early-stage cervical cancer can be effectively treated with radical surgery or definitive radiotherapy, which achieves similar survival outcomes. Concurrent chemoradiotherapy (CCRT) with a platinum-based agent is the recommended treatment for locally advanced cervical cancer. In this chapter, we summarize the findings of important clinical studies conducted in

S. Mabuchi (✉) • M. Kawano • T. Sasano • H. Kuroda
Department of Obstetrics and Gynecology, Osaka University Graduate School of Medicine, Suita, Osaka, Japan
e-mail: smabuchi@gyne.med.osaka-u.ac.jp;
tsukue1205@yahoo.co.jp; sasano106@gmail.com;
monjirota@hotmail.com

© Springer International Publishing AG 2017
D. Shoupe (ed.), *Handbook of Gynecology*,
DOI 10.1007/978-3-319-17798-4_34

845

the past few decades and review the current standard management strategies for early-stage and locally advanced cervical carcinoma.

1.1 Early-Stage Cervical Cancer

1.1.1 Stage IA

Historically, it was considered that FIGO stage IA1 or 1A2 adenocarcinoma of the cervix behaves more aggressively than FIGO stage IA1 or 1A2 squamous cell carcinoma. However, recent studies have demonstrated that the prognosis of FIGO stage IA1 or 1A2 adenocarcinoma of the cervix is comparable to that of squamous cell carcinoma of the cervix (Hirai et al. 2003; Ceballos et al. 2006).

Stage IA1

It has been reported that the risk of lymph node metastasis is generally very low (Table 1) in patients with stage IA1 cervical cancer (Elliott et al. 2000; Hirai et al. 2003; Kasamatsu et al. 2002; Lee et al. 2006). Moreover, as no parametrial involvement is observed in patients with stage IA1 cervical cancer (Hirai et al. 2003; Kasamatsu et al. 2002; Reynolds et al. 2010), the recommended treatment for such disease is extrafascial hysterectomy. However, a previous report found that 8.2% of patients that exhibited lymphovascular space invasion (LVSI) developed lymph node metastases, compared with 0.8% of the patients without LVSI (Benedet and Anderson 1996). Thus, in cases in which the patient's conization specimen demonstrates extensive LVSI, a more radical approach involving a modified radical hysterectomy (RH) and pelvic lymphadenectomy is recommended. Observation might be an appropriate option for patients that

exhibit negative margins and LVSI after cone biopsies and wish to preserve their fertility (Wright et al. 2010).

Stage IA2

According to previous studies, the risk of parametrial involvement is very low (~1%) in patients with stage IA2 cervical cancer (Table 2). As there is potential for lymph node metastasis to develop in patients with stage IA2 disease (Buckley et al. 1996; Lee et al. 2006; Poynor et al. 2006; van Meurs et al. 2009), the recommended treatment for stage IA2 cervical cancer is modified RH and pelvic lymphadenectomy. However, medically unfit patients can be treated with definitive radiotherapy consisting of pelvic external beam radiotherapy and brachytherapy. On the other hand, a combination of radical trachelectomy and pelvic lymphadenectomy is recommended for patients who wish to preserve their fertility.

1.1.2 Stage IB1–IIA

Surgery and Radiotherapy

FIGO stage IB1–IIA cervical cancer can be effectively treated with surgery or radiotherapy, which achieves similar survival outcomes. As pelvic node metastasis is common (frequency: >10%) in this patient population, the standard surgical management strategy is RH and bilateral pelvic lymph node dissection. For patients with stage IB1 disease who wish to preserve their fertility, radical trachelectomy combined with pelvic lymphadenectomy is an option, especially for those with tumors measuring ≤2 cm in diameter.

According to previous reports including a prospective randomized study, the 5-year survival

Table 1 Incidence of lymph node metastasis in patients with FIGO stage IA1 cervical cancer

Author	No. Patients	Nodal metastasis (%)
Hirai Y 2003	22	0 (0)
Kasamatsu T 2002	21	0 (0)
Lee KB 2006	174	1 (0.6)
Elliott P 2006	121	1 (0.8)

Table 2 Incidence of lymph node metastasis in patients with FIGO stage IA2 cervical cancer

Author	No. Patients	Nodal metastasis (%)
Buckley SL 1995	94	7 (7.4)
Lee KB 2006	28	1 (3.7)
Poynor EA 2006	12	0 (0)
van Meurs H 2009	48	0 (0)

rate of FIGO stage IB–IIA cervical cancer patients that are treated with radical surgery ranges from 83% to 91%, which is comparable to the 74–91% 5-year survival rate reported for those treated with radiotherapy alone (Landoni et al. 1997; Perez et al. 1987).

Neoadjuvant Chemotherapy Before Radical Surgery

Clinical trials of neoadjuvant chemotherapy (NACT) have been conducted in order to improve the prognosis of surgically treated cervical cancer patients; however, they obtained conflicting results (Rydzewska et al. 2012). The clinical benefit of NACT has recently been addressed in a meta-analysis of six phase III trials comparing NACT plus surgery with surgery alone (Rydzewska et al. 2012). The NACT regimens varied between the trials, but NACT achieved favorable clinical response rates ranging from 52% to 84%. The addition of NACT was associated with significantly improved local recurrence (odds ratio, 0.67; 95% confidence interval (CI), 0.45 to 0.99, $P = 0.04$), overall survival (OS) (hazard ratio (HR), 0.77; 95% CI, 0.62 to 0.96, $P = 0.02$), and progression-free survival (PFS) rates (HR, 0.75; 95% CI, 0.61 to 0.93, $P = 0.008$). However, only three of the trials included in this meta-analysis demonstrated a statistically significant benefit of NACT in terms of OS, whereas others found that NACT was of no benefit (Rydzewska et al. 2012). Thus, further studies involving the current standard chemotherapy (i.e., paclitaxel combined with cisplatin or carboplatin) should be conducted in the future to draw definitive conclusions regarding the benefits of NACT.

Risk Factors for Recurrence

A number of pathological risk factors that compromise the treatment outcomes of cervical cancer patients that are primarily treated with RH have been identified (Delgado et al. 1990; Fuller et al. 1989). For example, patients with positive pelvic lymph nodes, parametrial invasion, or positive surgical margins are regarded as being at high risk of recurrence. Moreover, patients with

tumors that are confined to the cervix and display risk factors for recurrence, such as a large tumor (≥ 4 cm), LVSI, or deep stromal invasion, are considered to be at intermediate risk of recurrence (Delgado et al. 1990; Fuller et al. 1989).

Among these prognostic factors, nodal metastasis remains the single most important prognostic factor in cervical cancer. It has been reported that pelvic lymph node metastasis is associated with a 30–50% reduction in the 5-year survival rate, and the survival of patients with positive pelvic lymph nodes is further affected by the number of positive pelvic lymph nodes (Delgado et al. 1990; Fuller et al. 1989). In addition, previous studies have found that the survival time of early-stage cervical cancer patients with ≥ 3 positive lymph nodes was significantly shorter than that of patients with 1 or 2 positive lymph nodes (Kamura et al. 1992; Okazawa et al. 2012).

In addition to the six risk factors mentioned above, the histological subtype of early-stage cervical cancer might also impact on survival. Previous case series have consistently suggested that small cell carcinoma has an unequivocally poor prognosis (Kuji et al. 2013; van Nagell et al. 1988). Some previous retrospective studies have found that patients with adenocarcinoma have a worse prognosis than those with squamous cell carcinoma, whereas others did not detect any survival differences between the two subtypes (Mabuchi et al. 2012a; Park et al. 2010). The prognostic significance of adenosquamous carcinoma is also disputed: some authors have reported that patients with adenosquamous carcinoma have comparable survival outcomes to those with adenocarcinoma, but have a worse prognosis than those with squamous cell carcinoma, whereas others have not detected any difference in survival between adenosquamous carcinoma and squamous cell carcinoma (Baek et al. 2014; Mabuchi et al. 2012b).

Tailored Postoperative Adjuvant Radiotherapy Based on Pathological Risk Assessments

For patients that exhibit intermediate-risk or high-risk prognostic factors, the administration of adjuvant external beam radiotherapy to the whole pelvis has been recommended as a way of reducing the risk of recurrence. In such regimens, the total radiation dose administered during the external beam radiotherapy has been reported to range from 46 to 50.4 Gy.

A Gynecologic Oncology Group phase III study (GOG 109/SWOG 8797) demonstrated that the addition of cisplatin-based concurrent chemotherapy to postoperative radiotherapy improved both PFS and OS in patients with high-risk factors (Peters et al. 2000).

As for patients with intermediate-risk factors, a GOG phase III study (GOG 92) found that adjuvant radiotherapy alone significantly reduced the risk of recurrence and prolonged PFS (Rotman et al. 2006). Although several retrospective studies have suggested that adjuvant CCRT produces superior outcomes to pelvic radiotherapy in patients with intermediate-risk factors, so far, the advantages of postoperative CCRT over radiotherapy alone in this patient population have never been demonstrated in a randomized prospective trial (Kim et al. 2009; Okazawa et al. 2013).

Minimally Invasive Approaches

Laparoscopic and Robotic Surgery
Minimally invasive surgery, including traditional laparoscopy and robotic-assisted laparoscopy, is being used increasingly and frequently in the surgical management of gynecological malignancies.

Laparoscopic RH (LRH) has been used for the management of uterine cervical cancer since the early 1990s. As for robotic RH (RRH), the Food and Drug Administration approved the use of this approach during gynecological surgery in 2005. Retrospective studies have shown that LRH and RRH are safe, feasible, and associated with less blood loss, fewer postoperative complications, and a shorter hospital stay than standard abdominal RH (ARH) in patients with cervical cancer (Nam et al. 2012). However, the feasibility and efficacy of LRH and RRH have not been demonstrated in the prospective setting.

In a recent meta-analysis evaluating the outcomes of LRH, RRH, and ARH, all three types of RH resulted in similar recurrence rates (Geetha and Nair 2012). The number of lymph nodes dissected and the frequencies of nodal metastasis

and positive margins were also similar in all three types of RH. However, ARH was associated with significantly greater blood loss and a significantly higher transfusion rate than both LRH and RRH. Postoperative infections were significantly more common among the patients who underwent ARH than among those that underwent the other two methods. In addition, the patients that underwent RRH stayed in hospital for significantly shorter periods than those treated with the other two methods. Although the long-term oncological outcomes of the LRH or RRH have not been fully investigated, the abovementioned results indicate that minimally invasive laparoscopic or robotic surgical procedures are appropriate options for radical surgery for early-stage cervical cancer.

Currently, a prospective randomized trial is underway to compare the roles of ARH, LRH, and RRH in the management of early-stage cervical cancer (Obermair et al. 2008).

Less Radical Surgery
As RH frequently results in serious complications, it is important to identify patients whose lesions are amenable to less radical surgery.

In 2012, the results of a randomized study comparing RH versus simple hysterectomy plus the removal of the upper one third of the vagina (SH) in patients with FIGO stage IB1 or IIA1 (≤ 4 cm) cervical cancer were reported (Landoni et al. 2001). Sixty-two patients were randomized to undergo a SH, while 63 patients were randomized to the RH group. Adjuvant radiotherapy was given to the patients that exhibited positive or close (<3 mm) surgical margins, LVSI close to the resection margin, or lymph node metastases. No significant differences in the recurrence rate or OS were observed between the two arms (Landoni et al. 2001, 2012). However, SH was found to be significantly superior to RH in terms of urological morbidities. When analyzed according to tumor size, the survival of patients with tumors measuring ≤ 3 cm did not differ significantly between the two groups (15-year OS, 76% vs. 80%, $p = 0.88$); however, in the patients with tumors measuring between 3.1 cm and 4 cm in diameter, radical surgery was associated with a significant improvement in survival (15-year OS, 74%

vs. 97%, $p = 0.03$). The results of this trial suggest that the surgical removal of the parametrium might not be necessary in some women with small cervical tumors and good prognostic factors.

Previous studies have tried to identify predictors of parametrial tumor spread and subsets of patients that are at low risk of parametrial disease. In one of these studies, it was noted that negative pelvic nodes, the absence of LVSI, and tumors that measure <2 cm in diameter are associated with a low risk of parametrial disease, i.e., an incidence of less than 1% (Kato et al. 2015). Of these, a tumor diameter of <2 cm was the most consistently reported factor in similar studies. In a recent large retrospective study, it was suggested that parametrial involvement was present in 1.9% (6/323) of tumors measuring ≤2 cm in diameter (Kato et al. 2015). These results indicate that less radical surgery might be a reasonable treatment option for early cervical carcinoma, especially for tumors measuring ≤2 cm in diameter.

Sentinel Lymph Node Biopsy

In early-stage cervical cancer patients, sentinel lymph node biopsy has been utilized to reduce the risk of postoperative complications after lymph node dissection and to precisely predict the status of regional lymph node metastasis. Two types of tracer are commonly available for the detection of sentinel lymph nodes: radioactive isotopes and vital dyes (Lécuru et al. 2011). A meta-analysis of 67 studies reported that the pooled detection rate of sentinel lymph nodes was 90.9, 80.9, and 92.3% when radioactive isotopes, vital dyes, and a combination of the two types of tracer were used, respectively (Kadkhodayan et al. 2015). Sentinel lymph node biopsy appears to be more accurate at determining lymph node status than commonly used imaging techniques, such as positron emission tomography (PET), magnetic resonance imaging (MRI), and computed tomography (CT). This was illustrated in a meta-analysis of 72 studies, involving 5,042 women with cervical cancer, that evaluated several approaches and found that the sensitivity and specificity of sentinel lymph node biopsy for detecting lymph node metastases were as high as 91% and 100%, respectively, whereas the

sensitivity and specificity values of the abovementioned imaging methods were as follows: PET, 75% and 98%, respectively; MRI, 56% and 93%, respectively; and CT, 58% and 92%, respectively (Selman et al. 2008). Further studies are required before sentinel lymph node mapping is routinely employed during the treatment of early-stage cervical cancer.

2 Locally Advanced Disease (IIB–IVA)

2.1 Primary Surgical Approach for FIGO Stage IIB Disease

The standard treatment for FIGO stage IIB–IVA cervical cancer is definitive pelvic radiotherapy. However, some European and Japanese institutions have treated stage IIB disease with radical surgery (Kasamatsu et al. 2009; Mabuchi et al. 2011). Retrospective studies of patients with FIGO stage IIB disease have suggested that patients that are treated with radical surgery and those that are treated with definitive radiotherapy exhibit similar treatment outcomes (estimated 5-year survival rates of 64–69%) (Kasamatsu et al. 2009; Mabuchi et al. 2011).

2.2 Radiotherapy

In patients with locally advanced cervical cancer who were free from para-aortic lymph node metastases, an earlier randomized trial conducted by the Radiation Therapy Oncology Group (RTOG 79–20) demonstrated an improvement in survival when prophylactic para-aortic radiotherapy was added to pelvic radiotherapy (Rotman et al. 1995). In a subsequent randomized trial (RTOG 90–01), it was found that pelvic CCRT improved OS and PFS compared with extended field radiotherapy alone in patients with locally advanced cervical cancer (Eifel et al. 2004). In the late 1990s, four other studies evaluated the survival benefit of adding concurrent chemotherapy to standard definitive radiotherapy (Keys et al. 1999; Morris et al. 1999; Rose et al. 1999; Whitney et al. 1999). Overall, when added to radiotherapy, cisplatin was demonstrated to reduce the risk of death from cervical cancer, with an absolute OS benefit of 10% (Keys et al. 1999; Morris et al. 1999; Rose et al. 1999; Whitney et al. 1999). Based on these findings, it is recommended that patients with stage IB2 or more advanced cervical cancer should receive platinum-based pelvic CCRT, except in cases where there are medical contraindications. The standard CCRT regimen involves the administration of single-agent cisplatin at a weekly dose of 40 mg/m^2 during external beam radiotherapy.

2.3   Prognostic Factors for Survival

Despite the overall improvement in patients' prognosis, the efficacy of the standard CCRT regimen is far from optimal in patients with locally advanced cervical cancer. According to an updated report from the RTOG (protocol 90–01), the 5-year survival rate of patients with stages IB–IIA that are treated with a combination of chemotherapy and radiotherapy is 78%, whereas the equivalent rate for patients with stages III–IVA disease is 59% (Eifel et al. 2004). In addition to an advanced clinical stage, larger tumors, nodal involvement, pretreatment hemoglobin levels of <12.0 mg/ml, pretreatment leukocytosis, an overall treatment time of >56 days, and adenocarcinoma histology have been identified as independent risk factors that compromise the treatment outcomes of radiotherapy (Grigiene et al. 2007; Serkies et al. 2006; Mabuchi et al. 2014; Perez et al. 1995; Rose et al. 2014).

3   Follow-up After Primary Treatment

The concept of posttreatment follow-up is based on the premise that early detection before the development of symptoms will result in decreased morbidity and mortality rates. As the follow-up programs employed after the treatment of uterine cervical cancer have never been evaluated in a prospective setting, the most appropriate modalities and the optimal timing of posttreatment

follow-up has not been established. However, as roughly 80% of recurrent lesions are diagnosed in the first 2 years after the initial therapy, careful posttreatment follow-up examinations should be performed frequently during this critical period.

4   Conclusion

Recent advances in surgery and radiotherapy have significantly improved the outcomes of both early-stage and locally advanced cervical cancer. However, a significant number of patients still suffer recurrence after the current standard primary treatments. As prognostic factors for recurrence are identified from analyses of clinical data, clinical studies of novel treatments should be conducted to improve the prognosis of high-risk cervical cancer patients.

References

Baek MH, Park JY, Kim D, Suh DS, Kim JH, Kim YM, Kim YT, Nam JH. Comparison of adenocarcinoma and adenosquamous carcinoma in patients with early-stage cervical cancer after radical surgery. Gynecol Oncol. 2014;135(3):462–7.

Benedet JL, Anderson GH. Stage IA carcinoma of the cervix revisited. Obstet Gynecol. 1996;87(6):1052–9.

Buckley SL, Tritz DM, Van Le L, Higgins R, Sevin BU, Ueland FR, DePriest PD, Gallion HH, Bailey CL, Kryscio RJ, Fowler W, Averette H, van Nagell JR. Lymph node metastases and prognosis in patients with stage IA2 cervical cancer. Gynecol Oncol. 1996;63(1):4–9.

Ceballos KM, Shaw D, Daya D. Microinvasive cervical adenocarcinoma (FIGO stage 1A tumors): results of surgical staging and outcome analysis. Am J Surg Pathol. 2006;30(3):370–4.

Delgado G, Bundy B, Zaino R, Sevin BU, Creasman WT, Major F. Prospective surgical-pathological study of disease-free interval in patients with stage IB squamous cell carcinoma of the cervix: a Gynecologic Oncology Group study. Gynecol Oncol. 1990;38(3):352–7.

Eifel PJ, Winter K, Morris M, Levenback C, Grigsby PW, Cooper J, Rotman M, Gershenson D, Mutch DG. Pelvic irradiation with concurrent chemotherapy versus pelvic and para-aortic irradiation for high-risk cervical cancer: an update of radiation therapy oncology group trial (RTOG) 90–01. J Clin Oncol. 2004;22(5):872–80.

Elliott P, Coppleson M, Russell P, Liouros P, Carter J, MacLeod C, Jones M. Early invasive (FIGO stage IA) carcinoma of the cervix: a clinico-pathologic study of 476 cases. Int J Gynecol Cancer. 2000;10(1):42–52.

Fuller AF, Elliott N, Kosloff C, Hoskins WJ, Lewis JL. Determinants of increased risk for recurrence in patients undergoing radical hysterectomy for stage IB and IIA carcinoma of the cervix. Gynecol Oncol. 1989;33(1):34–9.

Geetha P, Nair MK. Laparoscopic, robotic and open method of radical hysterectomy for cervical cancer: a systematic review. J Minim Access Surg. 2012;8(3):67–73.

Grigiene R, Valuckas KP, Aleknavicius E, Kurtinaitis J, Letautiene SR. The value of prognostic factors for uterine cervical cancer patients treated with irradiation alone. BMC Cancer. 2007;7(1):234.

Hirai Y, Takeshima N, Tate S, Akiyama F, Furuta R, Hasumi K. Early invasive cervical adenocarcinoma: its potential for nodal metastasis or recurrence. BJOG. 2003;110(3):241–6.

Kadkhodayan S, Hasanzadeh M, Treglia G, Azad A, Yousefi Z, Zarifmahmoudi L, Sadeghi R. Sentinel node biopsy for lymph nodal staging of uterine cervix cancer: a systematic review and meta-analysis of the pertinent literature. Eur J Surg Oncol. 2015;41 (1):1–20.

Kamura T, Tsukamoto N, Tsuruchi N, Saito T, Matsuyama T, Akazawa K, Nakano H. Multivariate analysis of the histopathologic prognostic factors of cervical cancer in patients undergoing radical hysterectomy. Cancer. 1992;69(1):181–6.

Kasamatsu T, Okada S, Tsuda H, Shiromizu K, Yamada T, Tsunematsu R, Ohmi K. Early invasive adenocarcinoma of the uterine cervix: criteria for nonradical surgical treatment. Gynecol Oncol. 2002;85(2):327–32.

Kasamatsu T, Onda T, Sawada M, Kato T, Ikeda S, Sasajima Y, Tsuda H. Radical hysterectomy for FIGO stage I-IIB adenocarcinoma of the uterine cervix. Br J Cancer. 2009;100(9):1400–5.

Kato T, Takashima A, Kasamatsu T, Nakamura K, Mizusawa J, Nakanishi T, Takeshima N, Kamiura S, Onda T, Sumi T, Takano M, Nakai H, Saito T, Fujiwara K, Yokoyama M, Itamochi H, Takehara K, Yokota H, Mizunoe T, Takeda S, Sonoda K, Shiozawa T, Kawabata T, Honma S, Fukuda H, Yaegashi N, Yoshikawa H, Konishi I, Kamura T, Group GOSGotJCO. Clinical tumor diameter and prognosis of patients with FIGO stage IB1 cervical cancer (JCOG0806-A). Gynecol Oncol. 2015;137(1):34–9.

Keys HM, Bundy BN, Stehman FB, Muderspach LI, Chafe WE, Suggs CL, Walker JL, Gersell D. Cisplatin, radiation, and adjuvant hysterectomy compared with radiation and adjuvant hysterectomy for bulky stage IB cervical carcinoma. N Engl J Med. 1999;340(15):1154–61.

Kim K, Kang SB, Chung HH, Kim JW, Park NH, Song YS. Comparison of chemoradiation with radiation as postoperative adjuvant therapy in cervical cancer patients with intermediate-risk factors. Eur J Surg Oncol. 2009;35(2):192–6.

Kuji S, Hirashima Y, Nakayama H, Nishio S, Otsuki T, Nagamitsu Y, Tanaka N, Ito K, Teramoto N, Yamada T. Diagnosis, clinicopathologic features, treatment, and prognosis of small cell carcinoma of the uterine cervix; Kansai Clinical Oncology Group/Intergroup study in Japan. Gynecol Oncol. 2013;129(3):522–7.

Landoni F, Maneo A, Colombo A, Placa F, Milani R, Perego P, Favini G, Ferri L, Mangioni C. Randomised study of radical surgery versus radiotherapy for stage Ib-IIa cervical cancer. Lancet. 1997;350(9077):535–40.

Landoni F, Maneo A, Cormio G, Perego P, Milani R, Caruso O, Mangioni C. Class II versus class III radical hysterectomy in stage IB-IIA cervical cancer: a prospective randomized study. Gynecol Oncol. 2001;80(1):3–12.

Landoni F, Maneo A, Zapardiel I, Zanagnolo V, Mangioni C. Class I versus class III radical hysterectomy in stage IB1-IIA cervical cancer. A prospective randomized study. Eur J Surg Oncol. 2012;38(3):203–9.

Lécuru F, Mathevet P, Querleu D, Leblanc E, Morice P, Daraï E, Marret H, Magaud L, Gillaizeau F, Chatellier G, Dargent D. Bilateral negative sentinel nodes accurately predict absence of lymph node metastasis in early cervical cancer: results of the SENTICOL study. J Clin Oncol. 2011;29(13):1686–91.

Lee KB, Lee JM, Park CY, Cho HY, Ha SY. Lymph node metastasis and lymph vascular space invasion in microinvasive squamous cell carcinoma of the uterine cervix. Int J Gynecol Cancer. 2006;16 (3):1184–7.

Mabuchi S, Okazawa M, Isohashi F, Matsuo K, Ohta Y, Suzuki O, Yoshioka Y, Enomoto T, Kamiura S, Kimura T. Radical hysterectomy with adjuvant radiotherapy versus definitive radiotherapy alone for FIGO stage IIB cervical cancer. Gynecol Oncol. 2011;123(2):241–7.

Mabuchi S, Okazawa M, Matsuo K, Kawano M, Suzuki O, Miyatake T, Enomoto T, Kamiura S, Ogawa K, Kimura T. Impact of histological subtype on survival of patients with surgically-treated stage IA2-IIB cervical cancer: adenocarcinoma versus squamous cell carcinoma. Gynecol Oncol. 2012a;127(2):114–20.

Mabuchi S, Okazawa M, Kinose Y, Matsuo K, Fujiwara M, Suzuki O, Morii E, Kamiura S, Ogawa K, Kimura T. Comparison of the prognoses of FIGO stage I to stage II adenosquamous carcinoma and adenocarcinoma of the uterine cervix treated with radical hysterectomy. Int J Gynecol Cancer. 2012b;22(8):1389–97.

Mabuchi S, Matsumoto Y, Kawano M, Minami K, Seo Y, Sasano T, Takahashi R, Kuroda H, Hisamatsu T, Kakigano A, Hayashi M, Sawada K, Hamasaki T, Morii E, Kurachi H, Matsuura N, Kimura T. Uterine cervical cancer displaying tumor-related leukocytosis: a distinct clinical entity with radioresistant feature. J Natl Cancer Inst. 2014;106(7):dju147.

Morris M, Eifel PJ, Lu J, Grigsby PW, Levenback C, Stevens RE, Rotman M, Gershenson DM, Mutch DG. Pelvic radiation with concurrent chemotherapy compared with pelvic and para-aortic radiation for high-risk cervical cancer. N Engl J Med. 1999;340(15):1137–43.

Nam JH, Park JY, Kim DY, Kim JH, Kim YM, Kim YT. Laparoscopic versus open radical hysterectomy in early-stage cervical cancer: long-term survival outcomes in a matched cohort study. Ann Oncol. 2012;23(4):903–11.

Obermair A, Gebski V, Frumovitz M, Soliman PT, Schmeler KM, Levenback C, Ramirez PT. A phase III randomized clinical trial comparing laparoscopic or robotic radical hysterectomy with abdominal radical hysterectomy in patients with early stage cervical cancer. J Minim Invasive Gynecol. 2008;15(5):584–8.

Okazawa M, Mabuchi S, Isohashi F, Suzuki O, Ohta Y, Fujita M, Yoshino K, Enomoto T, Kamiura S, Kimura T. The prognostic significance of multiple pelvic node metastases in cervical cancer patients treated with radical hysterectomy plus adjuvant chemoradiotherapy. Int J Gynecol Cancer. 2012;22(3):490–7.

Okazawa M, Mabuchi S, Isohashi F, Suzuki O, Yoshioka Y, Sasano T, Ohta Y, Kamiura S, Ogawa K, Kimura T. Impact of the addition of concurrent chemotherapy to pelvic radiotherapy in surgically treated stage IB1-IIB cervical cancer patients with intermediate-risk or high-risk factors: a 13-year experience. Int J Gynecol Cancer. 2013;23(3):567–75.

Park JY, Kim DY, Kim JH, Kim YM, Kim YT, Nam JH. Outcomes after radical hysterectomy in patients with early-stage adenocarcinoma of uterine cervix. Br J Cancer. 2010;102(12):1692–8.

Perez CA, Camel HM, Kao MS, Hederman MA. Randomized study of preoperative radiation and surgery or irradiation alone in the treatment of stage IB and IIA carcinoma of the uterine cervix: final report. Gynecol Oncol. 1987;27(2):129–40.

Perez CA, Grigsby PW, Castro-Vita H, Lockett MA. Carcinoma of the uterine cervix. I. Impact of prolongation of overall treatment time and timing of brachytherapy on outcome of radiation therapy. Int J Radiat Oncol Biol Phys. 1995;32(5):1275–88.

Peters WA, Liu PY, Barrett RJ, Stock RJ, Monk BJ, Berek JS, Souhami L, Grigsby P, Gordon W, Alberts DS. Concurrent chemotherapy and pelvic radiation therapy compared with pelvic radiation therapy alone as adjuvant therapy after radical surgery in high-risk early-stage cancer of the cervix. J Clin Oncol. 2000;18(8):1606–13.

Poynor EA, Marshall D, Sonoda Y, Slomovitz BM, Barakat RR, Soslow RA. Clinicopathologic features of early adenocarcinoma of the cervix initially managed with cervical conization. Gynecol Oncol. 2006;103(3):960–5.

Reynolds EA, Tierney K, Keeney GL, Felix JC, Weaver AL, Roman LD, Cliby WA. Analysis of outcomes of microinvasive adenocarcinoma of the uterine cervix by treatment type. Obstet Gynecol. 2010;116(5):1150–7.

Rose PG, Bundy BN, Watkins EB, Thigpen JT, Deppe G, Maiman MA, Clarke-Pearson DL, Insalaco S. Concurrent cisplatin-based radiotherapy and chemotherapy for locally advanced cervical cancer. N Engl J Med. 1999;340(15):1144–53.

Rose PG, Java JJ, Whitney CW, Stehman FB, Lanciano R, Thomas GM. Locally advanced adenocarcinoma and adenosquamous carcinomas of the cervix compared to squamous cell carcinomas of the cervix in gynecologic oncology group trials of cisplatin-based chemoradiation. Gynecol Oncol. 2014;135(2):208–12.

Rotman M, Pajak TF, Choi K, Clery M, Marcial V, Grigsby PW, Cooper J, John M. Prophylactic extended-field irradiation of para-aortic lymph nodes in stages IIB and bulky IB and IIA cervical carcinomas. Ten-year treatment results of RTOG 79–20. JAMA. 1995;274(5):387–93.

Rotman M, Sedlis A, Piedmonte MR, Bundy B, Lentz SS, Muderspach LI, Zaino RJ. A phase III randomized trial of postoperative pelvic irradiation in stage IB cervical carcinoma with poor prognostic features: follow-up of a gynecologic oncology group study. Int J Radiat Oncol Biol Phys. 2006;65(1):169–76.

Rydzewska L, Tierney J, Vale CL, Symonds PR. Neoadjuvant chemotherapy plus surgery versus surgery for cervical cancer. Cochrane Database Syst Rev. 2012;12:CD007406. doi:10.1002/14651858.CD007406.pub3.

Selman TJ, Mann C, Zamora J, Appleyard TL, Khan K. Diagnostic accuracy of tests for lymph node status in primary cervical cancer: a systematic review and meta-analysis. CMAJ. 2008;178(7):855–62.

Serkies K, Badzio A, Jassem J. Clinical relevance of hemoglobin level in cervical cancer patients administered definitive radiotherapy. Acta Oncol. 2006;45(6):695–701.

van Meurs H, Visser O, Buist MR, Ten Kate FJ, van der Velden J. Frequency of pelvic lymph node metastases and parametrial involvement in stage IA2 cervical cancer: a population-based study and literature review. Int J Gynecol Cancer. 2009;19(1):21–6.

van Nagell JR, Powell DE, Gallion HH, Elliott DG, Donaldson ES, Carpenter AE, Higgins RV, Kryscio R, Pavlik EJ. Small cell carcinoma of the uterine cervix. Cancer. 1988;62(8):1586–93.

Whitney CW, Sause W, Bundy BN, Malfetano JH, Hannigan EV, Fowler WC, Clarke-Pearson DL, Liao SY. Randomized comparison of fluorouracil plus cisplatin versus hydroxyurea as an adjunct to radiation therapy in stage IIB-IVA carcinoma of the cervix with negative para-aortic lymph nodes: a Gynecologic Oncology Group and Southwest Oncology Group study. J Clin Oncol. 1999;17(5):1339–48.

Wright JD, NathavithArana R, Nathavithrana R, Lewin SN, Sun X, Deutsch I, Burke WM, Herzog TJ. Fertility-conserving surgery for young women with stage IA1 cervical cancer: safety and access. Obstet Gynecol. 2010;115(3):585–90.

Management of Metastatic and Recurrent Cervical Cancer

Seiji Mabuchi, Mahiru Kawano, Ryoko Takahashi, and Hiromasa Kuroda

Abstract

Treatment guidelines for uterine cervical cancer have been established based on the findings of randomized clinical trials conducted in the past few decades. Although most cases of cervical cancer can be adequately managed with standard treatments, problems can arise in cases involving unusual presentations. Metastatic and recurrent cervical cancers are considered to be incurable. Although attempts have been made to treat patients with metastatic or recurrent cervical cancer with a variety of approaches including chemotherapy, radiotherapy, and surgery (as monotherapies or in combination), such patients have a dismal prognosis, with a reported 5-year survival rate of <10%. In this chapter, we first review the current management strategies for metastatic or recurrent cervical cancer. Then, we review the management strategies for unusual cases of cervical cancer, such as those involving the incidental detection of cervical cancer during pregnancy or in hysterectomy specimens, bulky lymph nodes, cervical stump cancer, cervical bleeding or ureteral obstruction, or unusual cervical cancer cell types.

S. Mabuchi (✉) • M. Kawano • R. Takahashi • H. Kuroda
Department of Obstetrics and Gynecology, Osaka University Graduate School of Medicine, Suita, Osaka, Japan
e-mail: smabuchi@gyne.med.osaka-u.ac.jp

Keywords

Metastatic cervical cancer • Recurrent cervical cancer • Chemotherapy • Cervical cancer in pregnancy • Unusual histology

Contents

1 Introduction

Although most cases of cervical cancer can be adequately managed with standard treatments, problems can arise in cases involving unusual presentations. In this chapter, we summarize the management strategies for such unusual conditions, including metastatic and recurrent cervical cancer, and cases of cervical cancer involving the incidental detection of the disease during pregnancy or in hysterectomy specimens, bulky lymph nodes, cervical stump cancer, cervical bleeding or ureteral obstruction, or unusual cancer cell types.

2 Stage IVB Cervical Cancer

Roughly 10% of newly diagnosed cervical cancer patients have distant metastases at the time of the initial diagnosis and, thus, are diagnosed with International Federation of Gynecology and Obstetrics (FIGO) stage IVB disease (SEER Stat Fact Sheets: Cervix Uteri Cancer). These patients represent a heterogeneous population, ranging from patients with nodal metastases to those with metastases to the visceral organs.

Due to the heterogeneity of such patients' symptoms at presentation, the optimal treatment varies according to the patient's symptoms, performance status, and disease characteristics.

Although no particular treatment has been demonstrated to be superior, a variety of therapeutic options are currently available for stage IVB cervical cancer: Platinum-based combination chemotherapy is recommended for patients with organ metastasis who are not candidates for definitive radiotherapy or exenterative surgery with the aim of achieving locoregional control (Monk et al. 2009; Tewari et al. 2014; Varia et al. 1998). To date, stage IVB and recurrent cervical cancer have been treated with the same chemotherapy regimens. Patients with limited distant nodal metastasis, such as metastasis to the para-aortic lymph nodes (PALN) or supraclavicular lymph nodes, might be candidates for radiotherapy with curative intent involving an extended radiation field (Grigsby et al. 1998; Monk et al. 2009; Tewari et al. 2014; Varia et al. 1998). Patients with poor performance statuses are usually treated with palliative treatment alone. However, these treatments only achieve limited improvements in survival, resulting in a 5-year survival rate of 10–20% (Monk et al. 2009; Tewari et al. 2014; Yoon et al. 2015).

3 Recurrent Cervical Cancer

3.1 Diagnosis

It is estimated that approximately 35% of patients with invasive cervical cancer will develop recurrent or persistent disease after the primary treatment, and recurrent cervical cancer patients have a dismal prognosis, with a reported 1-year survival rate of roughly 20%.

The diagnosis of recurrent cervical cancer is often difficult. The cytological evaluation of irradiated cervix tissue is particularly difficult because of the distortion produced in the exfoliated cells. Thus, the diagnosis of recurrent cervical cancer should be confirmed histologically whenever possible to avoid misdiagnosis and unnecessary treatment.

3.2 Treatment

The treatment of recurrent cervical cancer depends on the mode of the primary treatment and the site of recurrence. Single distant recurrent lesions, such as isolated recurrent lung or PALN lesions, are usually treated with surgery or radiotherapy. Patients that suffer recurrence in the central pelvis after primary surgery can be salvaged with radiotherapy. On the other hand, patients that develop central pelvic recurrence after primary radiotherapy can be treated with curative pelvic surgery (either pelvic exenteration (PE) or radical hysterectomy (RH)). Patients with pelvic sidewall disease or multiple recurrent lesions are usually treated with platinum-based chemotherapy.

3.2.1 Chemotherapy

A large proportion of patients with recurrent disease develop tumors in a previously irradiated area. As the irradiated field is usually fibrotic and avascular, it is difficult to obtain high blood flow and achieve the optimal tissue concentration of the administered anticancer agent. Moreover, as ureteral obstruction is common in patients with recurrent cervical cancer, platinum-based chemotherapy is sometimes avoided.

The findings of phase III trials that were conducted to establish the optimal chemotherapy regimen for uterine cervical cancer are summarized in Table 1 (Leath and Straughn 2013).

A previous study by the Gynecologic Oncology Group (GOG) showed that the i.v. administration of 50 mg/m^2 cisplatin every 3 weeks as a single agent is superior to all other single-agent options (GOG 43). Subsequent phase III trials have demonstrated that cisplatin-based doublet chemotherapies are superior to single-agent cisplatin. In a phase III study comparing four cisplatin-based doublet chemotherapies (cisplatin + paclitaxel, cisplatin + topotecan, cisplatin + gemcitabine, and cisplatin + vinorelbine), cisplatin + paclitaxel produced the longest progression-free survival (PFS) and overall survival (OS) periods, although the differences were not statistically significant (GOG 204). Based on these results, cisplatin + paclitaxel became the standard chemotherapy for patients with recurrent cervical cancer. Subsequently, in an effort to mitigate the nephrotoxicity encountered during the use of cisplatin and shorten the chemotherapy infusion interval in order to allow cisplatin + paclitaxel chemotherapy to be administered on an outpatient basis, the Japanese Clinical Oncology Group (JCOG) performed a prospective, non-inferiority, phase III trial comparing cisplatin + paclitaxel with carboplatin + paclitaxel. In the survival analysis, carboplatin + paclitaxel was not found to be inferior to cisplatin + paclitaxel. As anticipated, the cisplatin-containing regimen exhibited greater renal toxicity, while the carboplatin-containing regimen produced greater thrombocytopenia (JCOG 0505).

A recent randomized trial found that combining bevacizumab with cisplatin + paclitaxel or paclitaxel + topotecan was superior to either combination alone (GOG 240). In this study, although 75% of the enrolled patients had previously received platinum-based agents, the topotecan + paclitaxel arm was not demonstrated to be superior or inferior to the cisplatin + paclitaxel arm (hazard ratio: 1.20; 95% confidence interval: 0.82–1.76), indicating that non-platinum-based chemotherapy doublets are not more effective than cisplatin + paclitaxel in this patient population. Even when bevacizumab was used in combination with cisplatin + paclitaxel, it still only resulted in a median OS time of 17 months (Tewari et al. 2014). Accordingly, cost, convenience, and patient preference should be taken into consideration before offering this regimen to patients.

3.2.2 Surgical Treatments

Pelvic Exenteration

PE is a radical surgical procedure involving the en bloc resection of the pelvic organs, including the internal reproductive organs, the distal urinary tract (bilateral ureters, bladder, and urethra), and the anorectum. This procedure was first described by Alexander Brunschwig in 1948 (Brunschwig 1948). PE is a potentially curative option for selected patients with recurrent or persistent cervical cancer and results in a reported 5-year survival rate of 30–50% (Berek et al. 2005; Chiantera et al. 2014; Goldberg et al. 2006; Marnitz et al. 2006; Schmidt et al. 2012; Yoo et al. 2012). Major morbidities occur in 20–40% of cases and are mainly related to the urinary and digestive diversion procedures and the associated reconstructive surgery. Global mortality varies from 0% to 10%, depending on the study (Table 2).

Radical Hysterectomy

Selected patients that exhibit limited recurrent disease in the uterine cervix after primary radiotherapy might be suitable for RH. Although this procedure is associated with a high morbidity rate,

Table 1 Summary of phase III trials of chemotherapy for recurrent or advanced cervical cancer

Trial	Arms	Response rates (%)	PFS (months)	OS (months)	Comments
GOG 43	Arm 1: Cisplatin 50 mg/m^2/3 weeks Arm 2: Cisplatin 100 mg/m^2/3 weeks Arm 3: Cisplatin 20 mg/m^2×5 days/3 weeks	Arm 1: 20.7 Arm 2: 31.4 Arm 3: 25.0	Arm 1: 3.7 Arm 2: 4.6 Arm 3: 3.9	Arm 1: 7.1 Arm 2: 7.0 Arm 3: 6.1	Cisplatin 50 mg/m^2/3 weeks became standard
GOG 110	Arm 1: Cisplatin Arm 2: Cisplatin + Ifosfamide	Arm 1: 17.8 Arm 2: 31.1	Arm 1: 3.2 Arm 2: 4.6 *	Arm 1: 8.0 Arm 2: 8.3	*PFS was improved (p=0.003)
GOG 149	Arm 1: Cisplatin + Ifosfamide Arm 2: Cisplatin + Ifosfamide + Bleomycin	Arm 1: 32 Arm 2: 31.2	Arm 1: 4.5 Arm 2: 5.1	Arm 1: 8.5 Arm 2: 8.4	
GOG 169	Arm 1: Cisplatin Arm 2: Cisplatin + Paclitaxel	Arm 1: 19 Arm 2: 36	Arm 1: 2.8 Arm 2: 4.8 *	Arm 1: 8.8 Arm 2: 9.7	*PFS was improved (p<0.001)
GOG 179	Arm 1: Cisplatin Arm 2: Cisplatin + Topotecan	Arm 1: 13 Arm 2: 26.7	Arm 1: 2.9 Arm 2: 4.6 *	Arm 1: 6.5 Arm 2: 9.4 *	*Both PFS (p=0.014) and OS (p=0.017) were improved
GOG 204	Arm 1: Cisplatin + Paclitaxel Arm 2: Cisplatin + Topotecan Arm 3: Cisplatin + Gemcitabine Arm 4: Cisplatin + Vinorelbine	Arm 1: 29.1 Arm 2: 23.4 Arm 3: 22.3 Arm 4: 25.9	Arm 1: 5.8 Arm 2: 4.6 Arm 3: 4.7 Arm 4: 4.0	Arm 1: 12.9 Arm 2: 10.3 Arm 3: 10.3 Arm 4: 10.0	No significant differences were observed Cisplatin + Paclitaxel became standard
JGOG0505	Arm 1: Cisplatin + Paclitaxel Arm 2: Carboplatin + Paclitaxel	Arm 1: 58.8 Arm 2: 62.6	Arm 1: 6.9 Arm 2: 6.2	Arm 1: 18.3 Arm 2: 17.5	Non-inferiority of carboplatin + paclitaxel was demonstrated
GOG240	Arm 1: Cisplatin + Paclitaxel Arm 2: Cisplatin + Paclitaxel + Bevacizumab Arm 3: Topotecan + Paclitaxel Arm 4: Topotecan + Paclitaxel + Bevacizumab	Arm 1: 45 Arm 2: 50 Arm 3: 27 Arm 4: 47	Arm 1 + 3: 5.9 Arm 2 + 4: 8.2 * Arm 1 + 2: 7.6 Arm 3 + 4: 5.7	Arm 1: 14.3 Arm 2: 17.5 ** Arm 3: 12.7 Arm 4: 16.2 Arm 1 + 3: 13.3 Arm 2 + 4: 17 *** Arm 1 + 2: 15 Arm 3 + 4: 12.5	Addition of bevacizumab improved PFS and OS *Arm 1 + 3 versus Arm 2 + 4: p = 0.0002 **Arm 1 versus Arm 2: p = 0.04 ***Arm 1 + 3 versus Arm 2 + 4: p = 0.003

Table 2 Recent larger series of pelvic exenteration for cervical cancer

First author	N	Severe morbidity (%)	Operative mortality (%)	5-year survival (%)
Chiantera 2014	167	34,7	6	38
Yoo 2012	61	44	0	56
Schmidt 2012	212	51	5	41
Marnitz 2006	35	38	5.5	27
Goldberg 2006	103	25	1	48
Berek 2005	67	23	4.4	54

it can cure patients without the need for urinary and digestive diversion. According to a previous report, this procedure results in a 5-year survival rate of 49%, but major morbidities occur in 44% of cases (Maneo et al. 1999).

Radiotherapy

Recurrence outside of the irradiated field can be successfully treated with irradiation with or without concurrent chemotherapy. However, the utility of re-irradiation for pelvic recurrence, which might be an option for a selected group of patients, is disputed. Although re-irradiation is associated with little or no treatment-related mortality and preserves the structures and functions of the pelvic organs, it is often avoided due to concerns regarding severe late toxicities, such as fistula formation. Recent reports about re-irradiation involving interstitial brachytherapy alone have shown cure rates ranging from 20% to 50% and grade 3/4 late complication rates ranging from 10% to 40%. None of the patients in these studies died (Badakh and Grover 2009; Charra et al. 1998; Mabuchi et al. 2014; Prempree et al. 1979; Randall et al. 1993).

4 Invasive Cancer that is Detected After Simple Hysterectomy

In cases of invasive cancer that are found after simple hysterectomy, the treatment options include pelvic external beam radiotherapy or surgery consisting of radical parametrectomy, upper vaginectomy, and pelvic lymphadenectomy. It is generally more difficult to perform a reoperation than an RH, as the bladder and rectum firmly adhere to the vaginal vault and can also adhere to each other. In a previous study by Ayhan et al.,

operative complications occurred in 5 out of 27 patients (18.5%) (bladder perforation, intestinal perforation, ureteral injury, and external iliac vein injury), and the OS rate was 88.9% (Ayhan et al. 2006). In a case series in which postoperative radiotherapy was employed, Hopkins et al. reported that radiation therapy in the immediate postoperative period produced a survival of 88%, compared to observation only with a 69% survival (P = 0.10) (Hopkins et al. 1990).

5 Cancer of the Cervical Stump

In cases in which invasive cancer develops in a cervical stump, the treatment principles are the same as those employed for patients whose uteruses remain intact. When surgery is performed as an initial treatment, the bladder sometimes adheres firmly to the stump; therefore, dissection should be performed carefully. When radiotherapy is considered as an initial treatment, we have to recognize (1) that the ability to deliver an adequate dose of radiation to the primary tumor depends on the length of the cervical canal and (2) that it is difficult to accomplish this if the canal is less than 2 cm in length. Hellström et al. reported in their case–control study that the 5-year survival rate of patients with cervical stump cancer was similar to that observed in patients with intact uteruses (Hellström et al. 2001).

6 Cervical Bleeding

Cervical bleeding sometimes occurs after pelvic examinations or biopsies. When the bleeding cannot be controlled with gauze packing, embolization of the hypogastric or uterine arteries should be considered. However, there is a concern that such arterial embolization might increase tumor hypoxia and decrease the sensitivity of cervical cancer to radiotherapy.

7 Invasive Cervical Cancer with Bulky Lymph Nodes

Enlarged lymph nodes (>2 cm diameter) should be removed through an extraperitoneal approach before the initiation of radiotherapy, as they cannot be cured by external beam radiotherapy. Cosin et al. reported that the resecting of enlarged lymph nodes can improve a patient's prognosis so that it is similar to those of patients with micrometastasis without increasing the treatment-related morbidity or mortality rate (Cosin et al. 1998).

8 Ureteral Obstruction

Ureteral obstruction due to cervical cancer is an ominous sign and can occur due to compression by the primary or metastatic tumor, retroperitoneal adenopathy, or direct tumor invasion. Previous studies have indicated that hydronephrosis is an independent poor prognostic indicator in patients with advanced cervical cancer (Pradhan et al. 2011; Rose et al. 2010). Moreover, acute ureteral obstruction associated with renal failure, pain, or fever is an emergency that requires prompt evaluation and treatment. The current management options for this condition involve decompression by a cystoscopically inserted ureteral stent or a percutaneous nephrostomy tube. Generally, patients that are treated with stents experience significantly more urinary symptoms and require more assistance with nephrostomy care.

9 Cervical Cancer in Pregnancy

9.1 Incidence

Cervical cancer is the most commonly diagnosed gynecological malignancy during pregnancy. The incidence rate of the condition varies from 0.1 to 12 per 10,000 pregnancies (Al-Halal et al. 2013; Duggan et al. 1993; Takushi et al. 2002).

9.2 Symptoms

Although vaginal bleeding is the main symptom seen in pregnant patients with cervical cancer, abnormal bleeding is often mistakenly attributed to pregnancy-related complications. Pelvic pain and bowel or urinary symptoms can also be mistakenly linked to pregnancy-related complications. Thus, the diagnosis of cervical cancer is sometimes delayed, especially in cases in which cervical cancer is not initially suspected.

9.3 Diagnosis

In pregnant women, the diagnosis of cervical cancer should be based on colposcopy-directed punch biopsies, which can be performed safely during pregnancy. Endocervical curettage is contraindicated during pregnancy. Cone biopsies should be performed sparingly, as they are associated with hemorrhaging, abortion, and premature labor. In strictly indicated cases involving a strong suspicion of invasive disease, the optimal time to perform a conization during pregnancy is between 14 and 20 weeks' gestation.

9.4 Distribution by Stage

As pregnancy is associated with frequent obstetric examinations, most patients that are diagnosed with cervical cancer during pregnancy present with early-stage disease (Zemlickis et al. 1991).

9.5 Staging

The general rule when performing radiological and nuclear medicine examinations during pregnancy is that the radiation dose should be kept as low as possible and that such examinations should be avoided when possible. Thus, pelvic computed tomography (CT) and fluorodeoxyglucose positron emission tomography/CT are usually avoided. Magnetic resonance imaging (MRI) can be used safely during pregnancy to evaluate tumor size, stromal invasion, vaginal and parametrial invasion, and lymph node infiltration (Kanal et al. 2007). At present, there are no known deleterious effects of exposing a developing fetus to MRI.

9.6 Management

Decisions regarding the management strategy should be made after full discussions with both of the fetus' parents regarding the risks to both mother and fetus.

In cases in which pregnancy preservation is not included in the treatment aims, cervical cancer can be managed using a similar approach to that adopted for nonpregnant women. RH and pelvic lymphadenectomy can be performed during any trimester, either with the fetus in situ or after a classic cesarean section. In cases in which definitive radiotherapy is employed as a primary treatment, spontaneous abortion usually occurs after external beam radiotherapy. If it does not occur, hysterotomy and evacuation of the uterus should be performed before the initiation of intracavitary brachytherapy.

If pregnancy preservation is desired, the treatment choice is influenced by the gestational age of the fetus and the patient's disease stage. The mother must be informed and must understand that pregnancy-preserving management strategies for invasive cervical cancer remain experimental.

For patients that are diagnosed with cervical cancer before 20 weeks' gestation, pregnancy interruption and immediate treatment are usually recommended. However, in cases of stage IA1 disease that are diagnosed after conization and exhibit clear negative margins, it is reasonable to allow the pregnancy to proceed until term. Diagnostic conization should be performed at 12–20 weeks' gestation. A vaginal delivery should be chosen unless obstetric indications for cesarean section are present.

For patients that are diagnosed after 24 weeks' gestation, a watch and wait strategy should be employed until the fetus is viable. However, when progressive disease is observed before fetal maturity, early delivery or neoadjuvant chemotherapy (NACT) is advocated.

A dilemma arises when patients are diagnosed with cervical cancer between 20 and 24 weeks' gestation. Due to the limited number of such cases, it is impossible to offer a precise risk estimate for individual patients. In patients with stage IA2 or higher stage tumors, pelvic lymphadenectomy can be used to identify node-positive high-risk patients in whom it is necessary to terminate the pregnancy, although the therapeutic value of pelvic lymphadenectomy is unclear. A recent literature review reported that recurrence did not occur in pregnant women with stage IB1 tumors without lymph node metastasis (Morice et al. 2012; Zagouri et al. 2013). In those with stage IB2 and higher-stage tumors, NACT is the only way to prevent disease progression while allowing time for the fetus to achieve viability.

It has been reported that during pregnancy, NACT involving a platinum-based agent in combination with paclitaxel is superior to NACT involving a single platinum-based agent in terms of response rate (Amant et al. 2014). Thus, NACT involving paclitaxel (175 mg/m^2) in combination with cisplatin (75 mg/m^2) or carboplatin (AUC of 5–6) every 3 weeks is the currently recommended regimen.

Although several cases in which the patient was treated with pregnancy-preserving radical trachelectomy have been reported, in the absence of obstetric safety data, this procedure cannot be recommended at this time.

9.7 Prognosis

Previous studies have shown that pregnant and nonpregnant cervical cancer patients exhibit identical survival rates (Zemlickis et al. 1991). The favorable overall prognosis of pregnant patients with cervical cancer seems to be due to the greater proportion of pregnant patients that present with stage I disease.

10 Unusual Histological Types

10.1 Glassy Cell Carcinoma

Glassy cell carcinoma was first described in 1956. The latter study reported that the neoplastic cells found in glassy cell carcinoma exhibit the following features: a moderate amount of cytoplasm with a ground-glass appearance, distinct cell walls, and large nuclei with prominent nucleoli (Cherry and Glucksmann 1956). Glassy cell carcinoma is now regarded as a poorly differentiated form of mixed adenosquamous carcinoma. Previous studies have suggested that glassy cell carcinoma is associated with a high risk of distant failure and a worse prognosis than squamous cell carcinoma (Guitarte et al. 2014). However, due to the rarity of the disease and the lack of prospective studies examining it, no specific management strategy for glassy cell carcinoma has been developed. Thus, it is usually treated according to the management strategy for squamous cell carcinoma.

10.2 Small Cell Carcinoma

Small cell carcinoma is most frequently found in the lungs, with pulmonary small cell carcinoma accounting for 95% of all cases of the condition (van Meerbeeck et al. 2011). Small cell carcinoma of the uterine cervix is a rare histological entity, representing roughly 1% of cases of invasive cervical cancer (Satoh et al. 2014). Histologically, roughly one-third of small cell carcinomas are positive for the neuroendocrine markers chromogranin, synaptophysin, and CD56, whereas the remaining lesions only express epithelial markers, such as cytokeratin. Previous studies have suggested that small cell carcinoma is associated with higher incidences of lymphovascular space invasion, lymph node metastasis, and distant metastasis, even in the early stages of the disease, a higher rate of recurrence, and decreased survival compared with squamous cell carcinoma and adenocarcinoma (Chen et al. 2008; Kim et al. 2009; McCusker et al. 2003). Due to the rarity of this disease and the lack of a prospective study examining it, no specific management strategy for small

cell carcinoma has been established. Currently, early-stage small cell carcinoma is generally treated with surgery, and advanced disease is treated with concurrent chemoradiotherapy. However, previous retrospective studies have suggested that postoperative adjuvant therapy either with radiotherapy or chemotherapy did not improve the prognosis of patients with cervical small cell carcinoma (Cohen et al. 2010; Lee et al. 2008; Tian et al. 2012). In contrast, recent retrospective studies have indicated that the administration of adjuvant chemotherapy after RH or definitive radiotherapy is effective against the condition (Kuji et al. 2013; Wang et al. 2012). Etoposide and cisplatin were the most frequently used regimen in these trials. Given the propensity for early systemic spread and the high probability of distant treatment failure, the efficacy of adjuvant chemotherapy for cervical small cell carcinoma should be investigated in a prospective study (Kuji et al. 2013).

10.3 Sarcoma

Cervical sarcomas are rare tumors that constitute <1% of all cervical malignancies. The seven most common types of cervical sarcoma are embryonal rhabdomyosarcoma, leiomyosarcoma, undifferentiated endocervical sarcoma, alveolar soft part sarcoma, Ewing's sarcoma, primitive neuroectodermal tumor, and liposarcoma (Fadare et al. 2006). As the previously reported cases were treated using a wide variety of treatments and involved small numbers of patients as well as patients that presented with different disease stages, the assessment of the natural history and intrinsic biological behavior of cervical sarcoma remains difficult. International collaborative investigations need to be conducted to establish guidelines for the management of this condition.

10.4 Lymphoma

Primary lymphoma of the uterine cervix is an extremely rare disease. Approximately a quarter of malignant lymphomas arise in extranodal organs. The most common locations of extranodal lymphoma are the gastrointestinal tract and skin, and about 1.5% of extranodal lymphomas originate in the female genital tract, with the ovaries being the most commonly affected site (Upanal and Enjeti 2011).

Vaginal bleeding is the most common symptom at presentation. The Papanicolaou smear test is not useful for diagnosing uterine lymphoma. Instead, patients should be diagnosed based on histological and immunophenotypic evaluations of their biopsy samples. Histologically, B-cell lymphomas constitute the vast majority of uterine lymphomas, with the most frequent type being the diffuse large cell type (56%) followed by follicular lymphoma (15%).

Due to the rarity of uterine/cervical lymphoma, no standard treatment for primary uterine lymphoma has been established. In a recent review of 75 cases of malignant lymphoma (Upanal and Enjeti 2011), various treatment modalities were employed: surgery alone (25%); surgery and chemotherapy (25%); chemotherapy and radiotherapy (19%); chemotherapy alone (19%); chemotherapy, radiotherapy, and surgery (8%); and surgery combined with radiotherapy (3%). However, it remains unclear which primary treatment is the most advantageous. To preserve the reproductive function of young patients, combination chemotherapy alone has been advocated as a primary treatment in previous reports (Szánthó et al. 2003). In general, the overall prognosis of primary uterine lymphoma appears to be excellent and is comparable with those of other nodal lymphomas. In a study of 10 patients with uterine non-Hodgkin's lymphoma, Vang et al. reported a very good 5-year survival rate of 83% (Vang et al. 2000).

11   Conclusion

Although most cervical cancers can be adequately managed with standard treatments, problems can arise in cases involving unusual presentations. Due to the limited numbers of such patients, it is difficult to conduct randomized studies of their conditions. Further prospective, collaborative studies need to be conducted to establish standard evidence-based treatments for unusual types of cervical cancer.

References

Al-Halal H, Kezouh A, Abenhaim HA. Incidence and obstetrical outcomes of cervical intraepithelial neoplasia and cervical cancer in pregnancy: a population-based study on 8.8 million births. Arch Gynecol Obstet. 2013;287(2):245–50.

Amant F, Halaska MJ, Fumagalli M, Dahl Steffensen K, Lok C, Van Calsteren K, Han SN, Mir O, Fruscio R, Uzan C, Maxwell C, Dekrem J, Strauven G, Mhallem Gziri M, Kesic V, Berveiller P, van den Heuvel F, Ottevanger PB, Vergote I, Lishner M, Morice P, Nulman I, Pregnancy' EtfCi. Gynecologic cancers in pregnancy: guidelines of a second international consensus meeting. Int J Gynecol Cancer. 2014;24(3):394–403.

Ayhan A, Otegen U, Guven S, Kucukali T. Radical reoperation for invasive cervical cancer found in simple hysterectomy. J Surg Oncol. 2006;94(1):28–34.

Badakh DK, Grover AH. Reirradiation with high-dose-rate remote afterloading brachytherapy implant in patients with locally recurrent or residual cervical carcinoma. J Cancer Res Ther. 2009;5(1):24–30.

Berek JS, Howe C, Lagasse LD, Hacker NF. Pelvic exenteration for recurrent gynecologic malignancy: survival and morbidity analysis of the 45-year experience at UCLA. Gynecol Oncol. 2005;99(1):153–9.

Brunschwig A. Complete excision of pelvic viscera for advanced carcinoma; a one-stage abdominoperineal operation with end colostomy and bilateral ureteral implantation into the colon above the colostomy. Cancer. 1948;1(2):177–83.

Charra C, Roy P, Coquard R, Romestaing P, Ardiet JM, Gérard JP. Outcome of treatment of upper third vaginal recurrences of cervical and endometrial carcinomas with interstitial brachytherapy. Int J Radiat Oncol Biol Phys. 1998;40(2):421–6.

Chen J, Macdonald OK, Gaffney DK. Incidence, mortality, and prognostic factors of small cell carcinoma of the cervix. Obstet Gynecol. 2008;111(6):1394–402.

Cherry CP, Glucksmann A. Incidence, histology, and response to radiation of mixed carcinomas (adenoacanthomas) of the uterine cervix. Cancer. 1956;9(5):971–9.

Chiantera V, Rossi M, De Iaco P, Koehler C, Marnitz S, Ferrandina G, Legge F, Parazzini F, Scambia G, Schneider A, Vercellino GF. Survival after curative pelvic exenteration for primary or recurrent cervical cancer: a retrospective multicentric study of 167 patients. Int J Gynecol Cancer. 2014; 24(5):916–22.

Cohen JG, Kapp DS, Shin JY, Urban R, Sherman AE, Chen LM, Osann K, Chan JK. Small cell carcinoma of the cervix: treatment and survival outcomes of 188 patients. Am J Obstet Gynecol. 2010;203(4):347.e341–346.

Cosin JA, Fowler JM, Chen MD, Paley PJ, Carson LF, Twiggs LB. Pretreatment surgical staging of patients with cervical carcinoma: the case for lymph node debulking. Cancer. 1998;82(11):2241–8.

Duggan B, Muderspach LI, Roman LD, Curtin JP, d'Ablaing G, Morrow CP. Cervical cancer in pregnancy: reporting on planned delay in therapy. Obstet Gynecol. 1993;82(4 Pt 1):598–602.

Fadare O, Ghofrani M, Stamatakos MD, Tavassoli FA. Mesenchymal lesions of the uterine cervix. Pathol Case Rev. 2006;11(3):140–52.

Goldberg GL, Sukumvanich P, Einstein MH, Smith HO, Anderson PS, Fields AL. Total pelvic exenteration: the Albert Einstein College of Medicine/Montefiore Medical Center experience (1987 to 2003). Gynecol Oncol. 2006;101(2):261–8.

Grigsby PW, Lu JD, Mutch DG, Kim RY, Eifel PJ. Twice-daily fractionation of external irradiation with brachytherapy and chemotherapy in carcinoma of the cervix with positive para-aortic lymph nodes: phase II study of the Radiation Therapy Oncology Group 92–10. Int J Radiat Oncol Biol Phys. 1998;41(4):817–22.

Guitarte C, Alagkiozidis I, Mize B, Stevens E, Salame G, Lee YC. Glassy cell carcinoma of the cervix: a systematic review and meta-analysis. Gynecol Oncol. 2014;133(2):186–91.

Hellström AC, Sigurjonson T, Pettersson F. Carcinoma of the cervical stump. The radiumhemmet series 1959–1987. Treatment and prognosis. Acta Obstet Gynecol Scand. 2001;80(2):152–7.

Hopkins MP, Peters WA, Andersen W, Morley GW. Invasive cervical cancer treated initially by standard hysterectomy. Gynecol Oncol. 1990;36(1):7–12.

Kanal E, Barkovich AJ, Bell C, Borgstede JP, Bradley WG, Froelich JW, Gilk T, Gimbel JR, Gosbee J, Kuhni-Kaminski E, Lester JW, Nyenhuis J, Parag Y, Schaefer DJ, Sebek-Scoumis EA, Weinreb J, Zaremba LA, Wilcox P, Lucey L, Sass N, Safety ABRPoM. ACR guidance document for safe MR practices: 2007. AJR Am J Roentgenol. 2007;188(6):1447–74.

Kim YM, Jung MH, Kim DY, Kim JH, Kim YT, Nam JH. Small cell carcinoma of the uterine cervix: clinicopathologic study of 20 cases in a single center. Eur J Gynaecol Oncol. 2009;30(5):539–42.

Kuji S, Hirashima Y, Nakayama H, Nishio S, Otsuki T, Nagamitsu Y, Tanaka N, Ito K, Teramoto N, Yamada T. Diagnosis, clinicopathologic features, treatment, and prognosis of small cell carcinoma of the uterine cervix; Kansai Clinical Oncology Group/Intergroup study in Japan. Gynecol Oncol. 2013;129(3):522–7.

Leath CA, Straughn JM. Chemotherapy for advanced and recurrent cervical carcinoma: results from cooperative group trials. Gynecol Oncol. 2013;129(1):251–7.

Lee JM, Lee KB, Nam JH, Ryu SY, Bae DS, Park JT, Kim SC, Cha SD, Kim KR, Song SY, Kang SB. Prognostic factors in FIGO stage IB-IIA small cell neuroendocrine

carcinoma of the uterine cervix treated surgically: results of a multi-center retrospective Korean study. Ann Oncol. 2008;19(2):321–6.

Mabuchi S, Takahashi R, Isohashi F, Yokoi T, Okazawa M, Sasano T, Maruoka S, Anzai M, Yoshioka Y, Ogawa K, Kimura T. Reirradiation using high-dose-rate interstitial brachytherapy for locally recurrent cervical cancer: a single institutional experience. Int J Gynecol Cancer. 2014;24(1):141–8.

Maneo A, Landoni F, Cormio G, Colombo A, Mangioni C. Radical hysterectomy for recurrent or persistent cervical cancer following radiation therapy. Int J Gynecol Cancer. 1999;9(4):295–301.

Marnitz S, Köhler C, Müller M, Behrens K, Hasenbein K, Schneider A. Indications for primary and secondary exenterations in patients with cervical cancer. Gynecol Oncol. 2006;103(3):1023–30.

McCusker ME, Coté TR, Clegg LX, Tavassoli FJ. Endocrine tumors of the uterine cervix: incidence, demographics, and survival with comparison to squamous cell carcinoma. Gynecol Oncol. 2003;88(3):333–9.

Monk BJ, Sill MW, McMeekin DS, Cohn DE, Ramondetta LM, Boardman CH, Benda J, Cella D. Phase III trial of four cisplatin-containing doublet combinations in stage IVB, recurrent, or persistent cervical carcinoma: a Gynecologic Oncology Group study. J Clin Oncol. 2009;27(28):4649–55.

Morice P, Uzan C, Gouy S, Verschraegen C, Haie-Meder C. Gynaecological cancers in pregnancy. Lancet. 2012;379(9815):558–69.

Pradhan TS, Duan H, Katsoulakis E, Salame G, Lee YC, Abulafia O. Hydronephrosis as a prognostic indicator of survival in advanced cervix cancer. Int J Gynecol Cancer. 2011;21(6):1091–6.

Prempree T, Kwon T, VillaSanta U, Scott RM. Management of late second or late recurrent squamous cell carcinoma of the cervix uteri after successful initial radiation treatment. Int J Radiat Oncol Biol Phys. 1979;5(11–12):2053–7.

Randall ME, Evans L, Greven KM, McCunniff AJ, Doline RM. Interstitial reirradiation for recurrent gynecologic malignancies: results and analysis of prognostic factors. Gynecol Oncol. 1993;48(1):23–31.

Rose PG, Ali S, Whitney CW, Lanciano R, Stehman FB. Impact of hydronephrosis on outcome of stage IIIB cervical cancer patients with disease limited to the pelvis, treated with radiation and concurrent chemotherapy: a Gynecologic Oncology Group study. Gynecol Oncol. 2010;117(2):270–5.

Satoh T, Takei Y, Treilleux I, Devouassoux-Shisheboran M, Ledermann J, Viswanathan AN, Mahner S, Provencher DM, Mileshkin L, Åvall-Lundqvist E, Pautier P, Reed NS, Fujiwara K. Gynecologic Cancer InterGroup (GCIG) consensus review for small cell carcinoma of the cervix. Int J Gynecol Cancer. 2014;24(9 Suppl 3): S102–8.

Schmidt AM, Imesch P, Fink D, Egger H. Indications and long-term clinical outcomes in 282 patients with pelvic exenteration for advanced or recurrent cervical cancer. Gynecol Oncol. 2012;125(3):604–9.

SEER Stat Fact Sheets: Cervix Uteri Cancer. Available from http://seer.cancer.gov/statfacts/html/cervix.html

Szánthó A, Bálega JJ, Csapó Z, Sréter LL, Matolcsy A, Papp Z. Primary non-Hodgkin's lymphoma of the uterine cervix successfully treated by neoadjuvant chemotherapy: case report. Gynecol Oncol. 2003;89(1):171–4.

Takushi M, Moromizato H, Sakumoto K, Kanazawa K. Management of invasive carcinoma of the uterine cervix associated with pregnancy: outcome of intentional delay in treatment. Gynecol Oncol. 2002;87(2):185–9.

Tewari KS, Sill MW, Long HJ, Penson RT, Huang H, Ramondetta LM, Landrum LM, Oaknin A, Reid TJ, Leitao MM, Michael HE, Monk BJ. Improved survival with bevacizumab in advanced cervical cancer. N Engl J Med. 2014;370(8):734–43.

Tian WJ, Zhang MQ, Shui RH. Prognostic factors and treatment comparison in early-stage small cell carcinoma of the uterine cervix. Oncol Lett. 2012;3(1):125–30.

Upanal N, Enjeti A. Primary lymphoma of the uterus and cervix: two case reports and review of the literature. Aust N Z J Obstet Gynaecol. 2011;51(6):559–62.

van Meerbeeck JP, Fennell DA, De Ruysscher DK. Small-cell lung cancer. Lancet. 2011;378(9804):1741–55.

Vang R, Medeiros LJ, Ha CS, Deavers M. Non-Hodgkin's lymphomas involving the uterus: a clinicopathologic analysis of 26 cases. Mod Pathol. 2000;13(1):19–28.

Varia MA, Bundy BN, Deppe G, Mannel R, Averette HE, Rose PG, Connelly P. Cervical carcinoma metastatic to para-aortic nodes: extended field radiation therapy with concomitant 5-fluorouracil and cisplatin chemotherapy: a Gynecologic Oncology Group study. Int J Radiat Oncol Biol Phys. 1998;42(5):1015–23.

Wang KL, Chang TC, Jung SM, Chen CH, Cheng YM, Wu HH, Liou WS, Hsu ST, Ou YC, Yeh LS, Lai HC, Huang CY, Chen TC, Chang CJ, Lai CH. Primary treatment and prognostic factors of small cell neuroendocrine carcinoma of the uterine cervix: a Taiwanese Gynecologic Oncology Group study. Eur J Cancer. 2012;48(10):1484–94.

Yoo HJ, Lim MC, Seo SS, Kang S, Yoo CW, Kim JY, Park SY. Pelvic exenteration for recurrent cervical cancer: ten-year experience at National Cancer Center in Korea. J Gynecol Oncol. 2012;23(4):242–50.

Yoon HI, Cha J, Keum KC, Lee HY, Nam EJ, Kim SW, Kim S, Kim YT, Kim GE, Kim YB. Treatment outcomes of extended-field radiation therapy and the effect of concurrent chemotherapy on uterine cervical cancer with para-aortic lymph node metastasis. Radiat Oncol. 2015;10(1):18.

Zagouri F, Sergentanis TN, Chrysikos D, Bartsch R. Platinum derivatives during pregnancy in cervical cancer: a systematic review and meta-analysis. Obstet Gynecol. 2013;121(2 Pt 1):337–43.

Zemlickis D, Lishner M, Degendorfer P, Panzarella T, Sutcliffe SB, Koren G. Maternal and fetal outcome after invasive cervical cancer in pregnancy. J Clin Oncol. 1991;9(11):1956–61.

Management of Cervical Dysplasia

Katherine E. Tierney, Lynda D. Roman, and Koji Matsuo

Abstract

Abnormal cervical screening tests are diagnosed in millions of women each year in the United States. In some, the abnormality is indicative of cervical dysplasia or even invasive cervical cancer. The work-up of an abnormal cervical screening test includes colposcopy and cervical biopsies. Based on those results, treatment for cervical dysplasia can consist of observation or intervention with an excisional biopsy. In deciding to intervene aggressively, one must consider special circumstances including patient age, desire for future fertility, and concurrent pregnancy. Understanding the role human papillomavirus (HPV) plays in cancer development has led to advancements in detection and treatment of cervical dysplasia. Both preventative and therapeutic vaccinations against HPV provide promise in decreasing the number of women affected by this disease. This chapter highlights key changes in the recent ASCCP guidelines including the importance of conservative management among younger women as well as recommendations on the proper utilization of HPV cotesting. The rationale for HPV vaccination is also discussed.

Keywords

Human papillomavirus • Cervical intraepithelial neoplasia • Adenocarcinoma in situ • Loop electrosurgical excision procedure • Cold-knife cone

Contents

K.E. Tierney (✉)
Division of Gynecologic Oncology, Department of Obstetrics and Gynecology, Kaiser Permanente Orange County, California, Irvine, CA, USA
e-mail: Katherine.E.Tierney@kp.org; tierney.katherine@gmail.com

L.D. Roman (✉) • K. Matsuo (✉)
Division of Gynecologic Oncology, Department of Obstetrics and Gynecology, University of Southern California, Los Angeles, CA, USA
e-mail: Lroman@med.usc.edu; Koji.matsuo@med.usc.edu

© Springer International Publishing AG 2017
D. Shoupe (ed.), *Handbook of Gynecology*,
DOI 10.1007/978-3-319-17798-4_7

1   Introduction

Since the 1940s, the Pap smear has provided practitioners an opportunity to diagnose cervical dysplasia and prevent cancer development. From 1973 to 2007, invasive cervical cancer incidence declined by 54% in the United States (Adegoke et al. 2012). Furthermore, coordinated testing for human papillomavirus (HPV) has enabled healthcare providers the ability to appropriately triage patients based on risk. HPV infection is common and does not always cause cervical dysplasia; however, recognition and early intervention of high-risk HPV-related changes may prevent progression to cancer. In addition, early administration of vaccines against certain types of high-risk HPV could diminish the number of people diagnosed with cervical cancer precursors (Baldur-Felskov et al. 2014).

In the United States, there are an estimated two million abnormal cytology tests each year (Insinga et al. 2004). Among these women, 175,000 cervical intraepithelial neoplasia (CIN) 1 and 225,000 CIN 2/CIN 3 diagnoses are made. Progression from CIN to invasive cervical cancer is a slow process taking between 8.1 and 12.6 years for CIN 3 to progress to invasive cancer (ACOG Bulletin #140, December 2013). Despite advancements in the diagnosis and treatment of cervical dysplasia, cervical cancer continues to claim more than 4,000 lives each year in the United States http://seer.cancer.gov/statfacts/html/cervix.html. The body of knowledge on HPV, cervical dysplasia, and cervical cancer continues to grow bringing potential to decrease the number of deaths from cervical cancer each year.

The focus of this chapter is to provide readers with the most pertinent information on cervical dysplasia and, in turn, enable them to impart accurate and helpful information on their patients.

2   Cervical Cytology

Cervical cytology refers to cells that are obtained from the surface of the cervix and ideally include cells from the transformation zone of the cervix. Using a spatula and/or brush, cellular material from the cervix can be either spread and fixed directly onto a slide or transferred into a fixative liquid. In detecting precancerous lesions, the conventional Pap test using a slide- and liquid-based cytology proves to be equally sensitive and specific (Arbyn et al. 2008). Overall, sensitivity and specificity for cytologic testing for cervical dysplasia are about 60% and 70%, respectively (Nanda et al. 2000).

In an effort to standardize diagnosis and treatment, Bethesda 2001 developed terminology in the evaluation of cervical cytology. Management guidelines are based on these interpretations. The following information is adapted from the 2001 Bethesda system (Solomon et al. 2002). For any given cytologic sample, pathologists provide information on **specimen adequacy** and give an **interpretation/result**. Adequacy refers to whether the specimen is satisfactory for evaluation or unsatisfactory for evaluation. Interpretation can either reflect that the specimen is "negative for intraepithelial lesion or malignancy" or specify a type of epithelial cell abnormality. The most common cytologic abnormality is "atypical squamous cells" (ASC). Women with ASC have a 10–20% risk of underlying CIN 2–3 and 1 in 1000 risk of invasive cancer. The category is further subdivided between "atypical squamous cells of undetermined significance" (ASC-US) and "cannot exclude HSIL" (ASC-H) (Solomon et al. 2002).

Squamous intraepithelial lesions are categorized in a two-tier system. Low-grade squamous intraepithelial lesions (LSIL) refer to mild dysplastic or HPV-related changes and frequently correspond to a histologic diagnosis of CIN 1. High-grade squamous intraepithelial lesions (HSIL) refer to moderate and severe dysplasia and typically correspond to a histologic diagnosis of CIN 2 or CIN 3. Squamous cell carcinoma can be detected by cytology; however, confirmation should be pursued with a biopsy for histologic diagnosis (Solomon et al. 2002).

Atypical glandular cells (AGC) refer to a glandular abnormality that could be arising from the cervix, endocervix, or endometrium. This diagnosis reflects a high-grade abnormality in 10–39% of cases. "Atypical glandular cells, favor neoplastic," endocervical adenocarcinoma in situ (ACIS), and adenocarcinoma are other examples of diagnoses included in this standard terminology (Solomon et al. 2002).

According to the American College of Obstetricians and Gynecologists (ACOG), cervical cancer screening with cervical cytology should being at age 21 regardless of age at coitarche. Between the ages of 21 and 29, cytology testing alone can be done every 3 years. After age 30, cytology alone every 3 years or combined cytology and HPV cotesting every 5 years can be recommended. In the absence of a history of abnormal cytology, screening can stop at age 65. If a patient undergoes hysterectomy for a benign gynecologic indication without history of cervical dysplasia, cervical cancer screening can be stopped after hysterectomy.

3   Human Papillomavirus

Papillomaviruses are a double-stranded, circular DNA genome virus with more than 100 different described subtypes. The viral DNA is divided into three regions: upstream regulatory region, early region, and late region. The early region of the genome includes six open reading frames, and, of these, E6 and E7 are required for the development of invasive cervical cancer. The E7 protein binds to the tumor suppressor retinoblastoma (Rb) gene blocking suppression and allowing cell proliferation. The E6 protein binds and degrades tumor suppressor P53 resulting in blockage of apoptosis and increased cell proliferation (Wright 2009). HPV types 16 and 18 are present in 70% of diagnosed squamous cell carcinomas and over 80% of adenocarcinomas (de Sanjose et al. 2010).

Persistent HPV is essential for the development of cervical cancer precursors and invasive cancer. When compared to cytology, high-risk HPV testing has proven to have higher sensitivity and reproducibility but less specificity (ACOG Bulletin #140, December 2013). At this time, HPV panels only detect a finite number of high-risk HPV types. Not all tests specify the exact HPV type that is positive in the panel, i.e., genotype. According to the College of American

Pathologists, the most common indication for HPV testing remains reflex testing after ASC-US cytology; however, laboratories are reporting a general increase in the rate of cotesting (Zhao et al. 2015).

Transmission of HPV occurs via sexual exposure. Breaks in the skin and mucosal surfaces are susceptible to infection with the cervix being the most common site of transmission. Although condom use is still recommended for protection against HPV, external genitalia are susceptible to microtrauma and infection; thus, condom use is less protective than it is against other sexually transmitted infections. Vertical transmission from mother to infant is possible; however, the neonate can clear the vast majority of these infections within the first year of life (Erickson et al. 2013).

Overall prevalence of high-risk HPV is reported to be between 12% and 15% (Wright et al. 2012). The prevalence of HPV is highest in women 21–24 years old with a second spike occurring after menopause (Wright et al. 2012; Erickson et al. 2013). Most HPV infections will clear spontaneously; however, some infections will persist and cause cellular changes. Young women are more likely to clear HPV than older women. The clearance rate within 1 year of infection ranges from 40% to 70% and can reach a 2–5-year clearance rate of 100% in young women (Erickson et al. 2013). Certain types of HPV are more virulent and are more likely to be persistent than other types. HPV 16 and HPV 18 are the most common HPV subtypes found in carcinoma of the cervix and found to be the most persistent (Wheeler 2013). HPV types considered to be oncogenic include 16, 18, 31, 33, 35, 39, 45, 51, 52, 56, 58, and 59 (Erickson et al. 2013).

3.1   Risk Factors

Risk factors for the development of dysplasia and invasive cervical cancer are interlinked with HPV infection and clinical conditions that make patients more susceptible to infection with HPV. Risk factors associated with HPV infection in women include number of lifetime male sexual partners, early-onset sexual activity, coinfection with other sexually transmitted diseases, and current smoking (Erickson et al. 2013). Since HPV activity is dependent on the host immune system, immunosuppressed patients infected with HPV are at increased risk of developing cervical dysplasia and invasive cervical cancer. Immunosuppressed patients include patients with HIV, autoimmune disease, those who are status post organ transplant, and others who require chronic immunosuppressive therapies. These patients are recommended to have more frequent screening evaluation. Current recommendations are to screen these patients every 6 months for the first year after diagnosis of immunocompromised status followed by annual screening (Nguyen and Flowers 2013).

---

4   Management of Abnormal Screening Tests

The following management guidelines are based on the findings in the 2006 consensus guidelines for the management of women with abnormal cervical cancer screening tests and the ACOG Practice Bulletin on the management of abnormal cervical cancer screening test results and cervical cancer precursors (Wright 2007; ACOG Bulletin #140, December 2013; ASCCP guidelines). Most abnormal cytology results will require further evaluation of the cervix with **colposcopy**. The following are examples of abnormal results that do not require immediate colposcopy:

- For a woman older than 30 years of age with negative cervical cytology and her **first positive HPV** test, the ASCCP recommendation is to repeat cotesting in 1 year and proceed with colposcopy if cytology is abnormal or HPV remains positive at 1-year follow-up.
- For women with **ASC-US cytology and a negative HPV test**, ACOG recommends repeat cytology with HPV testing in 3 years.
- For women between the ages of **21 and 24 with ASC-US or LSIL**, HPV testing can be done. The patient should have repeat cytology 1 year after the test if positive and

repeat cytology in 3 years if the test is negative.
- Unsatisfactory cytology with negative or unknown HPV results can be repeated in 2–4 months. Two consecutive unsatisfactory cytology results warrant evaluation with colposcopy.

Algorithms for the management of specific screening test results are available at the ASCCP website (http://www.asccp.org/Guidelines) and can also be downloaded as an application for mobile devices.

4.1   Colposcopy

Colposcopy is microscopic examination of the cervix under low power magnification after application of acetic acid. The goal of this procedure is to visually detect any cervical changes suspicious for precancerous transformation. The procedure consists of a speculum exam during which gauze is soaked with 3–5% acetic acid and placed directly on the cervix for approximately 30 s to 1 min. After exposure to acetic acid, a reversible reaction occurs causing the abnormal cells to swell and turn white due to hyperchromatin within the nucleus of the dysplastic cells.

Identification of acetowhite epithelium (AWE) allows for directed biopsies of suspicious lesions. The transformation zone is identified, and a small cotton-tipped swab can be used to manipulate the cervical canal and identify whether the AWE extends into the canal. An endocervical speculum can be used for this part of the procedure. Other abnormal features to note include punctation, mosaic patterns that suggest underlying high-grade dysplasia, and abnormal neovascularization that could be an indication of possible invasive cancer.

In addition to the cervix, the upper vagina should be examined. Directed biopsies are performed with a sharp cervical biopsy device. A sharper device will lead to less manipulation and stretch of the cervical fibers and diminish pain. Bleeding is a risk of this procedure. Silver nitrate and Monsel solution can be used to hamper bleeding; however, spotting and brown discharge are common after biopsies. Excellent photographs and additional descriptions of colposcopic findings can be found in text by Baggish (2003).

Even if colposcopic examination is negative for any abnormal findings, a single random biopsy can increase detection of high-grade disease in high-risk HPV-positive patients (Huh et al. 2014). It remains unclear why some lesions are not visible colposcopically and whether this reflects a difference in the biological or clinical nature of non-visible lesions as compared with visible lesions. Ultimately, studies show that colposcopy has similar sensitivity and specificity when compared to cervical cytology in detecting high-grade lesions. Women with limited access to screening cytology in under-resourced countries that cannot afford to implement routine HPV testing may benefit from immediate colposcopic examination. The limitation of "see-and-treat" methodology remains the possibility of overtreating (Nooh et al. 2015).

5 Types of Cervical Dysplasia

5.1 Cervical Intraepithelial Neoplasia

Cervical intraepithelial neoplasia (CIN) is a term used to describe a continuum of dysplastic changes in cervical intraepithelial tissue. These changes are precursors to cervical cancer development. The continuum consists of mild, moderate, and severe cellular changes referred to as CIN 1, 2, and 3, respectively. A histopathologic diagnosis of CIN depends on the level of nuclear abnormality, mitotic activity, and level of differentiation (Robboy et al. 2002).

In **CIN 1**, extensive differentiation can be seen in the upper two-thirds of the cervical epithelium. There is minimal amount of nuclear atypia and few, if any, mitotic figures that are located in the **basal third** of the epithelium (Robboy et al. 2002). CIN 1 has a high rate of regression and can be managed conservatively with repeat

cytology and HPV testing 12 months after initial diagnosis. Patients should be counseled that this lesion usually represents a transient HPV infection and has very low premalignant potential. Over a period of 2 years, the risk of progression of CIN 1 to CIN 2 was 13%, and the risk of progression of CIN 1 to CIN 3 was 8.9% (ALTS 2003). If a patient has persistent CIN 1 for over 2 years, observation or excision is acceptable. Excision is recommended if the transformation zone cannot adequately be evaluated on colposcopy. In addition, if CIN 1 was found on endocervical curettage (ECC) at the time of colposcopy, ECC should be performed with the subsequent cytologic sampling (ACOG Bulletin #140, December 2013).

In **CIN 2**, mitotic figures are located in the **basal two-thirds** of the epithelium, differentiation can be seen in the upper half of the epithelium, and the nuclei are more atypical and larger than in CIN 1 (Robboy et al. 2002). Although CIN 2 can regress, patients should be counseled that 35% persist and 22% progress to CIN 3 (ACOG Bulletin #140, December 2013). Except in special populations, patients with CIN 2 are offered excision in an effort to prevent progression to CIN 3 and, ultimately, invasive cancer. In young age women, either close observation or ablation of the lesion can be considered.

In **CIN 3**, nuclear abnormalities and mitotic figures populate the **entire thickness** of the epithelium. The nuclei can occupy almost the entire cell and are bizarre in shape. Data on the natural history of CIN 3 revealed that 56% persist and 14% progress to invasive cancer (ACOG Bulletin #140, December 2013). The term carcinoma in situ (CIS) was included in prior terminology; however, this diagnosis is no longer used. Rather, that which was labeled as CIS is now considered CIN 3. Excisional biopsy is the preferred management for CIN 3.

5.2 Adenocarcinoma In Situ

Adenocarcinoma in situ (ACIS) describes a precursor lesion to invasive adenocarcinoma of the cervix. Pathologists describe ACIS as replacement of endocervical glandular cells with tall

Table 1 Recommendations for follow-up after cone biopsy for cervical dysplasia

Cone (LEEP or CKC)	Internal margin	ECC	Desiring future fertility	Risk of residual dysplasia	Risk of microinvasion	Risk of frank invasion	Follow-Up
CIN 3	neg	neg	n/a	18%	0%	0%	Cotesting in 1 year
CIN 3	neg	CIN 3	Yes	40%	0%	0%	4–6-month cotesting with ECC
CIN 3	neg	CIN 3	No	40%	0%	0%	4–6-month cotesting with ECC
CIN 3	CIN 3	neg	Yes	30%	0%	0%	4–6-month cotesting with ECC
CIN 3	CIN 3	neg	No	30%	0%	0%	4–6-month cotesting with ECC
CIN 3	CIN 3	CIN 3	Yes	44%	19%	11%	4–6-month cotesting with ECC preferred; repeat CKC acceptable
CIN 3	CIN 3	CIN 3	<50, neg FF	22–44%	Up to 17%	0%	4–6-month cotesting with ECC preferred; repeat CKC acceptable
CIN 3	CIN 3	CIN 3	>50/ postmenopausal	46%	9%	18%	CKC - > clear margins = follow as above; CKC - > positive margins/ ECC - > hyst v. MRH
ACIS	neg	neg	Yes	14%	0%	0%	6-month cotesting; recommend completion hyst after childbearing
ACIS	neg	neg	No	14%	0%	0%	Hyst
ACIS	+	neg	No	40%	7%	0%	CKC – > Hyst
ACIS	neg	+	No	80%	20%	0%	CKC – > Hyst
ACIS	+	+	No	77%	15%	0%	CKC – > Hyst
ACIS	Either +/−	Either +/−	Yes	59%	13%	0%	CKC until margins negative; recommend completion hyst after childbearing

columnar cells with nuclear atypia and elevated mitotic activity. Less prevalent than CIN, the management of ACIS has proven to be a challenge. Estimates for the risk of underlying malignancy can be up to 17%. After biopsy diagnosis, all patients should have a cone biopsy to exclude the diagnosis of underlying cancer. Standard treatment for ACIS is hysterectomy; however, fertility-sparing measures can be taken in special circumstances (Tierney et al. 2014). See *Special Considerations* for information of fertility preservation.

5.3 Management of Dysplasia

In managing a diagnosis of cervical dysplasia, the simple objectives are to prevent progression to invasive cervical cancer and to exclude the presence of concurrent carcinoma. Management decisions can only be made after thorough review of cytologic and colposcopic findings.

5.3.1 Observation

As previously mentioned, CIN 1 can safely be monitored without excision. Given the high likelihood of regression, ACOG recommends repeat cotesting 1 year from the diagnosis. For CIN 2, the risk of progression must be weighed against the risk to future pregnancies. Observation is preferred in women ages 21–24 and "young women." A "young woman" is considered someone in whom the risks to future pregnancies outweigh the risk of disease progression. Conservative management using serial cytologic sampling, HPV testing, and colposcopy at regular intervals appears to be appropriate in this population. Recommendations are for repeat exams every 6 months for at least the first year (ACOG Bulletin #140, December 2013).

5.3.2 Ablation

Ablative procedures for the treatment of cervical dysplasia include cryosurgery, CO_2 laser vaporization, and electrocoagulation. The primary benefits of these procedures are that they are cost-effective and simple. These methods are not commonly utilized secondary to their obvious disadvantages. Ablative procedures do not predictably destroy tissue and they do not provide a specimen. Therefore, diagnosis of an underlying cancer could be inadvertently overlooked (Morrow and Sideri 2013; Baggish 2003). Cryo for CIN 2 with follow-up is an acceptable option for women of reproductive age who desire future fertility.

5.3.3 Excision

The objective of an excisional procedure is to treat the existing precancerous lesion and, if present, diagnose any underlying microinvasive disease. If a cone is not feasible secondary to distorted anatomy, one may proceed with a hysterectomy. The patient must be informed of the risk of invasive cancer that may result in postoperative adjuvant therapy or additional surgery.

The specimen should be evaluable for the presence or absence of dysplasia at the margins (endocervical and ectocervical). Post-excisional endocervical curettage (ECC) should be performed routinely. Information on the margin status and ECC has been shown to predict the presence of residual disease for both squamous and glandular lesions (Kobak et al. 1996; Tierney et al. 2014). Positive endocervical margins and

positive ECC are more concerning than a positive ectocervical margin. Ectocervical lesions are more easily detected on Pap smear and colposcopy.

Follow-up recommendations are summarized in Table 1 (ACOG Bulletin #140, December 2013; Kobak et al. 1996; Tierney et al. 2014).

Following cone biopsy for CIN 3, ACOG recommends repeat cotesting in 1 year for those with negative margins and ECC. For those with positive margins and/or ECC, ACOG recommends closer follow-up with repeat cotesting in 4–6 months and repeat ECC at the time of cotesting. Providers and patients must understand that, although most who have positive margins and/or ECC will not have recurrent or persist cervical dysplasia, those with both positive margins and positive ECC are at the highest risk of recurrence/persistence. Some patients will find that the risk is unacceptable and will be more comfortable with a follow-up procedure such as a repeat cone.

Age should be considered when counseling patients on risk of persistent cervical dysplasia and invasive cervical cancer. Data suggests that women over 50 years of age (or postmenopausal women) who have a positive endocervical cone margin and a positive ECC have a 9–18% risk of having invasive cervical cancer. These women should have a repeat excisional procedure. If the margins and ECC are negative on the second conization, follow-up with cotesting and an ECC in 4–6 months is reasonable. If margins and/or ECC are positive on the second conization, recommendations are for repeat conization. If repeat conization is not feasible secondary to anatomy, the patient must be counseled on risk of concurrent cancer and consider a modified radical hysterectomy versus a simple hysterectomy (Kobak et al. 1996).

The following text will describe both cold-knife cone (CKC) and loop electrosurgical excision procedure (LEEP) as methods of excision. These methods have been found to be equivalent in treating dysplasia (Huang and Hwang 1999). An important risk of excisional procedures is the risk to future pregnancies. Women who undergo these procedures are at an increased risk of having cervical stenosis, cervical shortening, and preterm birth. Studies show about a 30% increased incidence of preterm birth in patients who have undergone an excisional procedure (Frey and Conner 2015).

Cold-knife cone (**CKC**), otherwise known as scalpel cone or sharp conization, is removal of a cone-shaped piece of tissue from the cervix. The specimen includes the transformation zone and a segment of the endocervical canal. The cone is typically 1.5–2.5 cm in height. The procedure is performed under anesthesia in the operating room. After colposcopy and/or Lugol application, the surgeon can determine the size and shape of the cone based on the extent of dysplasia. A sound should be used to determine the cervical length and direction of the canal. After traction sutures are placed and vasopressin is injected intracervically in select cases, a #15 or #11 blade is pushed into the cervical stroma at an angle that points toward the cervical canal. A single-tooth tenaculum can be applied to 12 and 6 o'clock to stabilize the cervix. An Allis clamp can be used to gently manipulate the specimen without losing orientation. After removal of the specimen from the cervix, suture is used to mark the 12 o'clock location to orient the specimen. An endocervical curettage follows the removal of the cone biopsy using a Kevorkian curette and endocervical cytobrush. Bleeding from the cone bed can usually be controlled with cautery. Monsel solution, Surgicel packing, and various suturing techniques can also be utilized (Morrow and Sideri 2013). The advantage of CKC is lack of thermal artifact allowing the pathologist to confidently comment on margin status. The disadvantage is that it requires anesthesia and an operating room to complete with possible increased risk of bleeding.

When compared with CKC, the **LEEP** procedure also provides a specimen for pathologic examination; however, it is an in-office procedure that is simple and inexpensive. In the office, the procedure is performed using local anesthetic with 1–2% lidocaine injected directly into the cervical stroma. Colposcopy with acetic acid application is performed followed by Lugol application if indicated. The appropriate loop electrode is selected based on the size of the lesion. Power is set at between 40 and 50 W using a blend of cutting and coagulation current. The loop is passed through the cervical stroma at a steady rate, careful to avoid both bleeding and thermal effect to the specimen. Endocervical curettage is performed after the specimen is obtained. Hemostasis can be achieved with the rollerball and Monsel solution (Morrow and Sideri 2013).

5.3.4   Pharmacological Agents

The utility of topical agents in the treatment of cervical dysplasia is under investigation. Both 5-flourouracil (5-FU) and imiquimod have been used as agents to treat vulvar dysplasia and are being considered in the treatment of cervical precancerous lesions. 5-FU is an antimetabolite that inhibits thymidylate synthase causing cell death. In young women, 5-FU used to treat CIN 2 was shown to cause regression in 93% of patients as compared to 56% regression among those who were observed. This data came from a randomized controlled trial of two groups (treatment with 5-FU versus observation) over a 6-month treatment period during which there were no reported moderate to severe side effects (Rahangdale et al. 2014). More common side effects include pain, burning, and dermatitis. Suggested treatment dosing is 2 g via transvaginal applicator every 2 weeks for a total of 8 doses. The use of 5-FU in this setting is considered off-label and should only be considered in young patients attempting to conserve fertility with informed consent.

The topical immune-response modulator imiquimod is another agent that could to be efficacious in treating cervical dysplasia. Imiquimod activates the innate immune system via a toll-like receptor (TLR-7) and recruits macrophages, natural killer cells, and B-lymphocytes to the treated site. In the treatment of CIN 2–3, remission rates in patients treated with imiquimod were higher when compared with those observed over time; 73% of those treated with imiquimod regressed while only 39% of those treated with placebo regressed (Grimm et al. 2012). Common side effects of imiquimod include mild pruritus, pain, and a systemic "flu-like" reaction. Long-term and larger studies are needed to determine the ideal therapeutic application of these agents. With more investigation, topical agents could prove to be a reasonable alternative to excisional biopsy in those who plan to reduce risk of preterm birth in future pregnancies.

5.3.5 Hysterectomy

Hysterectomy is not a standard treatment as primary therapy for CIN 2 or CIN 3 (ACOG Bulletin #140, December 2013). After diagnosis of recurrent disease, repeat excisional biopsy is preferred to exclude the presence of invasive cancer. Indications for hysterectomy include:

- Recurrent disease after evaluation with repeat excisional procedure
- Situations in which a repeat excisional procedure is not feasible due to distorted anatomy, i.e., minimal residual cervix or a flush cervix

For a diagnosis of ACIS, hysterectomy is standard of care in women who have completed childbearing. However, excisional biopsy needs to be preformed prior to hysterectomy to rule out concurrent invasive cancer.

5.4 Special Considerations

5.4.1 Dysplasia in Pregnancy

For women with dysplasia diagnosed during pregnancy, most dysplasia will regress, and evolution to cancer is extremely rare (Fader et al. 2010). Evidence-based guidelines for management of cervical dysplasia in pregnancy suggest cervical biopsies should only be performed if frank cancer is suspected on colposcopy. Repeat colposcopy at 6 weeks postpartum is recommended. If a biopsy is performed with a result of CIN 2 or CIN 3, colposcopy no sooner than every 12 weeks can be performed. A biopsy should only be done if the lesion appears to worsen (ACOG Bulletin #140, December 2013).

5.4.2 Fertility-Sparing and ACIS

For those who desire to maintain future fertility, patients with a diagnosis of ACIS should have a cone biopsy to exclude the diagnosis of underlying cancer. If cone margins or ECC is positive for ACIS, repeat cone can be performed in these patients. If both margins and ECC are negative,

data show that no patients had underlying cancer and about 14% had residual ACIS. Patients should be closely monitored with cotesting every 6 months (Tierney et al. 2014).

5.5 Human Papillomavirus Prevention

Vaccination against HPV has demonstrated efficacy in preventing development of cervical dysplasia. Additionally, therapeutic vaccines have emerged and may change the future treatment landscape for cervical dysplasia. HPV has two capsid proteins (L1 and L2), and the HPV vaccine is made with recombinant L1 protein (a virus-like particle) to target the L1 capsid protein (Erickson et al. 2013). Currently, there are three FDA-approved HPV vaccines available in the United States. Available vaccines include a bivalent vaccine targeting HPV 16 and HPV 18 (Cervarix by GlaxoSmithKline, Brentford, United Kingdom), quadrivalent (Gardasil by Merck & Co Inc., Kenilworth, NJ, USA), and 9-valent (9vHPV by Merck & Co Inc., Kenilworth, NI, USA) types.

The quadrivalent vaccine Gardasil protects against two high-risk types of HPV (16 and 18) and two low-risk types of HPV commonly seen in patients with genital warts (6 and 11). Administration is indicated to prevent HPV-related genital warts and precancerous and cancerous lesions in women and men for ages 9 through 26 years www.merckvaccines.com/products/gardisil. HPV vaccines have the secondary benefit of protection against all HPV-related cancers including some head and neck cancers and anal and penile cancer. In those who have been vaccinated, there is a 60% risk reduction for atypia, and the risk of CIN 2/CIN3 and CIN 3 is reduced up to 80% (Baldur-Felskov et al. 2014). Women vaccinated at an older age have been shown to have less of a risk reduction presumably because they have previously been exposed to HPV 16/HPV 18. Recommendations are to advocate for vaccination before sexual activity (Baldur-Felskov et al. 2014; Mahmud et al. 2014). However, current recommendations are to vaccinate all people between the ages of 9 and 26 regardless of sexual history or history of diagnosed cervical dysplasia. Indications for HPV vaccination in women older than 26 need to be developed in the future.

The 9-valent HPV (9vHPV) vaccine builds immunity against HPV types 6, 11, 16, 18, 31, 33, 45, 52, and 58. The efficacy against types 6, 11, 16, and 18 has been shown to be equivalent to the quadrivalent vaccine. 9vHPV has been shown to prevent disease associated with the HPV types covered by the vaccine (Joura et al. 2015).

For those who have been vaccinated, screening recommendations do not change (ACOG Bulletin #140, December 2013). Long-term follow-up is needed to see the effect these vaccines have on cervical and vulvar cancer prevalence as well as other HPV-related cancers such as head and neck and anal and penile cancer prevalence.

The use of therapeutic vaccinations in the treatment of infection-mediated precancerous and cancerous lesions is under investigation. For those patients with high-grade dysplasia, the efficacy of the available vaccines proves to be low (Mahmud et al. 2014). A therapeutic vaccine elicits an adaptive immune response against the lesion. A recent phase 2 trial shows promising results for a therapeutic vaccine, VGX-3100 (Inovio Pharmaceuticals, Inc, Plymouth Meeting, PA, USA), against cervical dysplasia (CIN 2/3). These findings lend hope for a nonsurgical treatment of cervical dysplasia (Trimble et al. 2015).

6　Conclusion

In conclusion, cervical cancer screening with cytology and HPV testing has decreased the overall incidence of cervical cancer over the last century. The standardization of dysplasia management has been facilitated by easily accessible ASCCP guidelines. Treatment of cervical dysplasia has remained relatively consistent; however, given the high rate of regression in certain populations, more conservative management has been recommended in younger patients and pregnant patients. Ultimately, ACOG and ASCCP give guidelines for the management of dysplasia;

however, care should still be individualized. Recommendations are based on "acceptable risk" meaning that negative screening does not guarantee the absence of an abnormality. Worrisome findings may warrant close follow-up and more frequent exams. Informed consent is key. Patients need to know the pathophysiology of HPV-related disease, risk of disease progression, and risks of invasive intervention. There are few preventative interventions for patients once they are diagnosed with HPV. Gynecologic and pediatric care providers should take every opportunity to discuss risk reduction and the benefits of HPV vaccination.

References

ACOG. Practice Bulletin Number 140: management of abnormal cervical cancer screening test results and cervical cancer precursors. Obstet Gynecol. 2013;122 (6):1338–67.

ASCUS-LSIL Triage Study (ALTS) Group. Results of a randomized trial on the management of cytology interpretations of atypical squamous cells of undetermined significance. Am J Obstet Gynecol. 2003;90:366–371.

Adegoke O, Kulasingam S, Virnig B. Cervical cancer trends in the United States: a 35-year population based analysis. J Women's Health. 2012; 21(10):1031–7.

Arbyn M, Bergeron C, et al. Liquid compared with conventional cervical cytology: a systemic review and meta-analysis. Obstet Gynecol. 2008;111(1):167–77.

ASCCP: http://www.asccp.org/Guidelines

Baggish MS. Colposcopy of the cervix, vagina and vulva: a comprehensive textbook. Philadelphia: Mosby; 2003. p. 79–97.

Baldur-Felskov B, Dehlendorff C, Munk C, Kjaer SK. Early impact of human papillomavirus vaccination on cervical neoplasia: nationwide follow-up of Young Danish women. JNCI J Natl Cancer Inst. 2014;106(3): djt460.

de Sanjose S, Quint WG, Alemany L, et al. Human papillomavirus genotype attribution in invasive cervical cancer: a retrospective cross-sectional worldwide study. Lancet Oncol. 2010;11:1048–56.

Erickson BK, Alvarez RD, Huh WK. Human papillomavirus: what every provider should know. Am J Obstet Gynecol. 2013;208(3):169–75.

Fader AN, Alward EK, Niederhauser A, et al. Cervical dysplasia in pregnancy: a multi-institutional evaluation. Am J Obstet Gynecol. 2010;203:113.e1–6.

Frey HA, Conner SN. Treatment of cervical dysplasia and the risk of preterm birth: understanding the association. Am J Obstet Gynecol. 2015;213(4):445–6.

Grimm C, Polterauer S, Natter C, et al. Treatment of cervical intraepithelial neoplasia with topical imiquimod: a randomized controlled trial. Obstet Gynecol. 2012;120:152–9.

Huang LW, Hwang JL. A comparison between loop electrosurgical excision procedure and cold knife conization for treatment of cervical dysplasia: residual disease in a subsequent hysterectomy specimen. Gynecol Oncol. 1999;73(1):12–5.

Huh W, Sideri M, et al. Relevance of random biopsy at the transformation zone when colposcopy is negative. Obstet Gynecol. 2014;124(4):670–8.

Insinga RP, Glass AG, Rush BB. Diagnoses and outcomes in cervical cancer screening: a population-based study. Am J Obstet Gynecol. 2004;191:105–13.

Joura EA, Giuliano AR, Iversen OE, et al. A 9-valent HPV vaccine against infection and intraepithelial neoplasia in women. N Engl J Med. 2015;372:711–23.

Kobak WH, Roman LD, et al. The role of endocervical curettage at cervical conization for high-grade dysplasia. Obstet Gynecol. 1996;85:197–201.

Mahmud SM, Kliewer EV, Lambert P, Bozat-Emre S, Demers AA. Effectiveness of the quadrivalent human papillomavirus vaccine against cervical dysplasia in Manitoba, Canada. J Clin Oncol. 2014;32:438–43.

Merck: www.merckvaccines.com/products/gardasil

Morrow CP, Sideri M. Surgery for cervical neoplasia. In: Gynecologic cancer surgery. Encinitas: South Coast Medical Publishing; 2013. p. 513–33.

Nanda K, McCrory DC, et al. Accuracy of the papanicolaou test in screening for and follow-up of cervical cytologic abnormalities: a systemic review. Ann Intern Med. 2000;132:810–9.

Nguyen ML, Flowers L. Cervical cancer screening in immunocompromised women. Obstet Gynecol Clin N Am. 2013;40(2):339–57.

Nooh AM, Mohamed ME, El-Alfy Y. Visual inspection of cervix with acetic acid as a screening modality for cervical cancer. J Low Genit Tract Dis. 2015;19:340–4.

Rahangdale L, Lippmann OK, Garcia K, et al. Topical 5-fluorouracil for treatment of cervical intraepithelial neoplasia 2: a randomized controlled trial. Am J Obstet Gynecol. 2014;210:314.e1–8.

Robboy SJ, Anderson MC, Russel P. Pathology of the female reproductive tract. Philadelphia: Churchill Livingstone; 2002. p. 165–93.

Seer database: http://seer.cancer.gov/statfacts/html/cervix.html

Solomon D, Darvy D, Kurman R, et al. The 2001 Bethesda system: terminology for reporting results of cervical cytology. JAMA. 2002;287:2114–9.

Tierney KE, Lin PS, Amezcua C, et al. Cervical conization of adenocarcinoma in situ: a predicting model of residual disease. Am J Obstet Gynecol. 2014;210:366.e1–5.

Trimble CL, Morrow MP, Kraynyak KA, et al. Safety, efficacy, and immunogenicity of VGX-3100, a therapeutic synthetic DNA vaccine targeting human papillomavirus 16 and 18 E6 and E7 proteins for cervical intraepithelial neoplasia 2/3: a randomized, double-blind, placebo-controlled phase 2b trial. Lancet. 2015;386:2078. Published online.

Wheeler CM. The natural history of cervical human papillomavirus infection and cervical cancer: gaps in knowledge and future horizons. Obstet Gynecol Clin N Am. 2013;40:165–76.

Wright TC Jr, Massad LS, et al. 2006 consensus guidelines for the management of women with abnormal cervical screening tests. J Low Genit Tract Dis. 2007;11(4):201–22.

Wright TC. Pathogenesis and diagnosis of preinvasive lesions of the lower genital tract. In: Principles and practice of gynecologic oncology. Philadelphia: Lippincott/Williams and Wilkins; 2009.

Wright TC, Stoler MH, et al. The ATHENA human papillomavirus study: design, methods, and baseline results. Am J Obstet Gynecol. 2012;206:46.e8–11.

Zhao C, et al. Human papillomavirus testing and reporting rates in 2012: results of a College of American Pathologists National Survey. Arch Pathol Lab Med. 2015;139:756–61.

Endometrial Hyperplasia

Kristina Williams and Emily Ko

Abstract

Endometrial hyperplasia (EH), a known precursor to endometrial adenocarcinoma, is a common gynecologic diagnosis among women, typically resulting from an increase in endogenous or exogenous unopposed estrogen. EH is a histologic diagnosis that is characterized by one of the two classification schemas: either the widely used WHO94 criteria or the more standardized endometrial intraepithelial neoplasia (EIN) criteria. The risk of progression to cancer varies and depends on the severity of the lesion. Lesions with atypia have the highest risk of progression to cancer and the diagnosis of concurrent endometrial cancer. EH mainly effects perimenopausal or postmenopausal women. Significant risk factors for EH include obesity, chronic anovulation as seen in disorders such as PCOS, estrogen only hormone replacement, tamoxifen use, and Lynch syndrome. Clinical manifestations include abnormal uterine bleeding, postmenopausal bleeding, or atypical endometrial glands on pap smear, which require a diagnostic workup in peri-/postmenopausal women. Transvaginal ultrasound (TVUS) is typically the first diagnostic study to be performed in a woman with abnormal uterine bleeding (AUB). Either office endometrial biopsy (EMB) or dilation and curettage (D&C) with or without hysteroscopy can be performed to diagnose EH. When EH is diagnosed, management includes surveillance, hormone therapy, or hysterectomy and choice of therapy depends on the type of EH, potential risk for endometrial cancer, and patient characteristics (i.e., desire to maintain fertility and surgical candidacy). There are no current recommendations for screening for endometrial hyperplasia in the general population.

Keywords

Endometrial hyperplasia • Endometrial intraepithelial neoplasia • Abnormal uterine bleeding • Postmenopausal bleeding • Unopposed estrogen • Endometrial cancer

Contents

K. Williams (✉)
Department of Obstetrics and Gynecology, Pennsylvania Hospital, Philadelphia, PA, USA
e-mail: Kristina.williams@uphs.upenn.edu

E. Ko
Division of Gynecologic Oncology, University of Pennsylvania Health System, Philadelphia, PA, USA
e-mail: Emily.ko@uphs.upenn.edu

© Springer International Publishing AG 2017
D. Shoupe (ed.), *Handbook of Gynecology*,
DOI 10.1007/978-3-319-17798-4_3

1   Introduction

Endometrial hyperplasia is a common condition defined histologically as an abnormal overgrowth of endometrial glands contained within the uterus. Clinically, it is important to recognize this condition as a precursor and marker for endometrial adenocarcinoma, the most common gynecologic cancer among American women (ACOG 2015; Armstrong et al. 2012; Trimble et al. 2012).

Normal endometrium changes throughout the menstrual cycle in response to estrogen and progesterone. Estrogen causes the endometrial lining to thicken by proliferation. After ovulation, the corpus luteum produces progesterone. If pregnancy is to occur, progesterone stabilizes the endometrium by inhibiting proliferation and stimulating differentiation. If pregnancy does not occur, progesterone production decreases and allows for shedding of the endometrial lining (Trimble et al. 2012).

Typically, in endometrial hyperplasia, unopposed estrogen (i.e., a lack of progesterone) causes the endometrial glands to proliferate such that there is an increase in gland to stroma ratio. Thus, endometrial hyperplasia affects those women that have intermittent or absence of ovulation (i.e., PCOS) or those women that have higher levels of circulating estrogens postmenopausally (i.e., HRT, obesity). The most common clinical manifestation of hyperplasia is abnormal uterine bleeding, which always requires diagnostic evaluation in a perimenopausal or postmenopausal woman. The mainstay of management of hyperplasia is the detection or prevention of endometrial cancer. This chapter will discuss the classification, epidemiology and risk factors, diagnosis, and management of endometrial hyperplasia.

2   Histology and Classification

The classification of endometrial hyperplasia is based on histology. There are currently two diagnostic classification systems used to categorize endometrial hyperplasia; the World Health Organization 1994 classification schema and the Endometrial Intraepithelial Neoplasia (EIN) diagnostic schema (Table 1).

2.1   WHO Classification

The WHO classification system divides endometrial hyperplasia into four subcategories based on glandular complexity and nuclear atypia (Fig. 1). The four subcategories include: (1) simple hyperplasia, (2) complex hyperplasia, (3) simple hyperplasia with atypia, and (4) complex hyperplasia with atypia. Simple hyperplasia is defined histologically as an overall increase in the number of endometrial glands with mild crowding. Frequently the glands exhibit dilation. Complex hyperplasia consists of a greater than 50% gland to stromal ratio ("crowding"), which is a much higher ratio than that seen for simple hyperplasia. Additionally, the glands typically appear disorganized with mitoses present. In either simple or complex hyperplasia, the glandular cells may also show features of nuclear atypia. Nuclear atypia refers to the presence of nuclear enlargement, prominent nucleoli, or rounded nuclei (normally elongated) with either evenly or irregularly dispersed chromatin.

The widespread use of this classification schema is based on retrospective data showing correlation of risk of endometrial cancer with the presence or absence of nuclear atypia. The risk of

Table 1 Classification systems used for defining precancerous endometrial lesions

World Health Organization 1994 (WHO 94) classification system		
Class	Risk of progression (%)	Treatment
Simple	1	Hormone therapy
Complex	3	Hormone therapy or surgical treatment
Simple with atypia	8	Surgical treatment or hormone therapy[a]
Complex with atypia	29	Surgical treatment or hormone therapy[a]

Endometrial intraepithelial neoplasia (EIN) classification system			
Class	Diagnostic criteria	Risk of malignancy	Treatment
Benign hyperplasia	Exclusion of EIN or cancer	0.60%	Hormone therapy or surveillance
Endometrial intraepithelial neoplasia	Topographically diffuse	19%	Hormone therapy or surgery
	Gland area > stromal area		
	Cells of lesion are cytologically different from background		
	Max linear dimension > 1 mm		
	Exclusion of carcinoma and "benign mimics"		
Endometrial cancer	N/A	N/A	Surgery

[a]Hormone therapy in these cases is reserved for women who desire to preserve fertility or for women who are poor surgical candidates or decline surgical treatment after being appropriately counseled References: (Armstrong et al. 2012; Committee on Gynecologic Practice and Society of Gynecologic Oncology 2015; Trimble et al. 2012)

progression to endometrial cancer in a woman with simple hyperplasia is exceedingly low (1%), while the risk of progression in a woman with complex atypical hyperplasia is as high as 29%, requiring invasive treatments (Table 1; Kurman et al. 1985; Lacey et al. 2010). In this sense, the WHO classification system correlates well with risk of progression and is currently the most commonly used schema by pathologists.

Although this classification system has been in use for many years, it has never been subjected to rigorous verification, putting into question the validity of this schema. Furthermore, two of the subcategories of classification are relatively rare in the population, simple EH with atypia and complex EH without atypia. Simple EH is thought to be a benign lesion resulting from estrogen effect, whereas atypical EH is thought to be a precancerous lesion resulting from the combination of estrogen effect and genetic effects; thus some experts question the biologic significance of simple hyperplasia as it is overall benign and may frequently spontaneously resolve. Additionally, some experts have questioned the WHO classification given that each of the subclasses fails to be

tied to a specific or different treatment option. Rather, largely the same treatments have been offered across EH subtypes.

The largest limitation of the WHO classification system is that there are no specific criteria for histologic diagnosis and thus interpretation is subjective and leads to high interobserver variability, especially when diagnosing cellular atypia. In a large prospective multicenter cohort study of complex EH with atypia, unanimous agreement of a diagnosis among three pathologists was observed in less than half of all diagnoses, and pathologists agreed with the initial diagnosis in only 38% of cases (Zaino et al. 2006). For this reason, many have recommended the use of the EIN classification system rather than the WHO system, although this has not been universally adopted.

2.2 EIN System

The EIN classification system, developed and introduced by the International Endometrial Collaborative Group, uses three subcategories to

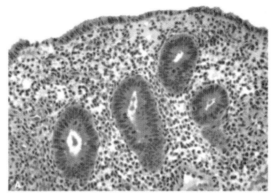

Normal proliferative endometrium

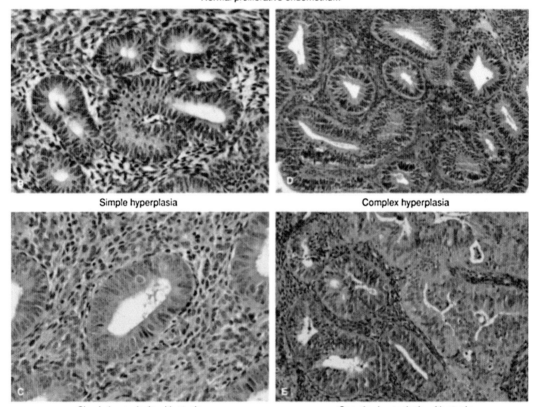

Simple hyperplasia

Complex hyperplasia

Simple hyperplasia with atypia

Complex hyperplasia with atypia

Fig. 1 Histology of endometrial hyperplasia (Originally published in Hoffman BL, Schorge JO, Schaffer JI, Halvorson LM, Bradshaw KD, Cunningham FG: *Williams Gynecology* , 2nd Edition' with kind permission of The McGraw-Hill Companies, Inc. All rights reserved. Photomicrographs display normal proliferative endometrium contrasted with different types of hyperplastic endometrium. (**a**). This high-power view of normal proliferative endometrium shows regularly spaced glands composed of stratified columnar epithelium with bland, slightly elongate nuclei and mitotic activity. (**b**). In simple hyperplasia, glands are modestly crowded and typically display normal tubular shape or mild gland-shape abnormalities. Nuclei are bland. (**c**). In this case, glands are only mildly crowded, but occasional glands, such as the one pictured in this high-power view, have nuclear atypia characterized by nuclear rounding and visible nucleoli. Cytologic atypia accompanies complex hyperplasia more often than it does simple hyperplasia. (**d**). In complex hyperplasia, glands are more markedly crowded and sometimes show architectural abnormalities such as papillary infoldings. In this case, gland profiles are fairly regular but the glands are markedly crowded. (**e**). Glands are markedly crowded and some show papillary infoldings. Nuclei show variable nuclear atypia. Some of the atypical glands have an eosinophilic cytoplasmic change (Photographs contributed by Dr. Kelley Carrick))

define abnormal endometrial tissue based on quantitative pathologic criteria (Committee on Gynecologic Practice and Society of Gynecologic Oncology 2015). The three subcategories include: (1) benign endometrial hyperplasia, (2) endometrial intraepithelial neoplasia, and (3) carcinoma. The pathologic diagnostic criteria of endometrial intraepithelial neoplasia include lesions that have a minimum dimension of 1 mm, increased gland to stroma ratio, a difference in cytology of the lesion as compared to the background tissue, and the exclusion of benign mimics (i.e., polyps, secretory endometrium, effects of exogenous estrogen), and cancerous lesions (Table 1). These criteria can be applied clinically by pathologists or by using formal computerized analysis to assign a D score, which correlates specifically to benign tissue versus EIN. The development of this specific criteria using histomorphologic, genetic, clinical, and biological data attempts to truly differentiate precancerous lesions from benign lesions while maintaining a high degree of sensitivity for detecting precancerous lesions. In a prospective multicenter study using the D score to assign a diagnosis of EIN, the classification system was shown to have a 100% sensitivity in detecting progression to cancer and a 38% positive predictive value, compared to the 91% sensitivity and 16% positive predictive value of the WHO classification system (Baak et al. 2001). In addition, the EIN system has shown that interobserver reproducibility of the EIN system is greater than the WHO94 (Hecht et al. 2005).

Although the EIN criteria represent a more quantitative classification system than the WHO94 criteria, the latter represent a more widely used classification system. Thus, most studies use the WHO94 classification system when performing analyses, and most of the current knowledge, including epidemiologic risk factors and management strategies, pertain specifically to the four-tier classification of EH. Epidemiology studies of EIN remain limited. The EIN nomenclature and system, however, falls in line with the nomenclature of other precancerous lesions of the gynecologic tract, for example, vulva intraepithelial neoplasia (VIN) or cervical intraepithelial neoplasia (CIN). Currently, the EIN classification system lumps all premalignant lesions into a single category. Current research is attempting to further divide the EIN category into grades or classes, to further delineate which lesions are more severe and to determine which lesions would be responsive to hormonal treatment versus require surgical management (Mutter 2000). Still, the EIN classification system is currently the preferred schema of the American Congress of Obstetricians and Gynecologists and the Society of Gynecologic Oncologists for classifying abnormal endometrial epithelium given the quantitative and reproducible nature of this classification system.

3 Epidemiology

Endometrial hyperplasia mainly effects postmenopausal women and women in their later reproductive years with irregular ovulation. This disorder has historically and most commonly been classified by the WHO criteria, and thus much of the epidemiologic data focus on the subcategories of this classification system. Endometrial hyperplasia affects approximately one out of 1000 women annually (Lacey et al. 2012). This condition is highest in women aged 50–54 and rare in women less than 30 years of age. The incidence of endometrial hyperplasia decreases after the age of 70. In asymptomatic postmenopausal women, the prevalence of endometrial hyperplasia with and without atypia is 0.54% and 4.86%, respectively (Gol et al. 2001).

4 Risk Factors

Risk factors for endometrial hyperplasia are generally similar to that of endometrial cancer. There is a strong association with disorders that involve exposure of the endometrium to an increase in either endogenous or exogenous unopposed estrogens. Thus, some of the most notable risk factors include Tamoxifen use, obesity, and polycystic ovarian syndrome (chronic anovulation). Other risk factors include Lynch syndrome, nulliparity and infertility, and diabetes.

4.1   Obesity

Obesity is associated with a higher level of circulating endogenous estrogens, which is secondary to the conversion of androstenedione from adipose tissue to estrone, increased rates of anovulation, and a decrease in circulating sex hormone globulins. There is a proportional relationship between BMI and risk of endometrial hyperplasia. Obese women have approximately six times the risk of endometrial hyperplasia compared to nonobese women (Balbi et al. 2012). In morbidly obese postmenopausal women (BMI > 40), the risk of endometrial hyperplasia with atypia is as high as eightfold. In morbidly obese premenopausal women, this risk is estimated to be as high as 13-fold, possibly suggesting an earlier age of diagnosis in women with obesity (Epplein et al. 2008).

4.2   Polycystic Ovarian Syndrome

Polycystic ovarian syndrome (PCOS), an endocrinologic disorder that is associated with chronic anovulation, affects approximately 8–12% of women of reproductive age (March et al. 2010). Women with PCOS have a threefold increased risk of endometrial cancer (Haoula et al. 2012). Among women with PCOS, the prevalence of endometrial hyperplasia is estimated to be approximately 35–49%, with a prevalence of approximately 13% for atypia (Cheung 2001; Tingthanatikul et al. 2006). The association of PCOS with endometrial hyperplasia is thought to be due to chronic anovulation. PCOS is also associated with obesity and diabetes, which are both independent risk factors for endometrial hyperplasia.

4.3   Hormone Replacement Therapy (HRT)

HRT, with either unopposed estrogen or estrogen and progesterone combinations, has been used for decades to combat the unacceptable effects of declining endogenous estrogens in women at the time of menopause. Long-term use of unopposed estrogen for the relief of vasomotor symptoms related to menopause is associated with a 10–20-fold increase risk of endometrial cancer (ACOG 2015). Use of unopposed estrogen as HRT is associated with a 5-fold to as high as 16-fold increase in the likelihood of developing endometrial hyperplasia with high doses or prolonged use (Lethaby et al. 2000). The estimated prevalence of women who use a moderate dose of estrogen alone for up to 3 years is 28% for simple endometrial hyperplasia, 23% for complex endometrial hyperplasia, and 11.8% for endometrial hyperplasia with atypia (Judd et al. 1996). The risk of progression is likely similar to that of any woman in the general population that carries the diagnosis of EH. Addition of progesterone to the HRT regimen greatly reduces the risk of endometrial hyperplasia. Thus, the recommended use of estrogen replacement therapy includes using the lowest dose for the shortest duration possible. In addition, the use of combined progesterone in continuous or cyclic fashion to counteract the proliferative effects of estrogen alone is recommended (ACOG 2015).

4.4   Tamoxifen Use

Tamoxifen is a selective estrogen receptor modulator (SERM), which acts as an estrogen antagonist in breast tissue and thus is used to prevent and treat breast cancer. Unlike other SERMs, such as raloxifene, tamoxifen acts as an estrogen receptor agonist in endometrial tissue, thus its use is associated with an increase in risk of EH and endometrial cancer (approx. 2.5-fold increase in risk) (ACOG 2015). This effect is evident in postmenopausal women rather than premenopausal women (Fisher et al. 2005). The incidence of EH among women with long-term use of tamoxifen is estimated to be 4.4 per 1000 women annually (Runowicz et al. 2011). In women with breast cancer who are treated with tamoxifen and also have a preexisting endometrial hyperplasia, the risk of progression to a higher grade of EH or endometrial cancer is approximately 20% (Garuti et al. 2006).

4.5   Lynch Syndrome

Lynch syndrome, also known as hereditary nonpolyposis colorectal cancer (HNPCC), is a highly penetrant autosomal-dominant condition associated with an increased risk of the early onset of a variety of cancers, including endometrial cancer and colon cancer. The syndrome is characterized by an inherited defect in mismatch repair genes. The lifetime risk of endometrial cancer in women with lynch syndrome is estimated to be as high as 60% and may exceed the risk of colorectal cancer (Committee on Practice Bulletins- Gynecology and Society of Gynecologic Oncology 2014). Up to 18% of women with lynch syndrome will develop endometrial cancer prior to the age of 40. Although the risk of endometrial hyperplasia in women with Lynch syndrome is unknown, studies have shown a prevalence of 2.8–4.5% of EH among women with Lynch syndrome undergoing surveillance screening with endometrial biopsy (Nebgen et al. 2014).

4.6   Reproductive Factors

Nulliparity and infertility have both been shown to be independent risk factors for EH in premenopausal women with abnormal uterine bleeding (Farquhar et al. 1999). Increasing parity is inversely proportional to the risk of EH among premenopausal women (Epplein et al. 2008).

5   Clinical Presentation

The most common clinical manifestation of endometrial hyperplasia is abnormal uterine bleeding (AUB). In women with postmenopausal bleeding, the prevalence of hyperplasia is as high as 15%, compared to a prevalence of <6% in asymptomatic women (Espindola et al. 2007). In perimenopausal women with AUB – characterized as prolonged, heavy, or irregular menstrual cycles – the prevalence of endometrial hyperplasia is estimated to be 10–36% (Ash et al. 1996; Jetley et al. 2013). Depending on the histologic findings,

the risk of endometrial hyperplasia progressing to cancer is as high as 29% and the risk of concomitant endometrial cancer is 42%. Thus, it is important to perform a diagnostic evaluation in any woman over the age of 45 with postmenopausal bleeding or AUB. In women under the age of 45 with AUB, whether or not to perform a diagnostic evaluation depends on risk factors and clinical suspicion (i.e., risk factors, persistence of symptoms). Occasionally, abnormal endometrial cells can be seen on cervical cytology in asymptomatic women. A finding of adenocarcinoma on cytology requires diagnostic evaluation in all women. Atypical glandular cells on cytology in women greater than 35 years of age or in women less than the age of 35 who are symptomatic (AUB) is a worrisome finding that requires evaluation of the endometrium. Postmenopausal women with endometrial cells on cervical cytology also require diagnostic evaluation of the endometrial cavity. Asymptomatic premenopausal women with findings of benign endometrial cells on cervical cytology do not require further workup (ACOG 2013).

6   Diagnostic Evaluation

The algorithm for diagnostic evaluation for women greater than the age of 45 with a clinical presentation concerning for endometrial hyperplasia is outlined in Fig. 2. Transvaginal ultrasound (TVUS) has a high negative predictive value for endometrial cancer and can be reliably used as the initial test in the diagnostic workup when evaluating a postmenopausal woman with bleeding. In a postmenopausal woman with a endometrial stripe less than or equal to 4 mm, the risk of cancer is less than 1%. In perimenopausal woman, ultrasound is less useful in ruling out endometrial carcinoma based on EMS; however, it can be used to detect any focal lesion or grossly thickened endometrial stripe (ACOG 2015). Any postmenopausal woman with an EMS of >4 mm or a focal lesion on TVUS requires endometrial sampling with either an endometrial biopsy (EMB) or dilation and curettage (D&C).

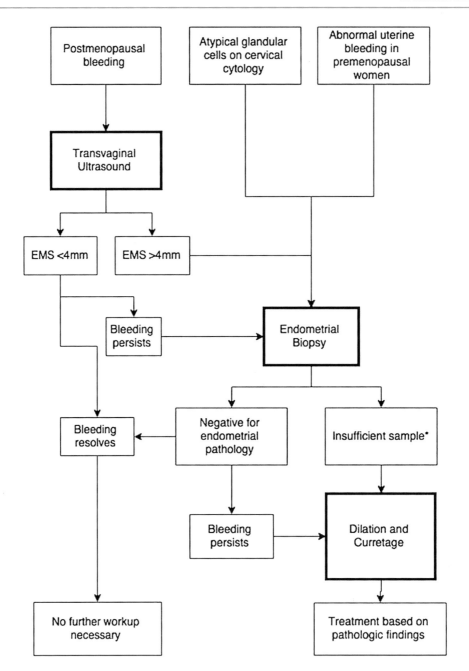

Fig. 2 Algorithm for the diagnostic evaluation for suspected endometrial hyperplasia (*It is reasonable to repeat EMB with one insufficient result. After two insufficient results, dilation and curettage is indicated)

EMB can be performed in the office setting and is the gold standard diagnostic test in the setting of abnormal uterine bleeding and/or abnormal ultra-sound findings. Because EMB can be done in an outpatient setting rather than in the OR, several advantages exist for an EMB over a D&C including less procedural time, minimal anesthe-sia (if any), less cost, need for minimal cervical dilation (if any), and decreased risk of uterine perforation. However, the ability for EMB to detect endometrial disease depends on whether the endometrial disease is focal or global. On average, EMB samples approximately 4% of the endometrial surface. Based on a metaanalysis, the endometrial pipelle technique of EMB has a sensitivity of 81% and a specificity of 98%, and the detection rates for endometrial cancer in postmenopausal and premenopausal women are 99.6% and 91%, respectively (Dijkhuizen et al. 2000). The negative predictive value for detecting endometrial cancer in women with complex atypical hyperplasia is higher for D&C than EMB (69% vs. 55%) (Suh-Burgmann et al. 2009). Thus it is not unreasonable to perform a D&C prior to hysterectomy, particularly if it would change surgical management regarding hysterectomy and possible staging strategies if concomitant endometrial cancer were known to exist.

In approximately 4–15% of women, an EMB will return with insufficient tissue for cytological evaluation. Postmenopausal women or women with a thin EMS have a higher likelihood of insufficient sampling (Elsandabesee and Greenwood 2005; Polena et al. 2007). If an insufficient result is obtained, it is reasonable to either repeat the EMB or proceed with D&C. After two insufficient results, endometrial sampling with D&C is indicated. In a postmenopausal woman, if the EMB is negative but the bleeding abnormality persists, D&C is indicated. The American Congress of Obstetricians and Gynecologists recommends a hysteroscopy with D&C for detection of any focal lesions that may be present (Committee on Gynecologic Practice and Society of Gynecologic Oncology 2015).

7   Management

In a patient who has been newly diagnosed with endometrial hyperplasia or endometrial intraepithelial neoplasia, after concurrent adenocarcinoma has been ruled out, the goal of treatment is prevention of progression to endometrial cancer. Generally, management options include surveillance, medical management, and surgical management. When choosing between these management options, the potential of concurrent malignancy or progression to endometrial cancer,

desire to preserve fertility, and surgical candidacy must all be considered. While surgical management is an effective and definitive means of treating higher-risk endometrial hyperplasia in women who have completed childbearing, nonsurgical treatment options are not as well defined for EH.

7.1   Surveillance

Surveillance by serial EMB is a management option for patients with either hyperplasia without atypia (WHO classification) or benign hyperplasia (based on EIN classification). The risk of progression to endometrial cancer for these entities is 1–3% for hyperplasia without atypia (based on WHO) or 0–2% for benign hyperplasia (based on EIN classification), respectively (Baak et al. 2005; Kurman et al. 1985). Furthermore, spontaneous regression has been estimated to be approximately 70% in women with hyperplasia without atypia (Reed et al. 2009). Although not the recommended management option, given the low risk of progression and high rate of regression, it is reasonable to monitor patients who either have a contraindication to progestin therapy or who decline medical/surgical management. These patients should be evaluated by EMB every 3–6 months until normal endometrium is found. There is not a defined time point for declaring failure to regress; however, most studies have shown median time to regression on hormonal management to be approximately 6 months, and therefore 6 months is likely a reasonable window for conservative management as well. Once regression is achieved, it is also worth considering repeat EMB to ensure stability of regression, and it is important to resample the endometrium in the future if abnormal uterine bleeding recurs.

7.2   Medical Management

Medical management involves the use of hormone therapy to reverse EH. It is the first-line treatment in women with hyperplasia without

Table 2 Progestin therapies commonly used for treatment of Endometrial Hyperplasia or EIN

Hormone	Route	Dosage	Comment	Common side effects
Medroxyprogesterone Acetate (MPA)[a]	Oral	10–20 mg daily or cyclic 12–14 days/month	First-line therapy for non-atypical hyperplasia. Cyclic therapy may be superior to continuous	Irregular bleeding, acne, abdominal pain/nausea
Megestrol Acetate (MA)[a]	Oral	40–320 mg daily	More potent than MPA thus usually reserved for women with atypical hyperplasia	Weight gain, abdominal pain/nausea/diarrhea, Insomnia/mood swings, hypertension, alopecia
Micronized progesterone	Vaginal	100–200 mg daily or cyclic 12–14 days/month	For use in women without atypia	
Depot medroxyprogesterone	Intramuscular	150 mg every 3 months	Regressions rates are likely similar to that of oral MPA	Amenorrhea, acne, Weight gain, headache
Levonorgestrel	Intrauterine	20 mcg/day releasing device	Estimated to be more effective than oral therapy.	Amenorrhea, abdominal pain, acne, irregular bleeding (first 90 days after insertion)

[a]Regression rates overall for oral progestin therapy based on systematic review is 66–69%. These regimens have been shown to have poor compliance compared to the IUD (Armstrong et al. 2012; Committee on Gynecologic Practice and Society of Gynecologic Oncology 2015; Gallos et al. 2010; Guven et al. 2001; Trimble et al. 2012)

atypia or benign hyperplasia as, again, the risk of progression to cancer is low. In women with atypical hyperplasia or EIN, medical management is acceptable in patients who wish to preserve fertility or who are poor surgical candidates. In women desiring to spare fertility, the goals of management are complete clearance of the disease, return of normal endometrial function, and prevention of invasive endometrial cancer. In patients who are poor surgical candidates (i.e., elderly patient with multiple comorbidities), the goals of management include disease stabilization and risk reduction of developing endometrial cancer.

Progestin is the most commonly used hormone to treat EH. In normal endometrium, progesterone counterbalances the endometrial proliferation caused by estrogen and stimulates secretory differentiation (Kim and Chapman-Davis 2010). In precancerous lesions, the mechanism by which progesterone is therapeutic involves apoptosis in neoplastic endometrial glands associated with tissue sloughing during withdrawal shedding, as well as activation of progestin receptors, which leads to stromal decidualization and thinning of

the endometrium (Kim and Chapman-Davis 2010). When used to treat EH, progestins have an impact on the endometrial lining as early as 10 weeks after initiation.

Progestin has been shown to be clinically effective in treating endometrial hyperplasia in a variety of routes, doses, and formulations (Table 2) A pooled analysis has estimated regression rates with use of oral therapy to be 66–69% (Gallos et al. 2010). Medroxyprogesterone acetate (MPA) and megestrol acetate (MA) are the most common progestin therapies. MA is known to be more potent than MPA, thus MA is typically used as first line in women with EH with atypia. In one prospective study, regression rates with the use of MA were as high as 90%. MPA may be administered via oral or intramuscular routes. Studies comparing various routes and formulations of oral progestin therapy have been inconclusive, thus an optimal regimen has not been determined. However, multiple single arm and retrospective studies of progestin-based therapies have been conducted and have been deemed acceptable for use (of any of the aforementioned regimens). Limited data exists for the use of vaginal progesterone in endometrial hyperplasia; however, the estimated regression rate is 90% in women with simple and complex hyperplasia without atypia (Affinito et al. 1994). For reproductive aged women without a contraindication to estrogen, combined oral contraceptives (COC) may be used, though these are typically used to manage women with EH without atypia. COCs are estimated to reduce the risk of endometrial cancer by approximately 50%.

In addition to systemic hormone therapy, the levonorgestrel-releasing intrauterine device (IUD) provides a feasible and possibly superior alternative to oral therapy. The local acting progesterone has a stronger effect on the endometrium while having lower systemic progesterone levels, reducing the incidence of side effects. The estimated regression rates for non-atypical and atypical hyperplasia with the use of the levonorgestrel IUD are 90% and 96%, respectively (Gallos et al. 2010). A recent metaanalysis comparing the levonorgestrel IUD with oral progesterone therapy suggest that the IUD is approximately three times as effective as oral progestin therapy with continual use for 6 months (Abu Hashim et al. 2015).

The median time to regression in most studies, defined by a biopsy revealing normal endometrium, is approximately 6 months, after which if abnormal endometrium still exists, treatment failure is probable (Mentrikoski et al. 2012). Progestin therapy should be continued for at least 12 months in women who do not desire pregnancy or until progression is identified. In women who desire pregnancy, oral progestins should be continued for 3–6 months or until EH is no longer found on endometrial biopsy.

Endometrial sampling can be performed via EMB and is usually performed at 3–6 month intervals. EMB can be performed with an IUD in place. D&C can also be performed for surveillance and is usually repeated every 3–6 months. EMBs generally can be done in the office whereas D&C's frequently require the operating room. For women who have a persistent or progressive lesion, surgical management should be considered on an individual basis.

7.3 Surgical Management

Total hysterectomy with or without bilateral salpingo-oophorectomy (BSO) is the most effective treatment for either atypical hyperplasia (AH) or EIN and provides definitive assessment of a possible occult carcinoma. Independent risk factors for concurrent endometrial cancer include age, obesity, and complex hyperplasia with atypia (Matsuo et al. 2015). Thus, this treatment option is the standard of care for EIN or AH in women who are done with childbearing, especially those with the aforementioned risk factors. Hysterectomy is also indicated in patients with EH with or without atypia if medical management has failed. Hysterectomy is curative for patients with a final postoperative diagnosis of endometrial hyperplasia.

Surgical approaches include abdominal, vaginal, and minimally invasive approaches with laparoscopic or robotic technique. All modalities are acceptable and depend on clinical and patient-specific factors, as well as the skill of the surgeon and the extent of the procedure. For example, clinical patient factors such as complex anatomy, uterine size, body mass index, and prior surgical history should all be considered when determining route of hysterectomy. Currently, vaginal hysterectomy is recommended as the preferred route for performing hysterectomy for nonmalignant conditions (Aarts et al. 2015). However, it is important to note that it may be technically difficult to perform a BSO from a vaginal approach, and surgical staging (i.e., retroperitoneal lymphadenectomy) cannot be performed. It is also preferred that the hysterectomy not require any form of morcellation or deconstruction of the uterus as it may disrupt proper evaluation of the endometrium, particularly when looking for occult cancer and may potentially cause iatrogenic metastases if cancer were present. Thus uterine size must be accounted for if considering a vaginal or minimally invasive approach (which typically requires delivering the uterus through the vagina).

If endometrial cancer is identified, one must also consider the strategy for surgical staging. In general, it may be challenging to diagnose occult endometrial cancer on intraoperative uterine analysis or frozen section. In one study, the negative predictive value for identifying endometrial cancer in patients with complex hyperplasia with atypia was only 73% (Morotti et al. 2012). Thus it is possible that over one quarter of patients who have endometrial cancer may not be detected by use of frozen section. Therefore, it is generally most effective to identify endometrial cancer in formalin fixed paraffin embedded tissue rather than by frozen section assessment. Surgeons may worry that the patients would then require a second surgery if endometrial cancer were identified on the permanent analysis of the hysterectomy specimen. However, the majority of these occult endometrial cancers are low grade, early stage cancers, which do not necessarily require lymphadenectomy; simple hysterectomy would be considered complete and definitive treatment. The premise of this staging strategy is based on a schema developed at the Mayo clinic, by which endometrial cancer cases of low grade (1–2), less than 2 cm tumor diameter on intraoperative evaluation and less than 50% myometrial invasion by frozen section, do not require lymphadenectomy, as the chance of identifying metastases is about 1% or less (Bogani et al. 2014; Mariani et al. 2000, 2008).

Whether or not to perform a bilateral salpingo-oophorectomy (BSO) depends on the presence or absence of endometrial cancer, patient characteristics, and presence of a primary indication for BSO. There is ovarian involvement in approximately 5% of endometrial cancer cases and BSO is indicated in known endometrial cancer cases. However, there are no current standardized recommendations about whether or not to perform a BSO for EH. In general, it has not been required. However, in most cases, there is relatively low surgical risk to performing a BSO. That being said, if a vaginal hysterectomy is performed, a separate abdominal approach either open or minimally invasive may be required to access the adnexa located high on the pelvic brim and complete the BSO. In postmenopausal women, it is reasonable to perform a BSO. In premenopausal women, however, risks of BSO including possible loss of bone density, increased cardiovascular events, and early onset of menopausal symptoms including hot flashes, decreased libido, and disrupted sleep patterns must be considered. Thus, in premenopausal women, BSO at the time of hysterectomy is not required unless there are other indications for removal of the ovaries. This must be considered against the risk of needing a separate surgery in the future for BSO.

Supracervical hysterectomy is contraindicated in patients with endometrial hyperplasia or EIN. The American Congress of Obstetricians and Gynecologists recommends against this approach because of concerns for underlying malignancy, which can reside in the lower uterine segment (ACOG 2007; Committee on Gynecologic Practice and Society of Gynecologic Oncology 2015). Hyperplasia can also reside in the lower uterine segment and there is risk of retained endometrium with supracervical hysterectomy. Morcellation and endometrial ablation are absolutely contraindicated in the surgical management of endometrial hyperplasia as morcellation has been associated with spread of occult cancers and endometrial ablation has an unknown effectiveness in treatment for hyperplasia because it is difficult to assess the endometrial lining after this procedure is performed.

8 Screening and Prevention

There currently are no recommendations for routine screening for endometrial hyperplasia (or endometrial cancer) in the asymptomatic general population. Lifestyle modifications, prophylactic medical management, and/or prophylactic surgery are indicated for some patients based on risk factors. In obese women or women with diabetes, lifestyle modifications such as diet, exercise, and weight loss, are recommended. In women with diabetes, glucose lowering agents such as metformin may decrease the risk of EH or endometrial cancer, although the evidence remains very preliminary and controversial and is limited to retrospective studies. In women with chronic amenorrhea or PCOS, progestin therapy can be used to lower the risk of development of EH or endometrial cancer. When hormone replacement therapy is indicated, the addition of progesterone to the estrogen regimen will reduce the risk of EH associated with HRT, and thus all women who retain a uterus should receive combination hormonal replacement therapy and not estrogen alone.

The prevalence of EH among women with ER positive breast cancer is estimated to be 7%. Therefore it is reasonable to screen women for preexisting endometrial pathology prior to the initiation of tamoxifen therapy (Garuti et al. 2006). Any woman that is to initiate tamoxifen therapy should be informed of the effects that tamoxifen may have on the uterus. They should be counseled appropriately and the importance of reporting any abnormal vaginal symptoms, specifically abnormal bleeding, should be evaluated (ACOG 2014). In women with lynch syndrome, endometrial biopsy every 1–2 years starting at age 30–35 years is recommended. In a multicenter, retrospective, case control study, the risk of endometrial cancer in women with lynch syndrome was significantly reduced from 33% to 0% with a prophylactic hysterectomy; therefore, risk-reducing surgery should be recommended to any woman with lynch syndrome that is done with childbearing (Committee on Practice Bulletins-Gynecology and Society of Gynecologic Oncology 2014; Schmeler et al. 2006).

9 Conclusion

It is critical for all gynecologic clinicians to understand diagnosis and management of EH. This precursor to endometrial cancer can be easily diagnosed based on clinical symptoms with minor gynecologic procedures. When detected, progression to invasive endometrial cancer can often be effectively reduced using progestin therapy with close follow-up and surveillance. Endometrial hyperplasia frequently resolves with hormonal treatment and is definitively cured with hysterectomy. In a small proportion of cases, concurrent endometrial cancer may be diagnosed on the final hysterectomy specimen. Fortunately, most cases of concurrent endometrial cancer are typically of early stage and low-grade

histology, which bears a very favorable prognosis even with hysterectomy alone. Treatment for EH should account for individualized characteristics (i.e., desire to preserve fertility, surgical candidacy), risk factors, severity of the lesion, and persistence or progression of the lesion or clinical symptoms. Patients and providers should discuss all these aspects of EH in order to manage the condition effectively.

10 Cross-References

▶ Conservative Management of Endometrial Cancer
▶ Diagnosis and Management of Postmenopausal Bleeding
▶ Impact of Obesity on Gynecological Diseases
▶ Management of Abnormal Uterine Bleeding: Later Reproductive Years

References

Aarts JW, Nieboer TE, Johnson N, Tavender E, Garry R, Mol BW, et al. Surgical approach to hysterectomy for benign gynaecological disease. Cochrane Database Syst Rev. 2015;8:CD003677.

Abu Hashim H, Ghayaty E, El Rakhawy M. Levonorgestrel-releasing intrauterine system vs oral progestins for non-atypical endometrial hyperplasia: a systematic review and metaanalysis of randomized trials. Am J Obstet Gynecol. 2015;213(4):469–78.

ACOG. ACOG Committee Opinion No. 388 388 November 2007: supracervical hysterectomy. Obstet Gynecol. 2007;110(5):1215–7.

ACOG. Practice Bulletin No. 140: management of abnormal cervical cancer screening test results and cervical cancer precursors. Obstet Gynecol. 2013;122 (6):1338–67.

ACOG. Tamoxifen and uterine cancer. Committee Opinion No. 601. Obstet Gynecol. 2014;123(6):1394–7.

ACOG. Practice Bulletin No. 149: endometrial cancer. Obstet Gynecol. 2015;125(4):1006–26.

Affinito P, Di Carlo C, Di Mauro P, Napolitano V, Nappi C. Endometrial hyperplasia: efficacy of a new treatment with a vaginal cream containing natural micronized progesterone. Maturitas. 1994;20(2–3):191–8.

Armstrong AJ, Hurd WW, Elguero S, Barker NM, Zanotti KM. Diagnosis and management of endometrial hyperplasia. J Minim Invasive Gynecol. 2012;19(5):562–71.

Ash SJ, Farrell SA, Flowerdew G. Endometrial biopsy in DUB. J Reprod Med. 1996;41(12):892–6.

Baak JP, Orbo A, van Diest PJ, Jiwa M, de Bruin P, Broeckaert M, et al. Prospective multicenter evaluation of the morphometric D-score for prediction of the outcome of endometrial hyperplasias. Am J Surg Pathol. 2001;25(7):930–5.

Baak JP, Mutter GL, Robboy S, van Diest PJ, Uyterlinde AM, Orbo A, et al. The molecular genetics and morphometry-based endometrial intraepithelial neoplasia classification system predicts disease progression in endometrial hyperplasia more accurately than the 1994 World Health Organization classification system. Cancer. 2005;103(11):2304–12.

Balbi G, Napolitano A, Seguino E, Scaravilli G, Gioia F, Di Martino L, et al. The role of hypertension, body mass index, and serum leptin levels in patients with endometrial hyperplasia during premenopausal period. Clin Exp Obstet Gynecol. 2012;39(3):321–5.

Bogani G, Dowdy SC, Cliby WA, Ghezzi F, Rossetti D, Mariani A. Role of pelvic and para-aortic lymphadenectomy in endometrial cancer: current evidence. J Obstet Gynaecol Res. 2014;40(2):301–11.

Cheung AP. Ultrasound and menstrual history in predicting endometrial hyperplasia in polycystic ovary syndrome. Obstet Gynecol. 2001;98(2):325–31.

Committee on Gynecologic Practice, Society of Gynecologic Oncology. Committee Opinion No. 631: endometrial intraepithelial neoplasia. Obstet Gynecol. 2015;125(5):1272–8.

Committee on Practice Bulletins- Gynecology, Society of Gynecologic Oncology. ACOG Practice Bulletin No. 147: lynch syndrome. Obstet Gynecol. 2014;124 (5):1042–54.

Dijkhuizen FP, Mol BW, Brolmann HA, Heintz AP. The accuracy of endometrial sampling in the diagnosis of patients with endometrial carcinoma and hyperplasia: a meta-analysis. Cancer. 2000;89(8):1765–72.

Elsandabesee D, Greenwood P. The performance of pipelle endometrial sampling in a dedicated postmenopausal bleeding clinic. J Obstet Gynaecol. 2005; 25(1):32–4.

Epplein M, Reed SD, Voigt LF, Newton KM, Holt VL, Weiss NS. Risk of complex and atypical endometrial hyperplasia in relation to anthropometric measures and reproductive history. Am J Epidemiol. 2008;168 (6):563–70; discussion 71–6.

Espindola D, Kennedy KA, Fischer EG. Management of abnormal uterine bleeding and the pathology of endometrial hyperplasia. Obstet Gynecol Clin N Am. 2007;34(4):717–37, ix.

Farquhar CM, Lethaby A, Sowter M, Verry J, Baranyai J. An evaluation of risk factors for endometrial hyperplasia in premenopausal women with abnormal menstrual bleeding. Am J Obstet Gynecol. 1999; 181(3):525–9.

Fisher B, Costantino JP, Wickerham DL, Cecchini RS, Cronin WM, Robidoux A, et al. Tamoxifen for the prevention of breast cancer: current status of the National Surgical Adjuvant Breast and Bowel Project P-1 study. J Natl Cancer Inst. 2005;97(22):1652–62.

Gallos ID, Shehmar M, Thangaratinam S, Papapostolou TK, Coomarasamy A, Gupta JK. Oral progestogens vs levonorgestrel-releasing intrauterine system for endometrial hyperplasia: a systematic review and metaanalysis. Am J Obstet Gynecol. 2010;203(6):547. e1–10.

Garuti G, Cellani F, Centinaio G, Sita G, Nalli G, Luerti M. Histopathologic behavior of endometrial hyperplasia during tamoxifen therapy for breast cancer. Gynecol Oncol. 2006;101(2):269–73.

Gol K, Saracoglu F, Ekici A, Sahin I. Endometrial patterns and endocrinologic characteristics of asymptomatic menopausal women. Gynecol Endocrinol. 2001; 15(1):63–7.

Guven M, Dikmen Y, Terek MC, Ozsaran AA, Itil IM, Erhan Y. Metabolic effects associated with high-dose continuous megestrol acetate administration in the treatment of endometrial pathology. Arch Gynecol Obstet. 2001;265(4):183–6.

Haoula Z, Salman M, Atiomo W. Evaluating the association between endometrial cancer and polycystic ovary syndrome. Hum Reprod. 2012;27(5):1327–31.

Hecht JL, Ince TA, Baak JP, Baker HE, Ogden MW, Mutter GL. Prediction of endometrial carcinoma by subjective endometrial intraepithelial neoplasia diagnosis. Mod Pathol. 2005;18(3):324–30.

Jetley S, Rana S, Jairajpuri ZS. Morphological spectrum of endometrial pathology in middle-aged women with atypical uterine bleeding: a study of 219 cases. J Midlife Health. 2013;4(4):216–20.

Judd HL, Mebane-Sims I, Legault C, Wasilauskas C, Merino SJM, Barrett-Connor E, et al. Effects of hormone replacement therapy on endometrial histology in postmenopausal women. The Postmenopausal Estrogen/Progestin Interventions (PEPI) trial. JAMA. 1996;275(5):370–5.

Kim JJ, Chapman-Davis E. Role of progesterone in endometrial cancer. Semin Reprod Med. 2010;28(1):81–90.

Kurman RJ, Kaminski PF, Norris HJ. The behavior of endometrial hyperplasia. A long-term study of "untreated" hyperplasia in 170 patients. Cancer. 1985;56(2):403–12.

Lacey Jr JV, Sherman ME, Rush BB, Ronnett BM, Ioffe OB, Duggan MA, et al. Absolute risk of endometrial carcinoma during 20-year follow-up among women with endometrial hyperplasia. J Clin Oncol. 2010; 28(5):788–92.

Lacey Jr JV, Chia VM, Rush BB, Carreon DJ, Richesson DA, Ioffe OB, et al. Incidence rates of endometrial hyperplasia, endometrial cancer and hysterectomy from 1980 to 2003 within a large prepaid health plan. Int J Cancer. 2012;131(8):1921–9.

Lethaby A, Farquhar C, Sarkis A, Roberts H, Jepson R, Barlow D. Hormone replacement therapy in postmenopausal women: endometrial hyperplasia and irregular bleeding. Cochrane Database Syst Rev. 2000;2: CD000402.

March WA, Moore VM, Willson KJ, Phillips DI, Norman RJ, Davies MJ. The prevalence of polycystic ovary syndrome in a community sample assessed under contrasting diagnostic criteria. Hum Reprod. 2010;25 (2):544–51.

Mariani A, Webb MJ, Keeney GL, Haddock MG, Calori G, Podratz KC. Low-risk corpus cancer: is lymphadenectomy or radiotherapy necessary? Am J Obstet Gynecol. 2000;182(6):1506–19.

Mariani A, Dowdy SC, Cliby WA, Gostout BS, Jones MB, Wilson TO, et al. Prospective assessment of lymphatic dissemination in endometrial cancer: a paradigm shift in surgical staging. Gynecol Oncol. 2008;109(1):11–8.

Matsuo K, Ramzan AA, Gualtieri MR, Mhawech-Fauceglia P, Machida H, Moeini A, et al. Prediction of concurrent endometrial carcinoma in women with endometrial hyperplasia. Gynecol Oncol. 2015;139 (2):261–7.

Mentrikoski MJ, Shah AA, Hanley KZ, Atkins KA. Assessing endometrial hyperplasia and carcinoma treated with progestin therapy. Am J Clin Pathol. 2012;138(4):524–34.

Morotti M, Menada MV, Moioli M, Sala P, Maffeo I, Abete L, et al. Frozen section pathology at time of hysterectomy accurately predicts endometrial cancer in patients with preoperative diagnosis of atypical endometrial hyperplasia. Gynecol Oncol. 2012;125 (3):536–40.

Mutter GL. Endometrial intraepithelial neoplasia (EIN): will it bring order to chaos? The Endometrial Collaborative Group. Gynecol Oncol. 2000;76(3):287–90.

Nebgen DR, Lu KH, Rimes S, Keeler E, Broaddus R, Munsell MF, et al. Combined colonoscopy and endometrial biopsy cancer screening results in women with Lynch syndrome. Gynecol Oncol. 2014;135(1):85–9.

Polena V, Mergui JL, Zerat L, Sananes S. The role of Pipelle Mark II sampling in endometrial disease diagnosis. Eur J Obstet Gynecol Reprod Biol. 2007;134 (2):233–7.

Reed SD, Voigt LF, Newton KM, Garcia RH, Allison HK, Epplein M, et al. Progestin therapy of complex endometrial hyperplasia with and without atypia. Obstet Gynecol. 2009;113(3):655–62.

Runowicz CD, Costantino JP, Wickerham DL, Cecchini RS, Cronin WM, Ford LG, et al. Gynecologic conditions in participants in the NSABP breast cancer prevention study of tamoxifen and raloxifene (STAR). Am J Obstet Gynecol. 2011;205(6):535.e1–5.

Schmeler KM, Lynch HT, Chen LM, Munsell MF, Soliman PT, Clark MB, et al. Prophylactic surgery to reduce the risk of gynecologic cancers in the Lynch syndrome. N Engl J Med. 2006;354(3):261–9.

Suh-Burgmann E, Hung YY, Armstrong MA. Complex atypical endometrial hyperplasia: the risk of unrecognized adenocarcinoma and value of preoperative dilation and curettage. Obstet Gynecol. 2009;114 (3):523–9.

Tingthanatikul Y, Choktanasiri W, Rochanawutanon M, Weerakeit S. Prevalence and clinical predictors of endometrial hyperplasiain anovulatory women presenting with amenorrhea. Gynecol Endocrinol. 2006;22(2):101–5.

Trimble CL, Method M, Leitao M, Lu K, Ioffe O, Hampton M, et al. Management of endometrial precancers. Obstet Gynecol. 2012;120(5):1160–75.

Zaino RJ, Kauderer J, Trimble CL, Silverberg SG, Curtin JP, Lim PC, et al. Reproducibility of the diagnosis of atypical endometrial hyperplasia: a Gynecologic Oncology Group study. Cancer. 2006;106(4):804–11.

Conservative Management of Endometrial Cancer

Lindsey Buckingham and Emily Ko

Abstract

Endometrial cancer is the most common gynecologic malignancy in the United States. Approximately 54,000 new cases will be diagnosed in 2015, and the incidence of endometrial cancer has increased by 1.5% per year among women younger than 50 years, and by 2.6% per year among women 50 years and older. Fortunately, the overall mortality due to endometrial cancer remains low (ACS. American Cancer Society facts & figures 2015. American Cancer Society; 2015). Endometrial cancer is standardly treated with surgical resection via total hysterectomy (removal of the uterine corpus and cervix) and bilateral salpingo-oophorectomy, with or without lymph node assessment. However, given the rise in incident endometrial cancers largely related to the obesity epidemic, increasing numbers of young women with endometrial cancer will desire to preserve the uterus for fertility, and opt for conservative management. At the other end of the spectrum, a subset of patients with endometrial cancer may be unsuitable surgical candidates largely due to obesity and its related comorbid conditions and physical dysfunction. Both of these patient populations present a challenging management dilemma because surgery may not be a primary treatment option. Instead, conservative management of endometrial cancer based largely on hormonal therapy may be considered. While this approach is not standard of care, there is increasing evidence supporting the safety and efficacy of conservative therapy, particularly for low-grade, early stage endometrial cancers. This evidence, however, must be tempered by the relative high recurrence rates and goal of subsequent hysterectomy when feasible.

Keywords

Fertility sparing • Conservative management • Hormonal therapy • Progesterone

L. Buckingham (✉)
Department of Obstetrics and Gynecology, Pennsylvania Hospital, Philadelphia, PA, USA
e-mail: Lindsey.Buckingham@uphs.upenn.edu

E. Ko
Division of Gynecologic Oncology, University of Pennsylvania Health System, Philadelphia, PA, USA
e-mail: Emily.ko@uphs.upenn.edu

Contents

© Springer International Publishing AG 2017
D. Shoupe (ed.), *Handbook of Gynecology*,
DOI 10.1007/978-3-319-17798-4_4

1   Introduction to Conservative Management

The most common reasons for conservative management of endometrial cancer are dichotomous: desire for fertility preservation or comorbidities and functional status that are not compatible with surgery. Primary conservative management of endometrial cancer with hormonal therapy is a newer concept; however, the biologic principle is not. Hormonal therapy has been utilized dating back to the 1960s for the management of metastatic endometrial cancer. Specifically, Drs. Kelley and Baker used progestins to treat patients with metastatic and/or symptomatic endometrial cancer. The majority of patients showed regression of disease, and most reported symptomatic relief. Responses were particularly seen in women with well-differentiated endometrial cancer (Kelley and Baker 1965). Using largely the same biologic principles, conservative treatment for endometrial cancer has been reported dating back to 1959 with use of different progesterone formulations (Kistner 1959). More recently, several small to moderate-sized studies have reported efficacy in hormone-based conservative

management of endometrial cancer (Gallos et al. 2012; Park et al. 2013; Ushijima et al. 2007; Park et al. 2013b). While surgery remains the mainstay of endometrial cancer treatment and primary medical management remains controversial, mounting evidence support these novel therapies.

2   Epidemiologic Considerations

2.1   Age: Young Women with Endometrial Cancer

Up to 14% of endometrial cancers occur in women of childbearing age, and the incidence of endometrial cancer continues to rise: recent data show 1.5% increase per year among women younger than 50 years, and 2.6% increase per year among women 50 years and older (ACS 2015). Younger women with endometrial cancer are typically obese, often nulliparous, and have history of menstrual irregularities including those related to polycystic ovarian syndrome, anovulation, or metabolic syndrome. These patients are usually detected due to infertility or bleeding complaints. While the youngest endometrial cancer patients are often better surgical candidates, their desire to maintain fertility, particularly to carry their own pregnancy, precludes hysterectomy. Fortunately, the majority of young women with endometrial cancer have the less aggressive subtypes, characterized by low-grade histology and early stage disease.

2.2   Age: Older Age and Comorbidities

Several differences exist in the clinical and pathologic profile of older compared to younger endometrial cancer patients. Not surprisingly a great majority of older women with endometrial cancer have one or more comorbidities, and comorbidities increase with age in the general adult population. In general, women with endometrial cancer have been found to have higher rates of comorbidities, namely, at least one and half times the risk for congestive heart failure, hypertension, or pulmonary disease; twice the risk of diabetes; and over three times the risk for obesity (Kurnit et al. 2015). Rates of hypertension and diabetes have been reported to be 25–58%, and 24–26%, respectively, in endometrial cancer patients (Ko et al. 2014; Kurnit et al. 2015). Furthermore, increased age at diagnosis has been associated with higher likelihood of hypertension and diabetes (Kennedy et al. 2000; Saltzman et al. 2008), and higher Charlson comorbidity scores (Truong et al. 2005). Somewhat paradoxically, the oldest women with endometrial cancer have been found to be less severely obese (Bittoni et al. 2013) which may be in part due to differences in the biology of disease, lending to a higher prevalence of more aggressive subtypes of endometrial cancer in women of older age.

2.3 Obesity and Endometrial Cancer

Obesity is a rising epidemic in many parts of the developed world. Current data drawn from the 2011–2012 United States NHANES (National Health and Nutrition Examination Survey) revealed that 58.5% of nonpregnant women aged 20–39 years were overweight or obese, 31.8% obese, and 8% extremely obese. Of women aged 40–59 years old, 71.7% were overweight or obese, 39.5% obese, and 9.8% extremely obese (Ogden et al. 2014). Given that well over half of all women in the United States are overweight or obese, obesity-related health conditions including endometrial cancer are only expected to increase (Fig. 1).

Renehan et al. showed that a 5 kg/m^2 increase in BMI was strongly associated with endometrial cancer (OR 1.59, $p < 0.001$) (Renehan et al. 2008). Accordingly, Reeves et al. predicted that up to 51% of endometrial cancer cases could be attributable to obesity (Reeves et al. 2007). Nevadunsky et al. report a strong correlation between obesity and younger age at diagnosis, and Duska et al. found that women aged 24–40 years and BMI >30 were associated with stage I, grade I disease (Duska et al. 2001; Nevadunsky et al. 2014). In general, obesity induces a hyperestrogenic state due to the conversion of adrostenedione to estrone in peripheral adipose tissue. Thus, obesity has been associated with estrogen-dependent endometrial cancers, classically referred to as the common, type I endometrial cancer. However, it appears that obesity may

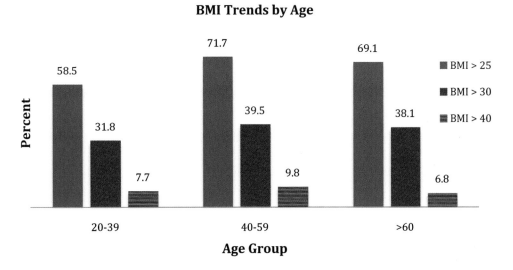

Fig. 1 Obesity category by age group in American women (Data adapted from Ogden et al. (2014))

also be associated with type II endometrial cancers. Drawing upon the pooled analysis by the Epidemiology of Endometrial Cancer Consortium, 75% of all type I and 61% of all type II patients were overweight or obese (Setiawan et al. 2013), and similar high rates were found in prospectively enrolled endometrial cancer patients in a national trial as well as smaller multi-institutional studies (Ko et al. 2014).

2.4 Special Populations: Hereditary Syndromes

While endometrial cancer has not been classically thought of as a heredity-based cancer, there is a subpopulation of endometrial cancer patients that do develop endometrial cancer as a result of a genetic syndrome. These include patients with Lynch syndrome, which may account for approximately 5% of endometrial cancer cases. Lynch syndrome, also referred to as hereditary nonpolyposis colorectal cancer, is an autosomal dominant condition characterized by having a germline mutation in one of four mismatch repair genes (MLH1, MSH2, MSH6, and PMS2) with an inherited propensity to develop colon, endometrial, ovarian, genitourinary, and gastric cancers. Women with Lynch syndrome have a lifetime risk of 15–66%, depending on the type of MMR mutation, for developing endometrial cancer and the risk increases sharply after age 40, with the median

Table 1 Amsterdam criteria

Amsterdam criteria: familial risk for Lynch syndrome or hereditary nonpolyposis colorectal cancer[a]
Minimum 3 relatives with an HNPCC-associated cancer
1. One first-degree relative of the other 2 relatives
2. At least 2 successive generations are affected
3. At least 1 relative diagnosed before age 50
4. Must exclude familial adenomatous polyposis
5. Tumors verified by pathological examination

[a]Approximately half of all patients meeting listed criteria will have Lynch syndrome. Importantly, many families with Lynch syndrome will not meet these criteria

age of diagnosis of 46 (Bonadona et al. 2011; Burke et al. 2014b). The identification of patients with Lynch syndrome has previously depended on clinical suspicion and inquiry into a detailed family history of a patient newly diagnosed with colon cancer based on the Bethesda and Amsterdam criteria (Matthews et al. 2008) (Table 1).

According to Lindor et al., approximately half of women meeting Amsterdam criteria will have Lynch syndrome (Lindor et al. 2006). While colorectal cancers are commonly expected sentinel events, more than 50% of women with Lynch syndrome will present with gynecologic malignancy first (Lu et al. 2005). For women with newly diagnosed endometrial cancer, immunohistochemistry (IHC)-based screening off of paraffin-embedded tissue has been found to have a higher detection rate of identifying Lynch syndrome affected patients than (especially in those age <60), compared to MSI testing, family history assessment, or tumor morphology testing (Ferguson et al. 2014). Subsequently, multiple other investigators have reported on the success of tissue-based screening algorithms using IHC assays for non-normal expression of mismatch repair genes in newly diagnosed endometrial cancer patients (Buchanan et al. 2014; Frolova et al. 2015; Mills et al. 2014). Dating back to 2007, the Society of Gynecologic Oncologists (SGO) had made formal recommendations to screen all women diagnosed with endometrial cancer under the age of 60 using IHC (Lancaster et al. 2007). Currently, the National Comprehensive Cancer Network Guidelines for the Management of Endometrial cancer suggests screening with IHC and microsatellite instability assays for inherited mismatch repair gene mutations in three patient populations: 1. Patients with newly diagnosed endometrial cancer under the age of 50, 2. Patients with a significant family history of endometrial and/or colorectal cancer, 3. Patients with epithelial tumors (rather than those with stromal/mesenchymal endometrial tumors) (NCCN 2015). Thus, patients diagnosed with endometrial cancer, particularly those who are premenopausal and of younger age, should be assessed for Lynch syndrome by IHC and/or referral to a genetic counselor. Determination of whether they are Lynch syndrome carriers may alter decisions about treatment and fertility desires.

Currently, the impact of the mismatch repair gene mutations in Lynch syndrome patients on cancer persistence, progression, and recurrence remains unknown. Conservative management of endometrial cancer in these cases may be considered using similar criteria as for non-Lynch syndrome patients; however, since Lynch syndrome patients also have an elevated lifetime risk for developing ovarian cancer of up to 24%, bilateral salpingo-oophorectomy at the time of definitive surgery for uterine cancer should be considered. The increased propensity to develop both uterine and ovarian cancer frequently sway both patients and physicians toward definitive surgical management sooner rather than later. Importantly, Lynch syndrome patients need expanded surveillance for other cancers including colorectal, genitourinary, and to a lesser extent, upper gastrointestinal.

Other genetic syndromes such as Cowden's and BRCA-associated hereditary syndromes contribute to fewer overall cases of endometrial cancer, but bear mentioning. Cowden's is an autosomal dominant condition characterized by a mutation in the PTEN tumor suppressor gene. The lifetime risk of endometrial cancer in women with Cowden's is 13–19%. The association between endometrial cancer and women with BRCA gene mutations remains controversial. While it is clear they have significantly increased lifetime risk of breast and ovarian cancer, data for endometrial cancer are mixed. One smaller case control study reported an association between BRCA2 mutation carriers and uterine serous carcinoma; however, other studies have not replicated these findings. More recently, a large prospective study of patients with BRCA1 and 2 mutations found an increased rate of endometrial cancer; however, this risk was attributable to Tamoxifen use, rather than the BRCA mutation itself (Beiner et al. 2007). Ultimately, a detailed family history should be taken for all cancer patients, and especially for patients diagnosed with premenopausal endometrial cancer.

3 Ideal Candidates for Conservative Management

3.1 Endometrial Cancer Classification

Endometrial cancer has classically been divided into two major categories: type I and type II, based on clinical pathologic differences. Type I endometrial cancers are typically associated hyperestrogenic or unopposed estrogenic states. Clinical characteristics of these patients frequently include obesity, nulliparity, and metabolic syndromes such as diabetes and PCOS (Bokhman 1983). Additionally, type I endometrial cancer typically presents with low-grade endometrioid histology (grade 1 and 2) and is diagnosed at early stage (stage I and II). As a result, women with type I endometrial cancer may be candidates for conservative management as these cancers are considered less aggressive, detected early, well differentiated, and sensitive to hormonal therapy.

In contrast, type II endometrial cancers are considered less driven by estrogen, less responsive to hormonal management, and generally more aggressive with higher grade histology and advanced stage at diagnosis. Patients with type II endometrial cancer are not typically offered conservative management as the risks of delayed surgical management almost always outweigh the benefits. Fortunately, type II endometrial cancers are typically diagnosed in older postmenopausal women and not frequently seen in women who are still seeking fertility-sparing procedures.

The abovementioned classification system is evolving, and there is a movement toward categorizing endometrial cancer into "low risk" versus "high risk" cases. Low risk has been defined by low-grade histology and early stage presentation, whereas "high risk" has been associated with high-grade histology (grade 3 histology of any histologic subtype: endometrioid, serous, clear cell, undifferentiated) (Brinton et al. 2013; Setiawan et al. 2013).

3.2   Selection of Low Risk Cases

Whereas conservative management was once geared toward patients with advanced disease or recurrence, fertility preservation for younger patients now represents a larger proportion of women diagnosed with endometrial cancer who do not undergo hysterectomy. One major principle exists for women desiring conservative management for endometrial cancer: they must carry a low risk diagnosis. Low risk is defined as having grade 1–2 histology, typically of the endometrioid subtype, less than 50% myometrial invasion based on MRI imaging, and no evidence of metastatic disease. Previous studies have shown that these patients carry a risk for pelvic and para-aortic lymph node involvement of less than 10% (Creasman et al. 1987). Various algorithms have been proposed for identifying individuals with low risk of having metastatic disease. One of the most common, proposed by Mariani et al., uses intraoperative frozen section protocol of hysterectomy-based pathology assessment. This study from the Mayo Clinic showed low incidence of nodal metastases (5%) in patients with <50% myometrial invasion, grade I/II preoperative histology, and endometrioid type endometrial cancer (Mariani et al. 2000). Obviously in conservative management of endometrial cancer, hysterectomy-based assessments cannot be used. However, many physicians have largely applied the same principles (minimal myometrial invasion, small tumor size, and low-grade histology) using imaging and biopsy results to select candidates for conservative management of endometrial cancer. The most ideal patient characteristics of women considering conservative management for fertility-sparing purposes are listed in Table 2.

The above parameters are minimum requirements for conservative management to be feasible. Other considerations include patient compliance and ability to follow-up for surveillance on at least biannual basis. The converse scenario involves inoperable patients whose advanced disease, distant metastases, and/or many comorbidities make them poor surgical candidates. Conservative management in these cases refers to palliative and symptom-controlling

Table 2 Ideal characteristics for patients electing to pursue conservative management of endometrial cancer

Ideal candidates for conservative management
Well-differentiated endometrial carcinoma – grade 1–2
No myometrial invasion
No extrauterine involvement (metastases, ovarian involvement, lymph nodes)
Strong desire for fertility sparing
Informed consent regarding standard of care (hysterectomy) and acceptance of risks

regimens involving radiation, chemotherapy, progestin therapy, or a combination of the three.

3.3   Pretreatment Evaluation: Diagnosis and Testing

The ability to provide medical management to an endometrial cancer patient hinges on accuracy in diagnosis. Tissue studies based on endometrial biopsy or dilation and curettage (D&C) samples are the primary sources for histology grading. With multiple methods of endometrial sampling available, however, a great deal of research has focused on utility of in-office versus surgical methods. A meta-analysis of more than 40 studies found that Pipelle EMB was the best device in both postmenopausal and premenopausal women, with a sensitivity of 99.6% and 91%, respectively (Dijkhuizen et al. 2000). A major shortcoming of this study, however, was that only 27% of studies compared their sampling method of choice to final pathology on hysterectomy. The remaining made comparisons to D&C histology. A more recent study showed that in patients with a preoperative diagnosis of FIGO grade 1, EMB using Pipelle had twice the rate of upgrade on final pathology (17.4% vs. 8.7%) (Leitao et al. 2009). Importantly and fortunately, the vast majority of upgrades were from grade 1 to 2 rather than 2 to 3 (16% vs. 1.7%); thus, these patients remained in the low or intermediate risk groups. Their group recommended that D&C be used in patients desiring fertility preservation as it offers more accurate diagnosis and is potentially therapeutic (15% had no residual carcinoma at hysterectomy) (Leitao et al. 2009).

3.4 Determining Extent of Disease

When selecting candidates for fertility-sparing conservative management of endometrial cancer, assessment for myometrial invasion is also extremely important, and this is dependent on imaging. Magnetic resonance imaging (MRI) is currently considered the most accurate tool for prediction myometrial invasion. T2-weighted imaging has a pooled sensitivity and specificity of 87% and 58%, respectively, while dynamic contrast-enhanced MRI has a pooled sensitivity and specificity of 81% and 72%, respectively, in the assessment of myometrial invasion (Kim et al. 1995). Transvaginal pelvic ultrasound has generally not been recommended for evaluation of myometrial invasion. Its greatest utility is to assess for abnormally thickened endometrial stripes (>4 mm) in postmenopausal women, but in premenopausal women the endometrial thickness is much harder to correlate to potential malignant pathology due to the extensive variation of endometrium through menstrual cycling (Burke et al. 2014b). Computed tomography (CT) shows greatest utility for detection of metastatic disease to the peritoneal cavity and abdominal and pelvic lymphadenopathy and is not recommended for assessment of myometrial invasion. In a meta-analysis of imaging techniques for endometrial cancer, the sensitivity for detecting myometrial invasion was best for contrast-enhanced MRI (80–100%), in comparison to 40–100% for CT and 50–100% for ultrasound (Kinkel et al. 1999). In summary, the National Cancer Center Network (NCCN) and Society of Gynecologic Oncology recommend MRI for evaluation of myometrial invasion in conservative management. Newer technologies including MRI combined with metabolomics and MR-PET are currently being evaluated in clinical trials.

Blood serum assays have not typically been used as selection criteria to identify candidates for conservative management of endometrial cancer. Some investigators have evaluated the utility of elevated CA-125 levels in the management of endometrial cancer, particularly to assess for metastatic disease with high-grade histologies, or as a factor in preoperative models to predict lymph node metastases (Kang et al. 2012). However, given the low specificity of CA-125 due to potentially abnormal values related to any number of conditions (gynecologic and nongynecologic, benign, or malignant), this test is unlikely to yield reliable results and not recommended.

Candidates for fertility-sparing conservative management of endometrial cancer are largely selected based on endometrial sampling, imaging, and clinical patient factors and do not require further surgical assessment. Some individuals, however, have preferred to also perform diagnostic laparoscopy to verify no extrauterine disease prior to initiation of conservative management (Mazzon et al. 2010; Minig et al. 2011; Shan et al. 2013).

4 Treatment Options

4.1 Hormonal Therapy

Conservative management is naturally divided into two groups: fertility-sparing candidates and patients whose medical comorbidities or advanced cancer stage have rendered them inoperable. Here we will focus on fertility-sparing treatment of endometrial cancer. The majority of low-grade endometrioid adenocarcinoma, characterized by well-differentiated tumor cells, are more likely to express progesterone receptors. The GOG 81 trial showed that progestins are more effective in differentiated (low-grade) endometrial cancers than in undifferentiated (high-grade) histologies (Lentz et al. 1996). As a result, most therapies for conservative management of endometrial cancer have been some form of progesterone. Progestin is the synthetic analog (generally administered by pill form) to the naturally synthesized progesterone in the body. The mechanism of action of progestins is downregulation of estrogen receptors, activation of enzymes involved in estrogen metabolism, and cell cycle regulation of cyclin-dependent kinase pathways (Park and Nam 2015).

Oral progesterone-based agents are the most widely studied therapy for conservative management, and the most commonly used agents include medroxyprogesterone acetate (MPA) and megestrol acetate (MA). MPA is typically dosed at 200–800 mg/day (in divided doses), but doses ranging from 2.5 to 1500 mg/day have been studied. MA is most often dosed at 160 mg/day (in divided doses) with reported doses ranging from 16 to 320 mg/day (Gallos et al. 2012). There remains no consensus on optimal dosing of oral progesterones. Park et al. compared high-dose MPA and MA ($\geq$500 mg/day) to low dose ($<$500 mg/day), and found no difference: 77% versus 79% complete response ($p = 0.775$) for low and high doses, respectively (Park et al. 2013a). The length of therapy is also a subject of debate. The reported minimum duration for oral therapy is generally 3 months, even if histologic response is documented prior to this time. Three to 6 months appears to be the most common duration of treatment, while 12 months duration is reported in several studies (Burke et al. 2014a; Gallos et al. 2012).

More recently, the levonorgestrel IUD (LNG-IUD) has also been used in fertility-sparing treatment of endometrial cancer with reported complete response rates ranging from 40% to 100%. Benefits of using the LNG-IUD include compliance (compared to daily pills), minimal side effects compared to oral progesterone (particularly gastrointestinal and mood), and direct delivery or higher dose progesterone directly to the endometrium. Minig et al. used the LNG-IUD in combination with monthly GnRH analog injections and showed a 57% complete response for endometrial cancer patients at 1 year of treatment (Minig et al. 2011). Pronin et al. showed even better results with 72% complete response using LNG-IUD and monthly goserelin injections (Pronin et al. 2015).

As with any intervention, side effect profile should be considered. Oral progestins and GnRH analogs have generally mild, though well-documented side effects including headache, menstrual prodrome symptoms, weight gain, and thrombophlebitis. The LNG-IUD carries a similarly mild profile including menstrual irregularities (amenorrhea or irregular uterine bleeding), pain at placement, and expulsion.

The newest agents under investigation include gonadotropin-releasing hormone agonists (Lupron), aromatase inhibitors (i.e., anastrazole), and inhibitors of mammalian target of rapamycin (mTOR) inhibitors (rapamycin, temsirolimus, everolimus). Additionally, inhibitors of phosphatidylinositol 3-kinase (PI3K), NDA-dependent protein kinase, and VEGF inhibitors (i.e., bevacizumab, aflibercept), and metformin are being investigated (Dedes et al. 2011; Park and Nam 2015). However, trials to date have been largely performed in women with recurrent or advanced EC, and these agents have not been investigated in frontline treatment for fertility-sparing therapy for EC except for a couple case reports. Current clinical trials include the following: LNG-IUD with MPA; MA with metformin versus MA alone; LNG-IUD with everolimus versus LNG-IUD alone; everolimus plus letrozole versus progestins; and the mTOR inhibitor temsirolimus.

4.2 Nonhormonal and Combination Modalities

Primary hysteroscopic resection followed by oral agents or LNG-IUS, though not studied extensively, is gaining attention. Results thus far have been promising with complete response rates ranging 57–100% and relapse rates which are often lower than with progestins alone (4–11%). These small series have all used similar surgical technique: resection of tumor, resection of endometrium adjacent to the tumor, and resection of the myometrium underlying the tumor. If no myometrial invasion was found on final pathology, the women were treated with hormonal therapy (Kalogera et al. 2014; Mazzon et al. 2010; Shan et al. 2013). Some have voiced concerns regarding potential intrauterine adhesions (with repeated instrumentation of the uterine cavity) leading to subsequent infertility; however, these small series have not been able to provide sufficient case numbers to make this assessment.

A novel regimen of photodynamic therapy (PDT) has been tried in endometrial cancer treatment. PDT uses a nontoxic light-sensitive compound that destroys cancer cells by producing active oxygen species when a light-sensitive compound applied to the tissues are exposed to a specific wavelength of light. Treatment of endometrial cancer with PDT has been reported in a small series of 16 patients (11 with primary treatment and 5 with secondary treatment after failure of hormonal therapy), with a response rate of 75% and a recurrence rate of 33% (Choi et al. 2013). Given these favorable results, PDT may represent a viable alternative to oral therapy which often requires several months of treatment to produce regression. This intervention, however, warrants significantly more research before it can be recommended as first line treatment.

4.3   Definition of Response

The definitions of response, failure, and progression are important to define. The literature separates responses into complete and partial: complete response is generally defined as reversion to normal endometrium with no hyperplastic or cancerous characteristics. Partial response has been defined as remaining hyperplasia or atypia with degeneration and atrophy of endometrial glands. Progressive disease is diagnosed when repeat sampling shows an upgraded histology (Ushijima et al. 2007). Durable complete response has been defined by some investigators as complete initial response with no later recurrence (Bakkum-Gamez et al. 2012). There is some variation in these definitions and some investigators have defined complete regression sufficient if simple hyperplasia or complex hyperplasia without atypia is found.

The time period for determining a patient's particular response is another topic for which there is no firm answer. Park et al. suggest that 3 months may be sufficient for diagnosis of treatment failure. Other investigators have reported a median treatment time needed for disease regression of 4–6 months, with potentially longer treatment needed in the more obese and anovulatory patients (Kalogera et al. 2014). A patient with no change in histology could continue treatment up to 12 months, while any patient with histologic

evidence of progression should proceed to surgical management (Park and Nam 2015).

5   Oncologic Outcomes

The majority of women who undergo fertility-preserving hormonal-based therapy for endometrial cancer respond to progesterone-based therapy. Data on fertility-sparing methods with grade 1 endometrial cancer show excellent response rates ranging from 55% to 100% (Table 3). This table summarizes the larger and/or prospective studies published for treatment of low-grade endometrial cancer. Response rates are favorable; however, recurrence rates range from 0% to 57%. Additionally, there have been two published meta-analyses on conservative treatments for endometrial cancer. The earlier reported on 32 studies published between 1985 and 2011, and reported a 76% regression rate (defined as no residual cancer or complex atypical hyperplasia). The recurrence rate was 40.6%, and median follow-up period ranged from 11 to 76 months (Gallos et al. 2012). Another contemporary meta-analysis published in 2012 on 38 studies from 2004 to 2011 reported an initial response rate of 74%. Overall however, 48.2% achieved a durable complete response and 35.4% experienced a recurrence; the median follow-up time ranged from 0 to 30 years (Gunderson et al. 2014). There has been no head-to-head trial comparing the efficacy of MPA versus MA, and overall response rates seem similar. One should note that the doses of MPA for treatment of endometrial cancer are typically high, unlike the low doses (10 mg) that are frequently administered for management of benign gynecologic conditions.

There is less information specifically regarding outcomes for potentially higher risk cases, which include grade 2 or 3 histology and those with myometrial invasion. Due to the understanding that more aggressive histologies have lower response rates, very few researchers have studied conservative management in women with grade 2 or 3 endometrial cancer or with myometrial invasion. In a more recent review article, Park (2015) summarized the available data on

Table 3 Selected reports of conservative management for endometrial carcinoma

Author	Number of patients	Therapy	Duration	Regression n/N (%)	Progression n/N (%)	Relapse n/N (%)	Surveillance	Complications
Ushijima, 2007	22	MPA 600 mg + ASA 81 mg then cyclic estrogen/progesterone	26 weeks then 6 months	12/22 (55)	0/22 (0)	8/14 (57)	TVUS and EMB at 8 and 16 weeks Hysteroscopy D&C at 26 weeks	Weight gain, liver dysfunction, abnormal coagulation factors
Park, 2013a	148	MPA 500 mg or MA 160 mg	Mean 8 months	115/148 (78)	0/148 (0)	35/115 (30)	Exam, US/MRI every 3–6 months	Not reported
Minig, 2011	14	LNG-IUD × 1y + GnRH analog × 6 m	1.5 years	8/14 (57)	4/14 (29)	2/14 (14)	TVUS and D&C or EMB at 6 months and 1 year	None
Pronin, 2015	32	LNG-IUD + goserelin monthly	Minimum 6 months	23/32 (72)	0/32 (0)	2/32 (6)	TVUS at 3 and 6 months, EMB at 3 months then TVUS/MRI and hysteroscopy D&C every 6 months	Not reported
Shan, 2013	26	D&C then MA 160 mg – increased dose for progression or no response	>/= 12 weeks	21/26 (81)	0/26 (0)	6/21 (29)	TVUS monthly until CR then every 3 months. D&C or EMB every 6 months	Weight gain, elevated GGT
Mazzon, 2010	6	Hysteroscopic resection followed by MA 160 mg	6 months	6/6 (100)	0/6 (0)	0/6 (0)	TVUS and D&C hysteroscopy every 3 months × 1 year then 6 months × 2 years	None

fertility-sparing management of grade 2–3 endometrial cancer or patients with myometrial invasion. The combined total included only 61 patients, with most studies reporting on only 1–3 patients. Response rates ranged from 0% to 100% (keeping in mind the sample size of 1–3). The largest series was reported by Park et al. (2013b) which included stage IA endometrial cancer of all histologic grades and some with myometrial invasion, treated with oral progestins. Overall, 77% (37/48) achieved complete response. Women with grade 2–3 histology and no myometrial invasion had a response rate of 76% (13/17), and recurrence rate of 23% (3/13), whereas those with grade 2–3 with superficial myometrial invasion had a complete response of 87% (7/8); however, recurrence rate was 71% (5/7). Those with stage IA, grade 1 with superficial myometrial invasion had a complete response of 73% (17/23) and recurrence rate of 47% (8/17) (Park et al. 2013a). Once a patient has achieved a complete response, the primary recommendation is for immediate attempt at pregnancy. If pregnancy is not desired or will be delayed, maintenance therapy is suggested via either oral progestin or LNG-IUD.

6 Risk of Recurrence

While many studies cited here report encouraging data on durable response to conservative management, lifetime remission is never a guarantee. According to Gallos et al., the recurrence rate for conservatively managed endometrial cancer in their large meta-analysis was 40.6% (Gallos et al. 2012). Conversely, in the comparison study of MA versus MPA, Park et al. showed a 55% durable response. Recurrence in this study was significantly associated with BMI >25. Protective factors included treatment with MPA, maintenance therapy after complete response, and pregnancy (Park et al. 2013a). Park et al. also examined the recurrence rates for women receiving infertility treatment compared to those who conceived without assistance and found no significant difference ($P = 0.335$). Again, pregnancy appeared to be protective as 76% of women who conceived were

disease free at 5-year follow-up versus 62% of women who did not conceive (Park et al. 2013d). Ichinose et al. report similar findings in a smaller cohort of women who had achieved complete response: 19% recurrence in the group achieving live birth versus 70% recurrence in the nulliparous group (Ichinose et al. 2013). In women with grade 2–3 disease or myometrial invasion, recurrence rises to 23–71% in Park's study, and the highest relapse rate was seen in the patients with evidence of myometrial invasion. On multivariate analysis, however, the group found that myometrial invasion itself was not an independent predictor of treatment failure (Park et al. 2013b).

Retreatment with oral progestins for recurrence after initial complete response continues to be studied. Park et al. have shown high complete (re)response rates with both MA and MPA (85%) as well as 85% durable complete response (Park et al. 2013c).

7 Fertility Outcomes

Pregnancy data after conservative management of endometrial cancer is relatively reassuring. In general, women who have achieved a complete response from endometrial cancer should be counseled to promptly pursue fertility if desired, as the reported recurrence rates are relatively high and frequently base-line risk factors for development of endometrial cancer have not changed. Referral to a reproductive endocrinologist is reasonable as many of these patients likely have underlying clinical risk factors for decreased fertility (PCOS, anovulation). Conversely, some patients have been diagnosed with EC while undergoing evaluation for infertility. The data on the safety of assisted reproductive therapies in the setting of prior endometrial cancer are limited. Most of the concern relates to the use of high-dose estrogen-based ovarian stimulation protocols, though a few studies have reported their relative safety. If patients do not seek immediate fertility, one should consider use of some type of hormonal maintenance therapy (progesterone-based, LNG-IUD, or combination oral contraceptive).

Reported pregnancy rates range from 25% to nearly 73% (Minig et al. 2011; Park et al. 2013d; Shan et al. 2013). In a large meta-analysis including 559 women, the live birth rate was approximately 28% (Gallos et al. 2012). Multiple studies have reported on nearly every form of assisted reproductive technology utilized by women achieving a complete response after conservative management. No studies have specifically compared the reported methods including ovulation induction with timed intercourse, hyperstimulation with intrauterine insemination, and in vitro fertilization.

The largest study to date by Park et al. followed 141 women who achieved remission with oral progestins. The overall live birth rate for the entire cohort was 26%, though if considering only those who attempted pregnancy, 73% conceived and 66% resulted in live births. Of those attempting pregnancy, one third had no assistance with reproduction, while two thirds underwent infertility treatments. Patients receiving infertility therapies were more successful at conceiving (86% vs. 50%) though both groups reported on patients who achieved multiple pregnancies. There were almost twice as many multiples in the treatment group compared to no treatment (11% vs. 6%). Out of a total 52 live births, only 2 anomalies were noted: one child with polydactyly and another with club foot. Ectopic and spontaneous abortion rates were similar in each group and approached population incidence. The preterm delivery rate was higher in the infertility treatment group (8% vs. 18%); however, this is likely related to higher incidence of multiple gestation pregnancies (Park et al. 2013d).

8   Surveillance

Upon achievement of remission, or complete response to therapy, surveillance measures must be performed thereafter, in order to monitor for potential recurrence and/or metastases. The National Comprehensive Cancer Network (NCCN) recommends surveillance with history, physical exam, and endometrial sampling every 3–6 months via D&C or in-office endometrial biopsy. Some investigators also have recommended checking serial CA-125, and use of imaging such as transvaginal ultrasound, MRI, or CT scans. These are not universally recommended but may be considered particularly if symptoms of potential metastases arise (pain, gastrointestinal, or genitourinary irregularities). Park et al. recommend against hysteroscopic biopsy during the follow-up period for women planning to conceive. The prevailing notion underlying this recommendation is that repetitive surgical disruption of the endometrium could negatively impact the basal layer and increase risk of intrauterine adhesions (Park and Nam 2015).

9   Definitive Management

In his review on conservative management of endometrial cancer, Park writes: "Surveillance after successful progestin therapy should include periodic interviews to explore any symptoms, physical examinations, and transvaginal ultrasonography at 3-month intervals. However, periodic pathologic evaluations of the endometrium, using office endometrial biopsy, D&C, or hysteroscopy, need not be recommended in patients who do not have symptoms or signs of recurrence"(Park and Nam 2015). The caveat to this recommendation is that once childbearing is complete, even in the absence of verified recurrence, hysterectomy should be performed. While some studies recommend hysterectomy if no response by 6–9 months, management and retreatment for up to 12 months without adverse effect has been reported (Park and Nam 2015).

While the discussion around ovarian preservation at the time of hysterectomy has been somewhat fraught, it appears this is a safe option especially in younger populations who stand to benefit from endogenous estrogens in their premenopausal years. Some studies have reported relatively high rates (19–25%) of concurrent ovarian malignancy in young patients undergoing hysterectomy and BSO for endometrial cancer (Soliman et al. 2005; Walsh et al. 2005). However, in a study of over 3000 women with endometrial cancer, 400 had ovarian preservation. In this large study, ovarian preservation had no effect on either cancer-specific or overall survival suggesting that ovarian preservation is safe (Wright et al. 2009).

10 Medically Inoperable Patients

Medically inoperable patients fall into two groups: low-grade/early stage whose medical comorbidities preclude surgical management, and advanced stage cases with diffuse metastatic disease that is considered unresectable. Data gathered in younger populations desiring fertility can be extrapolated to women with severe comorbidities who have low-grade endometrial cancers and provide good support for this option. A 2004 GOG study using MPA and Tamoxifen to treat advanced or recurrent endometrial cancer showed 33% response rate lending support to combinations of oral regimens (Whitney et al. 2004). The LNG-IUD has been more recently studied in populations whose multiple comorbidities prevent surgical management of endometrial cancer. Dhar et al. employed the IUD alone, while Montz et al. performed D&C with insertion of IUD. In each of these studies, complete response was observed in less than half of the study population (Dhar et al. 2005; Montz et al. 2002). Given favorable side effect profiles, progestins or the LNG-IUD may be preferable for early stage patients. Primary radiation and chemotherapy for medically inoperable patients are alternative methods which, though effective, carry high rates of side effects and toxicities. In a consensus statement from the American Brachytherapy Society, Schwarz et al. recommend dosing uterus, cervix, and upper 1–2 cm of vagina with brachytherapy and combining this treatment with external beam radiation (Schwarz et al. 2015). The Society of Gynecologic Oncology makes a Level A recommendation for chemotherapy in advanced endometrial cancer of any cell type. Moreover, chemotherapy in combination with radiotherapy provides improved response over either modality alone (Burke et al. 2014a). Finally, in a recent study conducted by Slomovitz et al., patients who had failed ≥ 2 chemotherapy regimens were treated with an mTOR inhibitor and aromatase inhibitor combination. The study population achieved 40% complete response with low toxicity (Slomovitz et al. 2015).

11 Conclusion

Conservative management of endometrial cancer, particularly in women with low-grade, early stage disease is a timely issue that is becoming more prominent with the rising obesity epidemic. There is increasing evidence in support of therapies that are largely hormone based; however, patients must be counseled in detail regarding the potential risk for cancer recurrence and that definitive treatment with hysterectomy is still recommended when feasible. With careful patient selection and adequate surveillance, fertility can be preserved for many young endometrial cancer patients, and those who achieve response are likely to be able to conceive and bear children. Conservative therapy may also be a very reasonable option for patients with severe comorbidities who are deemed nonsurgical candidates. Future studies may identify additional therapies in addition to progesterone-based agents for the conservative treatment of endometrial cancer.

12 Cross-References

▶ Diagnosis and Management of the Cancer of the Uterus
▶ Endometrial Hyperplasia
▶ Impact of Obesity on Gynecological Diseases
▶ Workup and Management of Polycystic Ovary Syndrome

References

ACS. American Cancer Society facts & figures 2015. American Cancer Society; 2015. Atlanta GA.
Bakkum-Gamez JN, Kalogera E, Keeney GL, Mariani A, Podratz KC, Dowdy SC. Conservative management of atypical hyperplasia and grade I endometrial carcinoma: review of the literature and presentation of a series. J Gynecol Surg. 2012;28(4):262–9.

Beiner ME, Finch A, Rosen B, Lubinski J, Moller P, Ghadirian P, et al. The risk of endometrial cancer in women with BRCA1 and BRCA2 mutations. A prospective study. Gynecol Oncol. 2007;104(1):7–10.

Bittoni MA, Fisher JL, Fowler JM, Maxwell GL, Paskett ED. Assessment of the effects of severe obesity and lifestyle risk factors on stage of endometrial cancer. Cancer Epidemiol Biomarkers Prev. 2013; 22(1):76–81.

Bokhman JV. Two pathogenetic types of endometrial carcinoma. Gynecol Oncol. 1983;15:10–7.

Bonadona V, Bonaiti B, Olschwang S, Grandjouan S, Huiart L, Longy M, et al. Cancer risks associated with germline mutations in MLH1, MSH2, and MSH6 genes in Lynch syndrome. JAMA. 2011;305(22):2304–10.

Brinton LA, Felix AS, McMeekin DS, Creasman WT, Sherman ME, Mutch D, et al. Etiologic heterogeneity in endometrial cancer: evidence from a Gynecologic Oncology Group trial. Gynecol Oncol. 2013;129(2):277–84.

Buchanan DD, Rosty C, Clendenning M, Spurdle AB, Win AK. Clinical problems of colorectal cancer and endometrial cancer cases with unknown cause of tumor mismatch repair deficiency (suspected Lynch syndrome). Appl Clin Genet. 2014;7:183–93.

Burke WM, Orr J, Leitao M, Salom E, Gehrig P, Olawaiye AB, et al. Endometrial cancer: a review and current management strategies: part II. Gynecol Oncol. 2014a;134(2):393–402.

Burke WM, Orr J, Leitao M, Salom E, Gehrig P, Olawaiye AB, et al. Endometrial cancer: a review and current management strategies: part I. Gynecol Oncol. 2014b;134(2):385–92.

Chen L-M, Berek J (2015) Endometrial carcinoma: epidemiology and risk factors. In: UpToDate, Post TW (ed) UpToDate, Waltham.

Choi MC, Jung SG, Park H, Cho YH, Lee C, Kim SJ. Fertility preservation via photodynamic therapy in young patients with early-stage uterine endometrial cancer: a long-term follow-up study. Int J Gynecol Cancer. 2013;23(4):698–704.

Creasman WT, Morrow CP, Bundy BN, Homesley HD, Graham JE, Heller PB. Surgical pathologic spread patterns of endometrial cancer. A Gynecologic Oncology Group Study. Cancer. 1987;60(8 Suppl):2035–41.

Dedes KJ, Wetterskog D, Ashworth A, Kaye SB, Reis-Filho JS. Emerging therapeutic targets in endometrial cancer. Nat Rev Clin Oncol. 2011;8(5):261–71.

Dhar KK, NeedhiRajan T, Koslowski M, Woolas RP. Is levonorgestrel intrauterine system effective for treatment of early endometrial cancer? Report of four cases and review of the literature. Gynecol Oncol. 2005;97(3):924–7.

Dijkhuizen FP, Mol BW, Brolmann HA, Heintz AP. The accuracy of endometrial sampling in the diagnosis of patients with endometrial carcinoma and hyperplasia: a meta-analysis. Cancer. 2000;89(8):1765–72.

Duska LR, Garrett A, Rueda BR, Haas J, Chang Y, Fuller AF. Endometrial cancer in women 40 years old or younger. Gynecol Oncol. 2001;83(2):388–93.

Ferguson SE, Aronson M, Pollett A, Eiriksson LR, Oza AM, Gallinger S, et al. Performance characteristics of screening strategies for Lynch syndrome in unselected women with newly diagnosed endometrial cancer who have undergone universal germline mutation testing. Cancer. 2014;120(24):3932–9.

Frolova AI, Babb SA, Zantow E, Hagemann AR, Powell MA, Thaker PH, et al. Impact of an immunohistochemistry-based universal screening protocol for Lynch syndrome in endometrial cancer on genetic counseling and testing. Gynecol Oncol. 2015;137(1):7–13.

Gallos ID, Yap J, Rajkhowa M, Luesley DM, Coomarasamy A, Gupta JK. Regression, relapse, and live birth rates with fertility-sparing therapy for endometrial cancer and atypical complex endometrial hyperplasia: a systematic review and metaanalysis. Am J Obstet Gynecol. 2012;207(4):266 e1–12.

Gunderson CC, Dutta S, Fader AN, Maniar KP, Nasseri-Nik N, Bristow RE, et al. Pathologic features associated with resolution of complex atypical hyperplasia and grade 1 endometrial adenocarcinoma after progestin therapy. Gynecol Oncol. 2014;132(1):33–7.

Ichinose M, Fujimoto A, Osuga Y, Minaguchi T, Kawana K, Yano T, et al. The influence of infertility treatment on the prognosis of endometrial cancer and atypical complex endometrial hyperplasia. Int J Gynecol Cancer. 2013;23(2):288–93.

Kalogera E, Dowdy SC, Bakkum-Gamez JN. Preserving fertility in young patients with endometrial cancer: current perspectives. Int J Womens Health. 2014;6:691–701.

Kang S, Kang WD, Chung HH, Jeong DH, Seo SS, Lee JM, et al. Preoperative identification of a low-risk group for lymph node metastasis in endometrial cancer: a Korean Gynecologic Oncology Group Study. J Clin Oncol. 2012;30(12):1329–34.

Kelley RM, Baker WH. The role of progesterone in human endometrial cancer. Cancer Res. 1965;25(7): 1190–2.

Kennedy AW, Austin Jr JM, Look KY, Munger CB. The Society of Gynecologic Oncologists Outcomes Task Force. Study of endometrical cancer: initial experiences. Gynecol Oncol. 2000;79(3):379–98.

Kim SH, Kim HD, Song YS, Kang SB, Lee HP. Detection of deep myometrial invasion in endometrial carcinoma: comparison of transvaginal ultrasound, CT, and MRI. J Comput Assist Tomogr. 1995;19(5):766–72.

Kinkel K, Kaji Y, Yu KK, Segal MR, Lu Y, Powell CB, et al. Radiologic staging in patients with endometrial cancer: a meta-analysis. Radiology. 1999;212(3): 711–8.

Kistner RW. Histological effects of progestins on hyperplasia and carcinoma in situ of the endometrium. Cancer. 1959;12:1106–22.

Ko EM, Walter P, Jackson A, Clark L, Franasiak J, Bolac C, et al. Metformin is associated with improved survival in endometrial cancer. Gynecol Oncol. 2014;132(2):438–42.

Kurnit KC, Ward KK, McHale MT, Saenz CC, Plaxe SC. Increased prevalence of comorbid conditions in women with uterine cancer. Gynecol Oncol. 2015;138 (3):731–4.

Lancaster JM, Powell CB, Kauff ND, Cass I, Chen LM, Lu KH, et al. Society of Gynecologic Oncologists Education Committee statement on risk assessment for inherited gynecologic cancer predispositions. Gynecol Oncol. 2007;107(2):159–62.

Leitao Jr MM, Kehoe S, Barakat RR, Alektiar K, Gattoc LP, Rabbitt C, et al. Comparison of D&C and office endometrial biopsy accuracy in patients with FIGO grade 1 endometrial adenocarcinoma. Gynecol Oncol. 2009;113(1):105–8.

Lentz SS, Brady MF, Major FJ, Reid GC, Soper JT. High-dose megestrol acetate in advanced or recurrent endometrial carcinoma: a Gynecologic Oncology Group Study. J Clin Oncol. 1996;14(2):357–61.

Lindor NM, Petersen GM, Hadley DW, Kinney AY, Miesfeldt S, Lu KH, et al. Recommendations for the care of individuals with an inherited predisposition to Lynch syndrome: a systematic review. JAMA. 2006;296(12):1507–17.

Lu KH, Dinh M, Kohlmann W, Watson P, Green J, Syngal S, et al. Gynecologic cancer as a "sentinel cancer" for women with hereditary nonpolyposis colorectal cancer syndrome. Obstet Gynecol. 2005;105 (3):569–74.

Mariani A, Webb MJ, Keeney GL, Haddock MG, Calori G, Podratz KC. Low-risk corpus cancer: is lymphadenectomy or radiotherapy necessary? Am J Obstet Gynecol. 2000;182(6):1506–19.

Matthews KS, Estes JM, Conner MG, Manne U, Whitworth JM, Huh WK, et al. Lynch syndrome in women less than 50 years of age with endometrial cancer. Obstet Gynecol. 2008;111(5):1161–6.

Mazzon I, Corrado G, Masciullo V, Morricone D, Ferrandina G, Scambia G. Conservative surgical management of stage IA endometrial carcinoma for fertility preservation. Fertil Steril. 2010;93(4):1286–9.

Mills AM, Liou S, Ford JM, Berek JS, Pai RK, Longacre TA. Lynch syndrome screening should be considered for all patients with newly diagnosed endometrial cancer. Am J Surg Pathol. 2014;38(11):1501–9.

Minig L, Franchi D, Boveri S, Casadio C, Bocciolone L, Sideri M. Progestin intrauterine device and GnRH analogue for uterus-sparing treatment of endometrial precancers and well-differentiated early endometrial carcinoma in young women. Ann Oncol. 2011; 22(3):643–9.

Montz FJ, Bristow RE, Bovicelli A, Tomacruz R, Kurman RJ. Intrauterine progesterone treatment of early endometrial cancer. Am J Obstet Gynecol. 2002;186 (4):651–7.

NCCN. National Comprehensive Cancer Network: uterine neoplasms (Version 2.2016). 2015 11/20/2015. Report No.: Contract No.: 11/24/2015.

Nevadunsky NS, Van Arsdale A, Strickler HD, Moadel A, Kaur G, Levitt J, et al. Obesity and age at diagnosis of endometrial cancer. Obstet Gynecol. 2014;124(2 Pt 1): 300–6.

Ogden CL, Carroll MD, Kit BK, Flegal KM. Prevalence of childhood and adult obesity in the United States, 2011–2012. JAMA. 2014;311(8):806–14.doi:10.1001/jama.2014.732.

Park JY, Nam JH. Progestins in the fertility-sparing treatment and retreatment of patients with primary and recurrent endometrial cancer. Oncologist. 2015; 20(3):270–8.

Park JY, Kim DY, Kim JH, Kim YM, Kim KR, Kim YT, et al. Long-term oncologic outcomes after fertility-sparing management using oral progestin for young women with endometrial cancer (KGOG 2002). Eur J Cancer. 2013a;49(4):868–74.

Park JY, Kim DY, Kim TJ, Kim JW, Kim JH, Kim YM, et al. Hormonal therapy for women with stage IA endometrial cancer of all grades. Obstet Gynecol. 2013b;122(1):7–14.

Park JY, Lee SH, Seong SJ, Kim DY, Kim TJ, Kim JW, et al. Progestin re-treatment in patients with recurrent endometrial adenocarcinoma after successful fertility-sparing management using progestin. Gynecol Oncol. 2013c;129(1):7–11.

Park JY, Seong SJ, Kim TJ, Kim JW, Kim SM, Bae DS, et al. Pregnancy outcomes after fertility-sparing management in young women with early endometrial cancer. Obstet Gynecol. 2013d;121(1):136–42.

Pronin SM, Novikova OV, Andreeva JY, Novikova EG. Fertility-sparing treatment of early endometrial cancer and complex atypical hyperplasia in young women of childbearing potential. Int J Gynecol Cancer. 2015;25(6):1010–4.

Reeves GK, Pirie K, Beral V, Green J, Spencer E, Bull D, et al. Cancer incidence and mortality in relation to body mass index in the Million Women Study: cohort study. BMJ. 2007;335(7630):1134.

Renehan AG, Tyson M, Egger M, Heller RF, Zwahlen M. Body-mass index and incidence of cancer: a systematic review and meta-analysis of prospective observational studies. Lancet. 2008;371(9612): 569–78.

Saltzman BS, Doherty JA, Hill DA, Beresford SA, Voigt LF, Chen C, et al. Diabetes and endometrial cancer: an evaluation of the modifying effects of other known risk factors. Am J Epidemiol. 2008;167(5):607–14.

Schwarz JK, Beriwal S, Esthappan J, Erickson B, Feltmate C, Fyles A, et al. Consensus statement for brachytherapy for the treatment of medically inoperable endometrial cancer. Brachytherapy. 2015; 14(5):587–99.

Setiawan VW, Yang HP, Pike MC, McCann SE, Yu H, Xiang YB, et al. Type I and II endometrial cancers: have they different risk factors? J Clin Oncol. 2013; 31(20):2607–18.

Shan BE, Ren YL, Sun JM, Tu XY, Jiang ZX, Ju XZ, et al. A prospective study of fertility-sparing treatment with megestrol acetate following hysteroscopic curettage for well-differentiated endometrioid carcinoma and atypical hyperplasia in young women. Arch Gynecol Obstet. 2013;288(5):1115–23.

Slomovitz BM, Jiang Y, Yates MS, Soliman PT, Johnston T, Nowakowski M, et al. Phase II study of everolimus and letrozole in patients with recurrent endometrial carcinoma. J Clin Oncol. 2015;33(8): 930–6.

Soliman PT, Oh JC, Schmeler KM, Sun CC, Slomovitz BM, Gershenson DM, et al. Risk factors for young premenopausal women with endometrial cancer. Obstet Gynecol. 2005;105(3):575–80.

Truong PT, Kader HA, Lacy B, Lesperance M, MacNeil MV, Berthelet E, et al. The effects of age and comorbidity on treatment and outcomes in women with endometrial cancer. Am J Clin Oncol. 2005;28(2):157–64.

Ushijima K, Yahata H, Yoshikawa H, Konishi I, Yasugi T, Saito T, et al. Multicenter phase II study of fertility-sparing treatment with medroxyprogesterone acetate for endometrial carcinoma and atypical hyperplasia in young women. J Clin Oncol. 2007;25(19):2798–803.

Walsh C, Holschneider C, Hoang Y, Tieu K, Karlan B, Cass I. Coexisting ovarian malignancy in young women with endometrial cancer. Obstet Gynecol. 2005;106(4):693–9.

Whitney CW, Brunetto VL, Zaino RJ, Lentz SS, Sorosky J, Armstrong DK, et al. Phase II study of medroxyprogesterone acetate plus tamoxifen in advanced endometrial carcinoma: a Gynecologic Oncology Group Study. Gynecol Oncol. 2004; 92(1):4–9.

Wright JD, Buck AM, Shah M, Burke WM, Schiff PB, Herzog TJ. Safety of ovarian preservation in premenopausal women with endometrial cancer. J Clin Oncol. 2009;27(8):1214–9.

Diagnosis and Management of Epithelial Ovarian Cancer

Katherine Nixon and Christina Fotopoulou

Abstract

Ovarian cancer is the fifth most common cancer among women after breast, bowel, lung, and endometrial and remains the leading cause of death due to gynecological malignancy (Cancer.org 2016). Epithelial ovarian cancer accounts for the vast majority of ovarian malignancies with figures of around 85%. Due to its insidious nature of presentation, it is often not diagnosed until the later stages leading to a high mortality rate. Five-year survival is very much influenced by stage at diagnosis. Over the last 20 years, incidence and mortality have remained fairly static, and much research is being undertaken looking for aids to diagnosis, possible screening methods, and improvement in treatment options, both surgical and medical. In this chapter we will discuss presentation, diagnostic tools, and possible management regimes for patients with epithelial ovarian cancer.

K. Nixon (✉)
Department of Gynecology, Imperial College NHS Trust, Queen Charlottes and Hammersmith Hospital, London, UK
e-mail: Katherine.nixon@hotmail.co.uk

C. Fotopoulou (✉)
Department of Gynaecological Oncology, West London Gynecological Cancer Centre, Imperial College NHS Trust, Queen Charlottes and Hammersmith Hospital, London, UK
e-mail: chfotopoulou@gmail.com

Keywords

Epithelial • Diagnosis • Imaging • Staging • Management

Contents

© Springer International Publishing AG 2017
D. Shoupe (ed.), *Handbook of Gynecology*,
DOI 10.1007/978-3-319-17798-4_1

1   Introduction

Epithelial ovarian cancer (EOC) is the second most common genital malignancy after uterine cancer in women and accounts for the majority of deaths from gynecological malignancies in Western countries (Jemal et al. 2007). Lifetime risk is about 1.6%; the latest data show that 1 in 43 women will develop EOC during their lifetime. Women with a mutated BRCA1 or BRCA2 gene are at increased risk ranging between 25% and 60% depending on the specific mutation.

Despite the continuous advances in diagnostics and imaging, more than 70% of the patients with newly diagnosed EOC will present with an advanced stage FIGO III and IV. This is mainly attributed to the unusual tumor biology and clinical behavior of the disease, which is typically associated with locoregional dissemination throughout the peritoneal cavity. This behavior results in a delay of symptoms until only at a later stage in a rather nonspecific pattern, including abdominal bloating and distention with pain, urinary frequency, postmenopausal bleeding, loss of appetite, and occasionally rectal bleeding (Goff 2012). This unusual natural history has therefore generated unique therapeutic strategies that highlight the important contribution of locoregional control to survival for this disease (Vaughn et al. 2011).

The last decades have brought a significant advance in the treatment of EOC, both in surgical and systemic aspects, with the development and addition to standard treatment of extensive cytoreductive techniques, refinement of surgical skills in the upper abdomen, dose-dense regimes, and novel targeted therapies. Nevertheless, the survival rate of women with EOC has changed little since the revolutionary platinum-

based treatment that was introduced more than 30 years ago (Omura 1986).

Only in the recent years, targeted therapies based on the principle of antiangiogenesis (Monk 2009) and homologous recombination repair mechanisms have brought a significant efficacy in the treatment of EOC: bevacizumab, pazopanib, and olaparib have proven in a maintenance regime during and/or after successful chemotherapy their efficacy in significantly prolonging progression-free survival (PFS), but failed to significantly influence the overall survival of the patients (Janczar et al. 2009). A possible mechanism discussed for this consistent discrepancy is the high rate of crossover in the subsequent lines that contaminate any survival benefit attributed to each agent.

Great changes in the way we understand ovarian cancers have occurred in the last decade. Traditionally ovarian cancers have been categorized based on their origin either from mesothelial epithelial cells, germ cells, or stromal cells, this being based on the theory that epithelial ovarian cancers arise from the ovarian epithelium. However it is now widely believed that high-grade serous ovarian cancers more likely arise from the epithelium of the fallopian tubes and ovarian deposits are therefore secondary implants. As such these are now investigated and managed as a group with primary peritoneal carcinomas (Kurman et al. 2010). Epithelial ovarian malignancies are histologically divided into serous carcinoma, mucinous carcinoma, endometrioid carcinoma, undifferentiated carcinoma, and clear cell carcinoma. These are further divided into low-grade and high-grade subtypes with low grade tending to be more stable and high grade behaving aggressively and usually presenting at an advanced stage (Doufekas 2014).

Management and prognosis are determined by stage at presentation and histological grading following biopsy or debulking surgery. The etiology of epithelial ovarian cancers has been studied at length. Factors found to increase risk include age, with most diagnoses made after 40 years, a steep curve after 50, and peak in the 80s. Around 10% of ovarian cancers have a hereditary component with the vast majority being BRCA1 and two mutations; there is also an association with hereditary non-polyposis colorectal cancer. Previous breast cancer, nulliparity, history of endometriosis, and long-term use of hormone replacement therapy have also all been shown to increase risk of ovarian cancer. Conversely, prolonged use of combined oral contraceptive medication, parity, and breastfeeding have been associated with risk reduction as well as history of tubal ligation and hysterectomy. Recent evidence even suggests that women who give birth to their first child in their mid-30s or later may have an even lower risk of ovarian cancer compared to those who gave birth to their first child earlier than that. Each 5-year increase in a woman's age at birth of their first child seems to correspond to a 16% lower risk of ovarian cancer. This association is not fully understood; however a possible mechanism is a progesterone-mediated effect which seems to be more prevalent and efficient in older women.

2   Presentation

Ovarian cancer often presents at a late stage and can be difficult to diagnose. This is because the signs and symptoms tend to be nonspecific and are sometimes put down to gastrointestinal upset. Common symptoms include bloating, loss of appetite, abdominal pain, disturbance in urinary or bowel habit, and weight loss. Patients may have increased abdominal girth, evidence of pelvic mass and ascites, bowel obstruction, and, depending on stage of presentation, a cachectic appearance.

Correct diagnosis is often delayed either because patients do not present to a medical professional or due to initial misdiagnosis of conditions such as irritable bowel disease, diverticular disease, and urinary tract infection.

3   Diagnosis

3.1   History and Assessment

If a diagnosis of ovarian cancer is suspected, a referral should be made to a specialist gynecological oncology center.

In clinic a full history should be taken including symptoms, age, parity, past medical history, and past surgical and gynecological history, especially focusing on risk factors, e.g., previous endometriosis or malignancies. Although the majority of patients will present postmenopausal, it is important to determine a patients' wishes with regard to fertility if premenopausal as this may influence management. Past surgical history is important as most treatment options for epithelial ovarian cancer will involve surgery and previous abdominal operations could complicate this. Different options for management will also be determined by the patients' performance status; therefore a full medical history is important to include, e.g., history of diabetes, respiratory or cardiac diseases, and smoking status. Social history should include who their support system is (family/friends), given the gravity of potential diagnosis being made. It will also contribute to the assessment of a patient's performance status; for example, someone requiring nursing home care will likely be a more complex surgical candidate than someone who is independent and living in their own home. Fragility scores predicting surgical outcome in older patients with comorbidities have not been well defined in ovarian cancer surgery; it is however the focus of various currently ongoing studies.

Examination in clinic should include patients' BMI, blood pressure, and heart rate. These simple observations will help indicate their current health status. Abdominal examination should assess for distension, presence of a mass or ascites, any tenderness, and previous scars. Vaginal examination will help with assessment of size and mobility of a pelvic mass, an indication of the likely difficulty of surgery. Rectal examination is helpful in determining any invasion of disease and to help instruct if rectal resection is likely to be necessary.

4   Bloods

Initial blood tests should include baseline full blood count, renal, and liver function and tumor markers to help determine the origin of the cancer.

Markers should be sent for cancer antigen 125 (Ca125) for ovarian pathology, carcinoembryonic antigen (CEA) for colorectal, carbohydrate antigen 19-9 (Ca 19-9) for pancreatic/gastrointestinal malignancies, and possibly alpha-fetoprotein if germ cell tumor is suspected. Ca 125 has a low sensitivity of 55% as it can be raised due to many processes in the pelvis, usually inflammation from infection or endometriosis. The ration of CA125 to CA199 could indicate a non-ovarian pathology and dictate the necessity of further investigations like colonoscopy. Some epithelial ovarian cancers will not express Ca125 and this makes them more difficult to follow-up posttreatment.

5   Imaging

Transvaginal ultrasound is the most commonly used modality for first-line imaging in epithelial ovarian cancer. It can demonstrate the presence of pelvic mass and the characteristics of the mass. It can also detect any free fluid in the pelvis and assess if the adnexal structures are fixed or mobile indicating the possible presence of adhesions. Features suggestive of malignancy include a multilocular mass, presence of papillary structures, solid areas, and a mass with increased vascularity on Doppler ultrasound. Risk of malignancy index can be used to help assess the likelihood of a mass being malignant. This is done by a simple calculation of a score given to the ultrasound findings, the menopausal status of the patient, and the Ca125 level (NICE 2011). The International Ovarian Tumor Analysis (IOTA) guidance may be used for premenopausal women (Timmerman 2010). Simple rules were applicable in 77% of adnexal masses and when inconclusive masses were considered as malignant, reporting a sensitivity of 91% and specificity of 93%. Guidance could consider supporting recruitment into ongoing trials that evaluate diagnostic tests and presurgical triage.

Magnetic resonance imaging (MRI) of the pelvis is used to correlate with USS to help further determine the nature of a mass in patients with the absence of metastatic sites and with fertility sparing wish, for additional guidance in regard to whether such an approach would be advisable or feasible.

Computerized tomography (CT) is used to evaluate stage and tumor dissemination pattern of the disease and especially identify distant intraparenchymatous metastases that would determine operability and course of optimal therapeutic approach. Additionally, chest pathology like pulmonary embolism, mediastinal lymphadenopathy, etc., can be identified and have impact on therapeutic decisions.

Epithelial ovarian cancer acts like a rash within the abdomen using the peritoneum as a vector; the disease is most commonly seen on the peritoneum covering the pelvis, bladder, para-colic areas, upper abdominal structures, and diaphragm. Omental disease can occur in deposits or forming one large "cake" of disease. Para-aortic and pelvic lymph nodes may be enlarged. CT can assess the presence of disease on the splenic surface and liver capsule plus any deposits on small/large bowel serosa, mesentery, and any more invasive lesions that may require a bowel resection to remove. CT PET (positron emission tomography) scans use a radioactive glucose solution which is injected into patients and the uptake monitored. The glucose solution is more readily taken up by cancerous cells, and therefore this imaging modality is useful in helping to locate areas of metastasis and also disease activity in lymph nodes. The rate of uptake can also advise on the potential grade of the cancer.

6   Pathology

Examination, blood results, and imaging may be sufficient to provide a working diagnosis of ovarian cancer, and even though histological diagnosis prior to primary surgery is not mandatory, it would be advisable to be available in borderline cases with atypical clinical pattern, in young women with fertility sparing wish – in which case a two-stage approach should be followed. If ascites is present, this can be drained and samples sent for both cytology and microscopy. Biopsies may be taken from tumor deposits demonstrated on imaging on the peritoneum or omentum or sometimes from the mass itself; this is usually done under USS or CT guidance. Occasionally the histology is already known from previous surgery such as an oophorectomy for ovarian cyst at another unit, and the patient is then referred to the specialist unit for ongoing management. If a CT- or US-guided biopsy is not technically possible, then a laparoscopic histological confirmation should be performed.

7   Staging

Using the imaging a provisional staging can be made. It should be noted that full staging will come after surgery, if this takes place, once the suspicious tissues have been removed and examined histologically. Imaging may indicate affected areas which turn out to be benign after excision and vice versa.

The staging for ovarian cancer as per FIGO 2014 is as follows (Helm 2014)

Stage I consists of tumor limited to the ovaries or fallopian tubes

Stage IA includes the following	
Tumor limited to one ovary (capsule intact) or fallopian tube	
No tumor on the external surface of the ovary or fallopian tube	
No malignant cells in ascites or peritoneal washings	
Stage IB includes the following	
Tumor limited to both ovaries (capsules intact) or fallopian tubes	
No tumor on the external surface of the ovaries or fallopian tubes	
No malignant cells in ascites or peritoneal washings	
Stage IC includes tumor limited to one or both ovaries or fallopian tubes, with any of the following:	
Stage IC1	Surgical spill
Stage IC2	Capsule ruptured before surgery, or tumor on ovarian or fallopian tube surface
Stage IC3	Malignant cells in the ascites or peritoneal washings

(continued)

Stage II tumor involves one or both ovaries or fallopian tubes, with pelvic extension (below pelvic brim) or primary peritoneal cancer

Stage IIA	Extension and/or implants on the uterus and/or ovaries and/or fallopian tubes
Stage IIB	Extension to other pelvic intraperitoneal tissues

Stage III tumor involves one or both ovaries or fallopian tubes, or primary peritoneal cancer, with cytologically or histologically confirmed spread to the peritoneum outside the pelvis and/or metastasis to the retroperitoneal lymph nodes

Stage IIIA1	Positive (cytologically or histologically proven) retroperitoneal lymph nodes only
Stage IIIA1(i)	Metastasis up to 10 mm in greatest dimension
Stage IIIA1(ii)	Metastasis more than 10 mm in greatest dimension
Stage IIIA2	Microscopic extrapelvic (above the pelvic brim) peritoneal involvement with or without positive retroperitoneal lymph nodes

Stage IIIB involves macroscopic peritoneal metastasis beyond the pelvis up to 2 cm in greatest dimension, with or without metastasis to the retroperitoneal lymph nodes

Stage IIIC involves macroscopic peritoneal metastasis beyond the pelvis more than 2 cm in greatest dimension, with or without metastasis to the retroperitoneal lymph nodes. Stage IIIC includes extension of tumor to the capsule of liver and spleen without parenchymal involvement of either organ

Stage IV

Stage IV consists of distant metastasis, excluding peritoneal metastases, and includes the following:

Stage IVA: Pleural effusion with positive cytology

Stage IVB: Parenchymal metastases and metastases to extra-abdominal organs (including inguinal lymph nodes and lymph nodes outside of the abdominal cavity)

8   Management

Treatment of epithelial ovarian cancer is from a multidisciplinary approach based on input from expert gynecological oncologists, medical oncologists, pathologists, and radiologists. In comprehensive cancer centers, patients should ideally be additionally supported by a specialist nurse to help them with their treatment journey (Vernooji 2007). The mainstay of treatment is surgical cytoreduction combined with systemic agents.

9   Definition of Surgery in EOC

The large differences in current practice nationally and internationally are also being reflected in the discrepancy in the terminology used to adequately characterize the different types of surgery at the different stages of the disease. A clarification of the various definitions used broadly is necessary before proceeding so that the context is clear:

- Exploratory surgery: usually laparoscopically to assess intraperitoneal dissemination patterns; the value of this in assessing operability is highly questionable and not standard practice, unless to set histological diagnosis or in cases of unclear ascites with absent ovarian mass or peritoneal disease at imaging.
- Primary or upfront cytoreduction: tumor debulking at initial diagnosis before any systemic treatment, aiming at maximal tumor reduction and ideally total macroscopic tumor clearance.
- Interval debulking: cytoreductive surgery after usually three cycles of neoadjuvant chemotherapy.
- Second look surgery: exploratory laparotomy or laparoscopy after completion of systemic treatment to confirm response; this method is obsolete, since it has no evidence of survival benefit.
- Secondary surgery: surgery due to the first relapse. Here definition is unclear in regard to aim; usually used to describe cytoreductive effort but can also be used for palliative surgery due to symptoms at first relapse.
- Tertiary surgery: the equivalent of secondary surgery at the second relapse.
- Quaternary surgery: the equivalent of secondary surgery at the third relapse.
- Palliative surgery: surgery aiming at palliation of tumor-induced symptoms, such as bowel obstruction and intestinal perforation, where conservative management has failed.

The maximum diameter of the postoperative residual tumor after cytoreductive surgery is considered the strongest independent clinical prognostic factor (Du Bois et al. 2009). Bristow et al. published for the first time a systematic meta-analysis on this subject based on a total of 53 studies with 6885 patients overall (period: 1989–1998).

They studied the influence of surgical tumor resection on overall survival. Published studies with surgically operated patients with FIGO stage III or IV and subsequent platinum-based chemotherapy were evaluated. According to this meta-analysis, patient cohorts that had had a maximum tumor reduction rate (<2 cm) of over 75% had a median overall survival of 36.8 months. By contrast, patient cohorts with a maximum tumor reduction rate of less than 25% had a median overall survival of only 23 months. Every 10% reduction in tumor was associated with a 6.3% prolongation of median overall survival (Bristow et al. 2002).

There is internationally ongoing debate as to the best timing of surgery, whether this should be done at the outset of treatment or following a course of neoadjuvant chemotherapy. However, the general recommended course of treatment for those patients with good performance status and resectable disease is primary debulking surgery followed by adjuvant chemotherapy (Colombo et al. 2009). Neoadjuvant chemotherapy can be used if the extent of the disease at the time of presentation is deemed to be not suitable for surgical resection; the patient is not fit enough to undergo a primary debulking due to advanced age, low performance status, and comorbidities, or for bridging acute events like thromboembolic episodes. Nevertheless, practice regarding the optimal upfront approach varies strongly between centers and countries and often depends on the gynecological oncology center and experience of surgeon. Two prospective randomized trials (Vergote et al. 2010; Kehoe et al. 2015) have demonstrated lower surgical morbidity and mortality in the neoadjuvant approach; however the oncologic safety is being doubted since both trials included mainly patients who had undergone in their majority suboptimal cytoreduction with much lower resection rates then anticipated in specialized centers for the disease. For that reason, future prospective randomized trials with strictly defined surgical quality are warranted in order to answer this question and establish optimal practice. These future trials will address additional issues such as management of fragile patients, assessment of short- and long-term quality of life scores, impact of ascites, and pleura effusion on hemodynamic management and would also have an additional translational portfolio in an attempt to identify valid biomarkers that would predict operability and clinical outcome. These are often extensive operations with the possibility of large volume shifts. Therefore, anesthetic involvement prior to proceeding is recommended and an ITU bed may be indicated. Surgery for ovarian cancer should always ideally be carried out by an experienced gynecological oncology surgeon (Eisenkop 1992; Paulsen 2006).

10 Tumor Dissemination Patterns at Relapse

A better understanding of the tumor dissemination patterns followed in the primary and subsequently in the recurrent situation of EOC is highly essential for the better understanding of the disease and may enhance the evolution and refinement of surgical and, by extension, systemic approach (Gabra 2010). Nevertheless, data correlating the tumor dissemination pattern and surgical outcome in primary and later recurrent situation at the same patient hardly exist. A prospectively maintained database evaluating the intraoperative tumor dissemination pattern and operative outcome of all women who underwent both primary and secondary tumor-debulking surgeries in the same institution within a 10-year period of time has been systematically analyzed (Braicu 2011). On the basis of 79 patients, it could be demonstrated that secondary cytoreduction appears to be associated with significantly lower optimal tumor-debulking rates compared to primary debulking, mainly attributed to less "accessible" recurring patterns such as gastrointestinal serosa, radix mesenterii, gastric serosa, and porta hepatis. Interestingly, no significant predictors of surgical outcome or tumor pattern, such as peritoneal carcinomatosis, intestinal tumor involvement, or positive lymph nodes, could be identified between

primary and relapse. It appeared that a different tumor "behavior" is followed in the primary compared to recurrent situation of the disease even in the same patient, while interestingly the primary tumor patterns do not appear to have any predictive value for the tumor patterns at recurrence, apart from the predictive value of initial tumor residuals which clearly correlate with the amount of postoperative tumor residuals at relapse. Venturing even beyond surgical borders, one could say that ovarian cancer reappears under a different dissemination profile than at its initial presentation in terms of a higher "aggressivity" and higher dissemination tendency. Any potential attempts to derive clinically relevant conclusions on the outcome of the forthcoming cytoreduction depending on the outcome and tumor dissemination at the outset of the disease would rather fail. Therefore, novel biomarkers are warranted in order to predict tumor patterns followed at recurrence and hence surgical outcome.

The role of imaging is also unclear in the characterization of peritoneal carcinosis as definite basis for indication for surgery at relapse, even though PET-CT appears to have higher accuracy indices than simple CT. Results suggest that PET/CT may prove a useful tool for presurgical staging of ovarian cancer with a sensitivity and specificity of 78% and 68%, respectively. In a prospective trial correlating the PET-CT results with laparoscopic findings, PET/CT showed an adequate correlation between SUVmax values and laparoscopy findings of lesions >5 mm, but a high rate of false negative results in lesions <5 mm such as in carcinomatosis (De Iaco 2010). Clinical decision-making processes should therefore be very carefully constructed around clinical findings and symptoms and history of the disease and not on imaging alone.

Interestingly, it appears that patterns of relapse may also be altered depending on the primary mode of treatment. In a retrospective evaluation of 175 stage IIIC-IV EOC patients who were operated in an Italian gynecology cancer center with diffuse peritoneal carcinosis, patterns of relapse were stratified according to whether the patient had upfront or interval debulking surgery at initial presentation (Petrillo et al. 2013). Forty patients received complete primary debulking surgery, and the remaining 135 were treated with neoadjuvant chemotherapy followed by interval debulking surgery with absent residual tumor after surgery. No differences were observed in the distribution of clinical pathological characteristics at the time of diagnosis between the two groups. In a median follow-up period of 31 months (range 9–150 months), the authors observed 20 (50.0%) recurrences in the upfront group compared to 103 (76.3%) in the interval debulking group. Duration of primary platinum-free interval was also significantly shorter in the interval debulking arm (13 vs. 21 months, respectively). A significantly higher percentage of patients in the interval debulking group experienced platinum-resistant recurrences and carcinomatosis at the time of relapse. Also the platinum-free interval of second relapse was significantly longer in favor of the upfront arm. This documented more "favorable behavior" of recurrent disease in EOC patients with diffuse peritoneal carcinomatosis treated with complete upfront surgical approach compared to women submitted to neoadjuvant chemotherapy needs to be prospectively validated in larger datasets; however it does give a clear signal about the highly significant impact of the quality of upfront treatment even in peritoneal disseminated disease.

11   Value of Secondary Cytoreduction

There is clear evidence that patients experiencing an early platinum resistant or even refractory EOC relapse are highly unlikely to benefit from secondary debulking surgery. Older reports could demonstrate very dismal overall survival rates of a mean value of 8 months, not adequately justifying a radical surgical approach but rather concentrating on palliation (Morris et al. 1989; Segna 1993). Anecdotal and empirical case reports may demonstrate a survival benefit in platinum-resistant patients who present with early lymph node relapse which rather represents a persistent lymph node metastasis not removed through lymph node dissection at primary surgery and

hence not representing a true relapse (Chan 2007). The selection of these patients however is very challenging and no randomized data will ever exist for this special subgroup of women. Caution should be awarded to adequately judge and evaluate situations always taking into consideration the quality of surgery at primary or interval debulk and the tumor dissemination pattern at relapse.

The first systematic data analysis for secondary debulking in a platinum-sensitive setting originates from the German AGO (Arbeitsgemeinschaft Gynaekologische Onkologie) within the DESKTOP I trial (Harter et al. 2006). This was a retrospective evaluation of 267 patients which showed that patients appeared to benefit from surgery in recurrent EOC only when total macroscopic clearance was achieved. Complete tumor resection was associated with significantly longer survival compared with surgery leaving any postoperative residuals. Hence, the challenge was to accurately preoperatively identify the optimal candidates for surgery, in order to avoid surgical procedures that would not have a prognosis benefit for the patients. Based on a multivariate model, three factors were identified as independently predicting resectability, building so the so-called AGO score: good performance status, complete resection at primary surgery, and absence of ascites. The value of the AGO score lies with others also in the simplicity to use, based on easy-to-assess clinical features and not on complicated mathematic algorithms that would make its use in the daily routine very challenging. An exploratory analysis of the DESKTOP results to evaluate the role of peritoneal carcinomatosis present in recurrent EOC clearly showed that even though peritoneal carcinomatosis was a negative predictor for complete resection in the recurrent situation of the disease, it appeared to have no negative impact on survival if total macroscopic clearance could be achieved. The authors concluded that improving surgical skills might increase the patient proportion that could benefit from surgery for recurrent disease (Harter et al. 2009).

A subsequent confirmation and validation of the AGO score followed within the prospective, multicenter DESKTOP II trial, in which the AGO score could be confirmed as a useful and reliable tool to predict complete tumor resection in more than two thirds of patients with platinum-sensitive relapsed EOC (Harter et al. 2011). Participating centers prospectively enrolled patients with platinum-sensitive first or second relapse. The AGO score was then applied to all patients, but each center was free to decide the therapeutic management. A total of 516 patients were screened within 19 months; of these, 261 patients (51%) were classified as score positive, and 129 patients with a positive score and first relapse received a secondary tumor debulking. The rate of complete resection was 76%, thus confirming the validity of this score regarding positive prediction of complete resectability in more than two thirds of patients. Interestingly on analysis poor correlation of imaging and intraoperative findings was found, both in terms of number of lesions identified and localization of tumor.

Perioperative morbidity and mortality appeared to be acceptable within the DESKTOP series with a mortality as low as 0.8% and an 11% relaparotomy rate mainly due to bowel leakage or fistula (7%). DVT rate was 2%, while 52% of the patients required a postoperative intensive care stay of a median 2 days (range: 1–20). Morbidity and mortality data of other equivalent series are in a similar level.

A subsequent multicenter randomized trial, the DESKTOP III (AGO-Ovar OP.4.), commenced in June 2010, to prospectively evaluate the impact of recurrent EOC-surgery in platinum-sensitive patients with positive AGO score (tumor-free initial surgery, good performance status, and ascites <500 ml). The study has completed recruiting all 409 preplanned patients and results are now awaited within the next 2–3 years. This very important study is anticipated to finally answer the question whether surgery at the relapse situation of the disease is truly associated with a benefit for survival and quality of life of the affected patients.

The equivalent American trial from the GOG (GOG 0213) has been recruiting for a longer period than the DESKTOP trial, however in a slower rhythm. A further difference is the additional randomization to systemic bevacizumab 15 mg/m^2 at maintenance. There are future plans to combine data of both trials together to achieve a larger cohort and more robust survival data.

The largest retrospective multicenter and multinational analysis worldwide showed equivalent results (Zang et al. 2011; Tian et al. 2012). Of the 1075 evaluated patients, 434 (40.4%) underwent complete resection. Total macroscopic tumor clearance was associated with a significant improvement in survival, from a median OS of 57.7 months, when compared with only 27.0 months in those with residual disease of 0.1–1 cm and 15.6 months in those with residual disease of >1 cm, respectively. Complete secondary cytoreduction was associated with six variables: FIGO stage, residual disease after primary cytoreduction, PFS, Eastern Cooperative Oncology Group (ECOG) performance status, CA125, and ascites at recurrence. These variables were entered into the risk model and assigned scores ranging from 0 to 11.9. Patients with total scores of 0–4.7 were categorized as the low-risk group, in which the proportion of complete cytoreduction was 53.4% compared with 20.1% in the high-risk group. In external validation, the sensitivity and specificity was 83.3% and 57.6%, respectively.

In one systematic meta-analysis by Bristow et al. where 40 cohorts of 2019 patients with recurrent EOC were identified over a period of 24 years, it could be clearly shown that, after controlling of all other disease-related factors, each 10% increase in the proportion of patients undergoing complete cytoreductive surgery was associated with a 3-month increase in median cohort survival time (Bristow 2009).

Despite the very encouraging retrospective data, it is still not clear if the actual tumor resection is significantly influencing survival or if it is just a surrogate marker of more "favorable" tumor biology and therefore associated with a better overall prognosis. The first two prospectively randomized surgical trials will definitely answer this question, change clinical practice worldwide, and set new evidence-based standards.

12   Value of Tertiary Cytoreduction

The scenery is even more vague and undefined in the second relapse of EOC. Obtaining palliation in cases of severe tumor-induced symptoms like bowel obstruction may often be the main purpose of tertiary cytoreduction (TCS); still, the potential prolongation of survival and improvement of quality of life may also constitute relevant goals even in a tertiary setting of this chronic disease. Experiences regarding TCS were recently only limited in six monocentric analyses including a small number of patients. All conclude mainly to the fact that TCS may indeed offer a survival benefit in a highly select group of recurrent EOC patients and that this benefit appears to be greatest in those patients in whom a complete gross resection can be achieved (Shih et al. 2010; Hizli et al. 2012). Leitao et al. was the first to report on 26 patients who had undergone TCS at a single institution (Leito et al. 2004). Treatment-free interval before TCS and current postoperative residual disease could be identified as independent prognostic factors for survival, whereas time to first recurrence failed to retain prognostic significance in the multivariate analysis. Interestingly, platinum resistance failed to be identified as being significantly associated with a more dismal outcome. No independent factors predicting optimal cytoreduction could be identified among common clinical factors such as advanced age, residual disease after initial surgery, time to first recurrence, time from second cytoreduction, platinum-sensitivity as well as size and site of tumor-recurrence.

A further retrospective report by Karam et al. (2007) evaluating the outcome of 47 EOC patients undergoing tertiary cytoreduction confirmed the statistically significant superior overall survival in patients with microscopic versus macroscopic residual disease (24 vs. 16 months). After controlling these analyses for age, time to progression, and optimal residual disease during TCS, the authors identified only the presence of diffuse peritoneal carcinosis, at tertiary exploration as significant predictor of a worse overall survival. In a subanalysis of patients with limited disease implants, multivariate analysis could indeed indicate that total macroscopic tumor clearance at TCS retains prognostic significance of overall survival, so that the authors concluded that size of disease implants on preoperative imaging may guide the selection of ideal candidates for TCS. Regarding the assessment of potential preoperative predictors of optimal TCS, the authors could identify only tumor size (<5 cm) as a statistically significant predictor of complete tumor resection at TCS. Other variables like presence of ascites, initial disease-free interval, age at TCS, and limited number of disease sites on preoperative imaging (i.e., <4) could not show any significant impact.

In a smaller analysis including only 20 patients, the authors concluded to opposing results, challenging the benefit of TCS in EOC (Gultekin et al. 2008). Multivariate analysis could identify neither any significant predictors for optimal cytoreduction nor any significant prognostic factors for survival. Major intrinsic pitfalls of this particular analysis are though, as emphasized by the authors themselves, the small sample of patients, rendering a multivariate analysis to have to be interpreted with caution. Furthermore, the authors defined as "optimal" cytoreduction residual disease of <2 cm, and not, as universally accepted, microscopic or <0.5 cm tumor residuals.

The largest monocentric TCS analysis evaluated 135 patients, and identified tumor involvement of the middle abdomen and peritoneal carcinomatosis as the two only parameters negatively affecting tumor resection (Fotopoulou et al. 2011).

A recent project published the largest multicentric analysis on TCS worldwide including 406 patients (median age, 55y; range,16–80) who underwent TCS between 1997 and 2011 in 12 centers across Europe, the USA, and Asia (Fotopoulou et al. Jan 2013). This represents the largest series so far in the tertiary setting of the disease and considering the fact that the conduction of any prospectively randomized trial in this advanced stage will be very challenging if not impossible, this constitutes currently the most valuable source of experience. The majority of the patients had an advanced initial FIGO stage

III/IV (69%), peritoneal carcinomatosis (51.7%), and absence of ascites (72.2%). Two hundred twenty-four (54.1%) patients underwent complete tumor resection. The most frequent tumor dissemination site was the pelvis (73%). This confirmed the knowledge from the previous results that even in the tertiary setting complete macroscopic tumor clearance plays a significant role both on overall and progression-free survival overruling the factor peritoneal carcinomatosis which failed to retain any prognostic significance on survival after controlling for tumor residual status. Median OS for patients without versus any tumor residuals was 49 versus 12 months. Most importantly, common clinicopathologic characteristics such as tumor stage, age, and histological subtype, which have been shown to be of significant predictive value at initial presentation of the disease, did not appear to be of any prognostic significance at the tertiary stage. A significant impact of third line postoperative systemic chemotherapy on overall survival was identified, emphasizing the importance of combinative systemic and surgical treatment in the fight against EOC even in this heavily pretreated patient collective. This may nevertheless constitute a selection bias since those patients who were fit enough and able to tolerate chemotherapy following radical surgery have theoretically also more favorable survival rates than patients too weak to tolerate any systemic treatment or even so advanced and multifocal metastasized that no chemotherapy was indicated. Rates of major operative morbidity and 30-day mortality were 25.9% and 3.2%, respectively, hence slightly higher than the equivalent data of secondary patients at the DESKTOP series; however here not only platinum-sensitive patients for cytoreduction were included but also palliative symptomatic patients who underwent surgery aiming at amelioration of symptoms. The most common complication was infection/sepsis by 13%, a 4.4% relaparotomy rate, but interestingly without any higher rates of thromboembolic events (2.5%).

Multivariate analysis identified platinum-resistant, tumor residuals at secondary surgery and peritoneal carcinomatosis to be of predictive significance for complete tumor resection, while tumor residuals at secondary and tertiary surgery, decreasing interval to second relapse, ascites, upper abdominal tumor involvement, and non-platinum third-line chemotherapy, significantly affected OS.

Again here, like at secondary surgery, correct selection of surgical candidates is crucial to minimize morbidity and maximizing benefit from this radical approach in a highly palliative patient cohort.

13 Beyond Tertiary Cytoreduction: Quaternary Surgery

Venturing even beyond tertiary cytoreduction, the evidence is very scarce. There are only two series internationally to systematically evaluate the results of quaternary surgery in EOC. The largest series of 49 recurrent EOC patients demonstrated that even in a quaternary setting, nearly 33% complete tumor resection rates are feasible in a highly specialized gynecologic oncologic center, despite the fact that the majority of the patients had peritoneal carcinomatosis (77.6%) (Fotopoulou et al. April 2013). According to prospectively documented intraoperative tumor mapping, patients presented with the following tumor pattern: lower abdomen 85.7%, middle abdomen 79.6%, and upper abdomen 42.9%. Median duration of surgery was 292 min and hence equivalent to the duration of primary and secondary cytoreduction. Rates of major operative morbidity and 30-day mortality were 28.6% and 2%, respectively. Also noted were highly significant differences in survival between tumor-free and not tumor-free patients. Mean OS for patients without any tumor residuals was 43 months as opposed to only 13.4 months for patients with any residual disease. Mean OS for patients who received postoperative chemotherapy (n = 18; 36.7%) was 40.5 months versus 12 months for those who did not, also highly a significant difference, corresponding so with the results of the TCS.

Multivariate analysis indentified multifocal tumor dissemination to be of predictive significance for incomplete tumor resection, higher operative morbidity, and more dismal survival.

Interestingly, otherwise established prognostic factors such as ascites, platinum resistance, high-grade histology, and advanced age appeared not to carry any significant impact on survival.

The second monocentric analysis includes 15 patients and originates from the Memorial Sloan Kettering Cancer Center (Shih et al. 2009). Their findings showed comparable results: the number of sites of recurrence and optimal tumor debulking were associated with a prolonged survival, especially when a total macroscopic tumor clearance could be obtained. They also reported that all other well-established predictive factors for primary ovarian cancer and first relapse such as time to recurrence and response to platinum failed to retain any prognostic value on survival.

Still, especially in this advanced situation of the disease indication for cytoreduction, aiming at a putative amelioration of survival should be done only with high caution, careful patient selection, and clear discussion with the patients about the chronic and palliative situation of the disease and weighing of risks and benefits.

14   Salvage Surgery in Acute Situations: Bowel Obstruction and Intestinal Perforation in the Era of Targeted Antiangiogenetic Agents

EOC appears to behave differently from other epithelial cancer types, since its constant, almost pathognomonic feature is its local and lymphatic dissemination to the peritoneal and pleural layers by a paucity of visceral distant metastases via hematogenous pathways. Locoregional peritoneal disease is what most patients die from, in terms of bowel obstruction, cachexia, hypoproteinemia from ascites, organ failure, and exhaustion. Attributed to this diffuse tumor dissemination pattern along the peritoneal layers, EOC patients often present with the clinical picture of impaired intestinal passage or even bowel obstruction in the advanced primary

and especially relapsed EOC. The newly emerging novel implementation of targeted therapies with antiangiogenetic potential may additionally favor fistula formation or intestinal perforation. EOC complicated by such severe and acute events constitutes a therapeutic dilemma. Massive systemic and surgical pretreatment and extensive tumor dissemination combined by acute systemic inflammatory immunologic response make any surgical intervention in this setting highly challenging, while associated with high morbidity and mortality rates (Sehouli et al. 2012). Appropriate balancing of risks and benefits is required to design the optimal treatment options tailored around the individual needs. The patient communication processes are currently based on rather scattered monocentric data series, since data from large multicenter analyses are broadly lacking. Surgical interventions include various surgical techniques and strategies, such as en bloc resections of the involved intestinal package and terminal proximal ileo- or jejunostomy, since due to the severe peritoneal carcinosis and inflammation, no plane dissection with anastomotic and repair techniques is feasible. Short bowel syndrome with subsequent total parenteral nutrition (TPN) is therefore in some cases inevitable and requires high institutional and physical resources.

In cases of acute intestinal complications such as perforation and peritonitis, therapeutic approaches are rather limited. The cancer-induced tissue alterations and the overall low patient reserve constitute a major challenge for both the patients themselves and the treating physicians so that often such acute situations provoke a therapeutic nihilism and overall hesitation of active surgical measures. Retrospective analyses have shown that patients operated on in acute situations had significantly higher rates of anastomotic insufficiency compared to those operated within a planned setting, as also that the anastomotic insufficiency rate seems to be higher at primary debulking with tumor residuals compared to those without. For these reasons, even though no randomized trials exist to prove the safety or not of a primary anastomosis in an acute setting with peritonitis, the high probability of an intestinal stoma should be preoperatively discussed with the affected patients.

EOC rarely develops true visceral metastases; organ involvement is mainly due to direct extension by continuous tumor growth of the visceral peritoneum. Based on this, tumor resection is best achieved by an extraperitoneal approach of the tumor mass and en block dissection of all the tumor-involved organs together with the adjacent peritoneum, following their dissection from the ureteric and blood vessel level in the lower abdomen and duodenum, pancreas, and biliary duct in the upper abdomen. Extensive multivisceral techniques are increasingly therefore being included in the surgical armamentarium of advanced disease management (Fotopoulou et al. 2010). This reflects also the optimal approach in acute situations. A simple local intestinal resection with reanastomosis or barrel loop ileostomy is often not feasible, since the combination of peritoneal carcinosis and peritonitis makes a dissection in the physiological planes impossible and of high risk of further injury.

A major issue is also the highly crucial role of psychosocial and nutritional support network to provide TPN at home. Multidisciplinary teams consisting of nutritional specialists, dieticians, gastroenterologists, and psycho-oncologists are therefore indispensable for the successful outcome of such surgeries.

---

15 Systemic Treatment of Epithelial Ovarian Cancer

15.1 Early-Stage Disease (FIGO I-IIb)

Adjuvant platinum-based chemotherapy should be discussed and offered in all cases of early ovarian cancer apart from Ia/Ib G1 not only in case of incomplete staging but also to optimally staged higher-risk early disease, such as higher grade or serous subtype (WHO 2014).

Two prospectively randomized trials examined the value of chemotherapy after surgery in early-stage ovarian cancer. ACTION and ICON1 included a broad range of early-stage patients with grade 2 and 3 stages IA/B and all grades of

stages IC/IIA, in order to recruit sufficient patients. The primary analysis of ICON1 on its own, with a median follow-up of 4-years demonstrated a significant improvement in both RFS and OS in favor of immediate adjuvant chemotherapy with six cycles of single agent carboplatin (AUC 5/6). Very similar findings were reported in the ACTION trial in which the majority of patients received a platinum-based combination chemotherapy.

A recent Cochrane meta-analysis of five large prospective clinical trials (four of ten with platinum-based chemotherapy) shows that chemotherapy is more beneficial than observation in patients with early-stage ovarian cancer. Patients who received platinum-based adjuvant chemotherapy had better OS and PFS than patients who did not receive adjuvant treatment. Nevertheless, in all abovementioned trials, only approximately one third of the patients were optimally staged, the remainder having a 30% chance of being understaged and harboring occult disease. Despite this, benefit for chemotherapy in optimally staged patients cannot be excluded and adjuvant chemotherapy should be discussed and offered to all patients with high-risk early-stage ovarian cancer.

The addition of targeted therapies such as bevacizumab and other VEGF inhibitors such as nintedanib and cediranib, tyrosine kinase inhibitors, or PARP inhibitors is not of any established evidence, so far, and should not be offered outside clinical trials.

15.2 Advanced Stage Disease (FIGO IIc – IV)

Platinum-based chemotherapy ± paclitaxel is the, as per national and international guidelines dictated, first-line chemotherapy. The standard of care for most is thus carboplatin (AUC5/6) and paclitaxel (175 mg/m^2) given 3 weekly for six cycles. Dose-dense scheduling of the paclitaxel (80 mg/m^2 days 1, 8, 15 every 21 days with carboplatin AUC 5/6 on day 1) has been shown to improve overall survival in a large prospective randomized Japanese trial where Paclitaxel was applied in the dose of 80 mg/m^2. These findings have not been confirmed yet in the Caucasian population. A similar Italian study by the MITO group has shown a better tolerability of the weekly arm; however, it failed to demonstrate any survival benefit by a paclitaxel dose of 60 mg/m^2 and hence lower to the Japanese equivalent study. The just completed UK-based ICON 8 trial will in a few years answer the question of value of dose density in first-line chemotherapy for ovarian cancer and hence potentially establish standards of care.

For those patients who develop allergy to or do not tolerate paclitaxel, the combination of docetaxel-carboplatin or pegylated liposomal doxorubicin-carboplatin can be considered as an alternative regime based on two randomized clinical trials that showed similar efficacy.

Addition of bevacizumab concurrently to chemotherapy as maintenance for up to 12 months afterward in the ICON 7 and for 15 months in the GOG 218 has been shown to significantly prolong PFS and OS in patients with documented residual disease and/or distant metastases (grade A). The antiangiogenic VEGF inhibitor, bevacizumab, has been shown to improve overall survival when given together with carboplatin and paclitaxel 3 weekly as maintenance for up to 12 months total, in a higher-risk subgroup of these patients, who have been suboptimally debulked (1 cm residual disease) or had no surgery or stage IV disease (ICON 7). However, in the GOG 262 study, no survival benefit was seen in the bevacizumab arm if patients received paclitaxel in a weekly regime, even though there was no prior randomization to bevacizumab versus placebo. The value and safety of bevacizumab in the neoadjuvant setting is currently the objective of various ongoing randomized trials.

The value of intraperitoneal (IP) chemotherapy continues to be strongly controversial despite the efficacy that has been shown in different prospective randomized trials; an effect that seems to pertain even decades later. The lack of broad acceptance seems to be due to the reported high toxicity and high drop-off rates in the IP arm, but also due to the fact that it is not clear whether the survival benefit is due to the dose-dense application of iv paclitaxel or to the IP application per se. Currently ongoing trials with dose regimes equivalent to the intravenous version will answer the question of value of IP chemotherapy.

Despite the initial high response rates to first-line platinum-based therapies, the majority of patients with EOC will experience relapse and die of the disease. Several therapeutic options are available and the decision as to which therapy to commence is dependent on the platinum-free interval (PFI), even though in the last Ovarian Cancer Consensus Conference (OCCC) in Tokyo, the consensus was to rather abandon the traditional 6-month cutoff as outdated and rather define treatment-free interval (TFI) of TFIp (platinum), TFInp (non-platinum), and TFIb (biological agent to be specified). Traditionally the platinum-free interval has been considered as a predictor of response to future platinum-based treatment, even though now-emerging theories support approaches of "platinum resensitization" by extending the platinum-free interval with agents like trabectedin.

15.3 Intermediate Platinum Response (PFS 6–12 Months)

Patients with an intermediate response to platinum (i.e., PFI between 6 and 12 months) represent a therapeutic challenge. Various trials exist addressing only this special patient subset. The Italian study group MANGO leads the OVATYON trial evaluating PLD 30 mg/m^2 1 h i.v. + carboplatin AUC 5 30–60 min i.v. on day 1 q4 weeks; treatment was allowed to six cycles or progression versus PLD 30 mg/m^2 1 h i.v. + trabectedin 1.1 mg/m^2 3 h i.v. on day 1 q3weeks, up to six cycles or progression in EOC relapse patients with a PFI of 6–12 months.

A further study is the phase III MITO-8-(Efficacy Study of Chemotherapy to Treat Ovarian Cancer Recurrence and to Prolong the Platinum Free Interval). This study aims to test the hypothesis that the artificial prolongation of the platinum-free interval with a non-platinum treatment will improve the effectiveness of overall therapy in patients with EOC progression occurring 6–12 months after first-line treatment with a platinum derivative. The study groups MANGO and AO-Ovar are also participating, and a total number of 46 patients of the overall estimated 253 have already been recruited. In the experimental arm patients are treated with stealth liposomal doxorubicin followed at a later progression by carboplatin and paclitaxel, while in the conventional arm patients receive carboplatin and paclitaxel followed at a later progression by stealth liposomal doxorubicin.

15.4 Platinum Resistant/Refractory EOC Relapse (PFI <6 Months)

This is a difficult group in which to demonstrate benefit. Sharma et al. reported recently their experience of extended weekly carboplatin and paclitaxel in an attempt to increase response to chemotherapy in this special population. Twenty patients with platinum-resistant/refractory ovarian cancer received carboplatin AUC 3 and paclitaxel 70 mg/m^2 on day weekly. The RECIST response rate was 60% by radiological criteria (RECIST) and 76% by CA125 assessment, comparably very high for this platinum-resistant situation. Despite the dose-dense regimen in this heavily pretreated patient collective, no grade 3/4 thrombocytopenia occurred. The dynamics of response to dose-dense therapy were as rapid as with front-line therapy within the same patient. The authors state that this dose-dense regimen is routinely extended to at least 18 weekly cycles over 6 months and that it forms a highly active and tolerable cytotoxic scaffold to which molecular-targeted therapies can be added in platinum-resistant ovarian cancer.

Like in the primary also in the recurrent situation of the disease, targeted therapies are being implicated into conventional cytotoxic regimens to enhance response. Various antiangiogenics and small molecules such as sorafenib, bevacizumab, cediranib, zibotentan (ZD4054), and farletuzumab (MORAb-003) are being evaluated.

The multicenter AURELIA trial showed a significant prolongation of PFS in platinum-resistant patients who were treated with bevacizumab additionally to non-platinum monotherapy (liposomal pegylated doxorubicin or paclitaxel weekly or topotecan); however equivalent to the platinum-sensitive trials, bevacizumab failed to show any significant effect on overall survival.

16 Follow-Up

The aim of follow-up is not only to detect relapse and direct patients toward future therapeutic approaches but also to help the patients cope with the chronic effects of the anticancer treatment they had such as polyneuropathy, gastrointestinal symptoms, etc.

Duration of follow-up and intervals between follow-up visits vary according to local practices, but generally every 3 months for the first years and then every 6 months, even though there is no randomized trial to prove survival benefit of strict follow-up protocols versus an individualized patient and symptom-led approach. Rises in CA125 can be used to document progressive disease in patients who achieve a normal CA125 after primary treatment but tend to precede symptomatic relapse by a median of 4.5 months (range 0.5–29.5 months). A recent MRC/EORTC trial demonstrated no difference in overall survival between patients who received chemotherapy based on a rising CA125 and those who did not receive chemotherapy until they were symptomatic. Although the value of routine CA125 measurements was negated by this randomized controlled trial (RCT), some patients prefer to know as accurately as possible what might lie ahead and can cope with the knowledge that a rising CA125 indicates that their cancer has returned and yet immediate treatment is not necessarily of any benefit.

Participation in first-line trials also generally requires regular CA125 measurements in order to accurately determine trial end points. But rising CA125 alone without clinical or radiographic evidence of recurrence is not sufficient enough to commence systemic chemotherapy.

The results of the upcoming prospectively randomized DESKTOP III and GOG 0213 will nevertheless newly define and potentially change follow-up practice if tumor-free secondary debulking will be shown to be associated with survival benefit, in which case tumor burden at the time of secondary surgery will impact on surgical complexity, morbidity, and overall outcome. Furthermore, in the increasingly emerging era of targeted agents and maintenance approaches, additional monitoring with CA125 may identify patients with early relapse (i.e., within 6 months) who may be suitable for phase 2 clinical trials with investigational new agents.

At follow-up visits, a careful history is imperative, together with clinical examination. CA125 measurement is not mandatory and has not been proven to be of prospective survival benefit. All patients should have the contact details of their key worker so that they can have early local review for unexpected symptoms.

17 Conclusion

To conclude, epithelial ovarian cancer is a complex disease which is difficult to detect in its early stages due to its vague symptom pattern and has a high mortality rate owing to the aggressive nature of the majority of tumors. No effective screening protocol has been designed as yet and so it continues to present at advanced stages. Work is ongoing, especially in proteomics, to discover a marker which can be used to detect cancer and then guide follow-up; however finding a universal marker is difficult due to the broad inter-tumor heterogeneity demonstrated by these cancers.

References

Braicu EI, Sehouli J, Richter R, Pietzner K, Lichtenegger W, Fotopoulou C. Primary versus secondary cytoreduction for epithelial ovarian cancer: a paired analysis of tumour pattern and surgical outcome. Eur J Cancer. 2012;48(5):687–94. Epub 2011 Jul 13.

Bristow RE, Tomacruz RS, Armstrong DK, Trimble EL, Montz FJ. Survival effect of maximal cytoreductive surgery for advanced ovarian carcinoma during the platinum era: a meta-analysis. J Clin Oncol. 2002; 20(5):1248–59.

Bristow RE, Puri I, Chi DS. Cytoreductive surgery for recurrent ovarian cancer: a meta- analysis. Gynecol Oncol. 2009;112(1):265–74.

Chan K, Urban R, Hu JM, Shin JY, Husain A, Teng NN, Berek JS, Osann K, Kapp DS. The potential therapeutic role of lymph node resection in epithelial ovarian cancer: a study of 13 918 patients. Br J Cancer. 2007; 96:1817–22.

Colombo PE, Mourregot A, Fabbro M, et al. Aggressive surgical strategies in advanced ovarian cancer: a monocentric study of 203 stage IIIC and IV patients. Eur J Surg Oncol. 2009;35(2):135–43.

De Iaco P, Musto A, Orazi L, Zamagni C, Rosati M, Allegri V, Cacciari N, Al-Nahhas A, Rubello D, Venturoli S, Fanti S. FDG-PET/CT in advanced ovarian cancer staging: value and pitfalls in detecting lesions in different abdominal and pelvic quadrants compared with laparoscopy. Eur J Radiol. 2011;80(2):e98–103. Epub 2010 Aug 4.

Doufekas K, Olaitan A. Clinical epidemiology of epithelial ovarian cancer in the UK. Int J Womens Health. 2014;6:537–45.

du Bois A, Reuss A, Pujade-Lauraine E, Harter P, Ray-Coquard I, Pfisterer J. Role of surgical outcome as prognostic factor in advanced epithelial ovarian cancer: a combined exploratory analysis of 3 prospectively randomized phase 3 multicenter trials: by the Arbeitsgemeinschaft Gynaekologische Onkologie Studiengruppe Ovarialkarzinom (AGO-OVAR) and the Groupe d'Investigateurs Nationaux Pour les Etudes des Cancers de l'Ovaire (GINECO). Cancer. 2009; 115(6):1234–44.

Eisenkop SM, Spirtos NM, Montag TW, et al. The impact of subspecialty training on the management of advanced ovarian cancer. Gynecol Oncol. 1992; 47:203–9.

Fotopoulou C, Richter R, Braicu EI, Schmidt SC, Lichtenegger W, Sehouli J. Can complete tumor resection be predicted in advanced primary epithelial ovarian cancer? A systematic evaluation of 360 consecutive patients. Eur J Surg Oncol. 2010;36(12):1202–10. Epub 2010 Sep 22.

Fotopoulou C, Richter R, Braicu IE, et al. Clinical outcome of tertiary surgical cytoreduction in patients with recurrent epithelial ovarian cancer. Ann Surg Oncol. 2011; 18:49–57.

Fotopoulou C, Zang R, Gultekin M, Cibula D, Ayhan A, Liu D, Richter R, Braicu I, Mahner S, Harter P, Trillsch F, Kumar S, Peiretti M, Dowdy SC, Maggioni A, Trope C, Sehouli J. Value of tertiary cytoreductive surgery in epithelial ovarian cancer: an international multicenter evaluation. Ann Surg Oncol. 2013a;20(4):1348–54. Epub 2012 Oct 2.

Fotopoulou C, Savvatis K, Kosian P, Braicu IE, Papanikolaou G, Pietzner K, Schmidt SC, Sehouli J. Quaternary cytoreductive surgery in ovarian cancer: does surgical effort still matter? Br J Cancer. 2013b; 108(1):32–8.

Gabra H. Back to the future: targeting molecular changes for platinum resistance reversal. Gynecol Oncol. 2010;118:210–1.

Goff B. Symptoms associated with ovarian cancer. Clin Obstet Gynecol. 2012;55(1):36–42.

Gultekin M, Velipaşaoğlu M, Aksan G, Dursun P, Dogan NU, Yuce K, Ayhan A. A third evaluation of tertiary cytoreduction. J Surg Oncol. 2008;98(7):530–4.

Harter P, du Bois A, Hahmann M, Hasenburg A, Burges A, Loibl S, Gropp M, Huober J, Fink D, Schröder W, Muenstedt K, Schmalfeldt B, Emons G, Pfisterer J, Wollschlaeger K, Meerpohl HG, Breitbach GP, Tanner B, Sehouli J, Arbeitsgemeinschaft Gynaekologische Onkologie Ovarian Committee, AGO Ovarian Cancer Study Group. Surgery in recurrent ovarian cancer: the Arbeitsgemeinschaft Gynaekologische Onkologie (AGO) DESKTOP OVAR trial. Ann Surg Oncol. 2006;13(12):1702–10.

Harter P, Hahmann M, Lueck HJ, Poelcher M, Wimberger P, Ortmann O, Canzler U, Richter B, Wagner U, Hasenburg A, Burges A, Loibl S, Meier W, Huober J, Fink D, Schroeder W, Muenstedt K, Schmalfeldt B, Emons G, du Bois A. Surgery for recurrent ovarian cancer: role of peritoneal carcinomatosis: exploratory analysis of the DESKTOP I trial about risk factors, surgical implications, and prognostic value of peritoneal carcinomatosis. Ann Surg Oncol. 2009;16(5):1324–30.

Harter P, Sehouli J, Reuss A, Hasenburg A, Scambia G, Cibula D, Mahner S, Vergote I, Reinthaller A, Burges A, Hanker L, Pölcher M, Kurzeder C, Canzler U, Petry KU, Obermair A, Petru E, Schmalfeldt B, Lorusso D, du Bois A. Prospective validation study of a predictive score for operability of recurrent ovarian cancer: the Multicenter Intergroup Study DESKTOP II. A project of the AGO Kommission OVAR, AGO Study Group, NOGGO, AGO-Austria, and MITO. Int J Gynecol Cancer. 2011;21(2):289–95.

Helm CW, Chief Editor: Harris JE. Ovarian cancer staging. http://emedicine.medscape.com/article/2007140-overview

Hızlı D, Boran N, Yılmaz S, Turan T, Altınbaş SK, Celik B, Köse MF. Best predictors of survival outcome after tertiary cytoreduction in patients with recurrent platinum-sensitive epithelial ovarian cancer. Eur J Obstet Gynecol Reprod Biol. 2012;163(1):71–5.

http://www.cancer.org/cancer/ovariancancer/overviewguide/ovarian-cancer-overview-survival

http://www.nice.org.uk/guidance/CG122/chapter/Appendix-D-Risk-of-malignancy-index-RMI-I

http://www.who.int/selection_medicines/committees/expert/20/applications/EpithelialOvarian.pdf?ua=1

Janczar S, Graham JS, Paige AJW, Gabra H. Targeting locoregional peritoneal dissemination in ovarian cancer. Expert Rev Obstet Gynecol. 2009;4(2):133–47.

Jemal A, et al. Cancer statistics. Cancer J Clin. 2007;57(1):43–66.

Karam AK, Santillan A, Bristow RE, Giuntoli 2nd R, Gardner GJ, Cass I, Karlan BY, Li AJ. Tertiary cytoreductive surgery in recurrent ovarian cancer: selection criteria and survival outcome. Gynecol Oncol. 2007;104(2):377–80. Epub 2006 Oct 2.

Kehoe S, et al. Primary chemotherapy versus primary surgery for newly diagnosed advanced ovarian cancer (CHORUS): an open-label, randomised, controlled, non-inferiority trial. Lancet. 2015;386(9990):249–57.

Kurman RJ, Shih I-M. The origin and pathogenesis of epithelial ovarian cancer- a proposed unifying theory. Am J Surg Pathol. 2010;34(3):433–43.

Leitao Jr MM, Kardos S, Barakat RR, Chi DS. Tertiary cytoreduction in patients with recurrent ovarian carcinoma. Gynecol Oncol. 2004;95:181–8.

Monk BJ, Coleman RL. Changing the paradigm in the treatment of platinum-sensitive recurrent ovarian cancer: from platinum doublets to nonplatinum doublets and adding antiangiogenesis compounds. Int J Gynecol Cancer. 2009;19 Suppl 2:S63–7. doi:10.1111/IGC.0b013e3181c104fa.

Morris M, Gershenson DM, Wharton JT. Secondary cytoreductive surgery in epithelial ovarian cancer: nonresponders to first-line therapy. Gynecol Oncol. 1989;33(1):1–5.

Omura G, et al. A randomized trial of cyclophosphamide and doxorubicin with or without cisplatin in advanced ovarian carcinoma. A Gynecologic Oncology Group Study. Cancer. 1986;57:1725–30.

Paulsen T, Kjaerheim K, Kaern J, et al. Improved short-term survival for advanced ovarian, tubal, and peritoneal cancer patients operated at teaching hospitals. Int J Gynecol Cancer. 2006;16 Suppl 1:11–7.

Petrillo M, Ferrandina G, Fagotti A, Vizzielli G, Margariti PA, Pedone AL, Nero C, Fanfani F, Scambia G. Timing and pattern of recurrence in ovarian cancer patients with high tumor dissemination treated with primary debulking surgery versus neoadjuvant chemotherapy. Ann Surg Oncol. 2013;20(12):3955–60.

Segna RA, Dottino PR, Mandeli JP, Konsker K, Cohen CJ. Secondary cytoreduction for ovarian cancer following cisplatin therapy. J Clin Oncol. 1993;11(3):434–9.

Sehouli J, Papanikolaou G, Braicu EI, Pietzner K, Neuhaus P, Fotopoulou C. Feasibility of surgery after systemic treatment with the humanized recombinant antibody bevacizumab in heavily pretreated patients with advanced epithelial ovarian cancer. Ann Surg Oncol. 2012;19(4):1326–33.

Shih KK, Chi DS, Barakat RR, Leitao Jr MM. Tertiary cytoreduction in patients with recurrent epithelial ovarian, fallopian tube, or primary peritoneal cancer: an updated series. Gynecol Oncol. 2010a;117:330–5.

Shih KK, Chi DS, Barakat RR, Leitao Jr MM. Beyond tertiary cytoreduction in patients with recurrent epithelial ovarian, fallopian tube, or primary peritoneal cancer. Gynecol Oncol. 2010b;116(3):364–9. Epub 2009 Nov 7.

Simple ultrasound rules to distinguish between benign and malignant adnexal masses before surgery: prospective validation by IOTA group. BMJ. 2010;341.

Tian WJ, Chi DS, Sehouli J, Tropé CG, Jiang R, Ayhan A, Cormio G, Xing Y, Breitbach GP, Braicu EI, Rabbitt CA, Oksefjell H, Fotopoulou C, Meerpohl HG, du Bois A, Berek JS, Zang RY, Harter P. A risk model for secondary cytoreductive surgery in recurrent ovarian cancer: an evidence-based proposal for patient selection. Ann Surg Oncol. 2012;19(2):597–604.

Timmerman D. Simple ultrasound rules to distinguish between benign and malignant adnexal masses before surgery: prospective validation by IOTA group. BMJ. 2010;341:c6839.

Vaughan S, Coward JI, Bast Jr RC, Berchuck A, Berek JS, Brenton JD, Coukos G, Crum CC, Drapkin R, Etemadmoghadam D, Friedlander M, Gabra H, Kaye SB, Lord CJ, Lengyel E, Levine DA, McNeish IA, Menon U, Mills GB, Nephew KP, Oza AM, Sood AK, Stronach EA, Walczak H, Bowtell DD,

Balkwill FR. Rethinking ovarian cancer: recommendations for improving outcomes. Nat Rev Cancer. 2011; 11(10):719–25.

Vergote et al. Neoadjuvant chemotherapy or primary surgery in stage IIIC or IV ovarian cancer. N Engl J Med. 2010;363:943–53.

Vernooij F, Heintz P, Witteveen E, et al. The outcomes of ovarian cancer treatment are better when provided by gynecologic oncologists and in specialized hospitals: a systematic review. Gynecol Oncol. 2007;105: 801–12.

Zang RY, Harter P, Chi DS, Sehouli J, Jiang R, Tropé CG, Ayhan A, Cormio G, Xing Y, Wollschlaeger KM, Braicu EI, Rabbitt CA, Oksefjell H, Tian WJ, Fotopoulou C, Pfisterer J, du Bois A, Berek JS. Predictors of survival in patients with recurrent ovarian cancer undergoing secondary cytoreductive surgery based on the pooled analysis of an international collaborative cohort. Br J Cancer. 2011;105(7):890–6. Epub 2011 Aug 30.

Fertility Sparing Treatment for Ovarian Cancer

Katherine Nixon and Christina Fotopoulou

Abstract

Consideration of fertility sparing options in the management of ovarian cancer is an increasing concern for gynecological oncologists. For various reasons, women are continuing to delay having children until later years when they may be more at risk of developing ovarian cancer. Preserving fertility in the presence of ovarian cancer diagnosis is a difficult scenario for all involved and creates a balancing act between patients' sometimes desperate wishes and maintaining safe clinical practice. There is obvious difficulty in researching the impact of fertility sparing surgery and alternative treatments for ovarian cancer, as a prospective analysis would be unethical; however, retrospective reviews of cases have been performed to aid guidelines regarding safest management options. We will consider the options available to patients who wish to preserve their fertility and the international guidance depending on types of cancer and method of treatment.

Keywords

Ovarian cancer • Fertility • Stage • Prognosis • Reproduction

Contents

1 Introduction

Annually in the UK, around 500 women under the age of 45 are diagnosed with ovarian cancer. Many of these women will be wishing to preserve their fertility potential and will need careful counseling regarding this. Approach to these, as with all gynecological oncology cases, should be with a multidisciplinary team. Being diagnosed with ovarian cancer at any stage of life is an extremely distressing situation for patients, but for younger women, adding in the possibility of losing the ability to conceive has the potential to make it much more devastating. The possibility of losing fertility potential as a result of ovarian

K. Nixon
Department of Gynecology, Imperial College NHS Trust, Queen Charlottes and Hammersmith Hospital, London, UK
e-mail: Katherine.nixon@hotmail.co.uk

C. Fotopoulou (✉)
Department of Gynaecological Oncology, West London Gynecological Cancer Centre, Imperial College NHS Trust, Queen Charlottes and Hammersmith Hospital, London, UK
e-mail: chfotopoulou@gmail.com

© Springer International Publishing AG 2017
D. Shoupe (ed.), *Handbook of Gynecology*,
DOI 10.1007/978-3-319-17798-4_13

cancer treatment has been shown to have a negative effect on quality of life for those patients who survive the disease (Duncan et al. 2011).

Management plans for patients with ovarian cancer are decided by teams of gynecological and medical oncologists with guidance from radiologists and pathologists. Most ovarian cancers will require surgery of some kind with the possibility of adjuvant chemotherapy, usually platinum based. Both the surgery and the chemotherapy have the potential to take away a patient's fertility. Surgery will usually involve removal of the affected ovary/tube, often with the necessity or advice of completion of staging by removing the uterus, contralateral tube plus other biopsies from around the abdomen, depending on the stage and grade of the cancer.

The stage and grade of the cancer are the most important factors guiding management advice, with early stage, low grade types proving to be more favorable for fertility sparing management options than high grade/stage. Retrospective trials that have been conducted show that fertility sparing surgery can represent a realistic alternative to the more traditional radical cytoreductive approach in women of child bearing age with early stage disease, without compromise to prognosis.

It is important that we clearly differentiate between the types of ovarian cancer when discussing surgical options. We know more about the potential impact on prognosis of fertility preserving surgery in early stage borderline, germ cell, and granulosa cell tumors (Fotopoulou et al. 2009). Epithelial ovarian cancers are more of a gray area; however, with greater understanding and surgical expertise less radical practices are being used for early stage disease.

2   Surgical Management

There are different treatment approaches depending on the type of ovarian cancer diagnosed. Long standing evidence exists for good outcomes with conservative surgical management

for early stage borderline, germ cell, and granulosa cell tumors. These cancers tend to follow predictable courses of progression. Preservation of fertility can be offered without compromising treatment of the disease, with 5-year survival rates of around 90% and no alteration in relapse rates. Fertility outcomes, measured by rates of conceptions and live births, have been good in these cases, both following surgery only management and also after chemotherapy regimes.

Clinical progression with epithelial ovarian cancer, the most common histological type, varies vastly with high levels of relapse. Therefore, conservative, potentially fertility sparing management regimes are adopted less frequently because of the concern over a poorer outcome. The diversity of presentation, spread, and relapse is attributed to the widespread intratumoral heterogeneity within these cancers. Despite great leaps in understanding the etiology of the disease over the last 20 years, prognosis has remained fairly constant. Due to concerns over endangering patients' lives by using more conservative measures, this approach is not one readily adopted by the specialty.

In terms of decisions based on staging, current international guidelines would not recommend fertility sparing techniques for ovarian cancer including and above stage II as defined by the International Federation of Gynecology Oncology (FIGO), as from this classification the disease has spread beyond the boundaries of the ovaries (Helm and Harris 2015). Furthermore, by FIGO staging, any ovarian cancers apart from stages Ia, Ic1, and Ic3 involve both ovaries or the surface of the affected ovary/tube and therefore these would not be suitable for a more conservative approach. There is limited data on outcomes of cases where macroscopic tumor deposits have been left in situ at the time of surgery in order to preserve fertility. Although still incredibly difficult, clinicians may find counseling for these higher stage cases relatively more straightforward as there are limited options, and guidance would generally be to opt for maximal cytoreductive surgery including bilateral salpingoophorectomy, hysterectomy, and following with adjuvant chemotherapy. Counseling, where fertility sparing surgery may be a safe option, can be more problematic as patients and their partners/families will have more considerations to take on board.

For stages 1a and 1c, it is less clear what the best course of treatment should be. Fertility sparing surgery requires leaving one ovary, tube, and the uterus in situ. There will always be concern regarding the chance of disease being present in these sites that is not visible macroscopically and about the risk of recurrence if they are not removed. To leave these structures in situ involves macroscopically staging the disease at the time of surgery and determining that the contralateral ovary/tube appear normal and there is no evidence of disease elsewhere. To aide staging, biopsies can be taken at the time of surgery from the pelvic and abdominal peritoneum, the omentum and lymph nodes, (the most common sites of dissemination). However without the resection of the contralateral ovary and tube staging is not complete (Mangili et al. 2011). New techniques are being adopted involving peritoneal resection from the pelvis and uterine serosa to aid staging (Rasool and Rose 2010). Uncertainty exists around the best management of Ic disease. This is regarding whether there is a difference between outcomes of patients who have had surgical spill of their disease from cyst rupture (Ic1) or those who have malignant cells present in peritoneal washings or ascites already before surgery, without evidence of other disease (Ic3).

The histological grade is also important in determining if fertility sparing is a safe option. In general, high grade, poorly differentiated, or clear cell histological cell types, irrespective of stage, are not deemed suitable for fertility sparing surgical techniques. Current evidence suggests that in stage 1a, low grade i.e., moderately or well-differentiated nonclear cell histology, it is appropriate to perform fertility sparing surgery without compromising the oncological outcome (Kajiyama et al. 2011). These patients may also not require adjuvant chemotherapy. There is an apparent discrepancy between stage 1c with surgical spill and those with noniatrogenic positive peritoneal cytology. Iatrogenic cases show better outcomes with fewer relapses and therefore a conservative course of action is not recommended for cases with preexisting malignant cells in ascites or peritoneal washings.

Average relapse rates in those undergoing fertility sparing surgery have been shown to be around 10% (Fotopoulou et al. 2012). While there is no significant difference in relapse rates between cases of stage 1a or 1c disease, the higher proportion of relapses tend to be in those with 1c or higher grade disease. Research has shown that in cases of low stage disease where fertility is not an issue and bilateral salpingoophorectomy has occurred, in order to complete staging, there is a low rate of tumor invasion in the contralateral ovary. This evidence supports the opinion for surgeons being capable of determining macroscopically if an ovary contains tumor at the time of surgery and therefore visually staging the disease; however, without biopsy this diagnostic strategy is not watertight.

International guidelines now recommend that a fertility sparing surgical approach is appropriate in cases of stage 1a or 1c1 low grade cases following discussion with the patient and fully informed consent.

3　Chemotherapy

Of the cases where fertility sparing surgery is deemed appropriate, those with stage Ia/Ic1 clear cell carcinoma or stage Ic3 are recommended to have adjuvant chemotherapy. Platinum-based chemotherapy agents are widely used in ovarian cancer and have the potential to cause ovarian failure and induce early menopause; this is more typical in older patients who may have been already approaching menopausal age. However studies have shown that the majority of patients, around 95%, receiving chemotherapy return to their normal menstrual cycle 6 months to a year following the end of their treatment (Satoh et al. 2010). Use of agents such as gonadotropin releasing hormone (GnRH) analogues or combined oral contraceptive pills (COCP) during chemotherapy have been investigated (Del Mastro et al. 2014). The aim of these medications is to downregulate the ovary during the treatment course and thus hope to reduce the toxic effect of the chemotherapy on the ovarian cells. This has been shown to be affective in some cases; however; there is insufficient conclusive data and no statistical significance has been demonstrated, hence use is still debated. Most of the research into this area has been performed in hematological and breast cancers and so understanding of its potential application to ovarian cancer management is limited.

Other options for fertility are cryopreservation of part of the ovary or oocytes; however, there is always a possible risk with this that part of the preserved tissue may contain malignant cells. Pregnancy rates following cryopreservation are reportedly low, and with this and the possibility of malignancy in the tissue, it is not a commonly used option.

4   Reproductive Outcomes

Both surgical management and chemotherapy treatment have the potential to affect fertility. Despite this, rates of successful conception following fertility sparing treatment have been good, reportedly around 66–100% in those who actively try to conceive. A minority of patients appear to require fertility assistance following treatment. There does not appear to be evidence of an increase in adverse pregnancy outcomes such as miscarriage, preterm labor, or congenital malformations in those who have undergone treatment. This information should be communicated to patients deemed suitable for fertility sparing measures to help with counseling and decision making.

5   Conclusion

Ovarian cancer has a huge impact on a patient's life no matter at what age the diagnosis is made. As society changes and women chose to have children at a later age, diagnoses and decisions on management are going to be increasingly difficult. Management regimes may seem more controversial in attempts to preserve fertility for those younger patients where this is a concern. There is well-acknowledged evidence of fertility preserving techniques in granulosa cell, germ cell, and borderline tumors without compromise in outcome. In the case of epithelial ovarian cancer, fertility sparing surgery is a reasonable course of action for those with stage 1a or 1c1 with low grade nonclear cell disease with no evidence of an impact on relapse rates or overall survival. Chemotherapy treatment used in ovarian cancer can lead to premature ovarian failure. In the majority of cases, however, ovarian function and menstruation will return to normal after the termination of treatment. In those aiming to conceive following the completion of treatment, rates of pregnancy and pregnancy outcomes are similar to a nonovarian cancer population. Careful counseling is required and all available facts should be given to the patient. This will enable them to make an informed decision regarding treatment options prior to commencement in cases where fertility sparing surgery is deemed appropriate. Gynecological oncologists have the responsibility to both adequately and safely treat the disease whilst also bearing in mind the patients' wishes for fertility preservation in ovarian cancer.

References

Del Mastro L et al. Gonadotropin-releasing hormone analogues for the prevention of chemotherapy-induced premature ovarian failure in cancer women: systematic review and meta-analysis of randomized trials. Cancer Treat Rev. 2014;40(5):675–83.

Duncan FE, Jozefik JK, Kim AM, Hirshfeld-Cytron J, Woodruff TK. The gynecologist has a unique role in providing oncofertility care to young cancer patients. US Obstet Gynecol. 2011;6(1):24–34.

Fotopoulou C, Schumacher G, Schefold JC, Denkert C, Lichtenegge W, Sehouli J. Systematic evaluation of the intraoperative tumor pattern in patients with borderline tumor of the ovary. Int J Gynecol Cancer. 2009;19 (9):1550–5.

Fotopoulou C, Braicu I, Sehouli J. Fertility-sparing surgery in early epithelial ovarian cancer: a viable option? Obstet Gynecol Int. 2012;2012, 238061.

https://www.rcog.org.uk/globalassets/documents/guidelines/1.2.13-sip35-fertility-sparing.pdf

Kajiyama H, Shibata K, Mizuno M, et al. Long-term survival of young women receiving fertility-sparing surgery for ovarian cancer in comparison with those undergoing radical surgery. Br J Cancer. 2011;105(9):1288–94.

Mangili G, Sigismondi C, Lorusso D, et al. Is surgical restaging indicated in apparent stage IA pure ovarian dysgerminoma? The MITO group retrospective experience. Gynecol Oncol. 2011;121(2):280–4.

Rasool N, Rose PG. Fertility-preserving surgical procedures for patients with gynecologic malignancies. Clin Obstet Gynecol. 2010;53(4):804–14.

Satoh T, Hatae M, Watanabe Y, et al. Outcomes of fertilitysparing surgery for stage I epithelial ovarian cancer: a proposal for patient selection. J Clin Oncol. 2010;28(10):1727–32.

William Helm C, Harris JE. Ovarian cancer staging. http://emedicine.medscape.com/article/2007140-overview (2015)

Diagnosis and Management of Nonepithelial Ovarian Cancer

Erin A. Blake, Saketh Guntupalli, and Koji Matsuo

Abstract

Nonepithelial ovarian cancers represent a small fraction of ovarian cancers. Malignancies in this category include sex cord-stromal tumors (SCST) and ovarian malignant germ cell tumors (OMGCT), and each of these classifications encompasses multiple histologic subtypes. The most common SCST include granulosa cell and Sertoli-Leydig cell tumors. Dysgerminomas, yolk sac tumors, and immature teratomas are the most frequently encountered OMGCT. The prognosis for these tumors is good; however, the survival outcome is dependent on factors such as tumor subtype and stage at diagnosis. Most patients with nonepithelial ovarian cancers present with low stage disease due to symptoms that occur early in the disease process. Surgery is the mainstay of treatment for all nonepithelial ovarian cancers. If desired, fertility sparing surgery is typically an appropriate management option for both SCST and OMGCT. Postoperative adjuvant chemotherapy is dependent on disease type and stage; however, due to the exquisite chemosensitivity of malignant germ cell tumors of the ovary, platinum-based combination chemotherapy is used for almost all cases. The most commonly used initial regimen for both SCST and OMGCT is combination of bleomycin, etoposide, and cisplatin. Surveillance for recurrent disease is mandated for all SCST and OMGCT, even those that present in early stages.

Keywords

Nonepithelial ovarian cancer • Sex cord-stromal tumors • Malignant germ cell tumors of the ovary • Granulosa • Sertoli-Leydig • Fibroma-thecoma • Gynandroblastoma • Dysgerminoma • Yolk sac • Teratoma

E.A. Blake
Department of Obstetrics and Gynecology, University of Colorado, Aurora, CO, USA
e-mail: Erin.blake@ucdenver.edu

S. Guntupalli
Division of Gynecologic Oncology, Department of Obstetrics and Gynecology, University of Colorado, Aurora, CO, USA
e-mail: Saketh.guntupalli@ucdenver.edu

K. Matsuo (✉)
Division of Gynecologic Oncology, Department of Obstetrics and Gynecology, University of Southern California, Los Angeles, CA, USA
e-mail: Koji.matsuo@med.usc.edu

© Springer International Publishing AG 2017
D. Shoupe (ed.), *Handbook of Gynecology*,
DOI 10.1007/978-3-319-17798-4_35

Contents

1 Introduction

Ovarian cancers are classified by their histological origin, and the majority of ovarian malignancies are of epithelial origin. Primary nonepithelial ovarian cancers most commonly include those originating from germ cells or sex cord-stromal cells, and there are extremely rare instances of alternative histological subtypes such as carcinosarcomas or lipoid cell tumors. Metastases from other primary sites can also be found on the ovaries; the most well-known example of this phenomenon is Krukenberg tumors. Nonepithelial ovarian cancers are relatively rare entities, composing only five to ten percent of all ovarian cancers (Quirk and Natarajan 2005). There are many similarities between different subtypes of nonepithelial ovarian cancer in epidemiologic presentation and treatment pattern; however, each specific type of tumor has individual clinical characteristics that are important to recognize. Nonepithelial ovarian cancers are often caught at an earlier stage than epithelial type because of more noticeable early symptoms; however, overall prognosis remains mainly dependent on histological subtype, tumor grade, and stage at presentation.

2 Sex Cord-Stromal Tumors

2.1 Pathogenesis

Sex cord-stromal tumors (SCSTs) are cancers that originate from the embryonal stromal or mesenchymal elements of the ovary. These matrix cell elements of the ovary are typically capable of producing sex hormones; so, patients with SCST often present with evidence of excessive estrogen or androgen phenotypes. The SCST subtypes consist of granulosa cell tumors, Sertoli-Leydig cell tumors, fibroma-thecoma tumors, steroid cell tumors, sex cord tumor with annular tubules, gynandroblastoma, and otherwise unclassified tumors. Mixed cell type tumors are relatively common. Refer Table 1 for SCST subtype classification. The typical age of presentation varies according to the subtype.

2.2 Granulosa Cell Tumors

Granulosa cell tumors (GCT) are the most common type of SCST, comprising approximately 75% of SCST (Chen et al. 2003). There are two types of granulosa cell tumor: adult type and juvenile type. Demographically, the age at

Table 1 World Health Organization histologic classification for sex cord-stromal tumors

WHO histologic classification	Pathology
Granulosa cell tumor	
Adult	Malignant
Juvenile	Malignant
Sertoli cell tumors	Malignant potential
Sertoli-Leydig cell tumors	
Well differentiated	Malignant potential
Intermediate differentiation	Malignant
Poorly differentiated	Malignant
Heterologous elements	Malignant
Leydig cell tumors	Benign
Stromal-Leydig cell tumors	Benign
SCTAT[a] without Peutz-Jaghers syndrome	Malignant
SCTAT[a] with Peutz-Jaghers syndrome	Benign
Gynandroblastoma	Malignant/malignant potential
Thecoma	
Typical	Benign
Luteinized	Malignant potential
Increased mitotic figures	Malignant potential
Fibroma	
Cellular	Malignant potential
Cellular with increased mitotic figures	Malignant potential
Fibrosarcoma	Malignant
Stromal tumor with minor sex cord elements	Benign
Sclerosing stromal tumor	Benign
Signet ring stromal tumor	Benign
Unclassified	Malignant potential
Steroid cell tumors	Malignant
Unclassified SCST[b]	Malignant potential

[a]Sex cord tumor with annular tubules
[b]Sex cord-stromal tumor

presentation for GCT is bimodal, with over 90% of juvenile type presenting prior to puberty, while the average age of presentation for adult type is 50 years (Schumer and Cannistra 2003).

2.3 Adult Type GCT

The presentation of a patient with adult type granulosa cell tumor often presents with signs of hyperestrogenization including heavy abnormal uterine bleeding or postmenopausal vaginal bleeding. Notably, due to the excess estrogen exposure encountered with these tumors, there is an increased risk of coincident endometrial hyperplasia, endometrial carcinoma, and breast cancer (Colombo et al. 2007). Endometrial adenocarcinoma is diagnosed in approximately 5–10% of patients with adult type GCT (Schumer and Cannistra 2003). Additionally, these tumors sometimes present with symptoms of torsion including acute visceral abdomino-pelvic pain and pressure, nausea, and vomiting. Adult GCT expand rapidly and are often 10–15 cm in diameter at the time of presentation; so, patients can also present with symptoms of mass effect including increasing abdominal girth, early satiety, decreasing appetite, nausea, vomiting, and vague abdominal or pelvic pain. It is not uncommon for women with adult type GCT to present with hemoperitoneum after rupture of one of these large vascular masses.

The most important prognostic factor for adult type GCT is stage at diagnosis. Although adult GCT is considered to be malignant, clinical aggressiveness is not defined by mitotic activity or nuclear atypia (Aboud 1997). The majority, 70–90%, of GCT is unilateral and diagnosed at stage I disease. For FIGO stage I disease, 5-year survival rate is reported to be 75–95%; however, that decreases to 55–75% for stage II disease. Stage III/IV disease has poor 5-year survival rates at 20–50% (Gurumurthy et al. 2014). Long-term recurrence is relatively high for patients with all stages of disease. Approximately 25% of patients experience a recurrence, with 30% recurrences occurring greater than 5 years after treatment and 20% after 10 years (Gurumurthy et al. 2014).

2.4 Juvenile Type GCT

Juvenile granulosa cell tumor also typically presents with the effects of hyperestrogenization. In prepubertal girls, these tumors can present with signs of isosexual precocious pseudopuberty, including premature breast and pubic hair development and other secondary sexual characteristics. Amenorrhea or menstrual irreg-ularities can present in young women who are closer to the expected chronologic age of puberty. Like adult type GCT, juvenile type can present with mass effect as described above or hemoperitoneum. Additionally, since these tumors potentially present in reproductive age women, they should be considered in the differential diagnosis of an adnexal mass during pregnancy. GCT are especially concerning as rupture during pregnancy can be catastrophic, with one review finding a 10% rate of rupture with resulting hemoperitoneum requiring emergent intervention during pregnancy (Blake et al. 2014).

Prognosis for juvenile type GCT is also dependent on stage at presentation, and these tumors exhibit more aggressiveness and worse outcome if initially diagnosed at an advanced stage. The juvenile form of GCT is also typically diagnosed early, with over 90% of cases being unilateral and stage I disease at diagnosis (Young et al. 1984). Survival has been noted to be approximately 25% for patients diagnosed with stage II–IV disease, and recurrences of juvenile type disease typically occur early, within 3 years or less from treatment (Young et al. 1984).

2.5   Diagnosis of GCT

Diagnosis of both types of GCT is similar. Clinical suspicion might be aroused by presentations as described above, specifically evidence of hyperestrogenization, mass effects, torsion, or more acute presentation of hemoperitoneum and hypotension indicating a surgical emergency. On physical exam, these clinicians will often encounter a palpable mass on bimanual pelvic exam. Other physical exam findings would be contingent on the patient's age at diagnosis, such as breast and pubic hair development in young girls or postmenopausal vaginal bleeding in older women.

Ultrasonography often demonstrates a large adnexal mass with semisolid or echogenic features, sometimes with septations. Additionally, thickened endometrial stripe is a concerning sign in postmenopausal women (Schumer and Cannistra 2003). Cystic adult GCT, a rare variant, can appear sonographically like a benign, simple cyst, thus causing delays in management and diagnosis. Cystic adult GCT are typically thin walled and can be loculated. There is no definitive diagnostic imaging modality for these or any other type of ovarian tumor.

Tumor markers are also not diagnostic but can contribute to clinical suspicion for and subsequent surveillance of GCT. Estradiol has not been found to be a reliable marker of disease progression. Inhibin A and B have been found to be useful markers for both adult and juvenile type disease; however, they are nonspecific and can also be elevated in epithelial ovarian cancers as well as other conditions (Colombo et al. 2007).

Other important diagnostic considerations include performing an endometrial biopsy and performing breast exam and imaging due to potential sequelae from elevated levels of serum estrogen.

Definitive diagnosis requires final pathological analysis. Gross analysis typically yields a large tumor measuring 10–15 cm with dense vascular solid components. Hemorrhage and necrosis are common macroscopic findings. The most characteristic microscopic features are the "coffee bean" nuclei within granulosa cells and the Call-Exner bodies, an eosinic cystic center surrounded by rosettes of cells. Microscopic images of granulosa cell and other ovarian sex cord-stromal tumors can be found in Fig. 1a. Microscopic nodular growth patterns can also be observed in juvenile type GCT (Fig. 1b).

2.6   Genetic Alteration of GCT

Recent advances have allowed for better elucidation of the molecular components of these rare tumors. A missense point mutation in a gene encoding a transcription factor, FOXL2, has been identified in adult granulosa cell tumors, and it is thought that this mutation is likely present

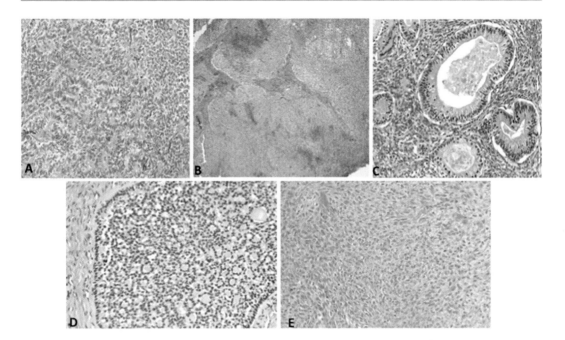

Fig. 1 Microscopic findings in sex cord-stromal tumors of the ovary ((**a**). Adult granulosa cell tumor with Call-Exner bodies (**b**). Juvenile granulose cell tumor with nodular growth (**c**). Sertoli-Leydig cell tumor with heterologous elements (**d**). Sex cord tumor with annular tubules (**e**). Fibrothecoma (Courtesy of Drs. Abby M Richmond and Miriam D Post, Department of Pathology, University of Colorado, Aurora, Colorado))

in all adult granulosa cell tumors (Gershenson 2012).

2.7   Sertoli-Stromal Cell Tumors

Sertoli-stromal cell tumors, or androblastomas, comprise approximately 5–10% of all diagnosed SCSTs. There are several subtypes of tumor that fall into this category, Sertoli cell tumors and Sertoli-Leydig cell tumors, which are then characterized by the degree of tumor differentiation. These tumors typically present in reproductive age women and are almost universally unilateral. Over 90% of Sertoli-stromal cell tumors are stage I at diagnosis (Colombo et al. 2007).

2.8   Sertoli-Leydig Cell Tumors

Sertoli-Leydig cell tumors are typically found in premenopausal women with an average age of presentation of 25. Histologically, they are formed of cells resembling stromal and epithelial testicular cells. They are frequently hormonally active, most commonly producing androgenic sex steroid hormones. Due to this, approximately 75% of patients present with clinical evidence of virilization including temporal balding, hirsuitism, voice changes, and even clitoromegaly in rare cases (Colombo et al. 2007).

There are five histological subtypes of Sertoli-Leydig tumor based on degree of differentiation: well, intermediate, poor, retiform, and heterologous. Sertoli-Leydig cell tumors are most likely to fall into the pathological category of low malignant potential; however, those that are poorly differentiated can demonstrate aggressive behavior. Multiple review articles have examined outcome based on histological subtype. Well-differentiated tumors have uniformly benign behavior, but poorly differentiated tumors have been shown to have malignant characteristics such as metastasis or invasion in up to 60% of the time (Young 2005; Zaloudek and Norris 1984). Grading is based on cellular differentiation; cytologic atypia, mitotic activity, and necrosis are markers of increased risk. Survival of patients with stage I disease is greater than 90% (Colombo et al. 2007). However, outcome is extremely poor for patients that present with disease beyond stage I with mortality being more than 90% (Chen et al. 2003).

2.9 Genetic Alteration of Sertoli-Leydig Cell Tumors

The recent identification of an important genetic alteration called the DICER1 somatic missense mutation will allow for future research on the molecular biology of these tumors. The DICER1 codes for a domain on a component of the RNase III family, and this mutation was identified on 60% of patients with Sertoli-Leydig cell tumors in one recent study (Gershenson 2012). The DICER1 mutation has also been identified in familial nontoxic multinodular goiter and pleuropulmonary blastoma, and both of these pathologies have been associated with increased frequency of Sertoli-Leydig cell tumors (Rio Frio et al. 2011).

2.10 Sertoli Cell Tumors

Sertoli cell tumors are formed from cellular proliferations that resemble the rete ovarii and rete testis and lack the Leydig component. The average age of presentation is 30 years. Only a quarter of these tumors demonstrate hormonal activity, which, if present, can be either estrogenic or androgenic. Sertoli cell tumors have been associated with Peutz-Jaghers syndrome (PJS) (Oliva et al. 2005). They are usually unilateral and stage I at presentation (Chen et al. 2003). Most of these tumors are well differentiated and clinically benign; however, those with atypical cytologic features are more likely to be clinically malignant (Young 2005). Pure Sertoli cell tumors are rare and there is little data on survival in patients with more advanced disease; however,

there is much higher risk for distant metastasis in tumors exhibiting cytologic atypia (Oliva et al. 2005).

2.11 Diagnosis of Sertoli-Stromal Cell Tumors

Clinical suspicion for Sertoli cell tumors should be aroused if an adnexal mass is detected in a young reproductive age woman with evidence of virilization. If evidence of masculinization is present, elevated serum testosterone-to-androstenedione ratio is concerning for Sertoli-Leydig tumor. Other serum markers for an androgenically active tumor includes serum testosterone levels >150 ng/dL or dehydroepiandrosterone sulfate (DHEAS) levels >8000 μg/L (Carmina et al. 2006). However, only one half of patients will present with evidence of androgenic change; presenting symptomatic complaints in most patients will be related to mass effects of a tumor. Inhibin A and B can be useful clinical markers to follow for Sertoli-stromal cell tumors if elevated prior to surgical management.

Pathological analysis of the excised tumor is the only way to definitively diagnose these tumors. Many of these tumors have notable eosinophilic cytoplasm that is sometimes strikingly vacuolated, similar to a seminoma (Young 2005). The predominant microscopic pattern noted is tubular cells. Immunohistochemical staining is important for correctly identifying different histologic subtypes of Sertoli cell tumors as they can appear visually similar (Young 2005). Sertoli-Leydig cell tumors, which are subclassified into five levels of differentiation, have significant overlap amongst these levels of differentiation (Fig. 1c). Sertoli-Leydig tumors are sometimes described as having a distinct retiform pattern (Young 2005).

2.12 Sex Cord Tumor with Annular Tubules

Sex cord tumors with annular tubules (SCTAT) are rare, encompassing only 5% of SCST. SCTAT are morphologically described as having components of both granulosa and Sertoli cell tumors (Fig. 1d). There are two distinct subtypes of SCTAT. Approximately one-third of SCTAT are associated with Peutz-Jaghers syndrome (PJS); these masses are typically small, bilateral, multifocal, and clinically benign.

SCTAT not associated with PJS tend to be larger and unilateral; approximately half of these tumors present with evidence of hyperestrogenization including postmenopausal vaginal bleeding, menstrual irregularities, or isosexual precocious puberty. Another distinctive characteristic is an association of SCTAT with adenoma malignum of the cervix. Adenoma malignum of the cervix, or minimal deviation adenocarcinoma, is an extremely rare well-differentiated adenocarcinoma of the cervix; this finding is only associated with SCTAT not found in conjunction with PJS. Although adenoma malignum of the cervix is a very rare finding, a review article of SCTAT found that of the four patients with this condition two of them died from it (Young et al. 1982). Approximately 20% of these tumors are malignant.

Diagnosis of SCTAT associated with PJS is typically incidental as they are not hormonally active nor large enough to cause mass effects. Diagnosis of SCTAT not associated with PJS is similar to that of other SCST. If there are signs of hyperestrogenism, endometrial sampling is recommended to evaluate for a coincident malignant process. Also, carefully evaluate the cervix prior to surgery due to the associated with adenoma malignum.

2.13 Fibroma-Thecomas

Fibromas are typically benign masses found incidentally as they are rarely hormonally active. They originate from collagen producing cells in the ovarian stroma. They typically present in women around the age of perimenopause. They are sometimes associated with ascites. Even more rarely, they present with a clinical triad including pleural effusion, typically right sided, ascites, and a solid ovarian mass. This triad is called Meigs syndrome and is present on only 1% of fibromas (Riker and Goba 2013). The mechanism surrounding Meigs

syndrome is unclear; however, it is likely due to a large volume transudative process involving the tumor which exceeds the pertinoeum's ability to resorb the fluid (Carson and Mazur 1982). While the vast majority of these tumors are benign, approximately 10% have nuclear characteristics, such as cytologic atypia or increased mitotic patterns, that characterize them as tumors of low malignant potential, and 1% show evidence of transformation into fibrosarcoma and therefore warrants further treatment.

Thecomas are called such due to their characteristic appearance which resembles the theca lutein cells surrounding ovarian follicles (Chen et al. 2003). They can present at any age but present most often in postmenopausal women. These tumors are often hormonally active and present with signs of hyperestrogenization. Much like granulosa cell tumors, patients presenting with signs of excess estrogen exposure are also at risk for endometrial hyperplasia or adenocarcinoma (Aboud 1997). Less commonly these tumors are either not hormonally active or androgenic luteinizing elements are present with resulting signs of masculinization. Notably, these are benign masses and are typically unilateral.

Sclerosing stromal tumors are rare masses that also fall under the classification of fibromathecomas. Their characteristic presentation is that of a unilateral mass in a woman under the age of 30. They are clinically benign. Sclerosing stromal tumors are typically hormonally inactive but can present with menstrual irregularities and pelvic pain (Marelli et al. 1998).

2.14 Diagnosis of Fibroma-Thecoma

Like other ovarian masses, fibromas and thecomas are definitely diagnosed histologically after surgical management (Fig. 1e). After initial clinical evaluation with a thorough history and physical, at which time an adnexal mass might be palpated, ultrasonography can be performed. Thecomas are uniformly solid appearing masses on ultrasound and can be mistaken as an extrauterine leiomyoma (Burandt and Young 2014). For fibromas, if the Meigs triad is present, a thoracentesis can help to evaluate for malignant pleural effusion prior to operative management. There are no specific serum markers that are relevant for fibroma-thecomas. However, cancer antigen 125 (CA125) is sometimes elevated, which can initially raise suspicion for epithelial ovarian carcinoma in the context of an adnexal mass. As with any patient presenting with postmenopausal vaginal bleeding, it is recommended that the endometrium be sampled prior to surgery if there is any concern for endometrial pathology.

2.15   Steroid Cell Tumor

Steroid cell tumors are rare, representing less than 5% of SCST. Histologically, they resemble either testicular Leydig cells (Leydig cell tumors), adrenal cells (stromal luteomas), or steroid cell tumors not otherwise specified (NOS). Both Leydig cell tumors and stromal luteomas typically present in older, postmenopausal women. Leydig cell tumors often present with evidence of virilization, while stromal luteomas are more likely to present with postmenopausal vaginal bleeding or other evidence of hyperestrogenization. These tumors are almost universally benign; however, as with other SCSTs that are hormonally active, evaluation of the endometrium is recommended if there is concern for excess estrogen exposure.

Steroid cell tumors NOS typically present in a younger demographic and are more likely to secrete adrenal hormones such as cortisol. Women with steroid cell tumors NOS might present with a clinical characteristics mimics to Cushing syndrome, signs of which include increased abdominal adiposity, violaceous striae, moon facies, and labile mood. Approximately one-fifth of these tumors behave in a malignant fashion (Chen et al. 2003).

2.16   Gynandroblastoma

Gynandroblastomas are extremely rare. Like many SCSTs they do not demonstrate uniform cellular patterns; they typically are composed of granulosa and Sertoli components. These tumors

can also present with signs of hormonal excess, and either evidence of hyperandrogenism or hyperestrogenism are possible depending on the histologic components of the tumor. The prognosis for gynandroblastoma is very good, although evidence regarding outcome is limited due to the extremely rare nature of this tumor.

2.17   Unclassified Sex Cord-Stromal Tumors

An additional category of SCST is otherwise unclassified. These are composed of an indistinct mixture of granulosa and Sertoli cells. Because they can have either ovarian or testicular cell predominance, their presentation is varied. Much like pure granulosa or Sertoli cell tumors, unclassified SCST can present with signs of virilization or hyperestrogenism. However, many of these tumors do not demonstrate hormonal activity. They behave clinically like their primary components, and outcome is typically based on the degree of morphological differentiation.

2.18   Management of Sex Cord-Stromal Tumor

Surgical resection is the foundation of treatment for SCST. However, while surgical management is the best method treatment and is often curative, it is important to tailor the treatment plan based on the patient and the specific tumor cell type. Typically, neoadjuvant chemotherapy does not have a role in treatment of SCST as these tumors are typically identified at an early stage and often aren't recognized as malignancies until intraoperative frozen section identifies them as such, especially in those tumors that are hormonally inactive.

2.19   Preoperative Management

Considerations prior to surgery include standard preoperative work-up. Serum labs, such as complete blood count, complete metabolic panel, and

Table 2 Tumor markers for sex cord-stromal tumor and malignant germ cell tumor of the ovary[a]

Serum marker	Associated nonepithelial ovarian tumor
Inhibin A and B	Granulosa cell tumor, Sertoli-Leydig cell tumor
Serum testosterone	Sertoli-Leydig cell tumor
Lactate dehydrogenase (LDH)	Dysgerminoma
Beta human chorionic gonadotropin (beta-hCG)	Choriocarcinoma, embryonal carcinoma
Alpha-fetoprotein (AFP)	Yolk sac tumor, embryonal carcinoma, immature teratoma
Serum squamous cell cancer antigen (SSCA)	Mature teratoma with malignant squamous transformation
Cancer antigen 25 (CA125)	Fibroma, struma ovarii, teratoma

[a]Markers will not be elevated in all cases of the associated malignancy

type and screen, are recommended. While the blood loss is typically minimal, a type and cross ought to be considered if granulosa cell tumor is suspected due to the possibility of highly vascular nature of these tumors and associated risk for rupture and hemoperitoneum. Other preoperative considerations include systemic imaging. If there is concern for metastasis beyond the ovary alone, chest radiography or computed tomography of the chest, abdomen, and pelvis can provide more insight regarding the presence of metastatic disease. Tumor markers can be drawn prior to resection, as these can be used in surveillance and can be predictive of increased risk for recurrent disease. See Table 2 for suggested tumor markers. CA125, which is a useful marker for many epithelial ovarian cancers, has no clinical utility for SCST (Stine et al. 2013). If the patient has multiple medical comorbidities, consider referral to a primary care physician and preanesthesia services to achieve the best medical optimization possible prior to surgery.

Another integral aspect of treatment planning that can be discussed with the patient and family preoperatively is desire for future fertility. Approximately, 15% of all ovarian cancers present in women of reproductive age, and, while the majority of SCST are diagnosed in

postmenopausal women, these tumors do present frequently in young women (Gershenson 2005). As detailed above, the vast majority of SCST present unilaterally at an early stage. In this context, it is possible to consider conservative surgery in those that desire future parity. While some fertility sparing options would require assisted reproductive technology, they would allow for the potential of future biological children. Oocyte cryopreservation can also be considered since recurrence in the contralateral ovary or premature ovarian failure following adjuvant chemotherapy can occur. A consultation with a specialist in oncofertility can be offered to young women wishing to discuss options for future fertility. While management of the malignancy must supersede considerations of future fertility, it is integral to discuss the subject of future fertility with younger women prior to proceeding with surgery. In addition, benefits of ovarian sex hormone for cardiovascular, bone, and cognitive health aspects in young premenopausal women need to be considered.

If a malignancy is suspected, a consultation with a gynecologic oncologist prior to operative management is suggested. Due to the rare nature of SCST and the fact that they are often not hormonally active, there are a significant number of these tumors that are identified intraoperatively or on pathology postoperatively. It is beneficial to have the potential for frozen pathology analysis if concerning tumor characteristics are encountered intraoperatively.

2.20 Surgical Management

Surgical management with complete cytoreduction if metastases are present will provide the patient with the best outcome (Gershenson 2012). Surgical approach will vary based on patient and disease characteristics. Minimally invasive approaches are often appropriate for presumed stage I disease; however, if there is tumor rupture this will result in upstaging and potentially necessitate further treatment. Open approaches allow more access for complete cytoreduction in more advanced stage disease, which can be anticipated based on clinical exam and imaging findings.

The decision to proceed with surgical staging will be based on frozen section results and intraoperative findings. If the tumor is not a malignant SCST, comprehensive staging can be omitted. Thus, if the pathology is positive for a benign lesion, then the surgery can be completed without further staging. However, it must be remembered that frozen pathology is not infallible, and accuracy may be decreased in the setting of rare tumors such as SCST (Covens et al. 2012). If staging was not performed at the time of an initial surgery, an additional staging procedure may be completed if indicated by malignancy results on permanent pathology and systemic imaging suggests suspicion for metastasis. Figure 2 provides recommendations for the initial surgical management of SCST.

Surgical staging can be completed via minimally invasive approach or open laparotomy.

Staging consists of a thorough exploration of the abdomen and pelvis, collection of pelvic washings, peritoneal biopsies and partial omentectomy as well as cytoreduction any visible tumor including hysterectomy and bilateral salpingo-oophorectomy in women not wishing to maintain reproductive potential. The role of routine lymphadenectomy in staging SCST has been debated. Lymphadenectomy has not been shown to improve survival in SCST, and the procedure can be associated with increased postoperative complications including lymphocele or lymphedema (Gershenson 2012). The National Comprehensive Cancer Network (NCCN), which articulates treatment guidelines for malignancies in the United States, specifies that routine lymphadenectomy can be omitted during the staging of SCST (Morgan 2015).

As above, the desire for future fertility can be discussed prior to proceeding with operative management. In the absence of advanced disease,

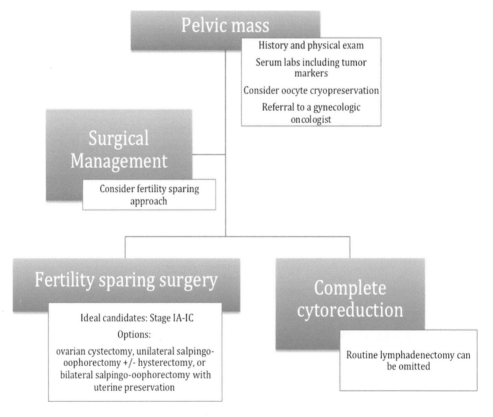

Fig. 2 Principles of surgical management for sex cord-stromal tumors of the ovary

fertility sparing surgery is an acceptable management option for women with stage IA to IC disease (Morgan 2015). Procedures considered fertility sparing include ovarian cystectomy, unilateral salpingo-oopherectomy with or without coincident hysterectomy, or bilateral salpingo-oopherectomy with uterine preservation (Gershenson 2005).

2.21 Postoperative Management

The decision to proceed with additional treatment versus expectant management is dependent on stage and, sometimes, tumor characteristics. Guidance on postoperative treatment is shown in Fig. 3. The most common postoperative treatment options utilized are either observation or platinum-based chemotherapy. Tumor markers, if elevated at the time of presentation, are a relatively noninvasive way to monitor for recurrence. Radiotherapy is of limited use for SCST but can be used for palliative purposes.

As with surgical management, fertility desires can be discussed prior to initiation of chemotherapy.

Cryopreservation can be considered before starting chemotherapy, especially since platinum-based modalities are known to be especially toxic to oocytes. Cryopreservation also allows for fertility in the context of recurrent disease on the contralateral ovary if fertility sparing surgery has been performed.

2.22 Low-Risk Disease

For stage IA disease, the prognosis is excellent; so, no further treatment is recommended (Morgan 2015). Surveillance, consisting of pelvic exams and serum tumor marking testing if initially elevated, should occur every 2–4 months for the first 2 years following surgery, then every 6 months thereafter (Salani et al. 2011). Systemic imaging is indicated if recurrence is suspected.

2.23 Intermediate-Risk Disease

For disease diagnosed at a higher stage, there is still debate over optimal management. Intermediate-risk

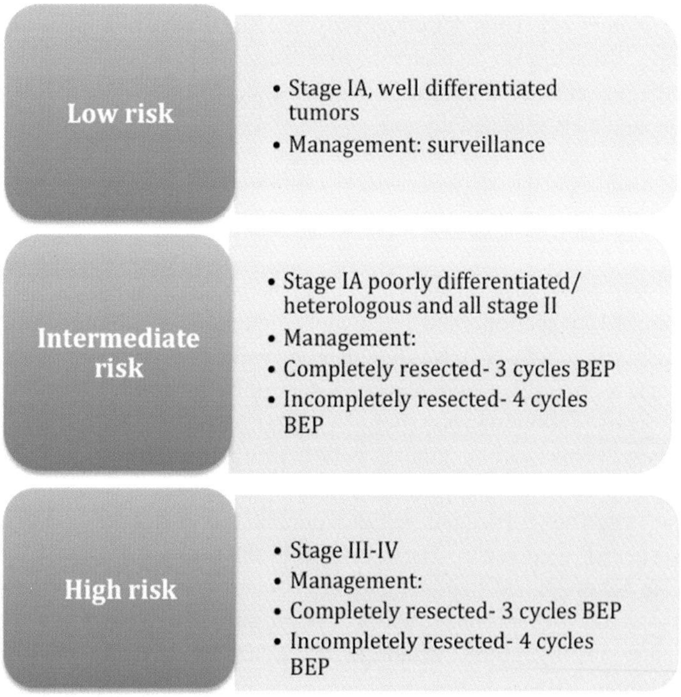

Fig. 3 Adjuvant therapy for sex cord-stromal tumors

Low risk
- Stage IA, well differentiated tumors
- Management: surveillance

Intermediate risk
- Stage IA poorly differentiated/ heterologous and all stage II
- Management:
- Completely resected- 3 cycles BEP
- Incompletely resected- 4 cycles BEP

High risk
- Stage III-IV
- Management:
- Completely resected- 3 cycles BEP
- Incompletely resected- 4 cycles BEP

stage I disease is classified based on characteristics such as tumor rupture, large tumor size, high mitotic rate, positive cytology, heterologous elements, poorly differentiated tumor, or incompletely staged disease (Morgan 2015). Any stage II disease also falls into the category of intermediate risk. The current consensus recommends either observation, with surveillance as detailed above, or platinum-based chemotherapy (Morgan 2015). The preferred adjuvant regimen is either platinum plus taxane or bleomycin, etoposide, and cisplatin (BEP). The most commonly used first line regimen is the 5-day BEP course because it has the highest known response rate (Homesley et al. 1999). Three cycles administered every 3 weeks is recommended for completely resected disease, but one additional cycle is recommended for patients with incompletely resected disease (Homesley et al. 1999).

2.24   High-Risk Disease

Adjuvant chemotherapy is definitely recommended for higher risk patients including stage III to IV disease. The same regimen of BEP as that detailed for intermediate-risk disease is recommended. Thus, for completely resected disease, three cycles is adequate treatment, while administering four cycles is recommended for incompletely resected disease.

2.25   Surveillance

Risk of recurrence remains high even years after surgical resection and adjuvant treatment. According to the NCCN guidelines, surveillance consists of office visits every 2–4 months for 2 years following completion of treatment. These visits will include a pelvic exam and serum tumor markers if initially elevated. Imaging can be performed in the context of a suspected recurrence. There is no role for routine serum tumor markers or imaging without suspicion for recurrence. After 2 years, surveillance visits should occur every 6 months (Morgan 2015).

2.26   Recurrent Disease

Disease can recur after long periods of remission, which is why continued surveillance at 6-month intervals is recommended after the initial 2-year period. Currently, there are no definitive guidelines for recurrent disease. Secondary cytoreduction is considered in cases with limited disease volume. Combination platinum-based chemotherapeutic regimens are typically considered first-line therapy whether or not secondary debulking is performed; BEP is administered most frequently due to its high response rate (Homesley et al. 1999). Other acceptable recurrence therapy options as designated by the NCCN include aromatase inhibitors, bevacizumab (for GCT), taxane, taxane plus ifosfamide, taxane plus carboplatin, tamoxifen, vincristine plus dactinomycin plus cyclophosphamide, radiation, or supportive care only (Morgan 2015). Possible novel strategies include hormonal therapy, such as aromatase inhibitors or the gonadotropin-releasing hormone agonist, leuprolide, for granulosa cell tumors (Morgan 2015). While promising, these treatment methodologies are still under investigation. The identification of germline mutations, such as FOXL2 mutations, may allow for exploration of targeted therapeutics. Thus far, there has been investigation of ketoconazole, the cytochrome P17 (CYP17) inhibitor, as a treatment modality for recurrent granulosa cell tumors due to the recognition that FOXL2 downregulates CYP17 (Garcia-Donas et al. 2013). Because this is based on case report, further studies are warranted. The antiangiogenic bevacizumab has been shown to have moderate activity against recurrent OSCST; more studies involving vascular endothelial growth factor inhibitors are currently underway (Gershenson 2012).

2.27   SCST in Pregnancy

Although a rare phenomenon, SCST does occur coincident with pregnancy. Mirroring the incidence of SCST outside of pregnancy, the most commonly encountered histological subtype is granulosa cell. Notably, a rate of serious adverse events including hemoperitoneum and maternal shock was observed to be greater than 40% in a recent review of pregnancies complicated by SCST (Blake et al. 2014). Therefore, pregnancy complicated by suspected SCST is characterized as a high-risk pregnancy and managed in conjunction with gynecologic oncology and maternal-fetal medicine specialists. Survival of patients with SCST diagnosed within the context of a pregnancy seems comparable to those diagnosed not related to pregnancy, even when managed conservatively (Blake et al. 2014). Management of pregnancy complicated by SCST is not standardized; however, fetal preservation surgery, especially if undertaken in the second trimester, is a reasonable option associated with good maternal and fetal outcomes.

3 Ovarian Malignant Germ Cell Tumors

3.1 Pathogenesis

Germ cell tumors are cancers that originate from primordial germinal cells. Germ cell tumors of the ovary are most often benign, with malignant tumors representing only 5% of germ cell diagnoses. Malignant germ cell tumors comprise only about 2–3% of all ovarian malignancies (Quirk and Natarajan 2005). Ovarian germ cell tumors can be further classified into primitive germ cell tumors, differentiated germ cell tumors, and mixed tumor types as described in Table 3. This chapter will address malignant variations of germ cell tumors including dysgerminoma, immature teratoma, yolk sac tumor, polyembryoma, choriocarcinoma, embryonal carcinoma, and mixed germ cell tumor. The most common germ cell tumor is the mature cystic teratoma, or dermoid cyst, and, while typically benign, cellular components of the dermoid can undergo malignant transformation. In general, ovarian malignant germ cell tumors (OMGCT) present in women under age 30. Depending on the subtype, malignant germ cell tumors can demonstrate hormonal activity.

Table 3 World Health Organization histologic classification for germ cell tumors of the ovary

Primitive germ cell tumors
Dysgerminoma
Yolk sac tumor
Embryonal carcinoma
Polyembryoma
Nongestational choriocarcinoma
Teratomas
Immature
Mature solid
Mature cystic (dermoid)
Monodermal
Mixed forms

The molecular pathogenesis of OMGCT is currently under investigation. Specific microRNA clusters were noted to be overexpressed in all OMGCT. Notably, after a patient with yolk sac tumor was successfully treated, these clusters returned to a normal level (Gershenson 2012). Additionally, the KIT oncogene, a tyrosine kinase receptor recognized as a proto-oncogene in multiple malignancies, has been identified in dysgerminomas, especially those at advanced stage (Gershenson 2012).

3.2 Dysgerminoma

Dysgerminomas are traditionally the most common malignant germ cell neoplasm, but incidence is reported to be decreasing proportionally to other germ cell malignancies in recent years (Smith et al. 2006). These tumors are the "prototypical" germ cell tumors, meaning they are composed of cells that resemble primordial germ cells and appear histologically very similar to seminomas originated from testicular cells. Unlike other types of germ cell tumors, dysgerminomas cannot further differentiate (Chen et al. 2003). These tumors present bilaterally in approximately 15% of cases.

Historically, the prognosis for dysgerminoma was dismal; however, due to their chemosensitivity, overall survival is now greater than 99% (Chan et al. 2008). Over two-thirds of patients present at stage I; however, even later stage disease has an excellent prognosis. Notably, dysgerminomas often spread lymphatically, and approximately one quarter of dysgerminomas are found to have metastasized to regional lymph nodes at the time of diagnosis (Kumar et al. 2008).

3.3 Diagnosis of Dysgerminoma

If an adnexal mass is identified in a young woman, malignant germ cell tumors can be considered in the differential diagnosis. Since these tumors occur bilaterally in approximately 15% of cases, careful attention during the exam of the contralateral ovary after a mass is appreciated. The most common presenting symptom is vague abdominal or pelvic pain due to mass effect. However, acute presentations can occur if the mass torses or ruptures causing hemoperitoneum.

Notably, dysgerminomas are found disproportionately in the context of gonadal dysgenesis. Females with karyotypically abnormal gonads, such as those with Turner syndrome (45X/46XY) or Swyer syndrome (46XY), are at risk for developing a gonadoblastoma. While gonadoblastomas are benign lesions, approximately 40% of these masses undergo malignant transformation, often into dysgerminomas (Pena-Alonso et al. 2005). Young women presenting with abnormal bleeding patterns and pelvic masses should be carefully evaluated for the presence of gonadal dysgenesis. If there is concern for gonadal dysgenesis, a karyotype can be performed.

Imaging via ultrasonography is another important component of the evaluation of a patient with an adnexal mass. Typically these present as solid masses on imaging. Ultrasound characteristics include a well-defined mass divided into component lobules with color Doppler demonstrating rich vascularization (Shaaban et al. 2014). Computed tomography (CT) also demonstrates a mass that is solid and potentially septated with scattered calcifications (Shaaban et al. 2014). CT can also demonstrate sequelae of advanced disease including ascites or evidence of distant metastases or lymphadenopathy.

Tumor markers can also be elevated in the presence of dysgerminoma. Typically these tumors are not hormonally active; they can contain syncytiotrophoblasts which cause serum beta-human chorionic gonadotropin (beta-hCG) elevations. Additionally, serum levels of lactate dehydrogenase (LDH) can also be elevated in the presence of dysgerminoma. While LDH is not specific, it can be a useful serum marker for recurrence if elevated initially.

As with any malignancy, definitive diagnosis cannot be made until final pathology is reviewed. These tumors are typically solid and white or gray in macroscopic appearance. Microscopically, these tumors resemble testicular cancers. Cells are round and uniform, usually surrounded by fibrous stranding or T lymphocyte infiltration (Fig. 4a).

3.4 Yolk Sac Tumors

Yolk sac tumors, previously called endodermal sinus tumors, are composed of remnants of the primitive yolk sac or vitelline elements. These tumors characteristically grow rapidly, and they typically present at a young age, rarely occurring in women over the age of 40. While yolk sac tumors are generally unilateral, they are more aggressive than most other germ cell tumors. Not only do yolk sac tumors demonstrate rapid growth, distant disease is often noted at presentation. The most common sites of metastasis include the lungs and local peritoneal spread (Chen et al. 2003).

Due to their aggressive characteristics, yolk sac tumors have the worst prognosis of all germ cell malignancies. Almost half of the cases of yolk sac tumor present after advancing beyond stage I disease. Even with appropriate treatment, survival rate for patients with stage III-IV disease is 50–75%. However, 5-year survival rate for patients with only stage I disease is greater than 90% (Chan et al. 2008). According to recent data, recurrences usually present within a year following treatment and are typically not responsive to further therapy (Cicin et al. 2009).

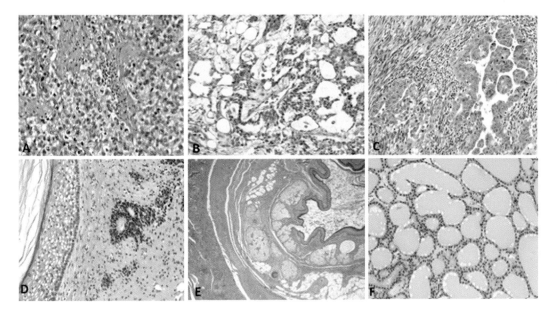

Fig. 4 Microscopic findings of malignant germ cell tumors of the ovary ((**a**). Dysgerminoma (**b**). Yolk sac tumor with Schiller-Duval bodies (**c**) Embryonal carcinoma (**d**). Immature teratoma with rosette (**e**). Mature cystic teratoma (**f**). struma ovarii (Courtesy of Drs. Abby M Richmond and Miriam D Post, Department of Pathology, University of Colorado, Aurora, Colorado))

3.5   Diagnosis of Yolk Sac Tumor

Since yolk sac tumors typically grow rapidly, women with these tumors often complain of relatively acute onset abdominal or pelvic pain. Review articles have noted several cases with growth of masses measuring greater than 20 cm over the course of weeks to months (Kurman and Norris 1976). Capsular rupture is fairly common, likely because of the rapid expansion of these tumors. These patients can also present with hemoperitoneum as these rapidly growing lesions are highly vascularized. If a large mass is palpable on pelvic exam, especially in a young premenopausal woman, suspicion for a yolk sac tumor is increased.

Imaging can be obtained after appreciation of a mass on exam. Ultrasound findings can include a unilateral mass with heterogenous echogenicity and septations. Computed tomographic images are often significant for enhancing foci in the tumor wall attributable to dilated blood vessels. Capsular tears can also sometimes be appreciated on imaging. None of these findings is pathognomonic for yolk sac tumors; however, they can help contribute to heightened preoperative suspicion for this entity (Shaaban et al. 2014).

Serum tumor markers can also be helpful in both preoperative evaluation for yolk sac tumors and for postoperative surveillance. These tumors produce alpha-fetoprotein (AFP). AFP is not specific for yolk sac tumors as other germ cell malignancies can produce this protein that is typically found in fetal circulation; however, yolk sac tumors will almost universally have elevated AFP level.

Pathological analysis is required for definitive diagnosis. Gross pathology will be significant for a large mass, on average measuring 15 cm, with mixed solid and cystic components. There are often focal areas of hemorrhage and necrosis in macroscopic appearance. Microscopically, these tumors can vary significantly in appearance; however, by definition they resemble the cellular structure of the primitive yolk sac. The appearance of an isolated papillary body containing a centralized vessel and surrounded by embryonic epithelial cells, called a Schiller-Duval body, is pathognomonic for yolk sac tumor but is not required for diagnosis (Fig. 4b).

3.6 Embryonal Carcinoma, Polyembryona, and Mixed Germ Cell Tumor

Other rare subtypes of primitive germ cell tumors include embryonal carcinoma, polyembryona, and mixed germ cell tumor. While all of these variants are likely to present in somewhat mixed form, they each have specific characteristics that allow them to be classified as individual entities.

Embryonal carcinoma is another malignant variant that can evolve from dysgenetic gonads. These tumors typically present in girls in their teenage years. Embryonal carcinoma typically produces beta-hCG and often produces AFP. On pathology, these tumors are noted to have solid sheets of anaplastic cells and distinctive papillary projections (Ulbright 2005; Fig. 4c).

Polyembryonas are extremely rare. These tumors have features of both primitive and differentiated germ cell tumor types, so are sometimes considered to be extremely immature teratomas (Ulbright 2005). Serum AFP and beta-hCG are often elevated in the presence of these tumors. Polyembryonas almost exclusively present as components of mixed germ cell tumor. Microscopically, these tumors have central "germ discs" surrounded by two cavities, one resembling the amniotic cavity and the other resembling the yolk sac cavity (Ulbright 2005).

Ovarian mixed germ cell tumors contain aspects of multiple types of germ cell tumors without one predominant component. Dysgerminoma is the most common component of mixed germ cell tumors, but they can contain elements of any histological subtype. The presence of higher risk malignant elements, such as high-grade immature teratoma, increases the likelihood of aggressive behavior.

3.7 Nongestational Choriocarcinoma

Nongestational choriocarcinoma in pure form is very rare, accounting for less than 5% of malignant germ cell tumors (Smith et al. 2006). These are aggressive tumors which can be confused with metastatic gestational choriocarcinoma. Gestational choriocarcinoma is associated with a proximate pregnancy and can metastasize to the ovaries. This distinction is important due to the poorer prognosis of nongestational choriocarcinoma (Corakci et al. 2005). The distinction between these two entities is made based on pathology findings; nongestational choriocarcinoma will be found in the presence of other germ cell components (Ulbright 2005).

These tumors are typically found in patients less than 20 years. Information on prognosis is limited due to the extremely rare nature of this tumor; however, prognosis is typically poor due to the frequency of distant metastasis at presentation (Corakci et al. 2005). Beta-hCG is often markedly elevated in these patients. The elevated beta-hCG can result in prominent symptoms such as isosexual precocious puberty or menstrual abnormalities in women who have undergone menarche.

3.8 Teratoma

All teratomas consist of components from all three germ cell layers: endoderm, mesoderm, and ectoderm. The malignant variation of teratoma is termed immature, but the majority of these tumors are classified as mature. Although rare, malignancy can develop within a mature cystic teratoma. The term dermoid is often used interchangeably with teratoma; however, there is a histological distinction between the two entities. Dermoids are composed of epidermal and dermal elements, while teratomas contain mesodermal and endodermal components. Teratomas can also be classified as monodermal or specialized when they consist predominantly of endodermal or ectodermal elements.

3.9 Immature Teratoma

Immature teratomas account for 30% of deaths from ovarian malignancy in women under age 20. They are now the most commonly detected malignant germ cell tumor (Smith et al. 2006). In addition to endodermal, mesodermal, and ectodermal components, they also contain embryonic tissue, thus qualifying them as immature. These tumors typically present in women in their teenage years and rarely occur in postmenopausal women. Immature teratomas are typically unilateral but often have spread via local peritoneal seeding or via lymphatics at the time of diagnosis. If bilateral, which occurs in about 10% of cases, the contralateral tumor is generally a mature teratoma. The typical size at presentation is 14–25 cm (Wisniewski and Deppisch 1973).

Despite immature teratomas having a propensity to disseminate early, approximately three-quarters of these tumors are detected at stage I. The 5-year overall survival for stage I disease is greater than 95%. Survival for later stage disease is associated with poorer prognosis, but overall survival is still relatively high, ranging from 73% to 88% (Chan et al. 2008). Recurrence is not uncommon, but recurrent disease typically remains chemosensitive.

A phenomenon specific to immature teratoma is that of growing teratoma syndrome, which refers to postoperative growth of mature teratoma elements implanted in the peritoneum. These implants are typically benign and chemoresistant and can continue enlarging so resection is required to exclude recurrent malignancy. The incidence is relatively low, approximately 12% (Zagame et al. 2006). Prognosis is generally not affected by the presence of growing teratoma syndrome.

3.10 Mature Teratoma with Malignant Transformation

Mature cystic teratomas are the most common benign ovarian neoplasm and typically present in women age 20–40. These masses typically measure approximately 7 cm at presentation (Wisniewski and Deppisch 1973). Malignant transformation occurs very rarely in mature cystic teratomas, and it typically presents in postmenopausal women. The incidence of malignant transformation is approximately 1–2% (Smith et al. 2006). The most commonly identified

malignancy is squamous cell carcinoma, which accounts for about 80% of malignant transformations. There is no clear mechanism of malignant transformation identified; however, it is notable that the average age of presentation is approximately 50 years, while most mature cystic teratomas are diagnosed in women several decades younger (Dos Santos et al. 2007). This finding has led to the hypothesis that prolonged presence of teratomas in situ increases the likelihood of malignant transformation; therefore, even though typically benign, it is important to surgically remove these masses. Unfortunately, the prognosis for squamous cell carcinoma within mature cystic teratoma is low as 48% overall; 5-year survival for stage IV disease is reported as 0% in one study (Chen et al. 2008). Other malignancies that have been reported within mature cystic teratomas include melanoma, basal cell carcinoma, thyroid carcinoma, carcinoid, chondrosarcoma, leiomyosarcoma, angiosarcoma, and intestinal adenocarcinoma (Chen et al. 2003).

3.11 Malignant Struma Ovarii

Struma ovarii refers to a type of monodermal teratoma that is composed of at least 50% thyroid tissue. Struma ovarii accounts for approximately 3% of mature teratomas (Roth and Talerman 2007). These tumors are typically benign, but a malignant component presents in less than 5% of cases of struma ovarii. Carcinomas that can occur within malignant struma ovarii include follicular or papillary variants. Additionally, struma ovarii can contain nonthyroid type neoplasms including carcinoid, Brenner tumor, or mucinous cystadenoma. These tumors typically present in postmenopausal women.

3.12 Paraneoplastic Encephalitis

Although not a malignancy, N-methyl-D-aspartate (NMDA) receptor antibody encephalitis is an important phenomenon associated with ovarian teratomas. NMDA receptor antibody encephalitis is a paraneoplastic neurologic syndrome characterized by psychiatric symptoms, seizures, amnesia, and semirepetitive dystonic movement abnormalities. While a mass is not always present, the syndrome is most classically associated with teratomas in young women. Positive serum NMDA receptor antibody titers in the presence of this constellation of symptoms is diagnostic, and typically a higher antibody titer correlates with more severe symptoms (Irani and Vincent 2011). The pathogenesis of this condition is not fully understood; however, it is thought that impaired immunomodulation in the context of a disrupted blood–brain barrier could be responsible for the paraneoplastic syndrome (Irani and Vincent 2011). Treatment is centered on decreasing antibody levels both via surgical resection and pharmacologic agents including corticosteroids, plasma exchange, and intravenous immunoglobulins. Early resection and treatment are noted to have the best outcomes; death or permanent neurological sequelae can occur in the absence of prompt recognition and treatment (Irani and Vincent 2011).

3.13 Diagnosis of Teratoma

Most teratomas will be diagnosed either incidentally or after palpation of an adnexal mass as there are typically few systemic sequelae. Some patients will present complaining of vague abdominal or pelvic pain. Mature teratomas also commonly present with symptoms of torsion including intermittent visceral abdominal pain or pressure and nausea or vomiting. Patients with struma ovarii present with clinical hyperthyroidism in approximately 5% of cases (Roth and Talerman 2007). Additionally, struma ovarii presents with ascites in one-third of cases and with Meigs syndrome in rare cases (Roth and Talerman 2007). Meigs syndrome is a clinical triad consisting of ascites, pleural effusion, and pelvic mass.

On imaging, teratomas appear as heterogenous solid adnexal masses, often described as a cystic mass with intratumoral fat. Classically, mature teratomas are described as having a "dot-dash" pattern on ultrasound. Small areas of cystic

calcifications or fatty elements can be appreciated on ultrasound. In immature teratomas, these calcified areas appear small, irregular, and scattered, while calcifications appear more well-defined or even tooth-like in mature teratomas (Shaaban et al. 2014). Another common ultrasound finding in mature teratomas is the Rokitansky nodule or dermoid plug, which is a nodule containing hair, teeth, and fat. If present, malignant transformation can occur in the region of the Rokitansky nodule and is seen as a heterogenous irregular solid mass that might demonstrate invasion into surrounding tissue (Shaaban et al. 2014). Cystic components have attenuation and signal intensity similar to that of simple fluid in immature teratomas but will appear more as fatty sebaceous material in mature teratomas on CT imaging (Shaaban et al. 2014).

Although no tumor marker is characteristic for teratomas, there are several that can be present depending on the predominant cell types contained within the teratoma. Serum markers such as AFP, CA125, cancer antigen 19-9 (CA19-9) can be elevated in immature teratomas (Li et al. 2002). If elevated, these markers can assist in postoperative surveillance. Another useful tumor marker evaluating for the presence of malignant transformation of a mature teratoma is serum squamous cell carcinoma antigen (SSCA). SSCA has been shown to be elevated in greater than 80% of patients that have foci of squamous cell carcinoma (Chen et al. 2008). Elevated CA125 can be found in the context of struma ovarii. While most patients with struma ovarii are chemically and clinically euthyroid, there can be abnormalities in thyroid hormone levels.

While the above factors can help assist in diagnosis and surveillance, final pathology is required for definitive diagnosis. Microscopically, components of all three germ cell layers can be observed in both immature and mature teratomas (Fig. 4d). Immature teratomas typically appear as disordered mixed tissue (Fig. 4e). Tumor grade or aggressiveness is dependent on the amount of immature neural tissue contained within the tumor. Teratomas grossly contain hair, fatty or sebaceous material, and calcifications or teeth; immature teratomas tend to be larger in diameter than mature teratomas. Struma ovarii is formed of mature thyroid tissue and grossly appears as brown- or amber-colored colloidal material with thick septations (Fig. 4f).

3.14 Management of Ovarian Malignant Germ Cell Tumors

Historically, malignant germ cell tumors were associated with an abysmal prognosis. However, the development of modern chemotherapeutic techniques has drastically improved outcomes for these tumors. Initial surgical cytoreduction remains the cornerstone of management for malignant germ cell tumors. Surgery and resulting pathology findings are both therapeutic and diagnostic. Neoadjuvant chemotherapy has little clinical utility in OMGCT.

3.15 Preoperative Evaluation

Thorough preoperative assessment includes a consideration of preoperative imaging to evaluate for evidence of distant metastasis and thus aid in surgical planning. Preoperative labs including complete blood count, complete metabolic panel, and type and screen can be drawn prior to any potential major abdominal surgery. Tumor markers including LDH, b-HCG, AFP, CA125, CA19-9, and SSCA can be considered. Appropriate tumor markers are to be selected based on presentation and clinical suspicion for specific subtypes of OMGCT. The age of incidence for OMGCT is typically younger than that of other malignancies, so medical comorbidities necessitating preoperative anesthesia clearance are less common in this demographic; however, preanesthesia evaluation can be taken into consideration.

It is important to discuss implications of surgery and subsequent chemotherapy with patients and their families prior to undertaking the procedure. Since OMGCT often presents in women of reproductive age, a discussion of future fertility desires is recommended. Although management of the present malignancy must take precedence over future fertility desires, current literature indicates that patients and their families appreciate this discussion and may even be unaware prior to the procedure that loss of fertility or changes in future hormonal status could be a result of treatment (Loren et al. 2013). Due to excellent outcomes, fertility sparing surgery is now considered standard of care for OMGCT (Gershenson 2012). Oocyte cryopreservation is also a potential option for patients wishing to preserve future fertility. Adjuvant chemotherapy and risk of relapse in the remaining ovary are concerns to potential future fertility; as such, oocyte harvesting can help to ensure better reproductive outcomes in the future. There are multiple options available for young women wishing to preserve their future fertility in the context of malignancy, and, if available, referral to a specialist in oncofertility can be offered.

There is a high rate of relapse after inadequate staging and follow-up of OMGCT (Gershenson 2012). Therefore, for cases in which there is high suspicion for one of these malignancies, a referral to a gynecologic oncologist for staging and management is recommended.

3.16 Surgical Management

Surgical approach is dictated based on tumor and patient characteristics. Whenever possible, surgical spill should be avoided in order to prevent iatrogenic upstaging of disease. Many OMGCT are large at the time of presentation and thus preclude minimally invasive surgical options. However, if possible, the reduced postoperative morbidity of laparoscopic surgery compared to laparotomy is favorable if adequate staging is allowed through this approach. Surgeons consider low threshold to convert from laparoscopy to laparotomy when surgical spill is concerned for tumor grossly confined in the ovary. See Fig. 5 for recommendations regarding surgical management for OMGCT.

The exact extent of appropriate surgical staging for apparent early stage OMGCT remains somewhat contentious. Procedures considered fertility sparing include ovarian cystectomy,

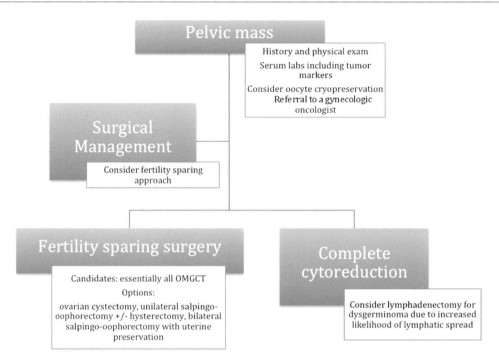

Fig. 5 Principles of surgical management for malignant germ cell tumors of the ovary

unilateral salpingo-oopherectomy with or without coincident hysterectomy, or bilateral salpingo-oopherectomy with uterine preservation (Gershenson 2005). Pediatric literature recommends conservative staging consisting of examination of peritoneal surfaces and collection of washings, palpation of retroperitoneal lymph nodes, and biopsy of abnormal appearing areas following resection of the affected ovary and visible mass (Billmire et al. 2004). A longitudinal review of oncologic and fertility outcomes for pediatric patients that underwent fertility sparing surgery and adjuvant chemotherapy found favorable outcomes regardless of histologic subtype and FIGO stage (Park et al. 2015). Additionally, fertility sparing surgery in the aforementioned study was conservatively defined as preservation of the unaffected ovary and uterus.

Bilateral tumors are present in less than 10% of OMGCT; however, they present a challenge to those wishing to preserve fertility. Although literature for the rare presentation of bilateral malignancies is minimal, available studies indicate that these tumors have a good prognosis and that fertility preservation can be considered, especially in

the setting of bilateral dysgerminoma (Sigismondi et al. 2015). In a small study examining outcomes of bilateral OMGCT of various subtypes, a unilateral salpingo-oophorectomy was performed along with either a biopsy or cystectomy on the contralateral ovary followed by treatment with chemotherapy. The small subset of four patients treated with ovarian preservation demonstrated resultant preservation of future fertility and similar survival outcomes to those patients that were completely staged (Sigismondi et al. 2015). This data is based on very limited case numbers and risks and benefits ought to be considered carefully before deciding to leave an affected ovary in situ.

Traditional practice endorses that, similar to those with epithelial ovarian cancers, patients receiving complete cytoreduction improves survival outcome (Suita et al. 2002). However, as supported by the data above, accumulating evidence endorses a less aggressive staging procedure even if fertility preservation is not a priority of management. A careful inspection of all intraabdominal and pelvic surfaces is necessary. If tumor histology is identified on frozen pathology, characteristic patterns of dissemination are to be taken into consideration. Dysgerminomas demonstrate lymphatic spread more frequently than other types of OMGCT, and this can be taken into consideration when deciding whether or not to perform staging with lymphadenectomy. Yolk sac tumors and immature teratomas are more likely to spread locally and have metastases present on the peritoneum and omentum. In advanced disease, the aim of surgery is maximally cytoreducing all accessible tumors.

4   Postoperative Management

4.1   Adjuvant Chemotherapy

OMGCT are typically notably chemosensitive. The responsiveness to chemotherapy allows surgical treatment to be less aggressive and allows for fertility sparing treatment as above. OMGCT, especially dysgerminoma, are often radiosensitive, and radiation was used in the past to treat these tumors but is no longer standard of care. Combination chemotherapy regimens including vincristine, dactinomcycin, cyclophosphamide (VAC) or cisplatin, vinblastine, bleomycin (PVB) were introduced in the 1970s with marked

improvement in outcomes for patients diagnosed with OMGCT. Currently, all histologic subtypes of these tumors are treated with a combination of bleomycin, etoposide, and cisplatin (BEP), as this regimen was found to be more active and had an acceptable toxicity in patients (Gershenson et al. 1990). BEP is now first line for adjuvant therapy. Figure 6 outlines basic principles of postoperative management of OMGCT.

Current standard of care includes postoperative chemotherapy for all patients except those with well staged stage IA, grade 1 pure immature teratoma or stage I pure dysgerminoma. BEP is typically administered every 3 weeks. Randomized control trials have demonstrated that three cycles is adequate to prevent recurrence in nearly all patients who have undergone staging with complete cytoreduction (Williams et al. 1994). NCCN guidelines recommend three cycles for patients considered low risk for recurrence and four cycles for higher risk disease (Morgan 2015). Pulmonary function tests are recommended prior to starting bleomycin. Alternatively, the NCCN specifies that three courses of carboplatinum and etoposide can be used to reduce toxicity if the diagnosis is stage IB-III dysgerminoma (Morgan 2015). This regimen is administered every 4 weeks for 3 cycles.

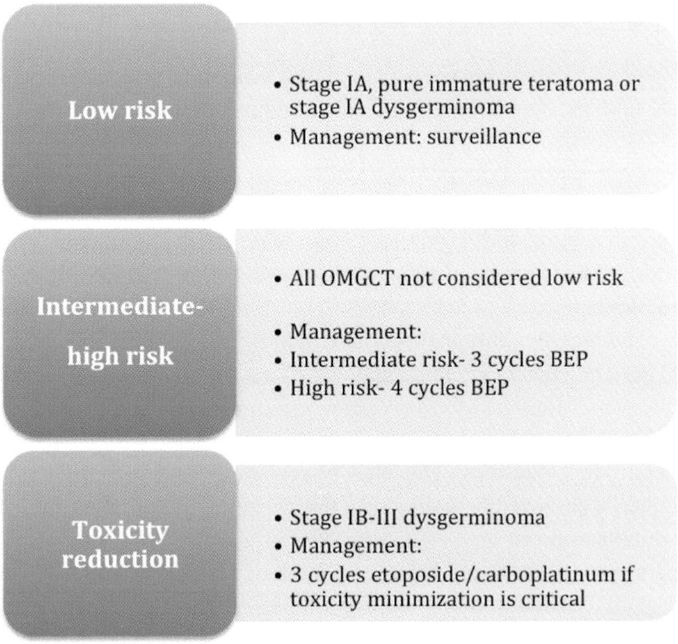

Fig. 6 Adjuvant therapy for malignant ovarian germ cell tumors

Low risk
- Stage IA, pure immature teratoma or stage IA dysgerminoma
- Management: surveillance

Intermediate-high risk
- All OMGCT not considered low risk
- Management:
- Intermediate risk- 3 cycles BEP
- High risk- 4 cycles BEP

Toxicity reduction
- Stage IB-III dysgerminoma
- Management:
- 3 cycles etoposide/carboplatinum if toxicity minimization is critical

Many patients and families will express concern about the effects of chemotherapy on future fertility. Unlike radiation treatment, the majority of patients receiving the standard BEP regimen resume normal menses and have successful future fertility outcomes (Weinberg et al. 2011). As above, oocyte cryopreservation will allow for improved fertility outcomes for the minority patients that experience premature ovarian failure following BEP.

4.2 Surveillance

Risk of recurrence is highest in the first few years following surgical resection. According to the NCCN guidelines, surveillance consists of office visits every 2–4 months for 2 years following completion of treatment (Morgan 2015). These visits include a pelvic exam and serum tumor markers if initially elevated. Imaging can be performed in the context of a suspected recurrence. There is no role for routine serum tumor markers or imaging without suspicion for recurrence. After 2 years, annual exams can be performed (Salani et al. 2011).

4.3 Recurrence

Rates of recurrence vary depending on histological subtype, disease stage, and extent of the initial cytoreduction. As above, there remains controversy about the extent of surgical staging that is recommended with the initial tumor reduction surgery. Fortunately, even in the event of recurrent disease, the overwhelming majority of patients are salvageable.

The NCCN guidelines recommend referral to a tertiary center for management of recurrent disease (Morgan 2015). There are multiple options for recurrent disease, but there are no definitive guidelines. The NCCN recommends either high-dose chemotherapy, the specifics of which can differ among institutions, or another choice of combination regimens, most of which include a platinum agent (Morgan 2015). Platinum agents are not recommended if the tumor is platinum resistant or recurrent within 6 months of completing initial treatment. There is negligible role for secondary cytoreduction if disease recurs unless it demonstrates growth or persistence following chemotherapy, thus demonstrating chemoresistance (Williams et al. 1994). Radiotherapy is another option for recurrent disease. KIT targeting in dysgerminoma has not been well studied and future studies are expected. Alternatively, for patients with advanced disease or otherwise poor prognosis, supportive care alone is an option.

4.4 Ovarian Malignant Germ Cell Tumor in Pregnancy

Although a rare event, the propensity for OMGCT to present in young reproductive aged women results in them accounting for 18–26% of all ovarian cancers recognized in pregnancy. Dysgerminoma is the most frequently encountered OMGCT in pregnancy. OMGCT diagnosed in pregnancy are usually unilateral and stage I, mirroring the typical presentation in nongravid women (Kodama et al. 2014). These tumors can sometimes be recognized in the context of a persistent adnexal mass due to markedly elevated tumor markers; however, this can sometimes be obscured by the expected presence of markers such as AFP during pregnancy.

Review of the literature indicates that, although rates of preterm birth are higher than those in the general population, the majority of these cases result in delivery of viable infants. Pregnancy preservation is in general a reasonable option. However, due to the tendency of OMGCT to disseminate rapidly, intervention should not be delayed until delivery. Surgical staging can be performed if suspicion for an ovarian malignancy is raised even during pregnancy. Although there are no randomized control trials to provide guidance, observational studies indicate that BEP is safe in pregnancy (Karimi Zarchi et al. 2008). Furthermore, advanced stage disease diagnosed during pregnancy has been identified as an independent predictor of decreased survival (Kodama et al. 2014). Therefore, although identification of a suspected OMGCT does not necessitate pregnancy termination, early intervention consistent with the standard of care is recommended if the patient desires continuation of the pregnancy.

5 Conclusion

Nonepithelial cell ovarian cancers are rare entities. Sex cord-stromal tumors and malignant germ cell tumors are the most common nonepithelial ovarian cancers. Although not encountered often, it is important to consider these tumors in differential diagnoses of adnexal masses. These tumors often, but not always, present with the sequelae of overproduction of either androgens or estrogens. It is important to diagnose these masses early, as overall prognosis is typically very good for early stage disease in all histological subtypes. Both sex cord-stromal tumors and malignant germ cell tumors of the ovary are treated with initial surgical resection. Fertility sparing surgery can be considered for both sex cord-stromal and malignant germ cell tumors of the ovary. Depending on the pathological diagnosis and disease stage, postoperative management consists of either expectant management or adjuvant chemotherapy. It is recommended that all patients with nonepithelial ovarian cancer be monitored for evidence of disease recurrence on a standardized schedule.

References

Aboud E. Adult granulosa cell tumours of the ovary. Eur J Gynaecol Oncol. 1997;18(6):520–2.

Billmire D, Vinocur C, Rescorla F, Cushing B, London W, Schlatter M, et al. Outcome and staging evaluation in malignant germ cell tumors of the ovary in children and adolescents: an intergroup study. J Pediatr Surg. 2004;39(3):424–9.

Blake EA, Carter CM, Kashani BN, Kodama M, Mabuchi S, Yoshino K, et al. Feto-maternal outcomes of pregnancy complicated by ovarian sex-cord stromal tumor: a systematic review of literature. Eur J Obstet Gynecol Reprod Biol. 2014;175:1–7.

Burandt E, Young RH. Thecoma of the ovary: a report of 70 cases emphasizing aspects of its histopathology different from those often portrayed and its differential diagnosis. Am J Surg Pathol. 2014;38(8):1023–32.

Carmina E, Rosato F, Janni A, Rizzo M, Longo RA. Extensive clinical experience: relative prevalence of different androgen excess disorders in 950 women referred because of clinical hyperandrogenism. J Clin Endocrinol Metab. 2006;91(1):2–6.

Carson SA, Mazur MT. Atypical endometrioid cystadenofibroma with Meigs syndrome: ultrastructure and S phase fraction. Cancer. 1982;49(3):472–9.

Chan JK, Tewari KS, Waller S, Cheung MK, Shin JY, Osann K, et al. The influence of conservative surgical practices for malignant ovarian germ cell tumors. J Surg Oncol. 2008;98(2):111–6.

Chen VW, Ruiz B, Killeen JL, Cote TR, Wu XC, Correa CN. Pathology and classification of ovarian tumors. Cancer. 2003;97(10 Suppl):2631–42.

Chen RJ, Chen KY, Chang TC, Sheu BC, Chow SN, Huang SC. Prognosis and treatment of squamous cell carcinoma from a mature cystic teratoma of the ovary. J Formos Med Assoc. 2008;107(11):857–68.

Cicin I, Saip P, Guney N, Eralp Y, Ayan I, Kebudi R, et al. Yolk sac tumours of the ovary: evaluation of clinicopathological features and prognostic factors. Eur J Obstet Gynecol Reprod Biol. 2009;146(2):210–4.

Colombo N, Parma G, Zanagnolo V, Insinga A. Management of ovarian stromal cell tumors. J Clin Oncol. 2007;25(20):2944–51.

Corakci A, Ozeren S, Ozkan S, Gurbuz Y, Ustun H, Yucesoy I. Pure nongestational choriocarcinoma of ovary. Arch Gynecol Obstet. 2005;271(2):176–7.

Covens AL, Dodge JE, Lacchetti C, Elit LM, Le T, Devries-Aboud M, et al. Surgical management of a suspicious adnexal mass: a systematic review. Gynecol Oncol. 2012;126(1):149–56.

Dos Santos L, Mok E, Iasonos A, Park K, Soslow RA, Aghajanian C, Kaled A, Barakat RR, Abu-Rustum NR. Squamous cell carcinoma arising in mature cystic teratoma of the ovary: a case series and review of the literature. Gynecol Oncol. 2007;105(2):321–4.

Garcia-Donas J, Hurtado A, Garcia-Casado Z, Albareda J, López-Guerrero JA, Alemany I, Grande E, Camara JC, Hernando S. Cytochrome P17 inhibition with ketoconazole as a treatment for advanced granulosa cell ovarian tumor. J Clin Oncol. 2013;31:165–6.

Gershenson DM. Fertility-sparing surgery for malignancies in women. J Natl Cancer Inst Monogr. 2005;34:43–7.

Gershenson DM. Current advances in the management of malignant germ cell and sex cord-stromal tumors of the ovary. Gynecol Oncol. 2012;125:515–7. United States.

Gershenson DM, Morris M, Cangir A, Kavanagh JJ, Stringer CA, Edwards CL, et al. Treatment of malignant germ cell tumors of the ovary with bleomycin, etoposide, and cisplatin. J Clin Oncol. 1990;8(4):715–20.

Gurumurthy M, Bryant A, Shanbhag S. Effectiveness of different treatment modalities for the management of adult-onset granulosa cell tumours of the ovary (primary and recurrent). Cochrane Database Syst Rev. 2014;4:Cd006912.

Homesley HD, Bundy BN, Hurteau JA, Roth LM. Bleomycin, etoposide, and cisplatin combination therapy of ovarian granulosa cell tumors and other stromal malignancies: a Gynecologic Oncology Group study. Gynecol Oncol. 1999;72(2):131–7.

Irani S, Vincent A. NMDA receptor anitbody encephalitis. Curr Neurol Neuosci Rep. 2011;11:298–304.

Karimi Zarchi M, Behtash N, Modares Gilani M. Good pregnancy outcome after prenatal exposure to bleomycin, etoposide and cisplatin for ovarian immature teratoma: a case report and literature review. Arch Gynecol Obstet. 2008;277(1):75–8. Gynecol Oncol. 1999;72:131–7.

Kodama M, Grubbs BH, Blake EA, Cahoon SS, Murakami R, Kimura T, et al. Feto-maternal outcomes of pregnancy complicated by ovarian malignant germ cell tumor: a systematic review of literature. Eur J Obstet Gynecol Reprod Biol. 2014;181:145–56.

Kumar S, Shah JP, Bryant CS, Imudia AN, Cote ML, Ali-Fehmi R, et al. The prevalence and prognostic impact of lymph node metastasis in malignant germ cell tumors of the ovary. Gynecol Oncol. 2008;110(2):125–32.

Kurman RJ, Norris HJ. Endodermal sinus tumor of the ovary: a clinical and pathologic analysis of 71 cases. Cancer. 1976;38(6):2404–19.

Li H, Hong W, Zhang R, Wu L, Liu L, Zhang W. Retrospective analysis of 67 consecutive cases of pure ovarian immature teratoma. Chin Med J (Engl). 2002;115(10):1496–500.

Loren AW, Mangu PB, Beck LN, Brennan L, Magdalinski AJ, Partridge AH, et al. Fertility preservation for patients with cancer: American Society of Clinical Oncology clinical practice guideline update. J Clin Oncol. 2013;31(19):2500–10.

Marelli G, Carinelli S, Mariani A, Frigerio L, Ferrari A. Sclerosing stromal tumor of the ovary. Report of eight cases and review of the literature. Eur J Obstet Gynecol Reprod Biol. 1998;76(1):85.

Morgan et al. [Internet]. NCCNOCV, updated Feb 2015, cited 15 Oct 2015. Available at http://www.nccn.org/professionals/physician_gls/pdf/ovarian.pdf

Oliva E, Alvarez T, Young RH. Sertoli cell tumors of the ovary: a clinicopathologic and immunohistochemical study of 54 cases. Am J Surg Pathol. 2005;29(2):143–56.

Park JY, Kim DY, Suh DS, Kim JH, Kim YM, Kim YT, et al. Outcomes of pediatric and adolescent girls with malignant ovarian germ cell tumors. Gynecol Oncol. 2015;137(3):418–22.

Pena-Alonso R, Nieto K, Alvarez R, Palma I, Najera N, Erana L, et al. Distribution of Y-chromosome-bearing cells in gonadoblastoma and dysgenetic testis in 45, X/46,XY infants. Mod Pathol. 2005;18(3):439–45.

Quirk JT, Natarajan N. Ovarian cancer incidence in the United States, 1992–1999. Gynecol Oncol. 2005;97(2):519–23.

Riker D, Goba D. Ovarian mass, pleural effusion, and ascites: revisiting Meigs syndrome. J Bronchology Interv Pulmonol. 2013;20(1):48–51.

Rio Frio T, Bahubeshi A, Kanellopoulou C, Hamel N, Niedziela M, Sabbaghian N, Pouchet C, Gilbert L, O'Brien PK, Serfas K, Broderick P, Houlston RS, Lesueur F, Bonora E, Muljo S, Schimke RN, Bouron-Dal Soglio D, Arseneau J, Schultz KA, Priest JR, Nguyen VH, Harach HR, Livingston DM, Foulkes WD, Tischkowitz M. DICER1 mutations in familial multinodular goiter with and without Sertoli-Leydig cell tumors. JAMA. 2011;305(1):68–77.

Roth LM, Talerman A. The enigma of struma ovarii. Pathology. 2007;39(1):139–46.

Salani R, Backes FJ, Fung MF, Holschneider CH, Parker LP, Bristow RE, et al. Posttreatment surveillance and diagnosis of recurrence in women with gynecologic malignancies: society of Gynecologic Oncologists recommendations. Am J Obstet Gynecol. 2011;204(6):466–78.

Schumer ST, Cannistra SA. Granulosa cell tumor of the ovary. J Clin Oncol. 2003;21(6):1180–9.

Shaaban AM, Rezvani M, Elsayes KM, Baskin Jr H, Mourad A, Foster BR, et al. Ovarian malignant germ cell tumors: cellular classification and clinical and imaging features. Radiographics. 2014;34(3):777–801.

Sigismondi C, Scollo P, Ferrandina G, Candiani M, Angioli R, Vigano R, et al. Management of bilateral malignant ovarian germ cell tumors: a MITO-9 retrospective study. Int J Gynecol Cancer. 2015;25(2):203–7.

Smith HO, Berwick M, Verschraegen CF, Wiggins C, Lansing L, Muller CY, et al. Incidence and survival rates for female malignant germ cell tumors. Obstet Gynecol. 2006;107(5):1075–85.

Stine JE, Suri A, Gehrig PA, Chiu M, Erickson BK, Huh WK, et al. Pre-operative imaging with CA125 is a poor predictor for granulosa cell tumors. Gynecol Oncol. 2013;131(1):59–62.

Suita S, Shono K, Tajiri T, Takamatsu T, Mizote H, Nagasaki A, et al. Malignant germ cell tumors: clinical characteristics, treatment, and outcome. A report from the study group for Pediatric Solid Malignant Tumors in the Kyushu Area, Japan. J Pediatr Surg. 2002;37(12):1703–6.

Ulbright TM. Germ cell tumors of the gonads: a selective review emphasizing problems in differential diagnosis, newly appreciated, and controversial issues. Mod Pathol. 2005;18 Suppl 2:S61–79.

Weinberg LE, Lurain JR, Singh DK, Schink JC. Survival and reproductive outcomes in women treated for malignant ovarian germ cell tumors. Gynecol Oncol. 2011;121(2):285–9.

Williams S, Blessing JA, Liao SY, Ball H, Hanjani P. Adjuvant therapy of ovarian germ cell tumors with cisplatin, etoposide, and bleomycin: a trial of the Gynecologic Oncology Group. J Clin Oncol. 1994;12(4): 701–6.

Wisniewski M, Deppisch LM. Solid teratomas of the ovary. Cancer. 1973;32(2):440–6.

Young RH. Sex cord-stromal tumors of the ovary and testis: their similarities and differences with consideration of selected problems. Mod Pathol. 2005;18 Suppl 2:S81–98.

Young RH, Welch WR, Dickersin GR, Scully RE. Ovarian sex cord tumor with annular tubules: review of 74 cases including 27 with Peutz-Jeghers syndrome and four with adenoma malignum of the cervix. Cancer. 1982;50(7):1384–402.

Young RH, Dickersin GR, Scully RE. Juvenile granulosa cell tumor of the ovary. A clinicopathological analysis of 125 cases. Am J Surg Pathol. 1984;8(8): 575–96.

Zagame L, Pautier P, Duvillard P, Castaigne D, Patte C, Lhomme C. Growing teratoma syndrome after ovarian germ cell tumors. Obstet Gynecol. 2006;108(3 Pt 1): 509–14.

Zaloudek C, Norris HJ. Sertoli-Leydig tumors of the ovary. A clinicopathologic study of 64 intermediate and poorly differentiated neoplasms. Am J Surg Pathol. 1984;8(6):405–18.

Diagnosis and Management of the Cancer of the Uterus

Kristy Ward and Amy R. Carroll

Abstract

Uterine cancer is the most common malignancy of the female genital tract. Treatment of uterine cancer is related to cell type, grade, and stage. However, the vast majority of uterine cancers will be low grade, early stage endometrial cancers with obesity being the primary risk factor associated with these cancers. Surgery is an important part of staging and management of uterine cancers.

Keywords

Uterine cancer • HNPCC • Lynch syndrome • Endometrial cancer • Sarcoma • Staging endometrial stromal cancer

Contents

K. Ward (✉)
Division of Gynecologic Oncology, Department of Obstetrics and Gynecology, University of Florida College of Medicine Jacksonville, Jacksonville, FL, USA
e-mail: Kristy.Ward@jax.ufl.edu

A.R. Carroll (✉)
WellStar Gynecologic Oncology, Austell, GA, USA
e-mail: gs11arc@yahoo.com

1   Introduction

As the most common gynecologic cancer seen in North America and Europe, uterine cancer can be encountered by anyone who provides healthcare to women. While the majority of these cancers will be cured with treatment, management can be controversial and confusing. This chapter will discuss the epidemiology, pathology, genetics, and treatment of this common malignancy.

© Springer International Publishing AG 2017
D. Shoupe (ed.), *Handbook of Gynecology*,
DOI 10.1007/978-3-319-17798-4_2

2   Epidemiology

Uterine cancer is the 6th most common cancer in women worldwide, with over 218,100 new cases diagnosed each year. In North America and Europe, endometrial cancer is the most common malignancy of the female reproductive tract, the 4th overall most common cancer diagnosed in women, and the 8th most likely cause of cancer death (Jemal et al. 2011). It is estimated that 49,560 US women will be diagnosed with uterine cancer in 2013 (age-adjusted incidence rate 24.5/100,000) and 8,190 will die of their disease (SEER 2013).

Ninety-five percent of cancers of the uterine corpus arise from the epithelial cells of the endometrium. Endometrial cancer is more common in postmenopausal women, with the mean age of diagnosis of 60 and the majority of patients being over the age of 50 (Sorosky 2012). The greatest risk factor for endometrial cancer is hyperestrogenic states including estrogen producing tumors, unopposed exogenous estrogen, and increased adiposity. Early menarche, late menopause, and nulliparity also increase exposure to estrogen and are associated with an increased risk of uterine cancer.

Among obesity-related cancers in women, endometrial cancer is most strongly associated with increasing body mass, with 49% of cases in the US attributable to obesity (Renehan et al. 2008). Regional and racial differences in rates of endometrial cancer are additionally linked to rates of obesity and hormone use. Conversely, factors that reduce estrogen levels such as smoking, physical activity, oral contraceptive usage, and multiparity are protective against endometrial cancer.

Uterine sarcomas originate from the muscle and connective tissue of the myometrium. They comprise 2–5% of uterine cancers and less than 1% of all gynecologic malignancies. In the USA, approximately 1,500 uterine sarcomas were diagnosed in 2013. Risk factors include a history of pelvic irradiation and black race. The peak incidence differs for the type of sarcoma. Leiomyosarcomas affect women at a mean age of 53, with many being premenopausal at diagnosis (SEER 2013; Pautier et al. 2014).

3   Genetics

The majority of uterine cancers are sporadic with approximately 1 in 10 associated with a genetic syndrome. Hereditary nonpolyposis colon cancer (HNPCC) syndrome is the most common genetic syndrome associated with endometrial cancer. The NCCN recommends genetic counseling should be considered in women diagnosed under the age of 55, and those who have a family history of colon cancer and endometrial cancer. HNPCC, also known as Lynch Syndrome, is associated with microsatellite instability in the mismatch repair genes MLH1, MSH2, MSH6, PMS2, or EPCAM, predisposing to cancers arising from the endometrium, colon, ovary, upper gastrointestinal tract, genitourinary tract, and other sites (ACOG 2014).

Approximately 50% of women with Lynch syndrome will present with endometrial cancer. Women with Lynch syndrome should be offered a risk reducing hysterectomy and bilateral salpingo-oophorectomy after child bearing is complete. For women who wish to maintain their fertility, there is no clear evidence that screening for uterine cancer is effective but annual pelvic ultrasound and/or endometrial sampling is common practice (ACOG 2014). The National Comprehensive Cancer Network (NCCN) states that annual endometrial biopsies are an option for cancer screening (NCCN 2012). The American College of Obstetricians and Gynecologists (ACOG) recommends endometrial sampling every 1–2 years starting at age 30–35 (ACOG 2014). Risk reduction via progestin-based contraception should also be considered in women that do not desire surgery. Surveillance for other cancers should be encouraged in these patients and genetic counseling should be considered for themselves and family members (Sorosky 2012; Lynch syndrome 2014).

Cowden Syndrome is associated with multiple hamartomas and increased risk of cancers including endometrial, breast, and thyroid. The most common mutation in Cowden Syndrome is PTEN, but mutations in SDHB, SDHD, and KLLN have also been seen. There is no evidence to support risk reducing hysterectomy, but this should be discussed with women with this syndrome (Cowden syndrome 2014).

Women with a history of retinoblastoma are at an increased risk for leiomyosarcoma. Retinoblastoma is associated with inactivation of the RB1 tumor suppressor gene. When the gene mutation involves all cells, there is increased risk for pinealoma, osteosarcoma, melanoma, and other muscle tumors (Retinoblastoma 2014).

4   Histology

Based on clinicopathological characteristics, Bokhman devised a dualistic classification of endometrial cancers. Type 1 lesions are the most common, comprising 80% of endometrial cancers. They include endometrioid cell type or variants (such as squamous differentiation, villoglandular, and secretory), are usually well to moderately differentiated, and are less likely to metastasize outside of the uterus. These tumors often occur in women with a history of anovulatory uterine bleeding and can be found in a background of endometrial hyperplasia. Women with a biopsy of complex endometrial hyperplasia with atypia have a 40% likelihood of having malignancy found in the hysterectomy specimen (Trimble et al. 2006).

Type II lesions include clear cell carcinoma, serous adenocarcinoma, and carcinosarcoma and are not associated with hyperestrogenism. These malignancies are poorly differentiated and more aggressive; deep myometrial invasion and metastic disease are more common than with type I tumors. Recurrence is more likely and survival is worse for type II uterine cancers. Serous carcinoma is characterized by papillae and has highly pleiomorphic tumor cells with necrosis and many mitoses. Endometrial intraepithelial carcinoma (EIC) is a rare finding, but it is thought to be the precursor lesion in serous tumors of the uterus. It involves pleiomorphic but noninvasive tumor cells (Trimble et al. 2012). Carcinosarcoma,

also known as malignant mullerian tumors, contain mixed components of sarcoma and adenocarcinoma. While it historically had been grouped with sarcomas, more recent evaluation has suggested that it is more similar to a dedifferentiated carcinoma than a sarcoma. Staging of carcinosarcoma is now included in the FIGO staging of endometrial carcinomas (Mutch 2009).

Uterine sarcomas include leiomyosarcomas, mixed epithelial and stromal tumors (carcinosarcoma and adenosarcoma), and endometrial stromal sarcomas. Leiomyosarcomas make up 30% of all uterine sarcomas. Sarcomas arising in the endometrial stroma account for 15% of all uterine sarcomas. Other sarcomas include mixed endometrial stromal and smooth muscle tumors, adenosarcomas, embryonal botryoides or rhabdomyosarcomas, and perivascular epithelial-cell tumors (PEComas) (D'Angelo and Prat 2009).

5   Diagnosis/Screening

Clinical features associated with uterine cancer include abnormal uterine bleeding, abnormal cervical cytology (e.g., atypical glandular cells on a cervical cytology), pelvic pain, and an enlarging pelvic mass. Approximately 90% of women with endometrial cancer present with abnormal bleeding. The diagnosis is obtained by pathological review of tissue, preferably obtained by endometrial biopsy, dilation and curettage, or hysteroscopy and biopsy. While these methods are very efficacious for detecting uterine cancers, if the lesion does not invade into the endometrial cavity, leiomyosarcoma may only be diagnosed after hysterectomy or myomectomy. Screening asymptomatic women for uterine cancer is not recommended (NCCN 2012).

6   Staging

The NCCN recommends a history and physical examination, chest x-ray, endometrial sampling, and cervical cytology for the initial workup for uterine cancer. Traditionally, staging of endometrial cancer involves an exploratory laparotomy, total

Table 1 2009 FIGO staging of endometrial carcinoma (Mutch 2009)

Stage 1	Tumor confined to the corpus uterus
1a	No or less than ½ myometrial invasion
1b	Invasion ≥ half of the myometrium
Stage 2	Tumor invades cervical stroma
Stage 3	Local and/or regional spread of tumor
3a	Tumor invades serosa of the uterus and/or adnexae
3b	Vaginal and/or parametrial involvement
3c	Metastases to pelvic and/or paraaortic lymph nodes C1: positive pelvic nodes C2: positive paraaortic nodes with/without positive pelvic nodes
4	Tumor invades bladder and/or bowel mucosa and/or distant metastases
4a	Tumor invasion of bladder and/or bowel mucosa
4b	Distant metastases including intra-abdominal metastases and/or inguinal lymph nodes

Table 2 2009 FIGO staging of uterine sarcoma (Mutch 2009)

Stage 1	Tumor confined to the corpus uterus
1a	Less than 5 cm
1b	≥5 cm
Stage 2	Tumor extends to the pelvis
2a	Adnexal involvement
2b	Tumor extends to extrauterine pelvic tissue
Stage 3	Tumor invades abdominal tissue
3a	One site
3b	More than one site
3c	Metastasis to pelvic and/or paraaortic lymph nodes
4	Tumor invades bladder and/or rectum and/or distant metastases
4a	Tumor invasion of bladder and/or rectum
4b	Distant metastases
*Endometrial stromal sarcoma	Simultaneous tumors of the uterine corpus and ovary/pelvis in association with ovarian/pelvic endometriosis should be classified as independent primary tumors
*Adenosarcoma Stage 1	1a: tumor limited to endometrium/endocervix (without myometrial invasion) 1b: tumor invades ≤ ½ of myometrium 1c: tumor invades > ½ of myometrium

abdominal hysterectomy, bilateral oophorectomy, and pelvic and paraaortic lymph node dissections (NCCN 2012).

Grade 1 tumors are well differentiated, with formed glands and no more than 5% of non-squamous solid components. Grade 2 contains 6–50% solid components and grade 3 has greater than 50% non-squamous solid components. If there is significant cytologic atypia, the tumor should be upgraded. Currently, nearly 70% of patients are diagnosed and treated at early stage with 5-year survival estimated at 95.8%, and an additional 20% are diagnosed with only regional disease with a 5-year survival estimated at 67.0% (SEER 2013) (Tables 1 and 2).

7 Management of Endometrial Cancer

Unless prohibited by patient comorbidities, surgery is usually the first step in the management of endometrial cancer. Comprehensive surgical staging traditionally includes a hysterectomy, bilateral salpingo-oophorectomy, lymph node assessment, and intraperitoneal cytology. However, much of the traditional recommendations for surgical management of endometrial cancer have been challenged recently.

While hysterectomy is indicated for women with endometrial cancer, the best surgical approach has been questioned. There have been multiple studies demonstrating the safety and efficacy of laparoscopic surgery for endometrial cancer staging. Proven benefits include improved quality of life, shorter hospital stay, and less blood loss than exploratory laparotomy. In addition, laparoscopy does not impact recurrence rates or survival (Zullo et al. 2012; Walker et al. 2012). Since the introduction of the DaVinci robotic surgical platform, its use has continued to climb. The literature demonstrating the safety and efficacy of robotic staging is growing. A clear benefit of utilizing the robot is the ability to stage obese patients minimally invasively (Seamon et al. 2009).

7.1 Lymphadenectomy

There continues to be significant debate regarding what population is at risk for nodal disease and warrants a lymphadenectomy. There is considerable variability in practice patterns amongst gynecologic oncologist with respect to indications for staging and extent of dissection. While lymphadenectomy guides staging and treatment, trials have failed to demonstrate either an overall survival or recurrence free survival benefit for pelvic lymphadenectomy (Mariani et al. 2000).

7.2 BSO

Several studies have retrospectively evaluated the outcomes of premenopausal women with ovarian preservation during surgery for endometrial cancer without finding any adverse survival impact. Given the impact on quality of life and increase in cardiovascular risk factors, it may be reasonable to forgo oophorectomy in premenopausal women with early-stage low-risk endometrial cancer (Lau et al. 2014; Lee et al. 2013; Wright et al. 2009). This should be carefully considered by the patient and her gynecologic oncologist. The benefit of retaining the ovaries in a postmenopausal woman has not been evaluated and bilateral salpingo-oophorectomy is recommended.

7.3 Cytologic Assessment

Pelvic washings were included in surgical staging for endometrial cancer prior to the 2009 FIGO staging. The findings of positive cytology are not correlated with clinical outcomes, and their utility has been questioned. As of the 2009 FIGO staging, pelvic washings are no longer required as part of surgical staging for endometrial cancer, and many gynecologic oncologists no longer include intraperitoneal cytology as part of their staging surgery (NCCN 2012).

8 Risk Assessment

Surgical stage and other significant pathologic risk factors are utilized to determine patients' risk for persistent disease or recurrence. This risk assessment is often utilized to determine the need for adjuvant therapy. Risk assessment and determination of adjuvant therapy can be complex and should be managed by an oncologist experienced in the treatment of uterine cancer.

8.1 Low Risk

Patients at low risk of recurrence have endometrioid histology with disease confined to the endometrium. This includes a subset of patients with stage IA and grade 1 or 2 endometrial cancer. Typically these patients are managed with close surveillance alone following surgery (NCCN 2012).

8.2 Intermediate Risk

Patients with an intermediate risk for recurrence have disease confined to the uterus, including the cervix (stage II) with myometrial invasion (stage IA or IB). Other prognostic factors such as deep myometrial invasion, grade 2 or 3 histology, and the presence of lymphovascular invasion can further subdivide this group into low or high intermediate risk. Recurrence rates range from 5% to 30% with or without radiation therapy. As such, consideration for adjuvant radiation therapy is warranted (NCCN 2012; Keys et al. 2004; Creutzberg et al. 2000) (Table 3).

Patients with a high risk for disease recurrence have advanced stage disease, and grade 3 carcinomas (including serous and clear cell) of any stage. This category is associated with a high rate of recurrence and death from endometrial cancer. As such, adjuvant chemotherapy is often utilized postoperatively (NCCN 2012).

Table 3 Risk assessment of local stage endometrial cancer (high intermediate risk (HIR)group determination)

Study	Risk factor	Determination of HIR
Gynecologic Oncology Group	Deep myometrial invasion Grade 2 or 3 Lymphovascular space invasion	Any age with all 3 50–69 with 2/3 70 or older with 1/3
PORTEC	Deep myometrial invasion Grade 3	Age > 60 with both risk factors

8.3 High Risk

Currently there is not a "standard" approach for high-risk disease. Often adjuvant therapy is dictated by surgical and pathologic factors such as uterine or extra uterine disease. Since multiple questions remain, enrollment on a clinical trial may be the most appropriate option for patients in this risk category.

In advanced stage disease, chemotherapy with carboplatin and paclitaxel is the most use regimen. Other active agents include doxorubicin, ifosfamide, topotecan, oxaliplatin, docetaxel, ixabepilone, and pegylated liposomal doxorubicin (NCCN 2012). The role of combined chemotherapy and radiation therapy has not been defined in advanced disease.

8.4 Recurrent or Metastatic Disease

Chemotherapeutic options for recurrent or metastatic disease are the same as for advanced disease. In localized recurrence in patients without prior radiation, radiation therapy can be utilized. For patients in whom radiation or cytotoxic therapy is not a reasonable option, hormonal therapy is an acceptable alternative for therapy in recurrent disease. In tumors that express estrogen and progesterone receptors, a favorable response to endocrine therapy is likely (Decruze and Green 2007). Tamoxifen is currently the only selective estrogen receptor modulator to demonstrate activity (Thigpen et al. 2001). Aromatase inhibitors are currently under investigation.

9 Non-Endometrioid Histologies

9.1 Uterine Papillary Serous Carcinoma (UPSC)

UPSC represents a histologically aggressive subtype of endometrial carcinoma that typically presents with extrauterine disease with a spread pattern similar to papillary serous ovarian cancer. Although this histology accounts for 10% of all endometrial cancers, it accounts for the majority of recurrences. Comprehensive staging for early stage UPSC is recommended in *all* patients. Multiple studies have clearly demonstrated that optimal resection of metastatic disease confers a survival benefit and should be the goal at the time of primary surgery. Any myometrial invasion is associated with higher risk of recurrence. Controversy also persists regarding the benefit of adjuvant therapy for disease confined to a polyp. Although the risk of recurrence is low in this population, it is not negligible (Rauh-Hain et al. 2010). Due to the propensity for uterine serous cancer to recur distantly, chemotherapy has been considered as an essential component of adjuvant therapy (Fader et al. 2009).

For advanced stage disease, following optimal cytoreduction, chemotherapy is the recommended adjuvant therapy due to high risk of distant recurrence. Currently, the combination of paclitaxel and carboplatin is an appropriate choice of cytotoxic therapy for advanced stage UPSC. The role of radiation therapy is limited and not typically recommended (NCCN 2012).

9.2 Uterine Carcinosarcoma

As with endometrial carcinoma, surgery is the primary management for carcinosarcoma. Surgical staging is recommended. For advanced stage disease confined to the abdomen, cytoreduction is also recommended (Tanner et al. 2011). For stage I and II uterine carcinosarcoma, there is a relative paucity of quality data to recommend adjuvant therapy. In the limited number of trials that do exist, there is a consistent improvement in progression free survival but not overall survival (Cantrell et al. 2012). Chemotherapy was associated with improved progression free survival compared to observation or radiation therapy (Omura et al. 1985). The role for radiation therapy or chemotherapy is questionable for early stage disease. Given the paucity of data, consideration should be given to enrollment on a clinical trial. For stage III and IV uterine carcinosarcoma, chemotherapy is recommended as adjuvant therapy. Ifosfamide, cisplatin, adriamycin, and paclitaxel have had the most significant evidence of activity (NCCN 2012).

10 Sarcomas

10.1 Leiomyosarcoma

Uterine leiomyosarcoma is often identified incidentally following a hysterectomy or myomectomy for presumed uterine leiomyomas. The standard surgical management for women with known leiomyosarcoma is a hysterectomy often coupled with a bilateral salpingo-oophorectomy (BSO) in postmenopausal women. The role of a BSO has been questioned due to a growing body of literature failing to demonstrate a survival benefit. For those with disease outside of the uterus, the role of cytoreduction is controversial and not clearly understood. The role of a lymphadenectomy is also uncertain. Any bulky nodes should be removed. Standard staging when disease is confined to the uterus is questionable since the risk of nodal metastasis is low (Kapp et al. 2008; Major et al. 1993). In patients with an incidental finding of leiomyosarcoma on final pathology, a return to the operating room for "staging" is not indicated. Imaging to identify extrauterine disease is recommended.

The role of chemotherapy, radiation therapy, or a combination of the two is undetermined. Adjuvant therapy for early stage disease is especially controversial. As such, enrollment on a clinical trial should be recommended. The NCCN recommends observation versus consideration for chemotherapy, with docetaxel and gemcitabine being the preferred regimen. Other suggested regimens are listed in the Uterine Cancer guidelines (NCCN 2012).

With respect to recurrent disease, leiomyosarcoma commonly recurs in the lungs, liver, abdomen, pelvis, and retroperitoneal lymph nodes. Local recurrences in patients with a prolonged progression free survival can be managed with surgical intervention. For patients with a local recurrence who are not ideal surgical candidates, radiation therapy can be considered. Chemotherapy is the recommended approach for women with recurrent metastatic disease. The combination of gemcitabine and docetaxel is supported by multiple clinical trials. In the setting of recurrent disease, the chemotherapeutic agent of choice is often dictated by performance status, medical history, and patient choice. In the setting of recurrent metastatic disease, palliation is the goal of chemotherapy (NCCN 2012).

10.2 Adenosarcoma

Treatment for adenosarcoma of the uterus is hysterectomy with bilateral salpingo-oophorectomy in postmenopausal women. As ovarian metastasis is uncommon, the ovaries can be left in premenopausal women. Lymphadenectomy is not required in disease confined to the uterus. As most adenosarcomas contain an endometrial stromal sarcoma component, adjuvant therapy should follow the ESS guidelines (Friedlander et al. 2014).

10.3 Endometrial Stromal Sarcoma

Hysterectomy is the primary treatment for early endometrial stromal sarcoma. Ovarian conservation may be considered in young women with small tumors. The role of lymphadenectomy is not well defined in this disease. In recurrent or advanced disease, cytoreductive surgery should be considered. As the rate of hormone receptor positivity is very high in endometrial stromal sarcoma, hormone therapy is recommended in advanced or recurrent low-grade disease. In high-grade disease, cytotoxic chemotherapy should be considered (NCCN 2012). Radiation therapy is often used for palliation as adjuvant pelvic radiation has not been shown to improve survival (Amant et al. 2014).

11 Conclusion

Uterine cancer is the most common gynecologic malignancy with a rising incidence in the United States. Endometrial cancers are associated with obesity and genetic syndromes such as HNPCC. They are histologically divided into type I and type II malignancies, with type I cancers usually being early stage and often curable. Type II cancers tend to be more aggressive and more often diagnosed at later stages of disease. Cancers of the uterine body include sarcomas such as leiomyosarcoma, adenosarcoma, and endometrial stromal sarcoma.

Abnormal uterine bleeding is the most common presenting symptom and should be evaluated with an endometrial biopsy. Following a diagnosis of uterine cancer, surgical staging is often performed. There are still many controversies regarding the need for a lymphadenectomy, and it is uncertain which patients need a complete lymph node dissection for prognostic information and guidance of therapy. Laparoscopic, robotic, and open approaches to staging are considered equivalent for cancer therapy and only differ in their operative risks.

The need for adjuvant therapy is determined by pathologic risk factors for recurrence. Patients at low risk for disease recurrence need no treatment after surgery. Those with an intermediate risk may benefit from chemotherapy and/or radiation. Patients with a high risk of recurrence need chemotherapy and radiation. All patients with a history of uterine cancer will need surveillance for recurrence of disease with frequent exams and biopsy of any suspicious lesion. Treatment of recurrent disease depends on the timing and location of recurrence.

References

Amant F, Floquet A, Friedlander M, Kristensen G, Mahner S, Nam EJ, Powell MA, Ray-Coquard I, Siddiqui N, Sykes P, Westermann AM, Seddon B. Gynecologic Cancer InterGroup (GCIG) consensus review for endometrial stromal sarcoma. Int J Gynecol Cancer. 2014;24(9 Suppl 3):S67–72.

American College of Obstetricians and Gynecologists. Lynch syndrome. Practice Bulletin No. 147. Obstet Gynecol. 2014;124:1042–54.

Cantrell LA, Havrilesky L, Moore DT, O'Malley D, Liotta M, Secord AA, Nagel CI, Cohn DE, Fader AN, Wallace AH, Rose P, Gehrig PA. A multi-institutional cohort study of adjuvant therapy in stage I-II uterine carcinosarcoma. Gynecol Oncol. 2012;127(1):22.

Cowden syndrome – Genetics Home Reference. 2014;1–7. http://ghr.nlm.nih.gov/condition/cowden-syndrome. Accessed 20 Jan 14.

Creutzberg CL, van Putten WL, Koper PC, Lybert ML, et al. Surgery and postoperative radiotherapy versus surgery alone for patients with stage-1 endometrial carcinoma: multicentre randomised trial. PORTEC Study Group. Post Operative Radiation Therapy in Endometrial Carcinoma. Lancet. 2000;355: 1404–11.

D'Angelo E, Prat J. Uterine sarcomas: a review. Gynecol Oncol. 2009;1–9. doi:10.1016/j.ygyno.2009.09.023.

Decruze SB, Green JA. Hormone therapy in advanced and recurrent endometrial cancer: a systematic review. Int J Gynecol Cancer. 2007;17:964.

Fader AN, Drake RD, O'Malley DM, Gibbons HE, Huh WK, Havrilesky LJ, et al. Platinum/taxane based chemotherapy with or without radiotherapy favorably impacts survival outcomes in stage I uterine papillary serous carcinoma. Cancer. 2009;115:2119–27.

Friedlander ML, Covens A, Glasspool RM, Hilpert F, Kristensen G, Kwon S, Selle F, Small W, Witteveen E, Russell P. Gynecologic Cancer InterGroup (GCIG) consensus review for mullerian adenosarcoma of the female genital tract. Int J Gynecol Cancer. 2014;24(9 Suppl 3): S78–82.

Jemal A, Bray F, Center MM, Ferlay J, Ward E, Forman D. Global cancer statistics. CA Cancer J Clin. 2011; 61(2):69–90. doi:10.3322/caac.20107.

Kapp DS, Shin JY, Chan JK. Prognostic factors and survival in 1396 patients with uterine leiomyosarcomas: emphasis on impact of lymphadenectomy and oophorectomy. Cancer. 2008;112(4):820.

Keys HM, Roberts JA, Brunetto VL, Zaino RJ, Spirtos NM, Bloss JD, Pearlman A, Bell JG. A phase III trial of surgery with or without adjunctive external pelvic radiation therapy in intermediate risk endometrial adenocarcinoma: a Gynecologic Oncology Group study. Gynecol Oncol. 2004;92(3):744–51.

Lau HY, Twu NF, Yen MS, Tsai HW, Wang PH, Chuang CM, Wu HH, Chao KC, Chen YJ. Impact of ovarian preservation in women with endometrial cancer. J Chin Med Assoc. 2014;77(7):379–84.

Lee TS, Lee JY, Kim JW, Oh S, Seong SJ, Lee JM, Kim TJ, Cho CH, Kim SM, Park CY. Outcomes of ovarian preservation in a cohort of premenopausal women with early-stage endometrial cancer: a Korean Gynecologic Oncology Group study. Gynecol Oncol. 2013; 131(2):289–93.

Lynch syndrome – Genetics Home Reference. 2014;1–7. http://ghr.nlm.nih.gov/condition/lynch-syndrome. Accessed 20 Jan 14.

Major FJ, Blessing JA, Silverberg SG, Morrow CP, Creasman WT, Currie JL, Yordan E, Brady MF. Prognostic factors in early-stage uterine sarcoma. A Gynecologic Oncology Group study. Cancer. 1993; 71 Suppl 4:1702.

Mariani A, Sebo TJ, Katzmann JA, Keeney GL, Roche PC, Lesnick TG, Podratz KC. Pretreatment assessment of prognostic indicators in endometrial cancer. Am J Obstet Gynecol. 2000;182(6):1535–44.

Mutch DG. The new FIGO staging system for cancers of the vulva, cervix, endometrium, and sarcomas. Gynecol Oncol. 2009;115:325–8.

NCCN. Uterine Neoplasm. 2012;1–63.

Omura GA, Blessing JA, Major F, Lifshitz S, Ehrlich CE, Mangan C, Beecham J, Park R, Silverberg S. A randomized clinical trial of adjuvant adriamycin in uterine sarcomas: a Gynecologic Oncology Group Study. J Clin Oncol. 1985;3(9):1240.

Pautier P, Nam EJ, Provencher DM, Hamilton AL, Mangili G, Siddiqui NA, Westermann AM, Reed NS, Harter P, Ray-Coquard I. Gynecologic Cancer InterGroup (GCIG) consensus review for high-grade undifferentiated sarcomas of the uterus. Int J Gynecol Cancer. 2014;24(9 Suppl 3):S73–7.

Rauh-Hain JA, Growdon WB, Schorge JO, Goodman AK, Boruta DM, McCAnn C, et al. Prognsotic determinants in patients with stage IIIC-Iv uterine papillary serous carcinoma. Gynecol Oncol. 2010;119:299–304.

Renehan AG, Tyson M, Egger M, Heller RF, Zwahlen M. Body-mass index and incidence of cancer: a systematic review and meta-analysis of prospective observational studies. Lancet. 2008;371(9612):569–78. doi:10.1016/S0140-6736(08)60269-X.

Retinoblastoma – Genetics Home Reference. 2014;1–4. http://ghr.nlm.nih.gov/condition/retinoblastoma. Accessed 20 Jan 14.

Seamon LG, Cohn DE, Henretta MS, Kim KH, Carlson MJ, Phillips GS, Fowler JM. Minimally invasive comprehensive surgical staging for endometrial cancer: robotics or laparoscopy? Gynecol Oncol. 2009;113(1):36–41.

SEER. Cancer of the Endometrium – SEER Stat Fact Sheets. 2013. 1–10 http://seer.cancer.gov/statfacts/html/corp.html. Accessed 20 Jan 14.

Sorosky JI. Endometrial cancer. Obstet Gynecol. 2012;120(2, Part 1):383–97. doi:10.1097/AOG.0b013e182605bf1.

Tanner EJ, Leitao Jr MM, Garg K, Chi DS, Sonoda Y, Gardner GJ, Barakat RR, Jewell EL. The role of cytoreductive surgery for newly diagnosed advanced-stage uterine carcinosarcoma. Gynecol Oncol. 2011; 123(3):548–52.

Thigpen T, Brady MF, Homesley HD, et al. Tamoxifen in the treatment of advanced or recurrent endometrial carcinoma: a Gynecologic Oncology Group Study. J Clin Oncol. 2001;19:364.

Trimble CL, Kauderer J, Zaino R, et al. Concurrent endometrial carcinoma in women with a biopsy diagnosis of atypical endometrial hyperplasia. Cancer. 2006;106(4): 812–9. doi:10.1002/cncr.21650.

Trimble CL, Method M, Leitao M, et al. Management of endometrial precancers. Obstet Gynecol. 2012;120(5): 1160. doi:10.1097/AOG.0b013e31826bb121.

Walker JL, Piedmonte MR, Spirtos NM, Eisenkop SM, Schlaerth JB, Mannel RS, Barakat R, Pearl ML, Sharma SK. Recurrence and survival after random assignment to laparoscopy versus laparotomy for comprehensive surgical staging of uterine cancer: Gynecologic Oncology Group LAP2 Study. J Clin Oncol. 2012;30(13):695–700.

Wright JD, Buck AM, Shah M, Burke WM, Schiff PB, Herzog TJ. Safety of ovarian preservation in premenopausal women with endometrial cancer. J Clin Oncol. 2009;27(8):1214–9.

Zullo F, Falbo A, Palomba S. Safety of laparoscopy vs laparotomy in the surgical staging of endometrial cancer: a systematic review and metaanalysis of randomized controlled trials. Am J Obstet Gynecol. 2012; 207(2):94–100.

Preinvasive Epithelial Disease of the Vulvar

Aida Moeini, Hiroko Machida, Sigita S. Cahoon, and Koji Matsuo

Abstract

Premalignant diseases of the vulva include disorders of epithelial growth and differentiation in the vulva. According to the latest classification from the International Society for the Study of Vulvar Disease, the three main categories for intraepithelial neoplasia include vulvar intraepithelial neoplasia (VIN), Paget's disease, and melanoma in situ (MIS). VIN is further divided into the two main categories: The most common one is VIN usual type or HPV related, and the second one is VIN differentiated type. The rate of progression of untreated high-grade VIN to invasive vulvar cancer is ranging from 9% to 18.5%. The diagnosis is usually carried out by visual inspection and biopsy is necessary for histologic confirmation. There is no useful screening test available for preinvasive vulvar disease, which highlights the importance of healthcare provider awareness for different existing premalignant vulvar lesions. Surgical excision remains the mainstay of the treatment for preinvasive epithelial vulvar disease. Alternative treatment options for VIN and Paget's disease include ablation and pharmacological treatment. Preinvasive epithelial vulvar disease can recur which warrants long-term patient monitoring. This review highlights epidemiological characteristics, histological patterns, clinical features, diagnostic studies, and management strategies for preinvasive vulvar diseases.

Keywords

Vulvar intraepithelial neoplasia • Paget's disease • Melanoma in situ

Contents

A. Moeini • H. Machida • K. Matsuo (⊠)
Division of Gynecologic Oncology, Department of Obstetrics and Gynecology, University of Southern California, Los Angeles, CA, USA
e-mail: aida.moeini@med.usc.edu; hiroko.machida@med.usc.edu; koji.matsuo@med.usc.edu

S.S. Cahoon
Department of Obstetrics and Gynecology, University of Southern California, Los Angeles, CA, USA
e-mail: sigita.cahoon@med.usc.edu

© Springer International Publishing AG (outside the USA) 2017
D. Shoupe (ed.), *Handbook of Gynecology*,
DOI 10.1007/978-3-319-17798-4_10

969

Table 1 Classification for epithelial vulvar disease from International Society for Study of Vulvar Disease (ISSVD)

I. Nonneoplastic epithelial disorders of the skin and mucosa (low malignant potential)
a. Lichen sclerosus
b. Squamous hyperplasia
c. Other dermatoses
II. Mixed nonneoplastic and neoplastic epithelial disorders
III. Intraepithelial neoplasia
a. Squamous intraepithelial neoplasia (VIN 1, VIN 2, and VIN 3)
b. Non-squamous intraepithelial neoplasia
i. Paget's disease
ii. Tumors of melanocytes
IV. Invasive tumors

1 Vulvar Intraepithelial Disease

Vulvar cancer is the fourth most common gynecologic cancer and encompasses 5% of all gynecologic malignancies. Some cases of vulvar cancer develop slowly through precancerous epithelial changes in the vulva, which highlights the importance of early diagnosis and treatment of these lesions. In 1966, Jeffcoate assigned chronic vulvar dystrophy to the entire group of disorders effecting vulvar epithelial growth and differentiation. In 1989 the International Society for the Study of Vulvar Disease (ISSVD) replaced the old dystrophy by a new classification shown in Table 1 and includes four different categories. This chapter is a review of third category including VIN, Paget's disease and MIS.

2 Squamous Vulvar Intraepithelial Neoplasia

2.1 Introduction

Vulvar intraepithelial neoplasia (VIN) refers to proliferation of atypical basal cells in the vulvar epithelium and characterized by disordered maturation and nuclear abnormalities. The incidence of

VIN has increased fourfold between 1973 and 2000 (ACOG 2011). The mean age at diagnosis is 43 years, and women younger than 50 years old account for 75% of cases (Jones et al. 2005; Judson et al. 2006).

2.2 Classification

The ISSVD classification in 1986 was based on cellular immaturity, nuclear abnormalities, and mitotic activity and defined to three grades, similar to the three-grade cervical intraepithelial neoplasia. In VIN 1, the basal one-third of the epithelium is involved, whereas in VIN 3 the whole thickness of the epithelium is involved. However, ISSVD modified this stance in 2004. The term VIN1 has been eliminated and flat lesions associated with koilocytic changes are consider condyloma, whereas VIN 2 and 3 have been combined and simply referred to as VIN.

ISSVD new classification (2004) (Sideri et al. 2005):

- **VIN usual type (uVIN)** is the most common, with three subtypes including warty, basaloid, and mixed VIN. These lesions are commonly associated with HPV infection.
- **VIN differentiated type (dVIN)** is more often associated with vulvar dermatoses, such as

Table 2 Summary of vulvar intraepithelial neoplasm

	Usual VIN (uVIN)	Differentiated VIN (dVIN)
Age	Young	Postmenopausal
Clinical features	Multifocal, multicentric[a], sharply defined, mostly elevated and involving labia minor	Less specific, mostly unicentric, hyperkeratotic plaques, treatment-resistant plaques
HPV infection	85%, predominantly HPV 16, 18, or 33	Rare
Risk factors	HPV, cigarette smoking, and immunosuppression	Lichen sclerosus
Pathogenesis	Deregulation of HPV E6-E7 oncoprotein causes suppression of p53, pRB, p21 which leads to inhibition of apoptosis and genomic instability	PTEN mutation, microsatellite instability, gene hypermethylation, p53 inhibition
Prevalence	>96%	<2–5%

[a]Multicentric disease means involving the cervix, vagina, anus, or vulva. It is age related, as it decreases from 59% in women aged 20–34 to 10% in women over 50 years of age

Lichen sclerosus and oncogenic HPV infection is uncommon.

- **VIN unclassified type (VIN NOS)** are rare Pagetoid lesions.

Clinical and molecular characteristics of usual and differentiated VIN are listed in Table 2.

2.3 Clinical Features

VIN can be asymptomatic and noted incidentally during gynecologic examination or may present with a mixed variety of symptoms such as pruritus, pain, vulvar soreness, discharge, bleeding, dyspareunia, or palpable lesions. Vulvar lesions can be any shade from white to red. If pigmented, coloration ranges from pale tan to black, depending on the degree of keratinization, patient race, and the type of lesion. They are usually on non-hair-bearing areas, sharply defined, and can be identified by unassisted vision.

2.4 Risk Factors for VIN

- **Usual type**: HPV, smoking, and immunosuppression
- **Differentiated type**: Lichen sclerosis (Conley et al. 2002)

2.5 Evaluation

- **History:** Medical history needs to be evaluated for risk factors associated with VIN. History of sexually transmitted infections, HPV infection, genital warts, and abnormal Pap test should be obtained.
- **Physical Exam:** The gynecologic examination requires complete exposure and includes inspection and palpation of the entire vulva, groin, and perianal area. The most common locations for VIN lesions are the labia minora and introitus between the positions 3 o'clock and 9 o'clock. Site, size, number of lesions, shape, color, and degree of thickness need to be reported. Lesions of particular concern include areas with marked hyperkeratosis which are elevated, roughened, nodular, or with an ulcerated surface. Sites most likely to harbor invasive disease are the posterior perineal and perianal areas.

Diagnostic Study: Management is based on histologic diagnosis, and biopsy is indicated for any suspicious lesion. Adequate biopsies can be obtained by using local anesthetic and a punch biopsy up to 6 mm.

- **Colposcopy:** Colposcopy can identify subclinical lesions and the extent of the lesion and detect other synchronous intraepithelial lesions. Evaluation of suspicious areas includes application of 3–5% acetic acid-soaked gauze pads to the vulva for 5 min (Barbara et al. 2008).

- **HPV detection:** Diagnosis of HPV infection with the VIN lesion is useful to differentiate uVIN from dVIN (koilocytosis, p16 and p53).
- It is mandatory to perform a careful examination of the entire lower anogenital tract, which also includes the cervix and vagina. Performing Pap smear is highly recommended.

Screening for VIN: No screening strategies have been developed for early detection of VIN. When HPV-related VIN is diagnosed in young sexually active women, full evaluation of sexually transmitted infections is recommended.

2.6 Management

Treatment is recommended for all women with VIN. As previously mentioned VIN1 has been eliminated in the new classification and lesions reported as VIN1 may be reassessed annually (ACOG 2011). The goal is to relieve patient symptoms, preserve vulvar anatomy and function, exclude concurrent invasive disease, and prevent progression to invasive cancer. Treatment strategies are based on either destroying affected cells or enhancing the host immune system's response and are selected based on patient and lesion characteristics as well as clinician expertise. Management options include surgery, ablative therapy, and pharmacological therapy.

2.7 Surgery

The mainstay of treatment for VIN remains surgical excision. For high-risk uVIN such as ulcerative lesions, dVIN, history of vulvar carcinoma, and in patients with immunosuppression, surgical excision is required. Preoperative counseling regarding expected anatomical changes especially after extensive surgeries and sexual function is necessary. Special attention has to be paid to the

psychosexual consequences and the quality of life of the patients. Surgical modalities include wide local excision, simple vulvectomy, and skinning vulvectomy.

- **Wide local excision (WLE):** WLE is the preferred initial intervention for women where clinical or pathologic findings suggest cancer. WLE is defined as excision of an individual lesion with 0.5–1 cm margin and can be performed with a knife, electrosurgery, or laser CO2 excision (Hart 2001). The margin may be altered to avoid injury to the clitoris, urethra, and anus. The resection depth is also important, in pilous areas, atypical cells can compromise skin appendages, and ideally the whole pilosebaceous complex needs to be resected (recommended resection up to 4 mm). In hairless areas, the resection depth does not need to extend more than 1 mm.

  Loop electrosurgical excision (LEEP) is another modality to perform WLE. LEEP is accomplished with the blend cutting mode, power output of 16 and 30 W using 0.2 mm microneedle, and 1×0.4 cm semicircle shape loop. Fulguration requires a 5 mm ball electrode or a 1 mm needle electrode (Terzakis et al. 2010). After finishing the procedure, the area needs to be carefully examined via colposcopy to rule out residual lesions.

  CO_2 laser excision is the other available option to perform WLE. The procedure is performed under colposcopic guidance, and the depth of tissue destruction is guided by colposcopy. Laser excision should be performed according to the Reid criteria (Reid et al. 1985). The laser device is set to continuous mode with power density ranging between 750 and 1250 w/cm. An excision is made at the periphery of the lesion in the third surgical plane; then, with the smallest sized laser spot, another excision should be made along the third surgical plane of the entire lesion, with up to 1 mm depth in hair-free epithelium to 3 mm depth in hairy areas to ablate the hair follicle. This requires special training as deep laser excision can lead to destruction of the skin appendage and hypertrophic scar formation. Consequently, large lesions over hair-bearing areas may be preferentially treated with other modalities.

- **Skinning Vulvectomy:** Skinning vulvectomy is a wide superficial vulvectomy, removing the skin and underlying structures while leaving the subcutaneous fat in place, and is rarely needed. It is indicated in confluent multifocal lesions or in patients for whom prior procedures have failed to control the disease.

2.8   Prognosis

Negative margins reduce the risk of recurrence at the same site and warrant the histologic evaluation of specimen margins with frozen sections intraoperatively (Barbara 2008; Jones et al. 2005). The recurrence rate of VIN after excision ranges from 20% to 40% (Hillemanns et al. 2006; Jones et al. 2005). In a recent study, the recurrence rate after vulvectomy, partial vulvectomy, local excision, laser ablation, and coagulation was 19, 18, 22, 23, and 56%, respectively (Van Seters et al. 2005). With regard to LEEP, studies are limited and have reported a recurrence rate between 13% and 20%. According to these studies, LEEP and cold knife excision are equivalent in their ability to achieve complete response (Ferenczy et al. 1994; Terzakis et al. 2010).

2.9   Ablative Therapy

Ablation therapy provides a cosmetically appealing treatment with a cure rate comparable to surgical excision but has the disadvantage of not providing a specimen for pathological analysis. It includes laser vaporization and ultrasonic surgical aspiration. It is essential to rule out the coexistence of invasive carcinoma by performing colposcopically directed biopsies.

- **CO_2 Laser vaporization:** Laser CO_2 vaporization combines the advantages of surgical excision in relation to cure rate with correct diagnosis and the advantages of laser vaporization with respect to cosmetic and functional results. A drawback of laser CO_2 vaporization is that there is no surgical specimen for histological evaluation. The procedure is performed under local or general anesthesia, and the laser device is on continuous mode with power density ranging between 750 and 1250 w/cm (ACOG 2011). Vaporization is usually carried out using a defocalized beam, 1–2 mm in diameter with the depth between 1–3 mm. The complete response rate for laser vaporization is almost 75% (Hillemanns et al. 2006; Jones et al. 2005).

- **Ultrasonic surgical aspiration (CUSA):** This technique uses ultrasound to cause cavitation and disruption of the tissues, which are then aspirated through a tube and collected as a specimen (Barbara et al. 2008). After detailed colposcopy, CUSA is used with a 20° angle hand piece, frequency 23 kHZ, aspiration up to 24 Hg, and irrigation up to 50 cc/min. The hand piece is used similar to a pencil. Recurrence rates up to 35% have been reported in studies (Miller 2002). The recent Cochrane study comparing CO_2 laser ablation and CUSA reported no significant difference in the recurrence rate (Kaushik et al. 2014).

2.10   Medical Treatment

As with ablative therapy, careful colposcopic examination is warranted to exclude invasive cancer. To date no medication is approved by US Food and Drug Administration for VIN treatment; however, several agents have been studied.

- **Imiquimod:** Imiquimod is an immune response modifier, which enhances cell-mediated immunity and was initially approved for genital condyloma acuminatum. Imiquimod used either alone or in conjunction with other therapies has been subjected to randomized clinical trials with promising results. Imiquimod elicits a strong antitumoral response by activating toll-like receptor on monocytes and dendritic cells. Activated dendritic cells release cytokines such as

INFα, TNFα, and IL-12, which induce and activate CD8(+) T cells.

Recommended regimens include topical application of a thin layer of imiquimod 5% cream to individual lesions that then remain uncovered overnight – 2–3 nights per week for a total of 12–20 weeks. Colposcopic assessments need to be performed at 4–6-week intervals during treatment. Side effects are common and include erythema, erosion, edema, and pain. A Cochrane review of four trials, comparing imiquimod to placebo, reported that the imiquimod arm achieved better results with either complete response (RR: 11.95) or significant reduction in size and histologic grade of residual lesion (RR: 9.10) in high-grade VIN (Pepas et al. 2015).

- **Cidofovir**: Cidofovir is a cytidine nucleotide analogue with in vitro and in vivo activity against HPV. A thin layer of 1% cidofovir is applied on the lesion with a gloved finger and then washed off 6–8 h later. The treatment can be applied 3 times a week for maximum 24 weeks. Evaluation is usually performed every 6 weeks after starting treatment. A recent clinical trial of cidofovir compared with imiquimod reported complete response in up to 46% of patients in the cidofovir group compared to 42% in the imiquimod group with high-grade VIN (Tristram and Fiander 2005).
- **Photodynamic therapy (PDT)**: PDT is based on light-induced oxidation reactions which lead to necrosis. A systemic or topical photosensitizing compound, usually 5-aminolevulinic acid (ALA), is used and is followed by the application of nonthermal light. Usually wavelength is matched to the absorption characteristics of the photosensitizer. The interaction generates oxygen radicals with high local cytotoxic effects. ALA gel or a patch is spread over the entire vulva, and then the vulva is covered by a nonadherent dressing. Mean time between drug application and light illumination is 3–6 h, and then the gel is washed off with saline. The fluorescence of ALA-induced protoporphyrin is evaluated with wood lamps, and PDT is performed with a non-laser light source. Studies have shown a treatment response rate between 40% and 70% (Fehr et al. 2001) with a recurrence rate around 48% (Hillemanns et al. 2006). Additional trials and long-term studies are required to evaluate the efficacy of this method.

- **Therapeutic HPV vaccines**: The therapeutic effect of HPV vaccines has been reported recently. Vaccines can enhance T-cell-mediated immunity in uVIN lesions. Most vaccines elicit a specific immunity against HPV E6 and E7 proteins (Preti et al. 2015). In a recent study, after injection of quadrivalent vaccine, up to 35% reduction in subsequent HPV-related disease was reported in patients diagnosed with genital warts, VIN, or VAIN (Joura et al. 2012). In another study, women with HPV-16-positive high-grade VIN were vaccinated with a mix of synthetic long peptides from HPV-16 viral oncoproteins E6 and E7, and complete response in up to 79% of cases has been reported after 12 months, and this effect was maintained for up to 24 months (Kenter et al. 2009). In a randomized clinical trial, imiquimod therapy followed by three injections of quadrivalent vaccine for VIN showed complete regression in up to 63% of cases in addition to a significant increase in the number of CD4 and CD8 T-cell counts in lesion responders (Daayana et al. 2010).

2.11 Follow-up

Recurrence of VIN occurs in 30–50% of cases (ACOG 2011). The true rate of progression with untreated high-grade lesions is not clear, ranging from 9% to 18.5% (Jones et al. 2005; Van Seters et al. 2005), whereas progression risk after treatment varied between 2% and 5% (Jones et al. 2005; Van Seters et al. 2005). In the majority of studies, follow-up has been limited; therefore, long-term surveillance is necessary. The risk factors for recurrence include multifocal or multicentric disease, high-risk HPV infection, positive margins after excision, immunosuppressant use, HIV, and smoking (Hillemanns et al. 2006; Wallbillich et al. 2012). The general follow-up schema is to repeat the exam at 3–4 month intervals during the first year, then every 6 months during the second and third years, and annually thereafter (Barakat et al. 2002). A recent American College of Obstetricians and Gynecologists (ACOG) committee suggested that women with complete response and no new lesions noted at follow-up are suggested to have a visit at 6 and 12 months after treatment and need to be monitored annually thereafter (ACOG 2011). Treatment for recurrent disease should be individualized and depends on the previous treatment method, location, and risk of occult disease.

2.12 Special Considerations

Pregnancy: Data about VIN in pregnancy is extremely rare. Any suspicious lesion warrants biopsy. If invasive carcinoma is ruled out, expectant management in the third trimester can be considered. Local excision and ablative therapy are available options for patients who are not close to delivery, and they follow the same principles as nonpregnant women (Tseng et al. 2012). Podofilox and sinecatechins should not be used during pregnancy. Imiquimod appears to pose low risk but is recommended to be avoided until more data are available. Management recommendations for pregnancy complicated by invasive vulvar cancer are discussed in the chapter for invasive vulvar cancer.

Immunocompromised: HIV-mediated immuno-suppression can result in exacerbation of HPV infection and impairment of the local immunity of lower genital tract (Conley et al. 2002). Therefore, this population has an increased risk for lower genitalia preinvasive and invasive neoplasia. Clinical manifestations are the same as for women without HIV infection, but lesions may be more extensive. A detailed pelvic examination needs to be performed at least once per year, and any suspicious lesions need to be biopsied. There are no established treatment guidelines; however, surgery is the mainstay of therapy. Medical treatment is the second option. There are a few studies reporting promising results using imiquimod and cidofovir for VIN treatment in HIV-infected

women (Tristram et al. 2014), and according to a recent study, HAART was associated with a one-third decrease in the incidence of VIN (Massad et al. 2004).

2.13 Prevention

The uVIN shows over 85% HPV positivity, with type 16 DNA being detected in 75% of high-grade VIN cases (de Sanjose et al. 2013; Preti et al. 2015). It has been demonstrated that immunization with quadrivalent vaccine will decrease the risk of VIN. The bivalent HPV vaccine is not approved for this indication, as this endpoint was not assessed in clinical trials (ACOG 2011).

2.14 Conclusion

The incidence of VIN is increasing in the past decades. There are two different types of VIN with distinct clinical features, etiology, pathology, and malignant potential. dVIN accounts for a smaller proportion of cases but has a higher risk of progression to malignancy, and surgical excision is the preferred treatment modality. uVIN occurs mostly in younger women, and HPV infection is the most important risk factor. Due to the low risk of malignant transformation in uVIN, conservative management is recommended. Due to high recurrence rates after treatment, long-term follow-up is crucial. HPV vaccination can potentially prevent and reduce the incidence of uVIN and related invasive vulvar cancer.

3 Vulvar Paget's Disease

3.1 Introduction

Extramammary Paget's disease (EMPD) is a rare noninvasive intraepithelial adenocarcinoma affecting areas rich in apocrine sweat glands. Whereas Paget's disease occurs most often in nipples, EMPD is prevalent to the vulva and accounts for up to 60% of EMPD and 1% of vulvar neoplasm cases (Parker et al. 2000). The origin of vulvar Paget's cell remains controversial. It may be viewed as a carcinoma of adnexal stem cells, as a sweat gland carcinoma arising from the intraepidermal portion of the gland, or as a carcinoma derived from the Toker cells of mammary-like glands of the vulva (Regauer 2006). Vulvar EMPD is mostly an intraepithelial lesion but has the potential to invade to the dermal layer. Up to 4–17% of vulvar EMPD are associated with underlying carcinoma of the vulva. In addition, in 11–20% of cases, other malignancies involving the vagina, uterus, cervix, breast, bladder, rectum, colon, and gallbladder have been reported (Karam and Dorigo 2012).

3.2   Classification

According to Wilkinson and Brown, vulvar Paget's disease can be subdivided into primary (cutaneous) and secondary. Primary vulvar Paget's disease is an intraepithelial adenocarcinoma arising within the epidermis, while the secondary is defined as involvement of vulvar skin by a noncutaneous internal neoplasm, either by direct extension or epidermotropic metastases (Wilkinson and Brown 2002):

Primary
- Paget's disease as a primary intraepithelial Paget's disease
- Paget's disease as an intraepithelial neoplasm with invasion
- Paget's disease as manifestation of an underlying primary adenocarcinoma of a skin appendage or a subcutaneous vulvar gland

Secondary
- Paget's disease secondary to anal or rectal adenocarcinoma
- Paget's disease secondary to urothelial neoplasm (PUN)
- PUN as a manifestation of intraepithelial urothelial neoplasia
- PUN as manifestation of urothelial carcinoma

- Paget's disease secondary to adenocarcinomas or related tumors of other sites

3.3   Clinical Features

Vulvar Paget's disease is common to postmenopausal Caucasian women. It can be asymptomatic or present with an erythematous, eczematoid, or pruriginous lesion. Many patients are treated for presumed eczema for years prior to a definitive diagnosis (Terlou et al. 2010). Vulvar Paget's disease is characterized by a multicentric nature and usually extends microscopically. Due to the occult fashion of spread beyond the margins, it has a chronic and relapsing course and is difficult to achieve complete elimination of disease. Nearly 10–20% of vulvar Paget's disease cases are associated with coexisting malignancies at other sites such as the breast, rectum, genitourinary tract, cervix, and skin (Parker et al. 2000; Tebes et al. 2002). Once vulvar Paget's disease is diagnosed, an underlying cancer needs to be ruled out in both vulva and other related areas such as the breast.

3.4   Evaluation

History: Patients with persistent pruritic eczematous lesions that fail to resolve within 6 weeks of appropriate treatment need to undergo further evaluation. This is important because diagnosis is frequently delayed and may result in the expansion of disease (Tebes et al. 2002).

Diagnostic Study: Diagnosis is based upon the characteristic histopathology. Vulvar biopsy needs to be performed in patients with suspicious lesions. Histologically, vulvar Paget's disease is characterized by the presence of Paget's cells, identified by typical pale vacuolated cytoplasm, high-grade nuclei, and prominent nucleoli. The differential diagnosis includes both benign etiologies such as leukoplakia, condyloma acuminata, contact dermatitis, psoriasis, lichen planus, and malignant conditions such as melanoma, basal cell, or squamous cell carcinoma (Hendi et al. 2004, Wilkinson and Brown 2002). Sometimes immunohistochemistry is required to exclude the differential diagnosis of melanoma and VIN. Paget's cells can express CA125 and Her-2/neu but do not express estrogen receptors (Lu and Chen 2014).

3.5   Management

An outline of various treatment modalities for vulvar Paget's disease is summarized in Table 3.

3.6   Surgery

Surgical resection remains the mainstay treatment of vulvar Paget's disease. Surgical interventions include wide local excision, Mohs micrographic surgery, and vulvectomy.

- **Wide local excision (WLE):** WLE is defined as an excision of the affected lesion to the depth of to 4–6 mm to include the pilosebaceous glands and skin adnexal structure. Margins up to 2 cm are preferred.

- **Mohs micrographic surgery (MMS):** MMS is a specialized surgical resection technique of skin tumors with highly accurate intraoperative mapping and histological assessment of the entire margin at the time of surgery. It allows maximal preservation of normal tissue (Hendi et al. 2004).

- **Vulvectomy (simple or radical):** Vulvectomy is an invasive management that may be required in cases of concurrent adenocarcinoma or deep invasion of EMPD. It often requires vulvar reconstructive surgery. Vulvectomy with skin graft placement has a 6.8% risk of having postoperative complications including physical or sexual dysfunction (Lavoue et al. 2013).

3.7   Prognosis of Surgical Resection

Response rates following surgical resection ranged from 33% to 70% (Edey et al. 2013; Lavoue et al. 2013; Parker et al. 2000; Tebes et al. 2002). The high recurrence rate is an important consideration for monitoring after surgical management. In a recent study of 529 cases, the

Table 3 Summary of management for vulvar Paget's disease

Treatment	Study size	Response rate	Recurrent rate	Side effect
Surgical resection[a]	40.5 (22–529)	33–70%	22–61%	Graft sloughing, dyspareunia Introital stenosis Sexual disorders
Radiotherapy	17 (2–92)	62–100%	0–35%	Acute reaction: radiation cystitis, nausea and vomiting, erythema, irritation, dermatitis Chronic reaction: bladder dysfunction, skin reactions (soreness, ulceration), chronic diarrhea, malabsorption, fistula
Chemotherapy				
Systemic[b]	3 (1–7)	33–50%	50%	Myelosuppression, neutropenia
Topical	1 (1–7)	57%	25%	Severe local pain, moist desquamation, allergic reaction
Photodynamic therapy	24 (16–32)	14–50%	38–56%	Photosensitivity reaction
CO_2 laser ablation	6 (1–6)	33%	67%	Severe local pain
Imiquimod	21 (10–31)	52–80%	19%	Skin irritation, erosion, pain, ulceration

[a]Surgical resection including wide local resection, vulvectomy (simple or radical), and Mohs micrographic surgery
[b]Systemic chemotherapy for metastatic or invasive vulvar Paget's disease. Sample size: (median, range)

recurrence rate after surgery was as high as 58% (Edey et al. 2013). Positive surgical margins were an important risk factor for recurrence. Patients with negative margins experienced rates of local recurrence between 18% and 38% (Edey et al. 2013; Lavoue et al. 2013) in comparison to 46–61% in patients with positive surgical margins (Edey et al. 2013; Lavoue et al. 2013).

3.8 Medical Treatment

Medical treatment is indicated if patient is not a candidate for surgical resection due to comorbidity or patient choice. Medical treatment can be also recommended for recurrent vulvar Paget's disease after multiple surgical resections.

- **Imiquimod**: Imiquimod is an immune response modifier, which enhances cell-mediated immunity. See the VIN section for the mechanism of action of imiquimod. It is a promising treatment modality especially for patients with recurrence and multiple surgical resections or in patients who are poor surgical candidates. In a small series, response rates of up to 52–80% have been reported. The recurrence rate is 6.5–19% regardless of primary versus recurrent disease status (Luyten et al. 2014). In a systematic review of 63 cases, complete response rates of 9.8%, 31.1%, and 71.6% were reported after 2, 4, and 6 months of imiquimod therapy (Machida et al. 2015). Based on this, a 6-month treatment course is suggested for vulvar Paget's disease.
- **Photodynamic therapy**: PDT is a technique using a tumor-localizing photoreactive drug such as 5-aminolevulinic acid with appropriate wavelengths to eliminate tumor cells. Response rates for PDT in vulvar Paget's disease range from 14% to 50%, and recurrence rates are 38–56% (Shieh et al. 2002). Photosensitivity reaction and burning sensation were reported as adverse effects for PDT.

3.9 Alternative Therapy

- **CO_2 laser ablation:** Laser ablation therapy has an advantage of preserving vulvar anatomy. However, the high recurrence rate of up to 67% is an important concern in vulvar Paget's disease. Laser ablation only penetrates the surface of the skin, and there is a high chance of leaving residual disease, especially in cases of deep dissemination (Louis-Sylvestre et al. 2001).
- **Radiotherapy**: Radiotherapy is an effective treatment in localized vulvar Paget's disease. The downside of radiotherapy is the dose limitation of radiation due to the concern for long-term side effects. Therefore, repeated irradiation to the vulva must be very limited. The response rate ranges from 62% to 100%, with a recurrence rate of 0–35% (Karam and Dorigo 2012; Oashi et al. 2014).
- **Systemic chemotherapy:** Systemic chemotherapy is indicated for disseminated metastatic Paget's disease. No standard chemotherapy guideline has been established. There are numerous case reports describing systemic chemotherapy for metastatic or invasive Paget's disease. Suggested chemotherapy regimens consist of epirubicin with mitomycin C, vincristine, carboplatin, and fluorouracil, mitomycin C plus etoposide and cisplatin, etoposide alone, cisplatin plus fluorouracil, or S1 plus carboplatin. The complete response rate is 33–50%, with partial response in up to 55–67% (Matsushita et al. 2011; Niikura et al. 2006; Oashi et al. 2014).
- **Topical chemotherapy**: Topical chemotherapy with fluorouracil or bleomycin monotherapy has been reported as an alternative treatment for local disease. Various adverse effects including severe pain, moist desquamation, and allergic reaction have been reported. According to studies, response rates are between 57% and 100% with a 25% recurrence rate (Del Castillo et al. 2000).

3.10 Follow-Up for Vulvar Paget's Disease

The overall recurrence rate after standard treatment modalities is up to 30%. (Luyten et al. 2014). Long-term follow-up is recommended, not only because of the high recurrence rate but also the higher risk of developing a secondary malignancy, which may occur many years after the initial diagnosis. According to a recent population-based study examining 1,439 patients with invasive EMPD that included 781 cases of vulvar Paget's diseases, 80.4% of cases were limited to local disease with a 5-year disease-free survival up to 94.9%. However, a significant increase in the rates of secondary vulvar or vaginal malignancy has been reported (Karam and Dorigo 2012). Despite the importance of long-term monitoring in vulvar EMPD cases, no established follow-up guidelines exist to date.

3.11 Conclusion

Vulvar Paget's disease is a rare noninvasive intraepithelial disease, which has a multifocal nature. Standard treatment for vulvar Paget's disease is surgical excision; however, positive margins with residual lesions are common. Because relapse occurs in over 30% of patients, medical treatment, especially imiquimod, can be an alternative treatment option in the management of vulvar Paget's disease.

4 Melanoma In Situ of the Vulva

4.1 Introduction

Vulvar melanoma is the second most common vulvar malignancy, and due to the poor prognosis, it is an important women's health issue. Vulvar melanoma represents 3.4% to 10% of vulvar neoplasms. Melanoma in situ (MIS) is the precursor of vulvar Melanoma which is confined to the epidermis and adnexal epithelium

(Kingston et al. 2004). Despite the slow nature of MIS, progression to invasive melanoma is definite (Terlou et al. 2010). Vulvo-vaginal melanoma appears to be biologically different from cutaneous melanoma and is more similar to mucosal melanoma. Pathologically, mucosal melanoma of female genital tract is subdivided into epithelioid, mixed spindle and epithelioid, and pure spindle. Up to 40% of mucosal melanomas of female genital tract are accompanied with MIS. Breslow thickness is the most significant prognostic factor of outcome in vulvar melanoma (Gru et al. 2014). Management of melanoma of the vulva is described in the chapter for vulvar cancer.

4.2 Clinical Features

Melanoma in situ appears as a pigmented vulvar lesion. Our understanding of MIS natural history is limited, and pure in situ lesions are seldom recognized. The ABCDE scheme (asymmetry, border irregularities, color variation, diameter >6 mm, enlargement or evolution of color change) needs to be considered for any pigmented lesions. In situ lesions appear to have good prognosis if completely excised.

4.3 Evaluation

History: Any change in size, shape, or color of the vulvar lesion is important. Personal or family history of dysplastic nevus syndrome is highly important. Exposure to excessive ultraviolet light can be considered as a risk factor for lesions arising on outer, non-hair-bearing portion of labia major.

Diagnostic study: Punch biopsy is the preferred method because assessing the depth of stromal invasion is important. The most significant histologic prognostic factors for vulvar melanoma are tumor thickness and depth of invasion. The biopsy needs to be performed from the thickest lesion (ACOG 2008). Small lesions can be completely excised. If melanoma is suspected, an excisional biopsy with 1–2 mm margin is necessary. On histologic examination, the in situ component is characterized by atypical melanocytes distributed predominantly along the dermoepidermal junction.

4.4   Management

Surgical resection is the standard approach for MIS. Studies support excision with 5 mm margins as the recommended surgical approach. Destruction by cryosurgery, laser, or cautery is contraindicated (Terlou et al. 2010).

4.5   Conclusion

When vulvar MIS is suspected in a vulvar lesion with changes in the ABCDE scheme, complete resection of a hyperpigmented vulvar lesion is recommended.

References

ACOG Committee Opinion No. 509: management of vulvar intraepithelial neoplasia. Obstet Gynecol. 2011; 118(5):1192–4.

ACOG Practice Bulletin No. 93: diagnosis and management of vulvar skin disorders. Obstet Gynecol. 2008;111(5):1243–53.

Barakat RR, Gershenson DM, Hoskins WJ. Handbook of gynecologic oncology: Marthin dunitz; 2002. Florida: CRC Press.

Barbara Hoffman JS, Schaffer J, Halvorson L, Bradshaw K, Cunningham Williams, F. Gynecology. 2nd ed. 2008;638–9. New York: McGraw-Hill Professional.

Conley LJ, Ellerbrock TV, Bush TJ, Chiasson MA, Sawo D, Wright TC. HIV-1 infection and risk of vulvovaginal and perianal condylomata acuminata and intraepithelial neoplasia: a prospective cohort study. Lancet. 2002;359(9301):108–13.

Daayana S, Elkord E, Winters U, Pawlita M, Roden R, Stern PL, et al. Phase II trial of imiquimod and HPV therapeutic vaccination in patients with vulvar intraepithelial neoplasia. Br J Cancer. 2010;102(7): 1129–36.

De Sanjose S, Alemany L, Ordi J, Tous S, Alejo M, Bigby SM, et al. Worldwide human papillomavirus genotype attribution in over 2000 cases of intraepithelial and invasive lesions of the vulva. European Journal of Cancer (Oxford, England : 1990). 2013;49(16): 3450–61.

Del Castillo LF, Garcia C, Schoendorff C, Garcia JF, Torres LM, Garcia AD. Spontaneous apparent clinical resolution with histologic persistence of a case of extramammary Paget's disease: response to topical 5-fluorouracil. Cutis. 2000;65(5):331–3.

Edey KA, Allan E, Murdoch JB, Cooper S, Bryant A. Interventions for the treatment of Paget's disease of the vulva. The Cochrane Database of Systematic Reviews. 2013;10, Cd009245.

Fehr MK, Hornung R, Schwarz VA, Simeon R, Haller U, Wyss P. Photodynamic therapy of vulvar intraepithelial neoplasia III using topically applied 5-aminolevulinic acid. Gynecol Oncol. 2001;80(1):62–6.

Ferenczy A, Wright TC, Richart RM. Comparison of CO_2 laser surgery and loop electrosurgical excision/fulguration procedure (LEEP) for the treatment of vulvar intraepithelial neoplasia (VIN). Int J Gynecol Cancer. 1994;4(1):22–8.

Gru AA, Becker N, Dehner LP, Pfeifer JD. Mucosal melanoma: correlation of clinicopathologic, prognostic, and molecular features. Melanoma Res. 2014;24(4): 360–70.

Hart WR. Vulvar intraepithelial neoplasia: historical aspects and current status. Int J Gynecol Pathol. 2001;20(1):16–30.

Hendi A, Brodland DG, Zitelli JA. Extramammary Paget's disease: surgical treatment with Mohs micrographic surgery. J Am Acad Dermatol. 2004;51(5):767–73.

Hillemanns P, Wang X, Staehle S, Michels W, Dannecker C. Evaluation of different treatment modalities for vulvar intraepithelial neoplasia (VIN): CO(2) laser vaporization, photodynamic therapy, excision and vulvectomy. Gynecol Oncol. 2006;100(2):271–5.

Jones RW, Rowan DM, Stewart AW. Vulvar intraepithelial neoplasia: aspects of the natural history and outcome in 405 women. Obstet Gynecol. 2005;106(6):1319–26.

Joura EA, Garland SM, Paavonen J, Ferris DG, Perez G, Ault KA, et al. Effect of the human papillomavirus (HPV) quadrivalent vaccine in a subgroup of women with cervical and vulvar disease: retrospective pooled analysis of trial data. BMJ. 2012; 344, e1401.

Judson PL, Habermann EB, Baxter NN, Durham SB, Virnig BA. Trends in the incidence of invasive and in situ vulvar carcinoma. Obstet Gynecol. 2006;107(5):1018–22.

Karam A, Dorigo O. Treatment outcomes in a large cohort of patients with invasive extramammary Paget's disease. Gynecol Oncol. 2012;125(2):346–51.

Kaushik S, Pepas L, Nordin A, Bryant A, Dickinson HO. Surgical interventions for high-grade vulval intraepithelial neoplasia. The Cochrane Database of Systematic Reviews. 2014;3, Cd007928.

Kenter GG, Welters MJ, Valentijn AR, Lowik MJ, Berends-van der Meer DM, Vloon AP, et al. Vaccination against HPV-16 oncoproteins for vulvar intraepithelial neoplasia. N Engl J Med. 2009;361(19): 1838–47.

Kingston NJ, Jones RW, Baranyai J. Recurrent primary vulvovaginal malignant melanoma arising in melanoma in situ – the natural history of lesions followed for 23 years. Int J Gynecol Cancer. 2004;14(4): 628–32.

Lavoue V, Lemarrec A, Bertheuil N, Henno S, Mesbah H, Watier E, et al. Quality of life and female sexual function after skinning vulvectomy with split-thickness skin graft in women with vulvar intraepithelial neoplasia or vulvar Paget disease. Eur J Surg Oncol. 2013;39(12): 1444–50.

Louis-Sylvestre C, Haddad B, Paniel BJ. Paget's disease of the vulva: results of different conservative treatments. Eur J Obstet Gynecol Reprod Biol. 2001;99(2):253–5.

Lu Z, Chen J. Introduction of WHO classification of tumours of female reproductive organs, fourth edition. Zhonghua bing li xue za zhi Chinese Journal of Pathology. 2014;43(10):649–50.

Luyten A, Sorgel P, Clad A, Gieseking F, Maass-Poppenhusen K, Lelle RJ, et al. Treatment of extramammary Paget disease of the vulva with imiquimod: a retrospective, multicenter study by the German Colposcopy Network. J Am Acad Dermatol. 2014;70(4):644–50.

Machida H, Moeini A, Roman LD, Matsuo K. Effects of imiquimod on vulvar Paget's disease: a systematic review of literature. Gynecol Oncol. 2015;139(1):165–71.

Massad LS, Silverberg MJ, Springer G, Minkoff H, Hessol N, Palefsky JM, et al. Effect of antiretroviral therapy on the incidence of genital warts and vulvar neoplasia among women with the human immunodeficiency virus. Am J Obstet Gynecol. 2004;190(5): 1241–8.

Matsushita S, Yonekura K, Mera K, Kawai K, Kanekura T. Successful treatment of metastatic extramammary Paget's disease with S-1 and docetaxel combination chemotherapy. J Dermatol. 2011;38(10):996–8.

Miller BE. Vulvar intraepithelial neoplasia treated with cavitational ultrasonic surgical aspiration. Gynecol Oncol. 2002;85(1):114–8.

Niikura H, Yoshida H, Ito K, Takano T, Watanabe H, Aiba S, et al. Paget's disease of the vulva: clinicopathologic study of type 1 cases treated at a single institution. Int J Gynecol Cancer. 2006;16(3):1212–5.

Oashi K, Tsutsumida A, Namikawa K, Tanaka R, Omata W, Yamamoto Y, et al. Combination chemotherapy for metastatic extramammary Paget disease. Br J Dermatol. 2014;170(6):1354–7.

Parker LP, Parker JR, Bodurka-Bevers D, Deavers M, Bevers MW, Shen-Gunther J, et al. Paget's disease of the vulva: pathology, pattern of involvement, and prognosis. Gynecol Oncol. 2000;77(1):183–9.

Pepas L, Kaushik S, Nordin A, Bryant A, Lawrie TA. Medical interventions for high-grade vulval intraepithelial neoplasia. The Cochrane Database of Systematic Reviews. 2015;8, Cd007924.

Preti M, Igidbashian S, Costa S, Cristoforoni P, Mariani L, Origoni M, et al. VIN usual type-from the past to the future. Ecancermedicalscience. 2015;9:531.

Regauer S. Extramammary Paget's disease – a proliferation of adnexal origin? Histopathology. 2006;48(6): 723–9.

Reid R, Elfont EA, Zirkin RM, Fuller TA. Superficial laser vulvectomy. II. The anatomic and biophysical principles permitting accurate control over the depth of dermal destruction with the carbon dioxide laser. Am J Obstet Gynecol. 1985;152(3): 261–71.

Shieh S, Dee AS, Cheney RT, Frawley NP, Zeitouni NC, Oseroff AR. Photodynamic therapy for the treatment of extramammary Paget's disease. Br J Dermatol. 2002;146(6):1000–5.

Sideri M, Jones RW, Wilkinson EJ, Preti M, Heller DS, Scurry J, et al. Squamous vulvar intraepithelial neoplasia: 2004 modified terminology, ISSVD Vulvar Oncology Subcommittee. J Reprod Med. 2005;50(11): 807–10.

Tebes S, Cardosi R, Hoffman M. Paget's disease of the vulva. Am J Obstet Gynecol. 2002;187(2):281–3; discussion 3–4.

Terlou A, Blok LJ, Helmerhorst TJ, van Beurden M. Premalignant epithelial disorders of the vulva: squamous vulvar intraepithelial neoplasia, vulvar Paget's disease and melanoma in situ. Acta Obstet Gynecol Scand. 2010;89(6):741–8.

Terzakis E, Androutsopoulos G, Zygouris D, Grigoriadis C, Derdelis G, Arnogiannaki N. Loop electrosurgical excision procedure in Greek patients with vaginal intraepithelial neoplasia. Eur J Gynaecol Oncol. 2010;31(4):392–4.

Tristram A, Fiander A. Clinical responses to Cidofovir applied topically to women with high grade vulval intraepithelial neoplasia. Gynecol Oncol. 2005;99(3): 652–5.

Tristram A, Hurt CN, Madden T, Powell N, Man S, Hibbitts S, et al. Activity, safety, and feasibility of cidofovir and imiquimod for treatment of vulval intraepithelial neoplasia (RT(3)VIN): a multicentre, open-label, randomised, phase 2 trial. Lancet Oncol. 2014;15(12):1361–8.

Tseng JY, Bastu E, Gungor-Ugurlucan F. Management of precancerous lesions prior to conception and during pregnancy: a narrative review of the literature. Eur J Cancer Care 2012;21(6):703–11.

Van Seters M, van Beurden M, de Craen AJ. Is the assumed natural history of vulvar intraepithelial neoplasia III based on enough evidence? A systematic review of 3322 published patients. Gynecol Oncol. 2005;97(2): 645–51.

Wallbillich JJ, Rhodes HE, Milbourne AM, Munsell MF, Frumovitz M, Brown J, et al. Vulvar intraepithelial neoplasia (VIN 2/3): comparing clinical outcomes and evaluating risk factors for recurrence. Gynecol Oncol. 2012;127(2):312–5.

Wilkinson EJ, Brown HM. Vulvar Paget disease of urothelial origin: a report of three cases and a proposed classification of vulvar Paget disease. Hum Pathol. 2002;33(5):549–54.

Sentinel Node Mapping in Vulva Cancer

Mamoru Kakuda, Eiji Kobayashi, Kiyoshi Yoshino, and
Tadashi Kimura

Abstract

The treatment of early-stage vulvar cancer previously included a complete inguinofemoral
lymph node dissection (IFLD). However,
IFLD is associated with a substantially high
probability of postoperative complications: up
to two-thirds of patients who have IFLD
performed experience wound infection or
breakdown, formation of lymphocytes, or
long-term lymphedema. For this reason, lymphatic mapping and sentinel lymph node
biopsy (SLNB) for early-stage vulvar cancer
have been studied. Compared to IFLD, SLNB
has significantly fewer complications and is
becoming a more common practice in treatment for selected patients with early-stage vulvar cancer. From our literature review, we
discuss SLNB as part of a standard treatment
for patients with early-stage vulvar cancer, and
we provide future considerations for its use in
the management of vulvar cancer.

Keywords

Vulvar   cancer   •   Sentinel   nodes   •
Inguinofemoral lymph node dissection • Early
stage • Complication

Contents

1   Introduction

Sentinel lymph node (SLN) identification and
lymphatic mapping for vulvar cancer have its
origins in cancers of other sites. In 1960, Gould
et al. first proposed the concept of a "sentinel
node" for head and neck cancer in their description of the key node which was identified at the
junction of the anterior and posterior facial vein

M. Kakuda • E. Kobayashi (✉) • K. Yoshino • T. Kimura
Department of Obstetrics and Gynecology, Osaka
University Graduate School of Medicine, Suita, Osaka,
Japan
e-mail: mamorukakuda@gmail.com;
kobachiroabiko@hotmail.com; yoshino@gyne.med.
osaka-u.ac.jp; tadashi@gyne.med.osaka-u.ac.jp

© Springer International Publishing AG 2017
D. Shoupe (ed.), *Handbook of Gynecology*,
DOI 10.1007/978-3-319-17798-4_37

(Gould et al. 1960). In the field of gynecologic cancers, DiSaia et al. first utilized the superficial inguinal lymph nodes as the "sentinel nodes" in the treatment of vulvar cancer to help them identify patients who would not benefit from a more morbidity-causing complete IFLD (DiSaia et al. 1979). In the 1990s, Morton et al. described what is now the new procedure lymphatic mapping in the treatment of melanoma, in which blue dye was used to identify the primary lymphatic drainage basin (Morton et al. 1992).

The premise of SLN biopsy (SNLB) is that tumor cells from the primary lesion will first migrate "downstream" in the lymphatic flow to one or a few key lymph nodes, prior to disseminating to other regional lymph nodes. These key lymph nodes can be identified by using either a vital blue dye (isosulfan blue/methylene blue), a radiocolloid, or indocyanine green (ICG). Key to the utilization of this technique is confidence that identification of the SLN accurately predicts the status of the remaining lymph nodes.

Surgery still remains the primary care for early-stage vulvar cancer, but in the past two decades, the standard treatment has made a transition from radical dissection to minimally invasive surgery. Primarily, the surgical treatment of early-stage vulvar cancer includes a complete inguinofemoral lymph node dissection (IFLD). However, IFLD is associated with a significantly high probability of postoperative complications; up to two-thirds of patients who have had extensive dissection of inguinal lymph node performed experienced wound infection or breakdown and lymphocyst formation or long-term lymphedema after surgery (Stehman et al. 1992; Gaarenstroom et al. 2003; Rouzier et al. 2003; Kirby et al. 2005). Because of this high morbidity, and since vulvar cancer is an excellent target for the SLN concept, the tumor is easy to inject with blue dye or radiocolloid. Because the lymph drainage is predictably to one or both of the groins, lymphatic mapping and SLNB for early-stage vulvar cancer have been widely studied as a possible alternative procedure to current IFLD procedures. As a result of those studies, SLNB has now become more common in the treatment for selected patients with early-stage vulvar cancer.

2 Patient Selection for SLNB Versus IFLD

As mentioned above, IFLD is associated with a high morbidity rate, including a 20–40% risk of wound complications and a 30–70% risk of lower extremity lymphedema. In addition, fewer than one-third of early-stage vulvar cancer patients have lymph node metastasis, which means that the routine application of IFLD exposes a large number of patients to potentially preventable surgical complications (Sedlis et al. 1987).

The most effective way to minimize morbidity in patients where surgical treatment of vulvar cancer is performed is to minimize damage of the lymphatic tracts by removing fewer lymph nodes. The benefits of dissecting fewer nodes, however, must outweigh the risk of failing to remove actual metastatic lymph nodes in the inguinofemoral region, as inguinal and pelvic recurrence of vulvar cancer is associated with a 27% 5-year survival rate (Maggino et al. 2000).

Two large trials have evaluated whether SLNB accurately detected positive lymph node and whether SLNB reduced morbidity as compared with IFLD in patients with early-stage vulvar cancer (Van der Zee et al. 2008; Levenback et al. 2012). The GROINSS-V study was an observational study of 276 patients with squamous cell cancer of the vulva, with T1/T2 (<4 cm) and no lymph node metastases detected on SLNB (Van der Zee et al. 2008). Study investigators found that patients with multifocal disease had a higher recurrence rate after SLNB (11.8%) compared with patients with unifocal disease (2.3%). The false-negative rate for SLNB of multifocal disease was 5.9% (4.6% for patients with unifocal disease), and the false-negative predictive value was 2.9%. This study suggested it was less common for surgical morbidity in patients who underwent only removal of SLN, compared with patients with a metastatic sentinel node who subsequently underwent IFLD. Wound breakdown, cellulitis, lymphedema, and recurrent erysipelas are also significantly less after SLNB compared to IFLD. A follow-up survey sent to patients after the GROINSS-V study found that no difference in overall quality of life was observed between the two procedure groups and that the major difference found was the increase in complaints of lower extremity lymphedema after IFLD (Oonk et al. 2009).

The Gynecologic Oncology Group (GOG) Protocol 173 was a multi-institutional observational study of 452 patients with early-stage vulvar cancer (Levenback et al. 2012). All patients underwent intraoperative lymphatic mapping and SLNB, followed by IFLD. The overall false-negative rate for SLNB was 3.7%. However, the false-negative rate for SLNB was much lower in women with tumors smaller than 4 cm than in women with tumors 4–6 cm (2.0% vs. 7.4%). In addition, the location of the tumor was another important factor found in a systematic review (Hassanzade et al. 2013). For lesions which were within 2 cm of the midline, the detection rate was considerably lower compared with more lateral lesions greater than 2 cm from the midline plane (73% vs. 95%).

From this evidence, we suggest that patients with early-stage vulvar cancer, with primary tumors that are unifocal and smaller than 4 cm and where the lesion(s) are located more than 2 cm from the midline, can be assured preoperatively that, if the SLNB is negative, the risk of a recurrence of the inguinal lesion is less than 3%. Given the cumulative results from these studies, we feel confident that the SLNB can be offered to patients carefully selected by skilled gynecologic oncologists. In clinical practices where vulvar cancer is rarely encountered and experience of the surgeon with the disease is negligible, referral to a high-volume center and a more experienced surgeon is recommended.

3   Drainage Tracer

In the GOG Protocol 173, the false-negative rates for SLNs identified by dye and radiocolloid, dye alone, and radiocolloid alone were 1.6%, 2.0%, and 7.8%, respectively (Levenback et al. 2012). A meta-analysis of 29 studies of SLNB for vulvar cancer found that the pooled SLN detection rates were 94.0% for 99mTc, 68.7% for blue dye alone, and 97.7% for combined 99mTc and blue dye

(Meads et al. 2014). These results demonstrate evidence that a combination of radiocolloid and blue dye is the most sensitive for detecting SLN. Because of the direct visualization of the lymphatic mapping for vulvar cancer provided by using blue dye, using the combination of radiocolloid and blue dye may also improve the learning curve for the SLNB procedure.

In recent years, near-infrared (NIR) fluorescence imaging has been introduced in lymphatic mapping and SLNB for vulvar cancer. The NIR technique has the potential for far more accurate and real-time intraoperative SLN mapping. A meta-analysis of SLNB with NIR fluorescence imaging in vulvar cancer has reported a good outcome, with a high detection rate of inguinal lymph node metastasis (91.4%) and a considerably higher negative predictive value (100%) (Handgraaf et al. 2014). However, the penetration capacity of NIR fluorescence is limited to approximately 8 mm. The use of radiotracers therefore remains indispensable, since it allows preoperative scintigraphy and intraoperative identification of deep SLN in the groin. Further studies will therefore be needed to compare the effectiveness of ICG with radiocolloid injection versus the traditional combination approach of blue dye and radiotracer.

4   Ultrastaging

Ultrastaging is the term used to describe intense histologic examination of the SLN samples. Ultrastaging is unrealistic in the daily practice setting and is thus rarely performed because it is an onerous task to examine the, on average, ten lymph nodes per groin removed by conventional IFLD. In contrast, ultrastaging is amenably performed on the 1–2 lymph nodes per groin obtained by SLNB. The combination of hematoxylin-eosin (H&E) and cytokeratin immunohistochemical (IHC) staining of paraffin-embedded SLN tissue that is sectioned every 0.4 to 0.5 mm intervals (as contrasted with the 2 to 3 mm section intervals used for traditional lymph node evaluations) has led to the identification of micrometastases in SLN otherwise thought to be void of lymph node metastasis by conventional pathologic examination. IHC staining should thus be added to H&E staining for more accurate identification of micrometastases.

In GOG Protocol 173, 23% of all SLN were detected to be positive by immunohistochemistry when the routine H&E staining did not reveal metastatic disease (Levenback et al. 2012). In the GROINSS-V study, the authors reported that, of 135 positive SLN in 403 patients, 80 (59%) were detected with routine sectioning and H&E staining, 19 (14%) were detected by ultrastage sectioning using H&E staining, and a further 36 (27%) positive SLN were detected by ultrastaging with immunohistochemical staining. The risk of a non-SLN metastases was higher when the SLN was found positive by routine histological assessment than by ultrastaging (27.1% vs. 5.4%) (Oonk et al. 2010). In patients with SLN metastasis identified by ultrastaging, the 5-year overall survival rate was higher than in patients with SLN metastasis identified by routine pathological examination (89% vs. 65%).

Without examination of the lymph nodes removed by SLNB or full IFLD by the same pathological evaluations, it will be difficult to confirm the true value of the detection of micrometastases by ultrastaging of SLN. A better consensus on the standards for pathological evaluations and the need for ultrastaging is required.

5   Recurrence Rate

Recurrence of vulvar cancer in the groin is usually a fatal event, making it an important outcome measurement for this patient population. IFLD patients were historically divided into two groups: superficial and complete resection. Complete resection was used to describe an inguinofemoral lymphadenectomy combined with removal of the deep femoral lymph nodes, while superficial resection was used to describe procedures without an attempt to remove the deep femoral lymph nodes. Using complete resection, the lowest

reported rate of groin recurrence following IFLD was about 1%. However, rates of surgical morbidity, especially wound breakdown and lymphedema, were excessively high (Stehman et al. 1992).

In the case of superficial resection, inguinal recurrence rates of 5–7% were seen and were considered less acceptable compared with historical controls (Robison et al. 2014). For SLNB, the groin recurrence rate was expected to be less than 3%. For well-selected patients with vulvar cancer, this result seems to be an acceptable compromise that minimizes surgical morbidity. Of course, for a tailored treatment in a clinical situation, the informed consent procedure for SLNB for vulvar cancer needs to include as a possible option a full IFLD. For patients with a 1 cm squamous cell carcinoma with less than 2 mm of stromal invasion, the risk of recurrence is approximately 1%, if the SLN is negative for metastasis. In contrast, for patients with a 4 cm or larger vulvar cancer, accompanied deep stromal invasion, the risk of recurrence is significantly higher, even if the SLN is negative for metastasis.

6   Survival Rate

Regardless of the type of lymphadenectomy, an inguinal recurrence of vulvar cancer worsens the survival rate (Martinez-Palones et al. 2006; Terada et al. 2006; Moore et al. 2008; Van der Zee et al. 2008; Oonk et al. 2010). Achimas-Cadariu et al. reported that the median overall survival period was 61.2 months but was only 16.2 months for patients who experienced a relapse (Achimas-Cadariu et al. 2009).

The GROINSS-V study is the largest investigation to date into the disease-specific survival rate among patients with no detected metastases by SLN (Van der Zee et al. 2008). At a median follow-up time of 35 months, the 3-year disease-specific survival rate among patients with unifocal vulvar disease and a negative SLN was 97.0%. The 3-year disease-specific survival for patients with sentinel node metastases larger than 2 mm was lower than for those with metastases 2 mm or smaller tumors (69.5% vs. 94.4%) (Oonk et al. 2010).

7 Complications

Surgical complications for vulvar cancer include wound infection, wound breakdown, lymphocele, and long-term lymphedema. However, wound complications have decreased dramatically since the implementation of the "separate groin incision" technique (Wills and Obermair 2013). A recent systematic review regarding complication rates of IFLD reported that lymphedema occurs in 14–48% of patients after groin dissection, lymphocele formation in 7–40%, wound infection in 21–39%, and wound breakdown in 17–39% (Wills and Obermair 2013). Estimates for complications following an SLNB and IFLD were reported in the GROINSS-V study. For SLNB and IFLD, the wound breakdown rate was 11.7% vs. 34%, cellulitis was 4.5% vs. 21.3%, and lymphedema was 1.9% vs. 25.2%, respectively (Van der Zee et al. 2008). The results of the Levenback et al. (2012) validation study (GOG Protocol 173) demonstrated similar results to the GROINSS-V study (Van der Zee et al. 2008).

8 Quality of Life

IFLD, particularly when it is followed by radiation or chemoradiation, can aggravate the patient's quality of life (QOL). One study (62 patients) investigating QOL with the European Organisation for Research and Treatment of Cancer Quality of Life Questionnaire (EORTC QLQ-C30) found few differences between SLNB and IFLD; only the score regarding financial difficulties was significantly worse in the IFLD group. For the FACT-V questionnaire, there were significantly worse results for the scales concerning contentment functional,

lymphedema, and complaints and stockings symptoms (Oonk et al. 2009).

Novackova et al. observed increased fatigue and more impaired lymphedema in patients with vulvar cancer after IFLD, compared with those after SLNB (Novackova et al. 2015). Forner et al. found that IFLD had a negative influence on the patients' sexual function (Forner et al. 2015). Additional studies are required to see how SLNB versus IFLD impact QOL in patients with vulvar cancer.

9 Cost-Effectiveness of SLNB

Erickson et al. compared the costs of SLNB with IFLD (Erickson et al. 2014). Their analysis concluded that SLNB is the most cost-effective strategy for the management of patients with early-stage vulvar cancer due to lower treatment costs and lower costs due to complications. Although there are additional costs associated with SLNB, including tracer injections, intraoperative mapping, imaging, and ultrastaging, these costs are offset by a shorter hospitalization. While both management strategies have similar disease-free survival estimates, the difference in treatment costs is approximately $4000 more for the IFLD per patient than for SLNB.

McCann et al. also reported a similar cost-effective analysis of SLNB and IFLD (McCann et al. 2015). Their analysis discovered that SLNB was less costly than IFLD ($13,449 vs. $14,261) and more effective for quality of life (4.16 quality-adjusted life years (QALYs) versus 4.00 QALYs). In this study, variations in the rate of positive SLNB and probability of lymphedema over clinically reasonable ranges did not alter the results. In their study, the increase in lymphedema associated with IFLD played a major role in the differences the costs between SLNB and IFLD.

SLNB is associated with shorter surgical time, fewer postoperative complications, and lower costs associated with postoperative complications. The incidence of lymphedema following IFLD are reported to be much higher, as high as

67% in one prospective study (Carlson et al. 2008). Among patients where only SLNB was performed, the morbidity rate was 1.9% (Van der Zee et al. 2008).

10 Learning Curve for Conducting SLNB

Vulvar cancer is a rare condition and the SLNB for it is a technically challenging procedure for surgeons. Acquiring experience in identifying the SLN accurately in patients with vulvar cancer is a very significant challenge. Schutter et al. describe the SLNB procedure as a complex interaction process between clinicians, specialists in nuclear medicine, and pathologists. So, if this interaction is ever inadequate, SLNB of vulvar cancer could have lethal consequences (Schutter and van der Sijde 2014). Given the strong potential for variations in operator skill in identifying SLN, an expert panel convened in 2008 recommended that a gynecologic oncologist performed at least ten consecutive cases with successful SLN identifications and no false-negative results before performing stand-alone SLNB without lymphadenectomy (Levenback et al. 2009).

While surgeons participating in the GOG Protocol 173 were not required to have a specific level of experience in conducting SLNB, surgeons participating in the GOG Protocol 270 were (GROINSS-V II study). Studies often define the first ten cases as part of the learning curve, after which SLNB without IFLD could be performed (Hampl et al. 2008; Van der Zee et al. 2008). Levenback et al. calculated that the rate of failure to identify an SLN was worse during the first 2 years of the study (16% in the first 2 years and then 7% for subsequent years) (Levenback et al. 2012).

Klapdor et al. reported that single-photon emission computed tomography (SPECT/CT) leads to higher SLN identification compared to lymphoscintigraphy in vulvar cancer (Klapdor et al. 2015). Due to its higher spatial resolution and three-dimensional anatomical localization of SLN, the number of cases required to become a skilled surgeon in SLNB for vulvar cancer may be

reduced by the use of preoperative SPECT/CT and by observing other surgical oncologists as they perform SLNB for breast cancer or melanoma (Chapman et al. 2016).

11 Conclusion

The development of SLNB in treatment for vulvar cancer has involved an unprecedented level of cooperation among investigators in Europe and the United States. SLNB is recommended for patients with early-stage vulvar cancer with primary tumors that are unifocal and smaller than 4 cm with clinically non-suspicious lymph nodes of metastasis in the groin, provided there is specific infrastructure with well-skilled surgeons. Some recommendations for appropriate techniques and procedures are also provided. Further recommendations on the management of patients with SLN metastasis are currently pending until the results are available from the GOG Protocol 270, which will incorporate the next phase of the GROINSS-V study (GROINSS-V II study). The purpose of this latter study is to investigate whether the dissection of SLN followed by chemotherapy and/or radiation is effective in managing early-stage vulvar cancer.

References

Achimas-Cadariu P, Harter P, Fisseler-Eckhoff A, Beutel B, Traut A, Du Bois A. Assessment of the sentinel lymph node in patients with invasive squamous carcinoma of the vulva. Acta Obstet Gynecol Scand. 2009;88(11):1209–14.

Carlson JW, Kauderer J, Walker JL, Gold MA, O'Malley D, Tuller E, Clarke-Pearson DL, Gynecologic Oncology G. A randomized phase III trial of VH fibrin sealant to reduce lymphedema after inguinal lymph node dissection: a Gynecologic Oncology Group study. Gynecol Oncol. 2008;110(1):76–82.

Chapman BC, Gleisner A, Kwak JJ, Hosokawa P, Paniccia A, Merkow JS, Koo PJ, Gajdos C, Pearlman NW, McCarter MD, Kounalakis N. SPECT/CT improves detection of metastatic sentinel lymph nodes in patients with head and neck melanoma. Ann Surg Oncol. 2016;23(8):2652–7.

DiSaia PJ, Creasman WT, Rich WM. An alternate approach to early cancer of the vulva. Am J Obstet Gynecol. 1979;133(7):825–32.

Erickson BK, Divine LM, Leath 3rd CA, Straughn Jr JM. Cost-effectiveness analysis of sentinel lymph node biopsy in the treatment of early-stage vulvar cancer. Int J Gynecol Cancer. 2014;24(8):1480–5.

Forner DM, Dakhil R, Lampe B. Quality of life and sexual function after surgery in early stage vulvar cancer. Eur J Surg Oncol. 2015;41(1):40–5.

Gaarenstroom KN, Kenter GG, Trimbos JB, Agous I, Amant F, Peters AAW, Vergote I. Postoperative complications after vulvectomy and inguinofemoral lymphadenectomy using separate groin incisions. Int J Gynecol Cancer. 2003;13(4):522–7.

Gould EA, Winship T, Philbin PH, Kerr HH. Observations on a sentinel node in cancer of the parotid. Cancer. 1960;13(1):77–8.

Hampl M, Hantschmann P, Michels W, Hillemanns P, German Multicenter Study Group. Validation of the accuracy of the sentinel lymph node procedure in patients with vulvar cancer: results of a multicenter study in Germany. Gynecol Oncol. 2008;111(2):282–8.

Handgraaf HJ, Verbeek FP, Tummers QR, Boogerd LS, van de Velde CJ, Vahrmeijer AL, Gaarenstroom KN. Real-time near-infrared fluorescence guided surgery in gynecologic oncology: a review of the current state of the art. Gynecol Oncol. 2014;135(3):606–13.

Hassanzade M, Attaran M, Treglia G, Yousefi Z, Sadeghi R. Lymphatic mapping and sentinel node biopsy in squamous cell carcinoma of the vulva: systematic review and meta-analysis of the literature. Gynecol Oncol. 2013;130(1):237–45.

Kirby TO, Rocconi RP, Numnum TM, Kendrick JE, Wright J, Fowler W, Mutch DG, Bhoola SM, Huh WK, Straughn Jr JM. Outcomes of stage I/II vulvar cancer patients after negative superficial inguinal lymphadenectomy. Gynecol Oncol. 2005;98(2): 309–12.

Klapdor R, Langer F, Gratz KF, Hillemanns P, Hertel H. SPECT/CT for SLN dissection in vulvar cancer: improved SLN detection and dissection by preoperative three-dimensional anatomical localisation. Gynecol Oncol. 2015;138(3):590–6.

Levenback CF, van der Zee AG, Rob L, Plante M, Covens A, Schneider A, Coleman R, Solima E, Hertel H, Barranger E, Obermair A, Roy M. Sentinel lymph node biopsy in patients with gynecologic cancers Expert panel statement from the International Sentinel Node Society Meeting, February 21, 2008. Gynecol Oncol. 2009;114(2):151–6.

Levenback CF, Ali S, Coleman RL, Gold MA, Fowler JM, Judson PL, Bell MC, De Geest K, Spirtos NM, Potkul RK, Leitao Jr MM, Bakkum-Gamez JN, Rossi EC, Lentz SS, Burke 2nd JJ, Van Le L, Trimble CL. Lymphatic mapping and sentinel lymph node biopsy in women with squamous cell carcinoma of the vulva: a gynecologic oncology group study. J Clin Oncol. 2012;30(31):3786–91.

Maggino T, Landoni F, Sartori E, Zola P, Gadducci A, Alessi C, Solda M, Coscio S, Spinetti G, Maneo A, Ferrero A, De Konishi GT. Patterns of recurrence in patients with squamous cell carcinoma of the vulva. A multicenter CTF Study. Cancer. 2000;89(1):116–22.

Martinez-Palones JM, Perez-Benavente MA, Gil-Moreno A, Diaz-Feijoo B, Roca I, Garcia-Jimenez-A, Aguilar-Martinez I, Xercavins J. Comparison of recurrence after vulvectomy and lymphadenectomy with and without sentinel node biopsy in early stage vulvar cancer. Gynecol Oncol. 2006;103(3):865–70.

McCann GA, Cohn DE, Jewell EL, Havrilesky LJ. Lymphatic mapping and sentinel lymph node dissection compared to complete lymphadenectomy in the management of early-stage vulvar cancer: a cost-utility analysis. Gynecol Oncol. 2015;136(2):300–4.

Meads C, Sutton AJ, Rosenthal AN, Malysiak S, Kowalska M, Zapalska A, Rogozinska E, Baldwin P, Ganesan R, Borowiack E, Barton P, Roberts T, Khan K, Sundar S. Sentinel lymph node biopsy in vulval cancer: systematic review and meta-analysis. Br J Cancer. 2014;110(12):2837–46.

Moore RG, Robison K, Brown AK, DiSilvestro P, Steinhoff M, Noto R, Brard L, Granai CO. Isolated sentinel lymph node dissection with conservative management in patients with squamous cell carcinoma of the vulva: a prospective trial. Gynecol Oncol. 2008; 109(1):65–70.

Morton DL, Wen DR, Wong JH, Economou JS, Cagle LA, Storm FK, Foshag LJ, Cochran AJ. Technical details of intraoperative lymphatic mapping for early stage melanoma. Arch Surg. 1992;127(4):392–9.

Novackova M, Halaska MJ, Robova H, Mala I, Pluta M, Chmel R, Rob L. A prospective study in the evaluation of quality of life after vulvar cancer surgery. Int J Gynecol Cancer. 2015;25(1):166–73.

Oonk MH, van Os MA, de Bock GH, de Hullu JA, Ansink AC, van der Zee AG. A comparison of quality of life between vulvar cancer patients after sentinel lymph node procedure only and inguinofemoral lymphadenectomy. Gynecol Oncol. 2009;113(3): 301–5.

Oonk MH, van Hemel BM, Hollema H, de Hullu JA, Ansink AC, Vergote I, Verheijen RH, Maggioni A, Gaarenstroom KN, Baldwin PJ, van Dorst EB, van der Velden J, Hermans RH, van der Putten HW, Drouin P, Runnebaum IB, Sluiter WJ, van der Zee AG. Size of sentinel-node metastasis and chances of non-sentinel-node involvement and survival in early stage vulvar cancer: results from GROINSS-V, a multicentre observational study. Lancet Oncol. 2010;11(7):646–52.

Robison K, Roque D, McCourt C, Stuckey A, DiSilvestro PA, Sung CJ, Steinhoff M, Granai CO, Moore RG. Long-term follow-up of vulvar cancer patients evaluated with sentinel lymph node biopsy alone. Gynecol Oncol. 2014;133(3):416–20.

Rouzier R, Haddad B, Dubernard G, Dubois P, Paniel BJ. Inguinofemoral dissection for carcinoma of the vulva: effect of modifications of extent and technique on morbidity and survival. J Am Coll Surg. 2003; 196(3):442–50.

Schutter EM, van der Sijde R. Evaluation of groin recurrence after sentinel node procedure in vulvar cancer is mandatory. Int J Gynecol Cancer. 2014;24(7):1138.

Sedlis A, Homesley H, Bundy BN, Marshall R, Yordan E, Hacker N, Lee JH, Whitney C. Positive groin lymph nodes in superficial squamous cell vulvar cancer. A Gynecologic Oncology Group Study. Am J Obstet Gynecol. 1987;156(5):1159–64.

Stehman FB, Bundy BN, Dvoretsky PM, Creasman WT. Early stage I carcinoma of the vulva treated with ipsilateral superficial inguinal lymphadenectomy and modified radical hemivulvectomy: a prospective study of the Gynecologic Oncology Group. Obstet Gynecol. 1992;79(4):490–7.

Terada KY, Shimizu DM, Jiang CS, Wong JH. Outcomes for patients with T1 squamous cell cancer of the vulva undergoing sentinel node biopsy. Gynecol Oncol. 2006;102(2):200–3.

Van der Zee AG, Oonk MH, De Hullu JA, Ansink AC, Vergote I, Verheijen RH, Maggioni A, Gaarenstroom KN, Baldwin PJ, Van Dorst EB, Van der Velden J, Hermans RH, van der Putten H, Drouin P, Schneider A, Sluiter WJ. Sentinel node dissection is safe in the treatment of early-stage vulvar cancer. J Clin Oncol. 2008;26(6):884–9.

Wills A, Obermair A. A review of complications associated with the surgical treatment of vulvar cancer. Gynecol Oncol. 2013;131(2):467–79.

Survivorship of Gynecologic Malignancy

Kristy Ward, Alexandra Walker, and Amy R. Carroll

Abstract

As screening and cancer treatment has improved, the number of women who are survivors of gynecologic malignancies is increasing. Gynecologic cancer survivors may present a unique challenge for gynecologists and practitioners who find themselves caring for these women. Understanding their unique psychosocial, sexual, and residual treatment symptoms as well as understanding surveillance and screening guidelines will help improve the care of this population.

Keywords

Survivorship • Cancer survivor • Gynecologic cancer • Women's cancer • Cancer follow-up

Contents

K. Ward (✉)
Division of Gynecologic Oncology, Department of Obstetrics and Gynecology, University of Florida College of Medicine Jacksonville, Jacksonville, FL, USA
e-mail: Kristy.Ward@jax.ufl.edu

A. Walker
Obstetrics and Gynecology, University of Florida College of Medicine, Jacksonville, FL, USA

A.R. Carroll
WellStar Gynecologic Oncology, Austell, GA, USA

1 Introduction

Advances in cancer diagnosis and treatment have led to a steady increase in the number of cancer survivors, a population with unique physical, psychosocial, and economic needs. In recent decades, coordinated efforts have focused on understanding this population and on enhancing the length and quality of life of survivors. In 1996, the National Cancer Institute created the Office of

© Springer International Publishing AG 2017
D. Shoupe (ed.), *Handbook of Gynecology*,
DOI 10.1007/978-3-319-17798-4_12

Cancer Survivorship, and in recent decades increasing research has investigated diverse aspects of survivorship (American Cancer Society 2014; National Institute of Cancer, Office of Cancer Survivorship; National Research Council 2005).

An individual is considered a survivor from the time of cancer diagnosis for the remainder of his or her life. The survivorship experience can be divided into phases including an acute treatment phase, an intermediate survivor phase, and a long-term survivor phase. Caregivers are also included as survivors, as their lives may be affected significantly by others' cancer diagnoses. General survivorship care encompasses surveillance of the primary malignancy, managing complications of the cancer or its treatment, risk reduction and screening for second malignancies, and assessment of overall quality of life and psychosocial well-being (American Cancer Society 2014; National Research Council 2005).

The number of gynecologic cancer survivors has grown substantially in recent decades, most notably among those diagnosed with early stage disease. In the United States, there are currently an estimated 625,000 survivors of endometrial cancer, 244,000 survivors of cervical cancer, and nearly 200,000 survivors of ovarian cancer, in total accounting for about 15% of all female cancer survivors (American Cancer Society 2014). As the number of cancer survivors increases, the general gynecologist can expect to care for women with a history of female genital cancers.

2 Effects of Gynecological Cancer and Treatment

2.1 Psychosocial Issues

Attempting to understand and address the psychosocial challenges faced by cancer survivors is an established and important aspect of survivorship care and research (National Research Council 2005). Proceeding with life after cancer can be a complicated, life-altering process.

The psychological evolution that occurs during this process can result potentially in both positive and negative outcomes among survivors (Thornton and Perez 2006).

Struggles commonly described by cancer survivors include fear, uncertainty, anxiety, depression, insomnia, relationship challenges, employment discrimination, financial concerns, and loss of insurance (Wenzel et al. 2002; Roland et al. 2013; Meyer and Mark 1995; Hodgkinson et al. 2007; Kirchhoff et al. 2012; Bodurka et al. 2005). Furthermore, due to disease and treatment specifics, gynecologic cancer survivors may frequently encounter issues with body image, sexuality, and fertility (Carter et al. 2005; Bukovic et al. 2008). Compared to other populations of cancer survivors, relatively few studies have specifically investigated the long-term psychosocial outcomes and needs of gynecologic cancer survivors. Caution must be emphasized when generalizing among survivors as each population faces unique challenges and has specific supportive care needs.

It has been recognized that medical variables, while important, seem to play a lesser role than psychological adjustment in predicting long-term psychological health among survivors (Hodgkinson et al. 2007; Carver et al. 2006). Studies have suggested that survivors with better social support systems experience less anxiety and depression (Kimmel et al. 2014; Carpenter et al. 2010) and that socioeconomic status may strongly contribute to overall wellbeing (Greenwald et al. 2014). A recent longitudinal study investigating long-term survivors of gynecologic cancers revealed overall normal levels of quality of life and relationship adjustment, however, increased levels of anxiety, and posttraumatic stress disorder among survivors (Hodgkinson et al. 2007). Overall, more research is needed in this area.

In general, cancer survivors as a whole have fortunately shown positive responses to psychosocial interventions (Meyer and Mark 1995). Unfortunately, many survivors do not receive psychosocial care (Forsythe et al. 2013), representing missed opportunities. Thus, we recommend routine psychological screening and emphasize that screening should continue throughout a survivor's life, as a longer survivorship period does not necessarily correlate with decreased psychosocial concerns (Hodgkinson et al. 2007). There are multiple brief psychosocial distress scales available for rapid in-office screening (National Cancer Institute). When psychological issues are identified, we recommend either treating or promptly referring for treatment.

Other interventions that have been associated with psychosocial well-being include healthy lifestyle interventions and management of menopausal symptoms. We recommend encouraging healthy lifestyle choices including healthy eating, regular exercise, and good sleep. Regular physical activity may positively affect survivors' psychosocial wellbeing and quality of life (Stevinson et al. 2007; Crawford et al. 2015). Menopausal symptoms, especially in premenopausal patients, have been associated with distress, depression, and sexual dysfunction (Carter et al. 2010). While most gynecologic cancer survivors can be treated with hormone replacement therapy (Biliatis et al. 2012), consult with the patient's oncologist if there is concern about tumor hormonal response. The American College of Obstetricians and Gynecologists also recommends several nonhormonal options for management of menopausal symptoms that may be of benefit to these women (American College of Obstetricians and Gynecologists 2014).

In addition, it is important to address survivors' supportive care needs, as increased unmet needs correlate with increased distress and decreased quality of life (Hodgkinson et al. 2007). Referral to a well-run local survivor support group may be helpful and can often be located through local chapters of the American Cancer Society (Sanson-Fisher et al.). Relationship counseling may be beneficial, especially among younger survivors (Kirchhoff et al. 2012). Finally, sexual dysfunction and infertility, to be discussed subsequently, may profoundly affect survivors' psychological health and social wellbeing (Carter et al. 2005, 2010).

2.2 Sexual Health

Among cancer survivors in general, sexual dysfunction has been broadly identified as a common and often untreated problem (Sadovsky et al. 2010). Women treated for gynecologic malignancies are at risk for sexual dysfunction due to the nature, location, and treatment of their disease. After all, patients with gynecological cancer often undergo pelvic surgery and/or pelvic radiation, which may have considerable effects on sexual function (Donovan et al. 2007). Research has indicated that sexual concerns among gynecologic cancer survivors may include physical, psychological, and social dysfunctions (Abbott-Anderson and Kwekkeboom 2012). A recent abstract presented at the 2015 American Society of Clinical Oncologists found that young, premenopausal women, those who underwent chemotherapy and those in committed relationships, may be at greater risk for sexual dysfunction, and among those with sexual dysfunction, a greater decline in sexual activity was seen after cancer treatment (Guntupalli et al. 2015).

Pelvic radiation therapy may contribute significantly to many of the physical effects described, including skin fibrosis, shortening and narrowing of the vagina, disruption in ovarian function and subsequent vaginal dryness, dyspareunia, and loss of interest in sexual activity (Donovan et al. 2007; Aerts et al. 2009; Bergmark et al. 1999; Amsterdam and Krychman 2006). Other concerns identified among gynecologic cancer survivors include altered body image, decreased libido, sexual performance anxiety, and perceived changes in partner interest (Bourgeois-Law and Lotocki 1999; Bukovic et al. 2008; Carmack Taylor et al. 2004; Corney et al. 1993; Juraskova et al. 2003; Lindaw et al. 2007).

When considering treatment options for cancer-related sexual dysfunction, it is important to recognize that normal sexual functioning can vary markedly and that sexual function may improve as time from treatment increases (Sadovsky et al. 2010; Vaz 2011). Therapies addressing sexual dysfunction may focus on physical or psychosocial components. Studies evaluating various interventions are few and have shown mixed results (Abbott-Anderson and Kwekkeboom 2012; Brotto et al. 2008; Robinson et al. 1994; Miles and Johnson 2014).

We recommend screening all gynecologic cancer survivors for sexual dysfunction and offering therapeutic suggestions to interested patients. Optimal evaluation and treatment often requires a multidisciplinary team. Physical concerns are often related to loss of ovarian function and anatomical changes resulting from treatment. Although conclusive evidence does not exist regarding the efficacy of vaginal dilator use (Miles and Johnson 2014), use of a graduated series of dilators with lubricant may improve vaginal compliance, dyspareunia, and sexual function. Vaginal dryness may be improved with use of a vaginal moisturizer or a local estrogen product (Carter et al. 2001). We also recommend screening for underlying psychological disorders. In addition, relationship counseling or consultation with a sexual therapist may benefit some patients.

2.3   Fertility Implications

While the majority of women diagnosed with gynecologic cancer are postmenopausal, a significant number are of reproductive age. Clinicians must be aware of the reproductive consequences of treatments, which can profoundly affect a woman's reproductive potential and overall wellbeing. Studies have shown that women with absent or impaired fertility resulting from gynecologic cancer treatment may experience depression, grief, and stress resulting from infertility (Carter et al. 2005; Stevinson et al. 2007).

Gynecologic cancers are treated with some combination of surgery, radiation, and chemotherapy, any of which may negatively affect fertility. While surgery may remove part or all of a woman's reproductive organs, radiation and chemotherapy can significantly hinder ovarian function and subsequent ability to conceive. Pelvic irradiation and alkylating chemotherapeutic agents pose the greatest threats to ovarian function, but other chemotherapeutics may contribute. In addition, pelvic irradiation affects the uterus and may hinder pregnancy implantation and appropriate growth (Stroud et al. 2009).

As fertility has emerged as such a significant quality of life issue among cancer survivors, fertility preservation in patients undergoing gynecologic cancer treatment is an emerging topic. Reproductive aged women with fertility desires and early stage endometrial, cervical, and ovarian cancers are increasingly being offered fertility-conserving treatment options (Ditto et al. 2014, 2015; Koskas et al. 2014). The complicated medical, ethical, and legal details of such are beyond the scope of this article; however, this trend will undoubtedly affect future gynecologic cancer survivors. Gynecologic cancer survivors with fertility concerns should be promptly evaluated by a reproductive specialist in conjunction with their oncologists.

2.4   Loss of Ovarian Function and Bone Health

As discussed previously, premenopausal women may lose ovarian function as a result of gynecologic cancer treatment. While this may be quite disruptive to a woman psychologically, sexually, and socially (Carter et al. 2010), early loss of ovarian function may also have significant long-term effects on bone health (Stavraka et al. 2013). While further study in this area is needed, it is important to regularly screen affected women and encourage healthy eating, calcium supplementation, and regular weight-bearing exercise. ACOG has published recommendations for management of osteoporosis (American College of Obstetricians and Gynecologists 2012).

Providers may be concerned with offering survivors of gynecologic malignancies hormone replacement therapy, especially survivors of ovarian and endometrial cancers. For women with a personal history of ovarian cancer, a recent meta-analysis showed no increased risk of recurrence of disease in users HRT (Li et al. 2015). As the data supports a negligible or no increased risk for women developing ovarian cancer on hormones and there is no added risk of recurrence in patients with a personal history of ovarian cancer, HRT should be considered safe for the management of menopause symptoms in these women.

Exogenous estrogen use is associated with an increased incidence of endometrial cancer while progesterone is protective against type I uterine malignancies. Multiple studies have demonstrated a regression of endometrial hyperplasia and low-grade endometrial cancers using various types of progestins (Santen et al. 2010). When estrogen is used in combination with progestin, there is no increased risk of uterine cancer over the general population. The Women's Health Initiative (WHI) investigated rates of endometrial cancer in postmenopausal women taking HRT to those taking a placebo. They found a small, non-significant decrease in the incidence of uterine malignancy, 56 versus 69 per 100,000 person-years compared to non-HRT users (Anderson et al. 2003). For women with a personal history of endometrial cancer, several trials have demonstrated no increased risk of recurrence of disease (Santen et al. 2010).

2.5 Lymphedema

Lower-extremity lymphedema is a late effect experienced by some gynecologic cancer survivors, especially those treated with surgery or radiation involving the pelvic or inguinal lymph nodes (Beesley et al. 2007). Onset may occur immediately after therapy or be delayed many years (Hareyama et al. 2015). Patients with lymphedema may complain of pain, heaviness, fullness, a tight sensation, or decreased flexibility in an affected limb. Simple activities of daily living may be affected, and ambulation may be difficult (International Society of Lymphology 2013). Physical exam findings may include nonpitting edema, and magnetic resonance imaging techniques are increasingly being used to diagnose early lymphedema (Brennan and Miller 1998).

Risk factors for developing lower extremity lymphedema include the extent of surgery or radiation to lymph nodes, removal of the circumflex iliac lymph nodes, cellulitis, and delayed wound healing (Brennan and Miller 1998; Abu-Rustum

and Barakat 2007). Lymphedema may be instigated by small traumas including cuts, bites, injections, and sunburns. It is important for patients with lymphedema to maintain good skin hygiene and to engage in simple, regular range of motion exercises (International Society of Lymphology 2013). Therapies which may help survivors suffering from lymphedema include: lymphedema hosiery, manual massage, compression bandages, or consultation with a lymphedema therapist. Severe cases may require hospitalization and intravenous antibiotics (Beesley et al. 2007; International Society of Lymphology 2013; Brennan and Miller 1998). Lymphedema therapists may be located through the Lymphology Association of North America.

2.6 Cognitive Dysfunction

Cancer patients may suffer from cognitive dysfunction, which may persist long after completion of treatment. The individual patient, type of cancer, and variety of treatment all combine to influence a survivor's cognitive state. Factors that may contribute to cognitive dysfunction include: indirect effects of the cancer itself, brain metastases, chemotherapy, radiation therapy, medication effects, preexisting conditions, and psychiatric issues (Andreotti et al. 2015). Research exploring cognitive-related cancer dysfunction in survivors of gynecologic cancers is scant, as most literature in this area has focused on general or breast cancer survivors. However, cognitive decline has been identified among gynecologic cancer survivors and must be considered in survivor care plans (Correa et al. 2010; Sleight 2015; Donovan et al. 2007).

Interestingly, the cognitive deficits commonly described by survivors tend to differ from those of neurodegenerative diseases. Cancer patients and survivors often describe problems with organization, attention, memory, multitasking, and efficiency, often causing problems with occupational or social responsibilities (Falleti et al. 2005; Boykoff et al. 2009). Standard tests such as the Mini Mental Status Exam are often not sensitive enough to detect the subtle cognitive deficits experienced by survivors, and perceived cognitive decline may be considered reason to explore potential intervention (Sleight 2015).

When assessing cancer survivors with perceived cognitive dysfunction, it is important to address and treat fatigue, assess psychological health, assess for anemia, and encourage healthy lifestyle habits. Potential interventions include cognitive behavior therapy, coping strategies such as assisted technology or memory aids, compensatory strategy training, stress management, and energy management (Sleight 2015; Ferguson et al. 2012; Goedendorp et al. 2014). It is also important to remember that a new cognitive deficit in a cancer survivor could be an indication of recurrence and requires prompt evaluation.

3 Long-Term Chemotherapy and Radiation Therapy Effects

Many different side effects of treatment can continue long after therapy is finished, sometimes lifelong. Some long-term side effects of radiation include vaginal narrowing and shortening, creating sexual dysfunction, radiation proctitis or cystitis, or skin break down. Long-term side effects of chemotherapy can include neuropathies, fertility issues, skin changes, and potential end-organ dysfunction. While many side effects can be treated symptomatically, specialty consultation should be sought for severe sequella.

4 Survivorship Issues by Gynecologic Cancer Type

4.1 Endometrial/Uterine Cancer

Endometrial cancer is both the most common and the most curable type of gynecologic cancer (Practice Bulletin 2015). Fortunately, among the nearly 55,000 women expected to be diagnosed with endometrial cancer in 2015, most will be diagnosed with early stage disease and given an excellent prognosis. Approximately 67% of women have localized disease at diagnosis, with

estimated 5-year survival at 95%. Overall 5-year survival for endometrial cancer patients is approximately 82%, the highest among gynecologic cancers (SEER Stat Fact Sheets – Cancer of the Endometrium). Thus it is important to understand and address the unique needs of this population.

When caring for endometrial cancer survivors, providers must address adverse treatment effects and screen for disease recurrence and second primary cancers. Equally important is addressing cardiovascular health and lifestyle factors. Overall morbidity among endometrial cancer survivors is high, despite favorable cancer prognoses. This has been attributed to the strong association of endometrial cancer with obesity and its related comorbidities including hypertension, diabetes, metabolic syndrome, and pulmonary disease (Von Gruenigen et al. 2006; Bjorge et al. 2010). Women with endometrial cancer are more likely to die from cardiovascular disease than from cancer (Ward et al. 2012), and obesity has been associated with increased morbidity and decreased quality of life in survivors (Courneya et al. 2005; Smits et al. 2014). Recent studies evaluating lifestyle programs that target endometrial cancer survivors have shown that various interventions may be able to increase physical activity levels, improve dietary habits, and influence weight loss in these patients (Basen-Engquist et al. 2014; Von Gruenigen et al. 2008, 2009, 2011, 2012; McCarrol et al. 2014). Further study is needed in this area.

While the majority of women diagnosed with endometrial cancer are postmenopausal, an estimated 25% are premenopausal. Since 1988, the standard treatment for endometrial cancer has been hysterectomy and bilateral salpingoophorectomy, making loss of ovarian function among premenopausal women treated for endometrial cancer an important issue (Practice Bulletin 2015; Sorosky 2008). These women experience abrupt onset menopausal symptoms, which may exacerbate psychological difficulties and sexual dysfunction.

Traditionally, estrogen replacement therapy in survivors of endometrial cancer has been avoided since most endometrial cancers are estrogen dependent. Review of limited evidence suggests that estrogen replacement may be a reasonable option in premenopausal patients with a history of early stage disease and may be considered with appropriate risk-benefit counseling and oncology consultation (Chapman et al. 1996; Barakat et al. 2006). Of note, some premenopausal women with endometrial cancer are choosing fertility-preserving or ovarian-preserving therapies (Erkanli and Ayhan 2010; Chaoyang et al.). The details of such treatments are beyond the scope of this review; however, it may influence the future composition of this population.

Furthermore, survivors of endometrial cancer are at increased risk for multiple subsequent cancers, including breast, colorectal, vulvar, vaginal, lung, and urologic cancers. Breast and colon cancers are the most commonly identified second primary cancers in endometrial cancer survivors and require regular screening. Patients with endometrial cancer may have a genetic predisposition for development of other cancers, such as in Lynch syndrome, and should be offered genetic screening when personal or family history indicates (Practice Bulletin 2015; Uccella et al. 2011; Re et al. 1997).

The majority of endometrial cancer recurrences will occur within 3 years of the completion of initial therapy (Fung-Kee-Fung et al. 2006; Salani et al. 2011; Sartori et al. 2010; Tjalma et al. 2004). Approximately 70% of recurrences are symptomatic (Fung-Kee-Fung et al. 2006; Sartori et al. 2010). Among the asymptomatic recurrences, most are detected by physical exam (Fung-Kee-Fung et al. 2006; Salani et al. 2011; Sartori et al. 2010). The NCCN recommends an exam every 3–6 months for 2–3 years then every 6–12 months. History and physical exam detects up to 100% of recurrent disease (range 52–100%) (Sartori et al. 2010; Tjalma et al. 2004).

CA-125 surveillance is optional and imaging should be performed only if clinically indicated according to both the NCCN and SGO (Salani et al. 2011). In patients with low-risk disease, CA-125 levels are only elevated in 0–5% of recurrences (Fung-Kee-Fung et al. 2006; Tjalma et al. 2004; Rose et al. 1994). Patients with advanced stage or high-grade histologies, however, will have an elevated CA-125 in >50% of recurrent disease (Rose et al. 1994).

Common practice has been to perform chest X-rays in surveillance. They diagnose up to 20% of all recurrences (Salani et al. 2011; Tjalma et al. 2004). The more relevant question, however, is if the diagnosis of distant disease will impact survival. Patients with pulmonary metastasis of recurrent uterine cancer have a poor prognosis as systemic chemotherapy is often ineffective. Other imaging modalities such as ultrasound, intravenous pyelogram, and computed tomography (CT) have also shown early detection of asymptomatic recurrences without a survival benefit (Salani et al. 2011; Tjalma et al. 2004). For these reasons, imaging is only indicated in patients with a history or exam concerning for recurrent disease.

Pap smears are not recommended for surveillance of uterine cancer. A restrospective review found that only 2.5% of all recurrent endometrial cancers were diagnosed with the help of cytology (Tjalma et al. 2004). Other retrospective studies showed only 0.5–0.7% of endometrial cancer patients had cytology that diagnosed an isolated vaginal recurrence at a cost of approximately $23,487 to $44,049 per recurrence detected (Bristow et al. 2006; Cooper et al. 2006). Additionally, 15% of patients with biopsy proven vaginal recurrence had a negative pap (Cooper et al. 2006). The opinion of the SGO is that vaginal cytology adds significant healthcare costs without added benefit and that most recurrences at the vaginal cuff can be found on exam (Salani et al. 2011).

Patients with uterine sarcomas may require closer monitoring. An exam every 3 months for 2 years then every 6–12 months is recommended by the NCCN. Additionally, they suggest consideration of CT imaging every 3–6 months for 2–3 years, then every 6 months for the next 2 years, and then annually.

We also recommend routine assessment of psychosocial wellbeing, sexual health, and adverse treatment-related effects, accompanied by treatment or referral as indicated. Furthermore, we recommend medical optimization of cardiovascular health and increased emphasis on healthy lifestyle choices. At minimum, obese endometrial cancer survivors should receive physician counseling regarding weight loss, physical activity, and healthy eating. Ideally, these patients should be referred to weight loss and lifestyle intervention programs available within their medical communities. Finally, in order to provide optimal care to endometrial cancer survivors, we recommend that these women follow with a gynecologist or gynecologic-oncologist as well as a primary care specialist familiar with the needs of this population.

4.2 Cervical Cancer

Cervical cancer is the third most common gynecologic cancer in the United States. Its incidence has decreased markedly in recent decades with the introduction of widespread screening and treatment of preinvasive disease. The recent introduction of the HPV vaccine will hopefully further decrease cervical cancer incidence in coming decades (American College of Obstetricians and Gynecologists 2013).

Despite improved screening, an estimated 13,000 women are expected to be diagnosed with this malignancy in 2015. Nearly half of these women will be diagnosed with local disease with 5-year survival at 90%. Overall, 5-year survival among cervical cancer patients is estimated at 68% (SEER Stat Fact Sheets – Cancer of the Cervix Uteri). Cervical cancer affects younger women when compared with other gynecologic cancers, with mean age at time of diagnosis approximately 50 years, resulting in longer posttreatment life expectancies. In addition, women of lower socioeconomic status and women of minority or immigrant groups are more likely to develop invasive cervical cancer (Ye et al. 2014; Akers et al. 2007).

Women diagnosed with very early stage disease are often treated exclusively with surgery. More advanced disease is generally treated with radiation and chemotherapy. Survivors may suffer from psychosocial difficulties, sexual dysfunction, long-term treatment side effects, and second primary malignancies. Studies have suggested

that survivors who received treatment with radiation therapy are at increased risk of suffering from long-term physical effects and sexual dysfunction when compared to those treated with radical surgery alone (Ye et al. 2014; Le Borgne et al. 2013; Harding et al. 2014).

Premenopausal women treated for cervical cancer may suffer from premature ovarian failure as a result of treatment. Estrogen replacement therapy is generally considered to be appropriate in this population and may be considered (Biliatis et al. 2012; Ploch 1987). Women who have not completed childbearing at the time of diagnosis may suffer from psychological and social difficulties resulting from treatment-induced infertility. Fortunately, fertility preservation is increasingly being offered to women with very early stage invasive disease (Abu-Rustum et al. 2008; Pareja et al. 2013; Ramirez et al. 2008), and ovarian-preserving efforts including pretreatment ovarian transposition have been investigated with promising results (Shou et al. 2015; Al-Badawi et al. 2010).

Furthermore, women with a history of cervical cancer are at increased risk of developing subsequent cancers of the vulva, vagina, and rectum as well as tobacco-related malignancies including lung, esophageal, stomach, urogenital, pancreatic, and leukemia in those with a tobacco use history (Balamurugan et al. 2008; Rodriguez et al. 2014; Underwood et al. 2012). Thus, it is important to screen for potential second malignancies and to routinely address tobacco use.

Most recurrences in patients with cervical cancer occur within the first 3 years, with a median of 7–36 months after completion of initial therapy (Elit et al. 2010; Salmal et al. 1998). Patients with isolated local recurrence have improved salvage rates over those with distant disease, so early detection of recurrence can be life-saving. The NCCN-recommended surveillance for cervical cancer includes an exam every 3–6 months for 2 years, then every 6–12 months for 3–5 years, and then annually. They also suggest annual cervical/vaginal cytology and imaging as indicated.

Cytologic evaluation of the vagina/cervix after treatment for cervical cancer is controversial.

Though it has been recommended as part of surveillance historically, several retrospective studies have shown that cytology alone is rarely the sole indicator of the presence of disease (Elit et al. 2010; Zanagnolo et al. 2009). One retrospective study calculated that 3,800 pap smears were performed on 271 patients in order to detect one asymptomatic recurrence (Salmal et al. 1998). SGO recommends elimination of cytologic testing or limiting its use to annually (Salani et al. 2011).

The role of imaging for surveillance of cervical cancer survivors is uncertain. Several studies have shown chest X-ray to detect distant disease in the absence of symptoms in 11–47% of patients with recurrence (Salmal et al. 1998; Bodurka-Bevers et al. 2000). Most patients with distant metastases are not salvageable so the early detection of chest lesions is unlikely to improve outcomes. PET scans for surveillance, on the other hand, may detect locoregional recurrence when salvage radiation or exenterative surgery is still an option. One retrospective study evaluated PET imaging in asymptomatic women after treatment of cervical cancer. Twelve percent of patients had a positive PET scan 15 months after completion of therapy and another 14% had a positive scan 21.5 months after treatment. Seven of the 13 patients with asymptomatic disease seen on PET had isolated recurrences amenable to curative therapy. They showed an improvement in 3-year survival over women with symptomatic disease that was not statistically significant (59 vs. 19%) (Brooks et al. 2009). In another retrospective study, 20 asymptomatic women were found to have recurrence on PET imaging. Eight of these patients had treatment with curative intent and five were cured of disease (Chung et al. 2006). Despite the potential for early detection of recurrence by PET imaging, the cost is high and there is a lack of prospective studies with clear evidence of improvements in outcomes. Radiography is often only employed in patients with a history or exam concerning for disease.

We encourage healthy lifestyle choices and regular tobacco prevention and cessation efforts, including referral to cessation programs for motivated patients. It is important to recognize that many of these patients may suffer from long-term psychological issues or have severe physical effects from cancer treatment. We also recommend educating these survivors on the importance of encouraging their family and community members to undergo routine cervical screening.

4.3 Ovarian Cancer

Ovarian cancer is the second most common gynecologic cancer in the United States, with an estimated 21,000 diagnoses expected in 2015. Significant survival differences exist between women diagnosed with early stage disease and those diagnosed with advanced disease. Unfortunately, 60% have distant spread at diagnosis and 5-year survival at 28%. However, women diagnosed with localized or regional spread have better prognoses with 5-year survival at 92% and 73%, respectively (SEER Stat Fact Sheets – Cancer of the Ovary; Bhoola and Hoskins 2006).

Ovarian cancer is generally treated with surgery and/or chemotherapy. Survivors may experience neuropathy, cognitive decline, psychosocial difficulties, and sexual dysfunction (Correa et al. 2010; Gutierrez-Gutierrez et al. 2010; Stavraka et al. 2012; Ezendam et al. 2014). Fear of recurrence is of particular concern in this population and may contribute to significant anxiety and decreased quality of life. Studies have shown that psychosocial wellbeing can have the greatest influence on overall quality of life among ovarian cancer survivors (Teng et al. 2014). Adequately powered longitudinal studies are needed to further qualify, quantify, and assess the specific survivorship needs of this population.

When compared to the general population, survivors of ovarian cancer are at greater risk of developing a second malignancy. Since most women treated for ovarian cancer have received a hysterectomy, the risk of a second gynecologic malignancy is less. However, these women are at increased risk of developing a multitude of cancers including breast, colorectal, and bladder cancers. Survivors may carry BRCA1, BRCA2, or HNPCC mutations and should be screened for such based on personal and family histories

(Gangi et al. 2014). Patients treated with chemo-therapeutic agents such as etoposide and platinum compounds are associated with an increased risk of a secondary leukemia later in life (Kollmannsberger et al. 1998).

Most women who achieve a complete clinical response to initial therapy for ovarian cancer will relapse. Approximately 75% of these women will recur, most within 2 years (Gadducci and Cosio 2003; Gadducci et al. 2009). The NCCN guidelines for monitoring for recurrence of ovarian, primary peritoneal, and fallopian tube cancer are for exams with CA-125 (if initially elevated) every 2–4 months for 2 years, then every 3–6 months for 3 years, and then annually after 5 years. They recommend imaging as clinically indicated. Women with borderline tumors or germ cell and sex-cord stromal tumors can have later recurrences, up to 20 years after treatment of the initial disease, and should have annual evaluations beyond 5 years (Salani et al. 2011).

Recently, the monitoring of CA-125 levels during remission has come into question. One randomized controlled trial evaluated the impact of starting therapy for ovarian cancer at the time of biochemical recurrence (Rustin 2010). They randomized 529 women with elevated CA-125 levels to early treatment or to delayed therapy (observation until the patient had clinical or symptomatic relapse of disease). The early treatment group started chemotherapy nearly 5 months earlier and experienced a significant decrease in quality of life compared to those assigned to delayed therapy. The early treatment group demonstrated no improvement in overall survival. Starting chemotherapy earlier in recurrence did not improve outcomes but it did negatively impact patients' quality of life. The dilemma of whether a serum CA-125 should be checked as part of surveillance for ovarian cancer recurrence should be discussed with and individualized for each patient.

Routine imaging for detection of disease recurrence is controversial. There is a paucity of data in the medical literature and no prospective studies to assess this issue. One study retrospectively evaluated patients surveilled with CT imaging every 6 months for 2 years then yearly. In the group of asymptomatic patients with disease found on imaging, 90% had an optimal secondary cytoreduction compared with 57% of patients with detection of recurrence based on symptoms. This resulted in an improved overall survival (72 vs. 51 months) compared with women who only had imaging after the onset of symptoms (Tanner et al. 2010). Another retrospective study, on the other hand, found that only 27% of 331 asymptomatic patients were diagnosed with recurrent disease based on imaging alone and that there was no difference in survival for patients among any of the modalities used to detect recurrence (Gadducci and Cosio 2003; Gadducci et al. 2009). Because of the significant cost of surveillance imaging without any prospective evidence of benefit, imaging is currently reserved for patients with suspected disease recurrence. For patients with symptoms concerning for recurrence, suspicious exam findings or an elevated CA-125, PET-CT scans have been shown in multiple studies to be more sensitive than CT at locating sites of disease. Additionally, PET-CT scans alter treatment in up to 60% of patients (Bhosale et al. 2010; Fulham et al. 2008; Risum et al. 2009; Thrall et al. 2007). Women who have had fertility-sparing surgery for ovarian cancer represent a special subgroup of patients. If their disease recurs, it is most likely to arise in their remaining gynecologic organs. SGO recommends serial ultrasound in these women every 6 months to evaluate their pelvic organs (Salani et al. 2011).

We recommend screening for neuropathy and cognitive difficulties, psychological and sexual dysfunction, and referral for treatment when indicated. Similar to endometrial cancer survivors, survivors of ovarian cancer benefit from a healthy diet, maintaining supportive relationships, regular physical activity, and maintaining a healthy weight.

4.4   Vulvar/Vaginal Cancer

Vulvar cancer is the fourth most common gynecologic cancer, with approximately 5,000 women expected to be diagnosed in 2015 (SEER Stat Fact Sheets – Cancer of the Vulva). Vulvar cancer diagnoses occur most frequently in women between the ages of 65–75; however, vulvar cancer has increased in younger populations, likely due to increasing HPV prevalence (SEER Stat Fact Sheets – Cancer of the Vulva). As with cervical cancer, the introduction of the HPV vaccine will hopefully decrease vulvar cancer incidence in the coming decades (Balamurugan et al. 2008). Women with vulvar cancer are generally treated with pelvic surgery and/or radiation therapy (Aerts et al. 2012). Vaginal cancer is considered very rare and often is metastatic from another site or related to HPV.

Overall, the literature assessing survivorship issues specific to vulvar cancer is limited. Patients treated with extensive surgery or radiation therapy seem to be at risk for decreased quality of life, including sexual dysfunction and psychosocial difficulties (Aerts et al. 2012; Gunther et al. 2014; Kunos et al. 2009). These patients may suffer from skin changes including changes in skin texture and color, thickening, contractures, fibrosis, decreased clitoral sensation, and painful intercourse. Patients treated with extensive lymph node surgery or radiation therapy often suffer from chronic lymphedema (Berger et al. 2015).

As vulvar cancer has increased among younger women who often present with less advanced disease, a trend toward less radical surgery has emerged. Wide local excision has been associated with higher quality of life among survivors when compared to radical vulvectomy (Gunther et al. 2014), and sophisticated sentinel node mapping techniques are decreasing the need for radical lymph node surgery and the associated risk of lymphedema (McCann et al. 2015). Overall, more research is needed to define and best meet the evolving needs of vulvar cancer survivors.

Due to the low incidence of vulvar and vaginal cancers, there is a paucity of information to guide surveillance recommendations. There are no guidelines published by NCCN and most strategies are extrapolated from practice patterns for cervical cancer. One report of 330 women with vulvar cancer reported that over 35% of recurrences or new sites of primary disease were found over 5 years after treatment for their primary cancer (Gonzalez Bosquet et al. 2005). This underscores the importance of long-term follow-up in vulvar cancer survivors. SGO recommends regular and long-term examinations of the vulvar, vaginal, cervical, and perianal tissue as well as assessment of the inguinal lymph nodes (Salani et al. 2011). Routine imaging is not recommended.

Continue with routine guideline-recommended screening for other cancers. In tobacco users we recommend an emphasis on cessation. Finally, we recommend approaching these patients with awareness that mental health or sexual counseling may be indicated, especially in patients with a history of extensive pelvic surgery or radiation therapy.

4.5 Gestational Trophoblastic Neoplasia

GTN is a rare malignant lesion arising from placental trophoblastic tissue. It encompasses invasive mole, choriocarcinoma, placental site trophoblastic tumor, and epithelioid trophoblastic tumor. Occurring in approximately 1: 40,000 pregnancies worldwide; it is most common in Asia. The majority of GTN is cured with chemotherapy, leaving relatively young survivors with concerns including long-term consequences of therapy, reproductive concerns, and concerns of recurrent disease.

Given that GTN is a tumor of women of reproductive age, concerns about future fertility is very important to this population. In women with a history of molar pregnancy, there is an approximately 1% risk of repeat molar pregnancy and this should be considered by the obstetrician-gynecologist seeing these patients. If treated with fertility-sparing treatment methods, which is common for these diseases, the majority of research looking at reproductive outcomes show pregnancy outcomes that are similar to the general population with a live birth rate of approximately 70% without increased risk of anomaly. However, it is important to note that women who have received chemotherapy for GTN have a slightly increased risk of stillbirth of approximately 1.3% and should be carefully monitored in later pregnancy (Gadducci et al. 2015; Vargas et al. 2014).

Other matters of concern involving these patients include need for contraception. Use of contraception, including hormonal contraception, is encouraged, especially during initial surveillance of GTN. Preventing pregnancy during this time is important as a pregnancy will alter the bHCG and may mask persistent disease. This should be managed with the aid of the treating oncologist. In addition, women who have received certain chemotherapies, especially platinum compounds, have an increased risk of secondary leukemia.

5   Conclusion

The number of gynecologic cancer survivors is expected to continue to increase in coming decades. While further research is warranted to better understand and meet the needs of this population, there are many things that the general gynecologists can do to manage the survivorship care of these women. Attention to the unique psychosocial symptoms, treatment-related sequella, cancer type specific issues, and management of general health maintenance and other health issues would improve the health and quality of life of gynecologic cancer survivors.

References

Abbott-Anderson K, Kwekkeboom K. A systematic review of sexual concerns reported by gynecological cancer survivors. Gynecol Oncol. 2012;124(3):477–89.

Abu-Rustum NR, Barakat RR. Observation on the role of circumflex iliac node resection and etiology of lower extremity lymphedema following pelvic lympadenectomy for gynecologic malignancy. Gynecol Oncol. 2007;106:4–5.

Abu-Rustum N, Neubauer N, Sonoda Y, Park K, et al. Surgical and pathologic outcomes of fertility-sparing radical abdominal trachelectomy for FIGO stage IB1 cervical cancer. Gynecol Oncol. 2008;111(2):261–4.

Aerts L, Enzlin P, Verhawghe I, Amant F. Sexual and psychological functioning in women after pelvic surgery for gynaecological cancer. Eur J Gynaecol Oncol. 2009;30(6):652–6.

Aerts L, Enzlin P, Vergote I, Verhaeghe J, Poppe W, Amant F. Sexual, psychological, and relational functioning in women after surgical treatment for vulvar malignancy. J Sex Med. 2012;9(2):361–71.

Akers AY, Newmann SJ, Smith JS. Factors underlying disparities in cervical cancer incidence, screening, and treatment in the United States. Curr Probl Cancer. 2007;31(3):157–81.

Al-Badawi I, Al-Aker M, AlSubhi J, et al. Laparoscopic ovarian transposition before pelvic irradiation: a Saudi tertiary center experience. Int J Gynecol Cancer. 2010;20(6):1082–6.

American Cancer Society. Cancer treatment and survivorship facts & figures 2014–2015. Atlanta: American Cancer Society; 2014.

American College of Obstetricians and Gynecologists. Practice Bulletin No. 129: osteoporosis. Obstet Gynecol. 2012;120(3):718–34.

American College of Obstetricians and Gynecologists. Practice Bulletin No. 140: management of abnormal cervical cancer screening test results and cervical cancer precursors. Obstet Gynecol. 2013;122(6):1338–67.

American College of Obstetricians and Gynecologists. Practice Bulletin No. 141: management of menopausal symptoms. Obstet Gynecol. 2014;123(1):202–16.

Amsterdam A, Krychman M. Sexual dysfunction in patients with gynecologic neoplasms: a retrospective pilot study. J Sex Med. 2006;3:646–9.

Anderson GL, Judd HL, Kaunitz AM, Barad DH, Beresford SAA, Pettinger M, Liu J, McNeeley SG, Lopez AM. Effects of estrogen plus progestin on gynecologic cancers and associated diagnostic procedures: the women's health initiative randomized trial. JAMA. 2003;290:1739–48.

Andreotti C, Root J, Ahles T, et al. Cancer, coping, and cognition: a model for the role of stress reactivity in cancer related cognitive decline. Psychooncology. 2015;24(6):617–23.

Balamurugan A, Ahmed F, Saraiya M, Kosary C, Schwenn M, Cokkinides V, Flowers L, Pollack LA. Potential role of HPV in the development of subsequent primary in situ and invasive cancers among cervical cancer survivors. Cancer. 2008; 113(10 Suppl):2919–25.

Barakat R, Bundy B, Spirtos N, Bell J, Mannel R, Gynecologic Oncology Group Study. Randomized double-blind trial of estrogen replacement therapy versus placebo in stage I or II endometrial cancer: a Gynecologic Oncology Group Study. J Clin Oncol. 2006;24(4):587–92.

Basen-Engquist K, Carmack C, Brown J, Jhingran A, Baum G, et al. Response to an exercise intervention after endometrial cancer: differences between obese and non-obese survivors. Gynecol Oncol. 2014;133(1):48–55.

Beesley V, Janda M, Eakin E, et al. Lymphedema after gynecological cancer treatment: prevalence, correlates, and supportive care needs. Cancer. 2007;109(12):2607–14.

Berger J, Scott E, Sukumvanich P, Smith A, Olawaiye A, Comerci J, Kelley JL, Beriwal S, Huang M. The effect of groin treatment modality and sequence on clinically significant chronic lymphedema in patients with vulvar carcinoma. Int J Gynecol Cancer. 2015; 25(1):119–24.

Bergmark K, Avall-Lundqvist E, Dickman P, Henningsohn L, Steineck G. Vaginal changes and sexuality in women with a history of cervical cancer. N Engl J Med. 1999;340(18):1383–9.

Bhoola S, Hoskins WJ. Diagnosis and management of epithelial ovarian cancer. Obstet Gynecol. 2006;107:1399–410.

Bhosale P, Peungjesada S, Wei W, Levenback CF, Schmeler K, Rohren E, Macapinlac HA, Iyer RB. Clinical utility of positron emission tomography/computed tomography in the evaluation of suspected recurrent ovarian cancer in the setting of normal CA-125 levels. Int J Gynecol Cancer. 2010;20:936–44.

Biliatis I, Thomakos N, Rodolakis A, Akrivos N. Safety of hormone replacement therapy in gynaecological cancer survivors. J Obstet Gynaecol. 2012;32(4):321–5.

Bjorge T, Stocks T, Lukanova A, et al. Metabolic syndrome and endometrial carcinoma. Am J Epidemiol. 2010;171:892–902.

Bodurka DC, Sun CC, Frumovitz MM. Quality of life in cervix cancer survivors – what matters the most in the long term? Gynecol Oncol. 2005;97:307–9.

Bodurka-Bevers D, Morris M, Eifel PJ, Levenback C, Bevers MW, Lucas KR, Wharton JT. Posttherapy surveillance of women with cervical cancer: an outcomes analysis. Gynecol Oncol. 2000;78(2):187–93.

Bourgeois-Law G, Lotocki R. Sexuality and gynecological cancer: a needs assessment. Can J Hum Sex. 1999;8(4): 231–40.

Boykoff N, Moieni M, Subramanian S. Confronting chemobrain: an in-depth look at survivors' reports of impact on work, social networks, and health care response. J Cancer Surviv. 2009;3:223–32.

Brennan M, Miller L. Overview of treatment options and review of the current role and use of compression garments, intermittent pumps, and exercise in the management of lymphedema. Cancer. 1998;83:2821–7.

Bristow RE, Purinton SC, Santillan A, Diaz-Montes TP, Gardner GJ, Giuntoli RL. Cost-effectiveness of routine vaginal cytology for endometrial cancer surveillance. Gynecol Oncol. 2006;103:709–13.

Brooks RA, Rader JS, Dehdashti F, Mutch DG, Powell MA, Thaker PH, Siegal BA, Grigsby PW. Surveillance FDG-PET detection of asymptomatic recurrences in patients with cervical cancer. Gynecol Oncol. 2009; 112:104–9.

Brotto L, Heiman J, Goff B, Greer B, Lentz G, Swisher E. A psychoeducational intervention for sexual dysfunction in women with gynecologic cancer. Arch Sex Behav. 2008;37(2):317–29.

Bukovic D, Silovski H, Silovski T, Hojsak I, Sakic K, Hrgovic Z. Sexual functioning and body image of patients treated for ovarian cancer. Sex Disabil. 2008;26:63–73.

Carmack Taylor C, Basen-Engquist K, Shinn E, Bodurka D. Predictors of sexual functioning in ovarian cancer patients. J Clin Oncol. 2004;22(5):881–9.

Carpenter KM, Fowler JM, Maxwell GL, Andersen BL. Direct and buffering effects of social support among gynecologic cancer survivors. Ann Behav Med. 2010;39(1):79–90.

Carter J, Goldfrank D, Schover LR. Simple strategies for vaginal health promotion in cancer survivors. J Sex Med. 2001;8:549–59.

Carter J, et al. Gynecologic cancer treatment and the impact of cancer-related infertility. Gynecol Oncol. 2005;97:90–5.

Carter J, Chi D, Brown C, Abu-Rustum N, Sonoda Y, et al. Cancer-related infertility in survivorship. Int J Gynecol Cancer. 2010;20(1):2–8.

Carver CS, Smith RG, Petonis VM, Antoni MH. Quality of life among long-tem survivors of breast cancer: different types of antecedents predict different classes of outcomes. Psycho-Oncology. 2006;15:749–58.

Chaoyang S, Chen G, Yang Z, et al. Safety of ovarian preservation in young patients with early-stage endometrial cancer: a retrospective study and meta-analysis.

Chapman J, DiSaia P, Osann K, Roth P, Gillotte D, Berman M. Estrogen replacement in surgical stage I and II endometrial cancer survivors. Am J Obstet Gynecol. 1996;175(5):1195–200.

Chung HH, Kim SK, Kim TH, Lee S, Kang KW, Kim JY, Park SY. Clinical impact of FDG-PET imaging in posttherapy surveillance of uterine cervical cancer: from diagnosis to prognosis. Gynecol Oncol. 2006;103:165–70.

Cooper AL, Dornfeld-Finke JM, Banks HW, Davey DD, Modestt SC. Is cytologic screening an effective surveillance method for detection of vaginal recurrence of uterine cancer? Obstet Gynecol. 2006;107:71–6.

Corney R, Crowther M, Everett H, Howells A, Shepherd J. Psychosexual dysfunction in women with gynaecological cancer following radical pelvic surgery. Br J Obstet Gynaecol. 1993;100:73–8.

Correa D, Zhou Q, Thaler H, et al. Cognitive functions in long-term survivors of ovarian cancer. Gynecol Oncol. 2010;119:366–9.

Courneya K, Karvinen K, Campbell K, Pearcey R, Dundas G, Capstick V, et al. Associations among exercise, body weight, and quality of life in a population-based sample of endometrial cancer survivors. Gynecol Oncol. 2005;97(2):422–30.

Crawford J, Vallance J, Holt N. Associations between exercise and posttraumatic growth in gynecologic cancer survivors. Support Care Cancer. 2015;23(3): 705–14.

Ditto A, Martinelli F, Lorusso D, Haeusler E, Carcangiu M, Raspagliesi F. Fertility sparing surgery in early state epithelial ovarian cancer. J Gynecol Oncol. 2014;25(4): 320–7.

Ditto A, Martinelli F, Bogani G, Fischetti M, Di Donato V, Lorusso D, Raspagliesi F. Fertility-sparing surgery in early-stage cervical cancer patients: oncologic and reproductive outcomes. Int J Gynecol Cancer. 2015;25(3):493–7.

Donovan K, Taliaferro L, Alvarez E, Jacobsen P, Roetzheim R, Wenham R. Sexual health in women treated for cervical cancer: characteristics and correlates. Gynecol Oncol. 2007;104:428–34.

Elit L, Fyles AW, Oliver TK, Devries-Aboud MC, Fung-Kee-Fung M. Follow-up for women after treatment for cervical cancer. Curr Oncol. 2010;17:65–9.

Erkanli S, Ayhan A. Fertility-sparing therapy in young women with endometrial cancer: 2010 update. Int J Gynecol Cancer. 2010;20:1170–87.

Ezendam NP, Pijlman B, Bhugwandass C, Pruijt JF, Mols F, Vos MC, Pijnenborg JM, van de Poll-Franse LV. Chemotherapy-induced peripheral neuropathy and its impact on health-related quality of life among ovarian cancer survivors: results from the population based PRO-FILES registry. Gynecol Oncol. 2014;135(3):510–7.

Falleti M, Maruff P, Weih L, Phillips K. The nature and severity of cognitive impairment associated with adjuvant chemotherapy in women with breast cancer: a meta-analysis of the current literature. Brain Cogn. 2005;59:60–70.

Ferguson RJ, McDonald BC, Rocque MA, et al. Development of CBT for chemotherapy-related cognitive change: results of a waitlist control trial. Psycho-Oncology. 2012;21:176–86.

Forsythe L, Kent E, Weaver K, et al. Receipt of psychosocial care among cancer survivors in the United States. J Clin Oncol. 2013;106:244–50.

Fulham MJ, Carter J, Baldey A, Hicks RJ, Ramshaw JE, Gibson M. The impact of PET-CT in suspected recurrent ovarian cancer: a prospective multi-centre study as part of the Australian PET data collection project. Gynecol Oncol. 2008;112:462–8.

Fung-Kee-Fung M, Dodge J, Elit L, Lukka H, Chambers A, Oliver T. Follow-up after primary therapy for endometrial cancer: a systematic review. Gynecol Oncol. 2006;101:520–9.

Gadducci A, Cosio S. Surveillance of patients after initial treatment of ovarian cancer. Crit Rev Oncol Hematol. 2003;30:401–12.

Gadducci A, Fuso L, Casio S, Landoni F, Maggino T, Perotto S, Sartori E, Testa A, Galletto L, Zola P. Are surveillance procedures of clinical benefit for patients treated for ovarian cancer? A retrospective Italian multicentric study. Int J Gynecol Oncol. 2009;19(3): 367–74.

Gadducci A, Lanfredini N, Cosio S. Reproductive outcomes after hydatiform mole and gestational trophoblastic neoplasia. Gynecol Endocrinol. 2015:1–6. Epub ahead of print.

Gangi A, Cass I, Paik D, Barmparas G, Karlan B, Dang C, Li A, Walsh C, Rimel BJ, Amersi F. Breast cancer following ovarian cancer in BRCA mutation carriers. JAMA Surg. 2014;149(12):1306–13.

Goedendorp M, Knoop H, Gielissen M, et al. The effects of cognitive behavioral therapy for postcancer fatigue on perceived cognitive disabilities and neuropsychological test performance. J Pain Symptom Manag. 2014; 47(1):35–44.

Gonzalez Bosquet J, Magrina JF, Gaffey TA, Hernandez JL, Webb MJ, Cliby WA, Podratz KC. Long-term survival and disease recurrence in patients with primary squamous cell carcinoma of the vulva. Gynecol Oncol. 2005;97(3):828–33.

Greenwald HP, McCorkle R, Baumgartner K, Gotay C, Neale AV. Quality of life and disparities among long-term cervical cancer survivors. J Cancer Surviv. 2014; 8(3):419–26.

Gunther V, Malchow B, Schubert M, et al. Impact of radical operative treatment on the quality of life in women with vulvar cancer – a retrospective study. Eur J Surg Oncol. 2014;40(7):875–82.

Guntupalli S, Flink D, Sheeder J, et al. Sexual and marital dysfunction in women with gynecologic cancer: a multi-institutional, cross-sectional trial. J Clin Oncol (Meeting Abstracts). 2015;33(15_suppl): 9592.

Gutierrez-Gutierrez G, Sereno M, Miralles A, Casado-Saenz E, Gutierrez-Rivas E. Chemotherapy-induced peripheral neuropathy: clinical features, diagnosis, prevention and treatment strategies. Clin Transl Oncol. 2010;12:81–91.

Harding Y, Ooyama T, Nakamoto T, Wakayama A, Kudaka W, Inamine M, Nagai Y, Ueda S, Aoki Y. Radiotherapy- or radical surgery-induced female sexual morbidity in stages IB and II cervical cancer. Int J Gynecol Cancer. 2014;24:800.

Hareyama H, Hada K, Goto K. Prevalence, classification, and risk factors for postoperative lower extremity lymphedema in women with gynecologic malignancies: a retrospective study. Int J Gynecol Cancer. 2015;25(4):751–7.

Hodgkinson K, Butow P, Fuchs A, et al. Long-term survival from fynecologic cancer: psychosocial outcomes, supportive care needs and positive outcomes. Gynecol Oncol. 2007;104:381–9.

International Society of Lymphology. The diagnosis and treatment of peripheral lymphedema: 2013 Consensus Document of the International Society of Lymphology. Lymphology. 2013;46(1):1–11.

Joura EA, Lösch A, Haider-Angeler MG. Trends in vulvar neoplasia. Increasing incidence of vulvar intraepithelial neoplasia and squamous cell carcinoma of the vulva in young women. J Reprod Med. 2000;45:613–5.

Juraskova I, Butow P, Robertson R, Sharpe L, McLeod C, Hacker N. Post-treatment sexual adjustment following cervical and endometrial cancer: a qualitative insight. Psychooncology. 2003;12(3):267–79.

Kimmel M, Fairbairn M, Giuntoli R, et al. The importance of social support for women with elevated anxiety undergoing care for gynecologic malignancies. Int J Gynecol Cancer. 2014;24(9):1700–8.

Kirchhoff AC, Yi J, Wright J, Warner EL, Smith KR. Marriage and divorce among young adult cancer survivors. J Cancer Surviv. 2012;6(4):441–50.

Kollmannsberger C, Beyer J, Droz JP, Harstrick A, Hartmann JT, Biron P, Fléchon A, Schöffski P, Kuczyk M, Schmoll HJ, Kanz L, Bokemeyer C. Secondary leukemia following high cumulative doses of etoposide in patients treated for advanced germ cell tumors. J Clin Oncol. 1998;16(10):3386–91.

Koskas M, Uzan J, Luton D, Rouzier R. Prognostic factors of oncologic and reproductive outcomes in fertility-sparing management of endometrial atypical hyperplasia and adenocarcinoma: systematic review and meta-analysis. Fertil Steril. 2014;101(3):785–94.

Kunos C, Simpkins F, Gibbons H, Tian C, Homesley H. Radiation therapy compared with pelic node resection for node-positive culcar cancer: a randomized controlled trial. Obstet Gynecol. 2009;114(3):537–46.

Le Borgne G, Mercier M, Woronoff AS, Guizard AV, Abeilard E, Caravati-Jouvenceaux A, Klein D, Velten M, Joly F. Quality of life in long-term cervical cancer survivors: a population-based study. Gynecol Oncol. 2013;129(1):222–8.

Li D, Ding CY, Qiu LH. Postoperative hormone replacement therapy for epithelial ovarian cancer patients: a systematic review and meta-analysis. Gynecol Oncol. 2015. pii: S0090-8258(15)30093-7. doi:10.1016/j.ygyno.2015.07.109. [Epub ahead of print].

Lindaw S, Gavrilova N, Anderson D. Sexual morbidity in very long term survivors of vaginal and cervical cancer; a comparison to national norms. Gynecol Oncol. 2007;106:413–8.

McCann GA, Cohn DE, Jewell EL, Havrilesky LJ. Lymphatic mapping and sentinel lymph node dissection compared to complete lymphadenectomy in the management of early-stage vulvar cancer: a cost utility analysis. Gynecol Oncol. 2015;136(2):300–4.

McCarrol M, Armbruster S, Frasure H, et al. Self-efficacy, quality of life, and weight loss in overweight/obese endometrial cancer survivors (SUCCEED): a randomized controlled trial. Gynecol Oncol. 2014;132(2):397–402.

Meyer TJ, Mark MM. Effects of psychosocial interventions with adult cancer patients: a meta-analysis of randomized experiments. Health Psychol. 1995;14:101–8.

Miles T, Johnson N. Vaginal dilator therapy for women receiving pelvic radiotherapy. Cochrane Database Syst Rev. 2014;9:CD007291.

National Cancer Institute. Adjustment to cancer: anxiety and distress–for health professionals (PDQ®). http://www.cancer.gov/about-cancer/coping/feelings/anxiety-distress-hp-pdq#link/stoc_h2_3. Accessed 28 June 2015.

National Institute of Cancer, Office of Cancer Survivorship. Definitions, statistics, and graphs. http://cancercontrol.cancer.gov/ocs/statistics/statistics.html. Accessed 1 June 2015.

National Research Council. From cancer patient to cancer survivor: lost in transition. Washington, DC: The National Academies Press; 2005.

Pareja R, Rendon G, Sanz-Lomana C. Surgical, oncological, and obstetrical outcomes after abdominal radical trachelectomy – a systematic literature review. Gynecol Oncol. 2013;131(1):77–82.

Ploch E. Hormone replacement therapy in patients after cervical cancer treatment. Gynecol Oncol. 1987;26:169–77.

Practice Bulletin No 149: endometrial cancer. Obstet Gynecol. 2015;125(4):1006–26.

Ramirez P, Schmeler K, Soliman P, Frumovitz M. Fertility preservation in patients with early cervical cancer: radical trachelectomy. Gynecol Oncol. 2008;110(3 Suppl 2):S25–8.

Re A, Taylor TH, DiSaia PJ, Anton-Culver H. Risk for breast and colorectal cancers subsequent to cancer of the endometrium in a population-based case series. Gynecol Oncol. 1997;66(2):255–7.

Risum S, Hogdall C, Markova E, Berthelsen AK, Loft A, Jensen F, Hogdall E, Roed H, Engelholm SA. Influence of 2-(18F) fluoro-2-deoxy-d-glucose positron emission tomography/computed tomography on recurrent ovarian cancer diagnosis and on selection of patients for secondary cytoreductive surgery. Int J Gynecol Cancer. 2009;19:600–4.

Robinson J, Scott C, Faris P. Sexual rehabilitation for women with gynecological cancer: information is not sufficient. Can J Hum Sex. 1994;3(2):131–42.

Rodriguez AM, Kuo YF, Goodwin JS. Risk of colorectal cancer among long-term cervical cancer survivors. Med Oncol. 2014;31(5):943.

Roland K, Rodriguez J, Patterson J, Trivers K. A literature review of the social and psychological needs of ovarian cancer survivors. Psychooncology. 2013;22(11):2408–18.

Rose PG, Sommers RM, Reale FR, Hunter RE, Fournier L, Nelson BE. Serial serum CA 125 measurements for evaluation of recurrence in patients with endometrial carcinoma. Obstet Gynecol. 1994;84(1):12–6.

Rustin GJ. What surveillance plan should be advised for patients in remission after completion of first-line therapy for advanced ovarian cancer? Int J Gynecol Cancer. 2010;20(11 Suppl 2):S27–8.

Sadovsky R, Basson R, Krychman M, et al. Cancer and sexual problems. J Sex Med. 2010;7:349–73.

Salani R, Backes FJ, Fung MFK, Holschneider CH, Parker LP, Bristow RE, Goff BA. Posttreatment surveillance and diagnosis of recurrence in women with gynecologic malignancies: Society of Gynecologic Oncologists recommendations. Am J Obstet Gynecol. 2011;204(6):466–78.

Salmal RAK, Van der Velden J, Van Ferden T, Schilthuis MS, Gonzalez DG, Lammes FB. Recurrent cervical carcinoma after radical hystetectomy: an analysis of clinical aspects and prognosis. Int J Gynecol Cancer. 1998;8(1):78–84.

Sanson-Fisher R, Girgis A, Boyes A, Bonevski B, Burton L, Cook P. The unmet supportive care needs of patients with cancer. Support Care Rev Group.

Santen RJ, Allred DC, Ardoin SP, Archer DF, Boyd N, Braunstein GD, Burger HG, Colditz GA, Davis SR, Gambacciani M, Gower BA, Henderson VW, Jarjour WN, Karas RH, Kleerekoper M, Lobo RA, Manson JE, Marsden J, Martin KA, Martin L, Pinkerton JV, Rubinow DR, Teede H, Thiboutot DM, Utian WH, Endocrine Society. Postmenopausal hormone therapy:

an Endocrine Society scientific statement. J Clin Endocrinol Metab. 2010;95(7 Suppl 1):s1.

Sartori E, Pasinetti B, Chiudinelli F, Gadducci A, Landoni F, Faggino T, Piovano E, Zola P. Surveillance procedures for patients treated for endometrial cancer: a review of the literature. Int J Gynecol Cancer. 2010; 20(6):985–92.

SEER Stat Fact Sheets – Cancer of the Cervix Uteri. Available http://seer.cancer.gov/statfacts/html/cervix. html. Accessed 3 June 2015.

SEER Stat Fact Sheets – Cancer of the Endometrium. http://seer.cancer.gov/statfacts/html/corp.html. Accessed 31 May 2015.

SEER Stat Fact Sheets – Cancer of the Ovary. Available http://seer.cancer.gov/statfacts/html/ovary. html. Accessed 28 May 2015.

SEER Stat Fact Sheets – Cancer of the Vulva. Available http://seer.cancer.gov/statfacts/html/vulva. html. Accessed 31 May 2015.

Shou H, Chen Y, Chen Z. Laparoscopic ovarian transposition in young women with cervical squamous cell carcinoma treated by primary pelvic irradiation. Eur J Gynaecol Oncol. 2015;36(1):25–9.

Sleight A. Coping with cancer-related cognitive dysfunction: a scoping review of the literature. Disabil Rehabil. 2015;17:1–9.

Smits A, Lopes A, Das N, Bekkers R, Galaal K. The impact of BMI on quality of life in obese endometrial cancer survivors: does size matter? Gynecol Oncol. 2014; 132:137–41.

Sorosky JI. Endometrial cancer. Obstet Gynecol. 2008; 111:436–47.

Stavraka C, Ford A, Ghaem-Maghami S, Crook T. A study of symptoms described by ovarian cancer survivors. Gynecol Oncol. 2012;125(1):59–64.

Stavraka C, Maclaran K, Gabra H, et al. A study to evaluate the cause of bone demineralization in gynecological cancer survivors. Oncologist. 2013;18(4): 423–9.

Stevinson C, Faught W, Steed H, Tonkin K, Ladha AB, Vallance JK, Capstick V, Schepansky A, Courneya KS. Associations between physical activity and quality of life in ovarian cancer survivors. Gynecol Oncol. 2007;106:244–50.

Stroud J, Mutch D, Rader J, Powell M, Thaker P. Effects of cancer treatment on ovarian function. Fertil Steril. 2009;92(2):417–27.

Tanner EJ, Chi DS, Eisenhauer EL, Diaz-Montes TP, Santillan A, Bristow RE. Surveillance for the detection of recurrent ovarian cancer: survival impact or lead-time bias? Gynecol Oncol. 2010;117:336–40.

Teng F, Kalloger S, Brotto L. Determinants of quality of life in ovarian cancer survivors: a pilot study. J Obstet Gynaecol Can. 2014;36(8):708–15.

Thornton A, Perez M. Posttraumatic growth in prostate cancer survivors and their partners. Psycho-Oncology. 2006;15:285–96.

Thrall MM, DeLoia JA, Gallion H, Avril N. Clinical use of combined positron emission tomography and computed tomography (FDG-PET/CT) in recurrent ovarian cancer. Gynecol Oncol. 2007;105:17–22.

Tjalma WAA, Van Dam PA, Makar AP, Cruickshanks DJ. The clinical value and the cost-effectiveness of follow-up in endometrial cancer patients. Int J Gynecol Cancer. 2004;14:931–7.

Uccella S, Cha S, Melton L. Risk factors for developing multiple malignancies in endometrial cancer patients. Int J Gynecol Cancer. 2011;21(5):896–901.

Underwood JM, Rim SH, Fairley TL, Tai E, Stewart SL. Cervical cancer survivors at increased risk of subsequent tobacco-related malignancies, United States 1992–2008. Cancer Causes Control. 2012;23(7):1009–16.

Vargas R, Barroilhet LM, Esselen K, Diver E, Bernstein M, Goldstein DP, Berkowitz RS. Subsequent pregnancy outcomes after complete and partial molar pregnancy, recurrent molar pregnancy, and gestational trophoblastic neoplasia: an update from the New England Trophoblastic Disease Center. J Reprod Med. 2014; 59(5–6):188–94.

Vaz AF. Quality of life and menopausal and sexual symptoms in gynecologic cancer survivors: a cohort study. Menopause. 2011;18(6):622–9.

Von Gruenigen V, Tian C, Frasure H. Treatment effects, disease recurrence, and survival in obese women with early endometrial carcinoma. Cancer. 2006;107:2786–91.

Von Gruenigen VE, Courneya KS, Gibbons HE, et al. Feasibility and effectiveness of a lifestyle intervention program in obese endometrial cancer patients: a randomized trial. Gynecol Oncol. 2008;109:19–26.

Von Gruenigen VE, Gibbons HE, Kavanagh MB, et al. A randomized trial of a lifestyle intervention in obese endometrial cancer survivors: quality of life outcomes and mediators of behavioral change. Health Qual Life Outcomes. 2009;7:17.

Von Gruenigen VE, Waggoner SE, Frasure HE, et al. Lifestye challenges in endometrial cancer survivorship. Obstet Gynecol. 2011;117:93–100.

Von Gruenigen V, Frasure H, Kavanagh MB, Janata J, Waggoner S, Rose P, Lerner E, Courneya KS. Survivors of uterine cancer empowered by exercise and healthy diet (SUCCEED): a randomized controlled trial. Gynecol Oncol. 2012;125(3):699–704.

Ward K, Shah N, Saenz C, McHale M, Alvarez E, Plaxe S. Cardiovascular disease is the leading cause of death among endometrial cancer patients. Gynecol Oncol. 2012;126(2):176–9.

Wenzel LB, Donnelly JP, Fowler JM, et al. Resilience, reflection, and residual stress in ovarian cancer survivorship: a gynecologic oncology group study. Psycho-Oncology. 2002;11:142–53.

Ye S, Yang J, Cao D, Lang J, Shen K. A systematic review of quality of life and sexual function of patients with cervical cancer after treatment. Int J Gynecol Cancer. 2014;24(7):1146–57.

Zanagnolo V, Minig LA, Gadducci A, Maggino T, Sartori E, Zola P, Landoni F. Surveillance procedures for patients for cervical carcinoma: a review of the literature. Int J Gynecol Cancer. 2009;19(3):306–13.

Part X

Pathology of the Female Gynecologic System (Paulette Mhawech-Fauceglia)

Benign Vulvar and Vaginal Pathology

Daman Samrao

Abstract

Benign vulvar and vaginal pathology is common, consisting of a wide variety of lesions which include inflammatory conditions, pigmented lesions, neoplastic and nonneoplastic masses, and cysts. Women of all ages are affected. The majority of these lesions are clinically insignificant unless symptomatic or when they mimic malignancy. Rare lesions with premalignant potential are also present.

Keywords

Lichen sclerosus • Papillary hidradenoma • Vulvar melanosis • Atypical melanocytic nevi of genital type • Fibroepithelial polyp • Dysplastic nevi • Bartholin's gland cyst • Mullerian cyst • Epithelial inclusion cyst

Contents

1   Introduction

The high prevalence of benign lesions of the vulva and vagina makes the clinical and pathologic recognition of these entities important. Some of these lesions can lead to significant morbidity, and some are even considered premalignant. Successful treatments are available for most all these lesions. We discuss the most common and clinically relevant of these in this chapter.

2   Lichen Sclerosus

2.1   Introduction

Lichen sclerosus (LS) is a chronic, progressive, and debilitating dermatosis which remains poorly understood despite its recognition in the late

D. Samrao (✉)
University of Southern California, Los Angeles, CA, USA

Laboratory Medicine Consultants, Las Vegas, NV, USA
e-mail: dsamraosidhu@gmail.com1; dsamrao@usc.edu

© Springer International Publishing AG 2017
D. Shoupe (ed.), *Handbook of Gynecology*,
DOI 10.1007/978-3-319-17798-4_60

nineteenth century. The hallmark of the disease is progressive scarring of the skin manifested grossly as white plaques and epidermal atrophy and histologically as dermal sclerosis with chronic inflammation. It affects males and females, adults and children, and all races but has a predilection for postmenopausal Caucasian women. It can involve any part of the skin but predominantly affects the anogenital region with only 6% of cases presenting as pure extragenital lesions. Of the vulvar dermatoses, it is the most common accounting for 39% of all cases. The prevalence of LS is estimated to be 0.1–1.7% but is likely an underestimate due to patient's presenting to numerous clinical settings, lack of clinical diagnosis, and underreporting by patients due to lack of symptoms or embarrassment.

The etiology of LS remains unknown and controversial. Interplay between immunologic alterations and chronic inflammation is believed to result in the formation of sclerosis. The development of LS in patients after surgery, trauma, instrumentation, and genital piercings supports this theory. Autoimmune and genetic components are strongly favored to play a part. Autoantibodies against extracellular matrix 1 (ECM1) protein and the basement membrane zone (BMZ) [BP180 and BP230] have been described in. *Borrelia burgdorferi* and Epstein Barr virus have been implicated as causative agents, but no strong evidence exists to support their involvement. Other possible causes include hormonal influences due to the presence of decreased dihydrotestosterone in affected females and the presentation of the disease at times of low estrogen (peak incidences in prepubertal and postmenopausal women).

2.2 Clinical Features

The diagnosis of LS is clinical, presenting as a constellation of symptoms, gross features, and clinical sequelae. In a prospective cohort study of 225 patients, the most common complaints were itching (90.2%), burning (74.3%), and dyspareunia (47.5%). On examination pallor, scarring sclerosis, and atrophy were seen in half the patients. Hyperkeratosis, purpura, itching related excoriations, and erythema were also present to a lesser degree (Virgili et al. 2014). Sites of involvement include the interlabial sulci, labia minora and majora, clitoris and hood, and perineum and perianal area; mucosal sites are spared.

LS usually starts as nonspecific erythema, edema, and fragility (erosions, fissuring, purpura, and ecchymoses) and progresses to large porcelain white plaques and papules. These evolve into dry, hypopigmented, sclerotic and atrophic lesions resulting in a crinkling or cellophane paper type appearance which is pathognomonic of LS. The progressive scarring of LS can result in fusion of the labia minora, obliteration of the clitoris, and stenosis of the introitus. Although controversial, LS is considered a risk factor for invasive squamous cell carcinoma (SCC) with a reported lifetime risk of 0.3–5%. It is not considered a premalignant lesion.

2.3 Histology

LS has been divided into an early and late stage clinically and histologically although this designation is debated due to lack of correlation between clinical duration and histologic findings. Early LS is histologically nonspecific. Findings include a lichenoid interface dermatitis and basement membrane thickening. Luminal hyperkeratosis and hypergranulosis of the adnexal structures; mild irregular, occasionally psoriasiform acanthosis; subepithelial edema; dermal homogenized collagen; and dilated blood vessels immediately under the basement membrane may also be seen. The differential includes lichen planus, psoriasis, and Zoon's vulvitis. Late LS has a classic histologic picture of hyperkeratosis, epidermal atrophy with flattening of the rete ridges, vacuolar interface changes, loss of elastic fibers, and hyalinization of the lamina propria with or without an underlying lymphocytic infiltrate. However, a not uncommon hyperplastic variant has been described and may increase risk of development of SCC (Scurry et al. 2001; Weyers 2013). An atypical variant that may be a precursor to differentiated vulvar intraepithelial neoplasia (VIN) has also been described (Chiesa-Vottero 2006). The nonspecific features of early LS and variants of more typical late LS often make histologic diagnosis of LS difficult; clinical correlation is a must.

3 Fibroepithelial Polyp

3.1 Clinical Features

Fibroepithelial polyps (FEP) are benign indolent lesions found most commonly in the genital region of premenopausal reproductive aged women. The most common site is the vagina followed by the vulva, cervix, and extragenital sites. In the vulva, they are usually present on hair-bearing skin but involvement of the labia minora has been described. The median age in one study was 32 years, (Nucci et al. 2000) but they have been reported in a wide age range of patients, including infants and the elderly. FEP typically presents as a polypoid or pedunculated exophytic mass that is usually solitary but can be multiple with multiple lesions being seen more often in pregnant patients (Nucci et al. 2000). Symptoms include bleeding, discharge, general discomfort, and sensation of a mass. Their clinical significance stems from their gross and clinical overlap with malignant neoplasms resulting in the alternative terminology of pseudosarcoma botyroides. Biopsy or excision with histologic examination is necessary to exclude malignancy.

FEP is thought to be a hyperplastic process rather than true neoplasm. Features supporting this theory are the presence of multinucleate cells in normal adjacent tissue and the presence of estrogen (ER) and progesterone receptors (PR) in normal stromal cells (see Sect. 3.2 below). The etiology is unknown and includes origin from a regressing nevus, irritation, skin aging, and hormones. Findings to support hormones as a cause include the fact that 20% of patients with FEP are pregnant, 10% are on hormone replacement therapy (HRT), multiple lesions are seen in pregnant patients, and spontaneous regression after birth has been reported.

The gross appearance of FEP is variable. It is often <5 cm in size, but the literature contains examples of 10, 15, and 18.5 cm lesions (Madueke-Laveaux et al. 2013; Navada et al. 2011). Gross features range from small fleshy colored to pigmented papillomatous resembling condyloma to large pedunculated lesions which are often hypopigmented. They have also been described as edematous, mucoid, rubbery, and hard with increased vascularity and as a gelatinous cyst. The differential includes numerous benign lesions such as sebaceous cyst, condyloma, fibroid, and hymenal ring as well as malignant neoplasms.

3.2 Histology

The typical histologic features of FEP include a fibrovascular core, loose edematous stroma, prominent dilated thick walled vessels, overlying intact squamous epithelium, multinucleate stromal cells throughout including at the epithelial stromal interface, and spindle or stellate stromal cells with tapering cytoplasmic processes. The squamous epithelium may be hyperplastic, acanthotic, parakeratotic, attenuated, and rarely even ulcerated (Navada et al. 2011; Nucci et al. 2000). The lesion lacks circumscription, merging with normal tissue at the margins. The constituent stromal cell is fibroblastic/myofibroblastic by immunohistochemistry and ultrastructurally and has been shown to be positive for ER, PR desmin, actin, and vimentin. The typical histologic appearance is easy to diagnose, but variants of these features pose diagnostic dilemmas. Focal myxoid stroma may lead to a misdiagnosis of aggressive angimyxoma (AA). However, AA is subcutaneous not exophytic and uniformly myxoid not focally. A cellular variant of FEP that has been described is particularly worrisome because it can be mistaken for sarcoma. It consists of a hypercellular stroma and can have cytologic pleomorphism, up to 10 mitoses per 10 high power fields, and atypical mitoses which can lead to a misdiagnosis of sarcoma. The presence of multinucleate cells should help exclude sarcoma as they are strictly a feature of FEP (Nucci et al. 2000).

4   Vulvar Melanosis

Vulvar melanosis (VM), also known as vulvar lentiginosis or vulvar melanotic macules, is the most common pigmented disorder of the vulva. It is a benign disorder that typically affects perimenopausal Caucasian women with a reported median age of 40–44 years in one study (Murzaku et al. 2014). It accounts for 68% of all pigmented lesions in reproductive aged women. The typical presentation is of single or multiple asymmetric macules or patches of varying shades of tan to black color that vary in size and have poorly demarcated irregular borders. The lesions can be longstanding and grow in size (Rudolph 1990). They arise most often on mucosal surfaces with the most common sites being the labia minora followed by the labia majora (Cengiz et al. 2015). Hair-bearing skin is spared. The etiology is unknown but lichen sclerosus, human papilloma virus, and hormones have all been implicated (Murzaku et al. 2014) although one study of 23 cases failed to demonstrate common strains of HPV (Jih et al. 1999).

The most common histologic finding in VM is increased melanin pigment in the basal layer of the epidermis. It is usually accompanied by no or mild proliferation of melanocytes. If proliferation is present, it is as single cells confined to the basal layer; nesting or confluent proliferation should not be seen. Other less common findings include acanthosis, pigment incontinence with melanophages in the papillary dermis, and dendritic melanocytes at the dermal-epidermal junction. Atypia is absent or very mild (Jackson 1984; Kanj et al. 1992; Rudolph 1990; Jih et al. 1999).

Despite its benign prognosis, VM is important clinically due to its gross similarity to malignant melanoma (MM). Conservative treatment consists of baseline photography followed by sequential imaging. If melanoma cannot be excluded biopsy must be performed. Dermoscopy can also help to determine the benign nature of the lesion (Murzaku et al. 2014). VM has been proposed as a risk factor for development of MM, but no strong evidence to support this has yet been identified.

5   Nevus

5.1   Clinical Features

Vulvar nevi are present in 2% of the female population and account for 23% of all pigmented vulvar lesions. The median age of diagnosis is 28–33 years although a significant number can be seen in the pediatric population (<18 years of age). The most common nevus diagnosed is the typical variant that is found at other sites in the body. It is most often acquired and can be junctional, compound, or intradermal. Other variants described are congenital, dysplastic, blue, and spitz nevus. An important variant due to its histologic similarity to malignant melanoma (MM) is atypical melanocytic nevi of genital type (AMNGT). AMNGT is considered a nevus with site specific features and accounts for 5% of vulvar nevi. Its median age of presentation is less than that of typical nevi and ranges from 17 to 26 years. A family history of dysplastic nevi or MM is more common in these patients.

Typical nevi present as symmetric macules or flat topped or dome-shaped papules with well-demarcated, regular borders. They are usually <1 cm in size and have uniform color ranging from pink, dark brown-black, and rarely blue. Common sites of involvement are the labia majora followed by the labia minora and clitoral hood. Involvement of hair-bearing sites is less common. AMNGT present with dark pigmentation, irregular borders, and larger size (up to 2 cm in diameter). They present more often on the labia minora and have an equal distribution between mucosal and hair-bearing sites. In children, AMNGT predominate at mucosal sites.

5.2   Histology

Typical nevi are histologically identical to typical nevi anywhere else on the body. They consist of nests of cytologically bland melanocytes at the dermal-epidermal junction (DEJ) (junctional nevus), in the dermis (intradermal nevus), or both (compound nevus). Confluent or merging nests, lentiginous or pagetoid spread, mitoses, and atypia are absent. Dermal components often show maturation. AMNGT, although worrisome to the unexperienced pathologist, has a characteristic histologic appearance enabling accurate diagnosis. It is a compound nevus with well-demarcated, symmetric contours. On low power it appears large, nodular, and has increased cellularity. The junctional component consists of florid, large, irregularly distributed nests of mild to moderately atypical melanocytes that may show confluence and often have retraction artifact. These nests often are fusiform or oval shaped with their long axis parallel to the DEJ (Brenn 2011). Lentiginous and pagetoid spread into the granular layer is usually a focal finding in the center of the lesion only (Ribe 2008). Hyperchromatic and multinucleate forms may be seen as well as mitotic activity up to 2 mitoses/HPF. If melanocytic atypia is random rather than uniform, deep dermal or atypical mitoses present or necrosis seen, a diagnosis of dysplastic nevus must be ruled out.

6 Papillary Hidradenoma

6.1 Clinical Features

Papillary hidradenoma (PH), also known as hidradenoma papilliferum, is a benign neoplasm that most often affects the vulva of postpubescent Caucasian women. Rare incidents of lesions in males, other races, and extragenital sites have been reported (Scurry et al. 2009; Duhan et al. 2011). The mean age in one study of 46 patients was 52 years with a reported age range in the literature of 20–89 years (Scurry et al. 2009). The most common sites of involvement in the vulva are the labia majora (38%) and labia minora (26%). PH usually presents as an asymptomatic, small (2 mm to 3 cm), solitary, slow growing, dome or spherical shaped freely movable mass. It can be solid or cystic; ulcerated; pedunculated; and blue, red, or skin colored. When symptoms are present they include a nodule

increasing in size, pruritus, bleeding, and very rarely tenderness. PH can rarely be multifocal; when it is, it is usually unilateral (Parks et al. 2012). The largest reported case is 8 × 5 cm (Kaufmann et al. 1987).

The histogenesis of PH was believed to be from apocrine and eccrine glands. Currently it is thought to be from mammary-like glands (MLG) in the vulva prompting some authors to advocate a name change to MLG adenoma (Scurry et al. 2009). Features supporting this theory are the analogous distribution of the lesion to vulvar MLGs, their immunophenotypic (see below) and histologic overlap, and the presence of MLGs adjacent to or in close proximity to PH on histologic sections. An association with human papilloma virus has been reported, but causation has not been proven (Vazmitel et al. 2008). PH is also thought to be a cause of Bartholin's cyst due to a reported and its typical anatomical proximity to Bartholin's duct (Docimo et al. 2008).

6.2 Histology

PH is an adenoma that arises in the dermis with no connection to the epidermis. At low power it can mimic adenocarcinoma due to the presence of a fibrotic pseudocapsule which entraps epithelium at the periphery mimicking an invasive pattern. High power shows anastomosing tubules and cystic spaces with papillary folds projecting into the lumen reminiscent of an intraductal papilloma of the breast. If tubules predominate, rare solid areas can also be seen (Scurry et al. 2009). The tubules and papillae are composed of two cell layers: an inner layer of tall, columnar ductal cells and outer layer of flat or cuboidal myoepithelial cells. Sometimes only a single layer is present. The ductal cells can have apical snouts and faint eosinophilic cytoplasm imparting an apocrine look. Rare examples of clear, mucinous and foam cells have also been described (Scurry et al. 2009). Pleomorphism and mitoses can be present but only mildly. Ductal cells are positive for estrogen receptor (ER), progesterone receptor (PR),

GCDFP-15, CK7, PanK, and EMA. Myopeithelial cells are positive for actin and p63 (Parks et al. 2012; Vazmitel et al. 2008; Shah et al. 2008).

7 Vaginal Cysts

7.1 Introduction

Vaginal cysts are clinically common lesions affecting an estimated 1/200 reproductive aged women. The cysts are often asymptomatic leading to an underestimate in not only prevalence but also a lack of pathologic examination and unfamiliarity with histologic designation. Although histologic distinction between the different cysts is not clinically important, it can be done with relative ease by understanding of embryogenesis of the vagina. The vagina is derived from mullerian, mesonephric, and urogenital sinus tissues. The common cysts can be divided into embryonic (Mullerian, Gartner's duct, and Bartholin's gland) and nonembryonic (epidermal inclusion cyst (EIC)).

7.2 Cysts of Embryonic Origin

7.2.1 Mullerian Cysts
Mullerian cysts are derived from the mullerian ducts which form the majority of the vagina. They are the most common of the benign vaginal cysts accounting for up to 44% of cysts. They can be located almost anywhere within the vagina but are usually found in the anterolateral aspect. They range in size from 1 to 7 cm and are often asymptomatic and clinically undetectable, especially if small.

Mullerian cysts can be comprised of any of the normal mullerian tissues including endocervical (mucinous), tubal, or endometrial. The most common finding is an admixture of endocervical and tubal with admixed squamous metaplasia. Endocervical epithelium consists of tall columnar cells, basally located nuclei, and cytoplasmic and

luminal mucin. Tubal epithelium consists of ciliated tubal cells with admixed tubal peg and secretory cells. Endometrial epithelium is rare and if present is usually focal. If abundant luminal mucin is present, the epithelium may become compressed or flattened making distinction between Gartner's duct cysts difficult. Confirmation of mucin with mucicarmine stain can help differentiate as Gartner's duct cysts are nonmucinous. Abundant squamous metaplasia can make distinction from EIC almost impossible but distinction is not clinically significant.

7.2.2 Gartner's Duct Cysts
Gartner's duct, or mesonephric, cysts arise from the Wolffian ducts. They are less common than their mullerian counterpart comprising approximately 10% of benign vaginal cysts. They are often smaller than mullerian cysts and usually found along the lateral wall of the vagina. They are lined by a nonmucinous low columnar or cuboidal epithelium. They can be distinguished from mullerian cysts by the lack of ciliated epithelium, squamous metaplasia, and negative mucicarmine confirming the absence of mucin.

7.2.3 Bartholin's Gland Cysts
Bartholin's gland cysts arise due to blockage of Bartholin's duct, a 2.5 cm duct which drains into the vaginal vestibule adjacent to the hymen posteriolaterally. The gland itself is located in the posteriolateral vulva beneath the labia majora and minora. Blockage is usually a result of infection or increased viscosity of the secreted mucin. The cysts are found in the lateral introitus, range in size from 1 to 4 cm, and are usually unilateral, nontender, and asymptomatic.

Bartholin's duct is comprised of three types of epithelium: mucinous proximally and in gland acini, transitional in the middle, and squamous distally and at the entrance into the vestibule. Following this pattern, Bartholin's gland cysts can contain one, two, or all three epithelial types depending on size and location along the duct. Luminal contents consist of a clear mucoid liquid. Acute and chronic inflammations are not uncommon, and infection with resultant abscess can also be seen.

7.3 Nonembryonic Cysts

7.3.1 Epithelial Inclusion Cysts

EICs are the most common of the nonembryonic vaginal cysts. They are most often located in areas of previous surgery or trauma and are believed to be a result of traumatic inclusion of the normal vaginal mucosa. They range in size from a few millimeters to several centimeters. They are lined by stratified nonkeratinizing squamous epithelium lacking rete ridges. The lumen contains keratinaceous debris and desquamated cells. Rupture of the cyst can result in an exuberant chronic inflammatory or granulomatous reaction.

7.3.2 Endometriosis

Endometriotic cysts of the vagina can be superficial or deep. When superficial, they are located in the vaginal vault, are not associated with pelvic endometriosis, and are usually present at a site of previous surgery. Deep cysts are more common, are associated with pelvic endometriosis, and are most often located in the posterior fornix. Endometriotic cysts present as friable erythematous masses ranging in color from red to blue. Histologically, they are lined by endometrioid epithelium surrounded by endometrial stroma, hemosiderin pigment, and hemosiderin-laden macrophages.

References

Baker G, et al. Vulvar adnexal lesions. A 32-year, single-institution review from Massachusetts General Hospital. Arch Pathol Lab Med. 2013;137(9):1237–46.

Brenn T. Atypical genital nevus. Arch Pathol Lab Med. 2011;135(3):317–20.

Carlson J, et al. Vulvar lichen sclerosus and squamous cell carcinoma: a cohort, case control, and investigational study with historical perspective; implications for chronic inflammation and sclerosis in the development of neoplasia. Hum Pathol. 1998;29(9):932–48.

Cengiz F, et al. Dermoscopic and clinical features of pigmented skin lesions of the genital area. An Bras Dermatol. 2015;90(2):178–83.

Chan M, Zimarowski MJ. Vulvar dermatoses: a histopathologic review and classification of 183 cases. J Cutan Pathol. 2015;42:510–8.

Chiesa-Vottero A. Histopathologic study of thin vulvar squamous cell carcinomas and associated cutaneous lesions: a correlative study of 48 tumors in 44 patients with analysis of adjacent vulvar intraepithelial neoplasia types and lichen sclerosus. Am J Surg Pathol. 2006;30(3):310–8.

Docimo Jr S, et al. Bartholin's abscess arising within hidradenoma papilliferum of the vulva: a case report. Cases J. 2008;1(1):282.

Duhan N, et al. Hidradenoma papilliferum of the vulva: case report and review of literature. Arch Gynecol Obstet. 2011;284(4):1015–7.

Fistarol S, Itin PH. Diagnosis and treatment of lichen sclerosus. An update. Am J Clin Dermatol. 2013; 14(1):27–47.

Jackson, RJ. Dermatol. Surg. Oncol. 1984;10:2.

Kanj et al. Journal of American Academy of Dermatology. 1992;27(5):Part 1:77.

Jih D, et al. A histopathologic evaluation of vulvar melanosis. Arch Dermatol. 1999;135(7):857–8.

Kaufmann T, et al. Cystic papillary hidradenoma of the vulva: case report and review of the literature. Gynecol Oncol. 1987;26(2):240–5.

Lee E, et al. Pseudoepitheliomatous hyperplasia in lichen sclerosus of the vulva. Int J Gynecol Pathol. 2003; 22(1):57–62.

Madueke-Laveaux O, et al. Giant fibroepithelial stromal polyp of the vulva: largest case reported. Ann Surg Innov Res. 2013;7:8.

McCluggage W, et al. Myogenin expression in vulvovaginal spindle cell lesions: analysis of a series of cases with an emphasis on diagnostic pitfalls. Histopathology. 2013;63(4):545–50.

Murphy R. Lichen sclerosus. Dermatol Clin. 2010; 28(4):707–15.

Murzaku E, et al. Vulvar nevi, melanosis, and melanoma: an epidemiologic, clinical, and histopathologic review. J Am Acad Dermatol. 2014;71(6):1241–9.

Navada M, et al. Large fibroepithelial polyp of vulva. Case Rep Dermatol Med. 2011;2011:273181.

Nielsen G, Young RH. Mesenchymal tumors and tumor-like lesions of the female genital tract: a selective review with emphasis on recently described entities. Int J Gynecol Pathol. 2001;20(2):105–27.

Nucci M, et al. Cellular pseudosarcomatous fibroe pithelial stromal polyps of the lower female genital tract: an underrecognized lesion often misdiagnosed as sarcoma. Am J Surg Pathol. 2000;24(2):231–40.

Ostor A, et al. Fibroepithelial polyps with atypical stromal cells (pseudosarcoma botryoides) of vulva and vagina. A report of 13 cases. Int J Gynecol Pathol. 1988;7(4): 351–60.

Parks A, et al. Hidradenoma papilliferum with mixed histopathologic features of syringocystadenoma papilliferum and anogenital mammary-like glands: report of a case and review of the literature. Am J Dermatopathol. 2012;34(1):104–9.

Ribe A. Melanocytic lesions of the genital area with attention given to atypical genital nevi. J Cutan Pathol. 2008;35 Suppl 2:24–7.

Rudolph R. Vulvar melanosis. J Am Acad Dermatol. 1990;23(5 Pt 2):982–4.

Scurry J, et al. Histology of lichen sclerosus varies according to site and proximity to carcinoma. Am J Dermatopathol. 2001;23(5):413–8.

Scurry J, et al. Mammary-like gland adenoma of the vulva: review of 46 cases. Pathology. 2009;41(4):372–8.

Shah S, et al. Adenocarcinoma in situ arising in vulvar papillary hidradenoma: report of 2 cases. Int J Gynecol Pathol. 2008;27(3):453–6.

Vazmitel M, et al. Hidradenoma papilliferum with a ductal carcinoma in situ component: case report and review of the literature. Am J Dermatopathol. 2008;30(4): 392–4.

Venkatesan A. Pigmented lesions of the vulva. Dermatol Clin. 2010;28(4):795–805.

Virgili A, et al. Prospective clinical and epidemiologic study of vulvar lichen sclerosus: analysis of prevalence and severity of clinical features, together with Historical and Demographic Associations. Dermatology. 2014;228(2):145–51.

Weyers W. Hypertrophic lichen sclerosus with dyskeratosis and parakeratosis – a common presentation of vulvar lichen sclerosus not associated with a significant risk of malignancy. Am J Dermatopathol. 2013;35(7):713–21.

Malignant Vulvar and Vaginal Pathology

Grace N. Kim

Abstract

Vulvar and vaginal malignant pathology are dominated by squamous cell carcinoma and its variants. In the vulva, the majority of squamous cell carcinomas are non-HPV driven (human papilloma virus), while in the vagina, HPV infection is a key driver. In both lower genital tract sites, HPV is the main cause for low and high grade squamous intraepithelial precursor lesions. Their multifocality and synchronus and metachronous existence with lesions elsewhere in the genital tract are well-established defining characteristics. Additionally, melanomas are disproportionately prevalent in the vulva when comparing the total vulvar skin surface area to that of the entire body. Melanomas can also rarely occur in the vagina. Lastly, there are four entities distinctively found in the vulvovaginal region of the female gynecologic tract: extramammary Paget disease, aggressive angiomyxomas, embryonal rhabdomyosarcomas, and DES-related clear cell adenocarcinomas. An extensive list of different malignant entities that may occur in the vulvovaginal region are not reviewed here, but rather merely the most common.

Keywords

Human papilloma virus (HPV) • Low grade squamous lesion • Koilocyte • High grade squamous lesion • Squamous dysplasia • Differentiated-type VIN • Usual type VIN • Well-differentiated squamous cell carcinoma • Conventional squamous cell carcinoma • Melanoma • Basal cell carcinoma • Extramammary Paget disease • Merkel cell carcinoma • Aggressive angiomyxoma • Clear cell adenocarcinoma • Diethylstilbestrol (DES) • Embryonal rhabdomyosarcoma

Contents

G.N. Kim (✉)
Department of Pathology, University of Texas MD Anderson Cancer Center, Houston, TX, USA
e-mail: GNKim@mdanderson.org

© Springer International Publishing AG 2017
D. Shoupe (ed.), *Handbook of Gynecology*,
DOI 10.1007/978-3-319-17798-4_61

1   Introduction

Vulvar cancer comprises merely 0.3% of all new cancer cases in the United States, with an estimated 5,150 new cases in 2015. It contributes to 0.2% of all cancer deaths with 0.3% of women being diagnosed with vulvar cancer during their lifetime (Howlader et al. 2015). Albeit a rare malignancy of the female genital tract, vulvar cancer poses a significant clinical challenge due to its critical anatomic site at the junction of the urinary, gynecologic, and gastrointestinal systems. The associated complications, high morbidity, and multifocal recurrence are accredited to several factors, primarily the lack of effective treatment modalities which are limited currently to surgical excision, radiation, and chemotherapy. No single or combination treatment is entirely curative. Additionally, despite the well-established role of HPV infection as a driver of lower genital tract gynecologic pathology, non-HPV-driven vulvar malignancies are poorly understood and remain an area of continuing investigation.

Vaginal pathology, in comparison to the vulva, is a rare site for primary cancers. The majority of vaginal malignancies are secondary to direct extension or metastasis from nearby gynecologic sites, and merely 10–20% of tumors involving the vagina are in fact classified as primary vaginal disease (Kurman et al. 2011). Nonetheless, HPV-driven squamous cell carcinoma is the most common primary vaginal malignancy, as it is for the vulva.

2   Vulva

The most common vulvar malignancies are squamous cell carcinomas (approximately 95%) (Kurman et al. 2011), followed by malignant melanoma. The remainder of malignant tumors is comprised of adenocarcinomas and rarely neuroendocrine, soft tissue, and hematopoietic malignancies (Crum 2014a).

Vulvar squamous cell malignancies can be largely divided into HPV-driven and non-HPV-driven carcinomas. The HPV-driven malignancies and precursors occur in younger women (mean age 50 years), whereas non-HPV-driven carcinomas occur in an older age population (mean age 77 years). Different histologic subtypes and precursors are characteristic of each group (Kurman et al. 2011).

2.1   HPV-Driven Squamous Cell Carcinoma

HPV-driven squamous cell carcinomas of the vulva are largely associated with high risk HPV type 16. In adjacent areas, precursor lesions of intraepithelial squamous dysplasia are often seen. The precursor lesions of HPV-driven carcinomas are divided into low grade squamous intraepithelial lesion (LGSIL, historically vulvar intraepithelial neoplasia grade 1, VIN 1) and high grade squamous intraepithelial lesion (HGSIL, historically VIN 2 or 3), and both have identical histology as those found not only in the vagina, but rather the entire lower anogenital tract in both women and men. This nomenclature was widely published in 2012 through the work of The Lower Anogenital Squamous Terminology (LAST) Project and has since been recommended by the World Health Organization (WHO) for the vulva, vagina, and cervix (Darragh 2015).

Low grade squamous intraepithelial lesions can be associated with both low and high risk HPV types and tend to regress without further progression to cancer. Conversely, high grade squamous intraepithelial lesions carry a significant risk of progression to invasive carcinoma, which is three times amplified in patients who are immunosuppressed, in particular, with HIV infection. Synchronous or metachronous disease in other genital sites are not uncommon. Despite complete excision, 15% can recur and if excisional margins are positive, the recurrence rate increases to 50% (Crum 2014a).

Histologically, low grade and high grade squamous intraepithelial lesions are similar across all organ sites. Low grade squamous dysplasia is classically characterized by koilocytic atypia, which is most often found in the middle to upper portions of the squamous epithelium. Koilocytes are enlarged keratinocytes with hyperchromatic (dark), wrinkled, or raisinoid

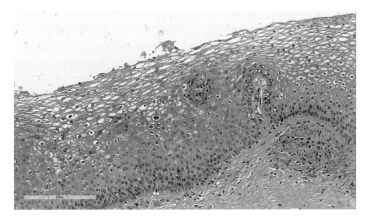

Fig. 1 Low grade squamous intraepithelial lesion (VAIN 1). Dysplastic keratinocytes involve the lower one-third of the squamous epithelium and are characterized by cellular enlargement, crowding, hyperchromasia, and increased mitoses. Koilocytes are most frequently found in the superficial third of the epithelium and have dark raisinoid or wrinkled nuclei with a well-demarcated perinuclear halo

nuclei surrounded by a well-demarcated perinuclear halo. The basal layer of the squamous epithelium is also hypercellular or crowded with dysplastic keratinocytes that are enlarged and hyperchromatic. These changes in the basal layer do not extend above the bottom one-third of the squamous epithelium (Fig. 1). On the contrary, high grade squamous intraepithelial lesions have dysplastic changes occupying a greater thickness of the epithelium (at least half or more). Historically, moderate dysplasia is confined to the bottom two-thirds of the epithelium and demonstrates a superficial layer of normal squamous maturation. Severe dysplasia extends the full thickness of the epithelium and may have overlying parakeratosis (retention of nuclei in stratum corneum) or a thickened granular layer. It however lacks normal keratinization or maturation of the top layers. Additionally, mitotic figures that are normally confined to the basal layer in normal epithelium and low grade dysplasia are seen throughout the upper half of the epithelium in high grade dysplasia. Atypical forms can also be seen (Fig. 2).

When the squamous dysplasia once contained within the squamous epithelium breaks through the basement membrane into the underlying stroma, the lesion meets criteria for an invasive squamous cell carcinoma. Squamous cell carcinomas in the vulva are characterized by a variable degree of maturation or differentiation and are classified on a spectrum of well to poorly differentiated. As a general rule, less differentiation correlates with fewer areas of keratinization. Of importance, the precise terminology of well-differentiated, *keratinizing* squamous cell carcinoma in the vulva is reserved for non-HPV-related carcinomas as discussed later in this chapter. Well-differentiated keratinizing squamous cell carcinomas can be deceiving on superficial biopsies due to its histologic similarity to benign or reactive squamous epithelium, despite its deeply invasive portions. Conventional squamous cell carcinomas can be subtyped into a variety of histologic variants, including basaloid, warty, verrucous, giant cell, spindle cell, acantholytic, papillary squamous, lymphoepithelioma-like, and plasmacytoid. Basaloid carcinomas (squamous cell carcinomas of the usual type) are commonly HPV 16 related and resemble the basal, non-mature cells of the squamous epithelium often seen in the classic type of squamous high grade dysplasia. These cells have scant cytoplasm and the tumor infiltrates the stroma as irregular nests and broad bands, cords, or cells (Fig. 3). Warty and verrucous carcinomas histologically resemble more mature squamous cells, often associated with keratinization. Warty type is characterized by areas of koilocytosis and fibrovascular cores, while the

Fig. 2 High grade squamous intraepithelial lesion (VAIN 3). Dysplastic keratinocytes involve the full thickness of the squamous epithelium. The cells are crowded, hyperchromatic, and enlarged with mitoses seen in the upper two-thirds of the epithelium

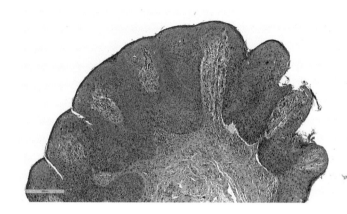

Fig. 3 Invasive moderately differentiated squamous cell carcinoma (conventional type). This basaloid subtype of invasive squamous cell carcinoma is associated with an overlying high grade squamous intraepithelial lesion (VIN 3). Nests of cells infiltrate the superficial stroma and a focus of lymph-vascular space invasion is seen on the *left*

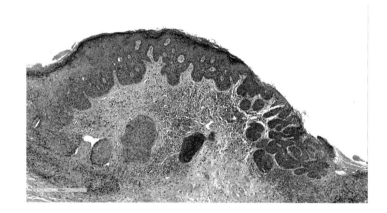

verrucous type lacks koilocytosis and fibrovascular cores, and has an exophytic papillary surface and association with HPV 6. Of importance, the verrucous type is composed of well-differentiated neoplastic cells with keratinization and absence of significant atypia or pleomorphism. Verrucous carcinoma has the best prognosis, followed by warty, and finally the basaloid type.

2.2 Non-HPV-Driven Squamous Cell Carcinoma

The most prevalent type of invasive squamous cell carcinoma of the vulva is the well-differentiated keratinizing squamous cell carcinoma. It comprises approximately 65–80% of vulvar cases. Characteristically, keratinizing squamous cell carcinoma occurs in older women (70s) and is associated with chronic vulvar disease or vulvar dystrophy, such as lichen sclerosus and less commonly, lichen planus. Keratinizing squamous cell carcinoma is not associated with HPV infection nor the usual vulvar intraepithelial neoplasia (uVIN), but rather a vulva-specific precursor lesion termed differentiated-type VIN (D-VIN) or VIN simplex. The risk of progression to cancer in differentiated-type VIN increases with age and the duration of the preceding chronic skin disease, and is more frequent compared to uVIN (33% vs. 5.7%) (Reyes and Cooper 2014).

D-VIN is a difficult histologic diagnosis, vastly different from the features of usual VIN or squamous dysplasia. D-VIN has a mitotically active basal layer with nuclear atypia characterized by

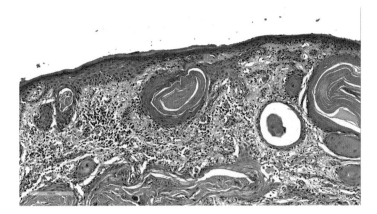

Fig. 4 Differentiated VIN (D-VIN). This precursor of non-HPV-driven squamous cell carcinoma of the vulva is a difficult histologic diagnosis. Enlarged dysplastic keratinocytes with prominent nucleoli, significant intercellular edema (spongiosis), abundant eosinophilic cytoplasm, and occasional mitoses can be seen in the parabasal and basal layers. Keratin pearls at the base of rete ridges is a characteristic finding

dyskeratosis (abnormal keratinization), prominent nucleoli, abundant eosinophilic cytoplasm, and spongiosis (intercellular edema). These features can be seen throughout enlarged keratinocytes of the basal and parabasal layers. Distinctively, squamous keratin pearls are present at the inferior portion of the elongated and anastomosing rete ridges. Hyperkeratosis is nearly always present (Fig. 4). P53 mutations have been associated with D-VIN; however, concordance with the p53 immunostain is variable. The surrogate marker for HPV, the p16 immunohistochemical stain, would be invariably negative. Of note, HPV-driven and non-HPV-driven precursor and invasive lesions can occur simultaneously, and thus the usual type of VIN can occur alongside D-VIN or in the background of a well-differentiated keratinizing squamous cell carcinoma in 5% of cases (Kurman et al. 2011).

Well-differentiated keratinizing squamous cell carcinoma is best characterized by dyskeratosis (abundant eosinophilic cytoplasm) and extensive keratinization that manifests as keratin pearls within the tumor. The tumor cells are large, crowded, and dark, forming invasive islands and nests, often with an irregular invasive border. In keeping with a well-differentiated squamous malignancy, intercellular bridges are well formed and histologically recognizable (Fig. 5).

2.3 Malignant Melanoma

The second most common malignant neoplasm of the vulva after squamous cell carcinoma is malignant melanoma, comprising nearly 9% of all vulvar malignancies (Kurman et al. 2011). The vulvar skin comprises merely 1–2% of the human body's total skin surface area; however, 3–7% of melanomas ailing female patients occur in the vulva. Therefore, although vulvar melanomas and melanomas of the lower female genital tract are rare, there is a notable predilection of melanomas for the vulvar region. Vulvar melanomas follow an aggressive clinical course. (Mert et al. 2013; Rouzbahman et al. 2015).

Akin to melanomas elsewhere, melanomas of the vulva are most prevalent in women with fair skin and can be associated with precursor pigmented lesions with or without atypia. They tend to occur in an older age population (median age of 67 years at diagnosis) compared to melanomas involving cutaneous skin and are less commonly driven by BRAF mutations (Rouzbahman et al. 2015). Additionally, in contrast to cutaneous melanomas, melanomas of the vulva are not driven by exposure to UV light, and hence the incidence of vulvar melanomas has been consistent over time (Mert et al. 2013). Prognostic factors of vulvar melanoma have been studied to be

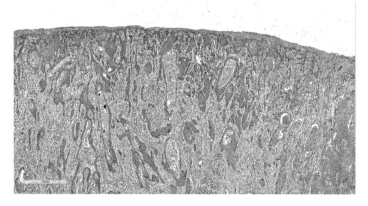

Fig. 5 Well-differentiated keratinizing squamous cell carcinoma is characterized by keratinization in the form of squamous pearls, dyskeratosis (abundant eosinophilic cytoplasm), and prominent intercellular bridges. The tumor forms islands and nests of enlarged, crowded cells with hyperchromatic nuclei and an irregular invasive border. Mitoses are common

similar across melanomas of different anatomic sites and include level of invasion (Clark level) and tumor thickness (Breslow). The most critical prognostic marker is lymph node involvement. Despite these analogous characteristics between cutaneous and vulvar melanomas, an optimal staging system for vulvar melanoma has yet to be consolidated (Mert et al. 2013). Additionally, histologic features that influence survival include mitotic count, surface ulceration, inflammatory response, tumor necrosis, lymph-vascular space invasion, and recurrence. Recurrences can occur in neighboring vulvar sites such as the urethra, vagina, cervix, and rectum, or metastasize to distant locations. Prognosis after recurrence is poor (Kurman et al. 2011).

Melanomas occur equally across anatomic sites of the vulva including the labia minora, labia majora, and clitoris; however, they frequently occur at the junction of the mucosa and skin in glabrous skin (smooth, non-hair bearing). The three major histologic types of melanomas arising in the vulva include the most common mucosal/lentiginous type, followed by nodular and superficial spreading types (Reichert 2012) (Fig. 6). Patterns of dermal invasion include single cells or nests and cords of atypical melanocytes with variable degrees of epithelioid, spindled, or nevoid morphology. A lymphocytic infiltrate often accompanies the invasion and an increased mitotic count signals a malignant process. With extensive variation in the histology of malignant melanocytes, melanomas have been coined as the "great mimicker," with an ability to recapitulate the histologic features of any malignant tumor at any site. Hence, a combination of melanocytic markers such as a S-100, HMB-45, Melan-A, tyrosinase, and MiTF can be employed to render the correct diagnosis. Additionally, molecular testing is currently advancing not only diagnosis, but also therapeutic options.

2.4 Basal Cell Carcinoma

This common carcinoma of the skin can also be found on the vulva, most frequently the labia majora. They account for approximately 3–5% of vulvar malignancies unlike the very prevalent cutaneous form (Reichert, 2012), and the infiltrative type comprises nearly one-half of all cases. The histologic features are identical to basal cell carcinomas found elsewhere with a small basaloid cell population and classic peripheral palisading pattern. Wide local excision is the most common treatment modality in this often low grade lesion, although local recurrence can certainly occur.

Fig. 6 Malignant melanoma. Melanoma is characterized by an increase in atypical melanocytes lining the basal layer of the epithelium with budding nests into the stroma. These lesions can be melanotic or amelanotic and can exhibit various patterns of growth, most commonly mucosal/lentiginous in the vulva. In the vagina, the nodular type is the most common.

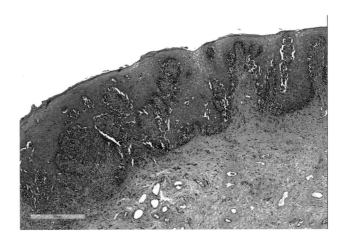

2.5 Adenocarcinoma

Adenocarcinoma of the vulva is the rarest type of carcinoma arising in the vulva. Most adenocarcinomas of the vulva are derived from the Bartholin gland; however, due to the presence of skin appendages in the vulvar skin, adenocarcinomas of adnexal structures (sweat glands) and other vulvar components (Skene's glands) can be seen. Bartholin gland adenocarcinomas often present as a painless swelling in the area of the Bartholin glands (4 and 8 o'clock position of vulva) and can have mucinous, papillary, or rarely clear cell morphology. Of note, the Bartholin gland can harbor adenocarcinomas (40%), but also squamous cell carcinomas (40%), adenosquamous carcinomas (5%), adenoid cystic carcinomas, transitional cell carcinomas, neuroendocrine carcinomas, and Merkel cell carcinoma (Crum 2014b).

Rarely, an adenocarcinoma of the vulva can be associated with an overlying extramammary Paget disease. The more common finding is that of Paget disease in isolation. Paget disease is often associated with pruritus and eczematous change and is most commonly found on the labia majora or minora. Recurrences frequently occur after local resection (33%); however, invasion is less common. "Paget cells" are large round cells with ample cytoplasm and prominent nucleoli that are scattered as single cells or in clusters throughout the epithelium. with a greater density of cells in the basal layer. Single cells tend to float upwards towards the stratum corneum in a percolating fashion, a process traditionally described as pagetoid spread. Paget cells can often also infiltrate neighboring adnexal structures. Characteristically, Paget cells contain PAS-D positive material and immunohistochemically are positive for CK7, CAM 5.2, GCDFP-15, and carcinoembryonic antigen (CEA). In the case of S-100 positivity, melanoma must be excluded with additional immunohistochemical studies. P53 positivity in vulvar Paget cells has also been linked to metastatic disease in lymph nodes (Crum 2014a) (Fig. 7).

2.6 Neuroendocrine Carcinoma

The predominance of the already rare vulvar neuroendocrine carcinoma is mainly attributed to Merkel cell carcinoma, a neuroendocrine carcinoma of the skin. The incidence of Merkel cell carcinomas tends to increase with age and immunosuppression. Often times they present clinically as a single surface nodule or multiple nodules and can be associated with a squamous cell carcinoma or usual type VIN.

Histologically, Merkel cell carcinoma resembles neuroendocrine tumors elsewhere (small cell carcinoma of the lung) and are comprised of small ovoid cells with scant cytoplasm and stippled

Fig. 7 Extramammary
Paget disease.
Extramammary Paget
disease is most frequently
an intraepidermal process of
single cells or clusters of
Paget cells. The malignant
cells are round and large
with abundant cytoplasm. A
higher density of cells is
often found at the basal
layer with cells percolating
to the surface. Paget disease
can be associated with an
underlying adenocarcinoma

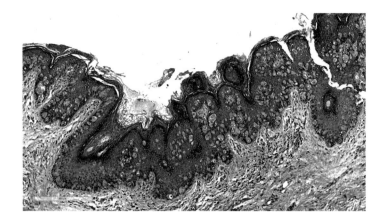

chromatin to small cell carcinoma of the lung. Small polygonal cells with scant cytoplasm, granular chromatin, and small nucleoli characterize a second histologic type that resembles a low grade or well-differentiated neuroendocrine tumor previously known as carcinoid tumor. Foci of secondary glandular or squamous differentiation and adjacent intraepidermal pagetoid spread can also be seen. The prognosis of Merkel cell carcinoma is largely driven by tumor size and stage. In keeping with the universally guarded prognosis of neuroendocrine carcinomas, one-third of vulvar neuroendocrine carcinomas are linked to tumor-related mortality (Crum 2014b).

2.7   Aggressive Angiomyxoma

This low grade lesion is often found in the reproductive women involving the deep soft tissues of the vulva, vagina, or perineum and is commonly clinically mistaken for a Bartholin gland cyst. Contrary to its benign mimicker, aggressive angiomyxomas have infiltrative borders that complicate its accurate excision and propagate local recurrence. These lesions are usually large and gelatinous with histologically hypocellular and abundant, Alcian blue positive, myxoid material. Small, innocuous-appearing spindle to stellate cells are dispersed throughout, and variably sized vessels with widely patent lumens are frequently seen in a patternless, random distribution. Entrapped smooth muscle fibers and nerve twigs, extravasated red blood cells, and

mast cells can be seen. Absence of certain features, such as multinucleation, mitoses, and necrosis are also characteristic. Most importantly, the edges of the tumor are poorly circumscribed and infiltrative into surrounding adipose tissue. Aggressive angiomyxomas are positive for vimentin, estrogen receptor (ER), progesterone receptor (PR), and HMGA2 (Fig. 8).

3   Vagina

The vagina is largely a rare site of primary malignant pathology. There is no one malignant tumor that is unique to the vagina, and most vaginal malignancies are either more commonly found elsewhere in the female lower genital tract or are contributable to field effect (HPV-related), metastasis, or tumor recurrences of adjacent sites. For example, the vagina is the most common site of recurrence for endometrial carcinomas after hysterectomy. Consequentially, a few of the most common vaginal malignancies will be mentioned here, albeit the majority have been more thoroughly discussed elsewhere.

3.1   Vaginal Squamous Intraepithelial Lesions

In line with the recommendation of The Lower Anogenital Squamous Terminology (LAST) Project, all HPV-driven squamous precursor lesions

Fig. 8 Aggressive angiomyxoma. Vulvar aggressive angiomyxomas are deep soft tissue neoplasms that have infiltrative borders and vessels of varying wall thickness. The stroma is hypocellular with bland, spindle cells embedded in a background of abundant and homogenous, loose myxoid stroma

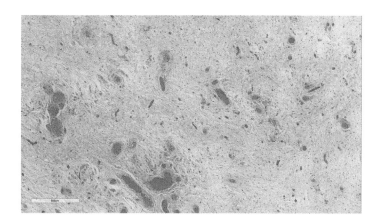

regardless of site of involvement are classified as low grade squamous intraepithelial lesion (LGSIL, historically vaginal intraepithelial neoplasia or VAIN 1) or high grade squamous intraepithelial lesion (HGSIL, historically VAIN 2 or 3). The vagina, compared to the cervix and vulva, is the least common site for LGSIL and HGSIL, and vaginal lesions are most often multifocal and found in the company of other cervical or vulvar lesions, synchronous or metachronous. The majority of vaginal lesions (80–90%) occur in the upper vagina and are associated with high risk HPV types, in particular HPV 16, regardless of the degree of dysplasia (Reichert 2012). The risk of progression in these lesions to invasive carcinoma is 5% (Sillman et al. 1997). The histologic findings of squamous dysplasia in the vagina are no different from those found in the vulva and cervix (Fig. 2).

3.2 Squamous Cell Carcinoma

The World Health Organization (WHO) definition of primary vaginal squamous cell carcinoma includes only those carcinomas with exclusive disease in the vagina. Prior and/or concurrent invasive squamous cell carcinoma of the cervix or vulva, or any other carcinomas of adjacent sites preclude a diagnosis of primary vaginal squamous cell carcinoma. As such, vaginal squamous cell carcinoma is rare, with an incidence of 0.69/ 100,000 women (age-adjusted). Nevertheless, it

is the most common malignant tumor of the vagina with higher incidence in black versus white women (Ferenczy et al. 2014). A predominance of vaginal squamous cell carcinomas is associated with high risk HPV infection; although, analogous to the vulva, a non-HPV-driven etiology of some squamous carcinomas is noted particularly in the lower parts of the vagina. The most common site of occurrence for squamous cell carcinoma however is the posterior, upper third vagina. Histologically, the most common variant of squamous cell carcinoma is of moderate differentiation with absence of keratinization. Other rare types, including verrucous, basaloid, warty, and papillary have been reported. Verrucous carcinoma is associated with the most favorable survival rate.

3.3 Adenocarcinomas

Adenocarcinomas comprise the majority, if not all, of the vaginal malignancies that occur in women under the age of 20 years. The most well-known adenocarcinoma is clear cell carcinoma, due to its association with diethylstilbestrol (DES) exposure in utero. DES was historically utilized in pregnant mothers from 1940 to 1971. The daughters of mothers having taken DES during the first trimester of pregnancy have the highest risk of developing clear cell carcinoma at a young age ranging from 7 to 33 years. The risk in these women through the age of 34 is

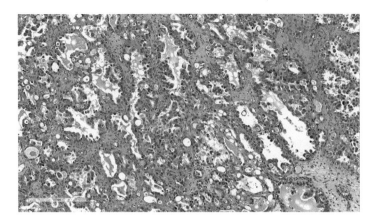

Fig. 9 Clear cell carcinoma. Clear cell carcinomas in the gynecologic tract are similar regardless of the site of involvement. These tumors are heterogeneous, with areas of papillary, solid, and tubulocystic patterns. Common histologic findings include cytoplasmic eosinophilic hyaline globules, hobnailing of atypical nuclei, fibrotic stroma, and ample clear or eosinophilic

about 1 in 1000 (Melnick et al. 1987). A second risk factor for clear cell carcinoma is increased endogenous estrogen levels. Due to the widely publicized risk of DES exposure in utero, the rate of clear cell carcinoma of both the vagina and cervix has declined, and DES is no longer used under the therapeutic misconception of reducing pregnancy-related complications and miscarriages.

Clear cell carcinoma is most often found in the upper third of the anterior vaginal wall. The histology is identical to the clear cell carcinomas found elsewhere in the female gynecologic tract. Briefly, the three main patterns are papillary, tubulocystic, and solid, often with nuclear hobnailing (protrusion of nuclei from the cytoplasm), hyperchromatic nuclei, hyalinized stroma, and abundant clear to eosinophilic cytoplasm. Intracytoplasmic eosinophilic hyaline globules are characteristic, and mitotic activity and nuclear pleomorphism are underwhelming compared to other high grade carcinomas (Fig. 9).

Endometrioid adenocarcinoma is another adenocarcinoma that can be found in the vagina, with identical histologic features as those in the endometrium and ovary. They have been associated with DES exposure and also endometriosis similar to clear cell adenocarcinomas.

Lastly, mucinous carcinomas similar to the intestinal and endocervical types of the cervix can also be seen in the vagina. Little is known about the prognosis or histogenesis of this tumor in the vagina due to its rarity. Classic histomorphologic features are deferred to the description of mucinous carcinomas of the cervix.

3.4 Sarcoma

Sarcomas of the vagina are rare; however, one malignant sarcoma is of notable mention as the most common vaginal sarcoma – rhabdomyosarcoma. The three variants of rhabdomyosarcoma are as follows: embryonal, alveolar, and pleomorphic. The most common variant in the vagina is the embryonal rhabdomyosarcoma, the majority (90%) occurring in young patients, mainly infants and children under the age of 5 years. However, these sarcomas can rarely occur in the older population.

Classically, embryonal rhabdomyosarcomas are clinically described as "grape-like" polypoid extrusions from the vagina, and are appropriately named sarcoma botryoides from the Greek term "botryose" meaning "bunch of grapes." Histologically, these polypoid projections are covered by squamous epithelium, with or without surface ulceration, and a cambium layer immediately underneath the epithelium. The cambium layer is an area of cellular density beneath the squamous

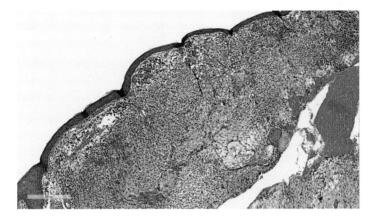

Fig. 10 Embryonal rhabdomyosarcoma. Embryonal rhabdomyosarcoma is the most common subtype of rhabdomyosarcoma found in the vagina. Clinically and histologically, they are polypoid with a densely cellular region beneath the epithelium (cambium layer). A population of hyperchromatic malignant rhabdoid cells infiltrates the deeper layers in alternating areas of cellularity in a background of myxoid material

epithelium comprised of hyperchromatic nuclei. The remainder of the lesion exhibits areas of alternating hypo- and hypercellularity with round to spindle cells and scant cytoplasm. Typical rhabdoid features of an eccentrically located nucleus with abundant pink or eosinophilic cytoplasm can be seen. Cross striations of mature skeletal muscle are less common. Mitotic figures are easily found and the background stroma is usually loose and myxoid in nature. Despite historically poor clinical outcomes in young patients, current therapy combinations are highly effective with cure rates of greater than 90% (Nucci 2014a) (Fig. 10).

3.5 Malignant Melanoma

Malignant melanomas comprise 4% of malignancies occurring in the vagina and merely comprise 0.4% of all melanomas. As opposed to the most common vulvar melanoma subtype, mucosal/lentiginous, melanomas of the vagina are frequently nodular. Most are pigmented with high mitotic rates, although less commonly there is absence of pigmentation or a lymphocytic response. The usual melanocytic immunohistochemical markers confirm the diagnosis. The prognosis of vaginal melanomas is extremely poor (5-year survival rate of 0–21%), and the most significant prognostic factor is tumor size (Cao and Hirschowitz 2014).

4 Cross-References

▶ Benign Vulvar and Vaginal Pathology

References

Cao D, Hirschowitz L. Melanocytic tumours. In: Kurman RJ et al., editors. WHO classification of tumours of female reproductive o. 4th ed. Lyon: IARC; 2014.

Crum CP, et al. Neuroendocrine tumours. In: Kurman RJ et al., editors. WHO classification of tumours of female reproductive organs. 4th ed. Lyon: IARC; 2014a.

Crum CP, et al. Tumours of the vulva: epithelial tumours. In: Kurman RJ et al., editors. WHO classification of tumours of female reproductive organs. 4th ed. Lyon: IARC; 2014b.

Darragh TM. The LAST project and the diagnostic bottom line. Cytopathology. 2015;26:343–5.

Ferenczy AS, et al. Tumours of the vagina: epithelial tumours. In: Kurman RJ et al., editors. WHO classification of tumours of female reproductive organs. 4th ed. Lyon: IARC; 2014.

Howlader N, Noone AM, Krapcho M, Garshell J, Miller D, Altekruse SF, Kosary CL, Yu M, Ruhl J, Tatalovich Z, Mariotto A, Lewis DR, Chen HS, Feuer EJ, Cronin KA, editors. SEER cancer statistics review, 1975–2012. Bethesda: National Cancer Institute; 2015. http://seer.cancer.gov/csr/1975_2012/. Based on November 2014 SEER data submission, posted to the SEER web site, Apr 2015.

Kurman RJ, et al. Blaustein's pathology of the female genital tract. New York: Springer; 2011.

Melnick S, et al. Rates and risks of diethylstilbestrol-related clear-cell adenocarcinoma of the vagina and cervix. N Engl J Med. 1987;316(9):514–6.

Mert I, et al. Vulvar/vaginal melanoma: an updated surveillance epidemiology and end results database review. Comparison with cutaneous melanoma and significant of racial disparities. Int J Gynecol Cancer. 2013; 23(6):1118–25.

Nucci MR, et al. Mesenchymal tumours. In: Kurman RJ et al., editors. WHO classification of tumours of female reproductive organs. 4th ed. Lyon: IARC; 2014a.

Nucci MR, et al. Melanocytic tumours. In: Kurman RJ et al., editors. WHO classification of tumours of female reproductive organs. 4th ed. Lyon: IARC; 2014b.

Reichert RA. Diagnostic gynecologic and obstetric pathology: an atlas and text. Philadelphia: Lippincott Williams & Wilkins; 2012.

Reyes MC, Cooper K. An update on vulvar intraepithelial neoplasia: terminology and a practical approach to diagnosis. J Clin Pathol. 2014;67:290–4.

Rouzbahman M, et al. Malignant Melanoma of Vulva and Vagina: a histomorphological review and mutation analysis – a single-center study. J Low Genit Tract Dis. 2015;19(4):350–3.

Sillman FH, et al. Vaginal intraepithelial neoplasia: risk factors for persistence, recurrence, and invasion and its management. Am J Obstet Gynecol. 1997;176(1):93–9.

Lesions of the Uterine Cervix

Saloni Walia and Paulette Mhawech-Fauceglia

Abstract

The fact that cervical epithelium is prone to microtrauma and its proliferation is hormonally influenced by estrogen and progesterone leads to a wide spectrum of cervical epithelial lesions. These lesions include repair, atrophy, metaplasia, infection, and inflammatory processes, as well as malignant tumors and their precursors. The uterine cervix is also unique as it is accessible to screening by Pap smears thus allowing early diagnoses of lesions. Epithelial tumors such as squamous and glandular tumors have well-characterized precursor lesions, including cervical intraepithelial neoplasia and adenocarcinoma in situ. These precursor lesions as well as epithelial malignancies are mainly caused by human papillomavirus (HPV) infection, and screening algorithms include co-testing by Pap test and HPV DNA detection. Cervical lesions are broadly classified into epithelial and mesenchymal subtypes. Epithelial tumors are by far the most common, and they are further subclassified as squamous cell carcinoma, adenocarcinoma, and neuroendocrine carcinomas. Mesenchymal tumors (sarcomas) are rare, and they are classified based on the cell of origin of the tumor. Tumors with mixed phenotypes are rare occurrences. This chapter provides a brief overview of the histological patterns of the common cervical lesions with a focus on epithelial malignant tumors and their precursors.

Keywords

Uterine cervix • Human papillomavirus (HPV) • Epithelial tumors and precursors • Mesenchymal tumors

Contents

S. Walia
Department of Pathology and Laboratory Medicine, Los Angeles County and University of Southern California Medical Center, Los Angeles, CA, USA
e-mail: saloni.b.walia@gmail.com

P. Mhawech-Fauceglia (✉)
Division of Gynecologic Oncologic Pathology, Department of Pathology, Keck School of Medicine, University of Southern California, Los Angeles, CA, USA
e-mail: pfauceglia@hotmail.com; mhawechf@usc.edu

© Springer International Publishing AG 2017
D. Shoupe (ed.), *Handbook of Gynecology*,
DOI 10.1007/978-3-319-17798-4_62

1   Introduction

Uterine cervix is anatomically divided into the ectocervix lined by squamous epithelium and the endocervix lined by columnar epithelium. The transformation zone is the transition zone between the ectocervix and endocervix and is the region of high cell turnover. Precursor lesions have been identified in the uterine cervix most commonly in the transformation zone. Clinically, many benign or reactive epithelial lesions might visually mimic malignancy, and definitive diagnosis can be made only by biopsy and histologic evaluation. In addition, the uterine cervix is amenable to cytologic screening by Pap test, which has proved to be an important public health strategy leading to a decline in the overall incidence of cervical cancer. However, cervical cancer is still the fourth most common cancer among women worldwide (Ferlay et al. 2015). Cervical cancer causes significant morbidity and mortality in the developing world where universal screening by Pap test is not available. Underlying the epithelium is cervical stroma, which is composed mainly of fibroelastic tissue laced by few smooth muscle fibers. Additionally, vessels, nerves, and remnants of the Wolffian mesonephric ducts are present in the stroma. Rarely, proliferation of these mesenchymal elements leads to development of benign or malignant tumors. This chapter provides a brief overview of the cytologic and histopathologic changes characteristics of the common lesions affecting the cervix.

2   Epithelial Lesions/Tumors

2.1   Benign Lesions

Squamous Metaplasia Squamous metaplasia is the replacement of benign endocervical epithelium by benign squamous epithelium. This occurs by proliferation of the reserve cells forming immature squamous epithelium followed by maturation to benign squamous epithelium that cannot be distinguished from ectocervical epithelium (Wright et al. 2011a).

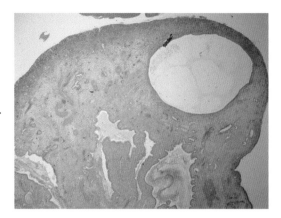

Fig. 1 Endocervical polyp: Polypoid lesion covered by endocervical mucinous epithelium and containing dilated endocervical glands, fibrotic stroma, and increased numbers of thick-walled blood vessels

Squamous Atrophy Squamous atrophy is seen during childhood and postmenopausal years due to the absence of estrogen stimulation. It is characterized by absence of glycogen in cells and lack of surface epithelial maturation. While the cells may lose their polarity, there is residual cohesion and absence of atypia distinguishing it from in situ premalignant lesions.

Endocervical Polyps Endocervical polyps are the most common benign tumors of the cervix. They most commonly occur in women in the fourth to sixth decades of life. The initial presentation includes leukorrhea or abnormal bleeding (Wright et al. 2011a). Histologically, the most common presentation is crypts and glands lined by endocervical mucinous epithelium surrounded by fibrotic stroma containing thick-walled blood vessels (Fig. 1). Dysplastic and malignant changes are very rarely seen in endocervical polyps (Long et al. 2013).

2.2   Premalignant Squamous Cell Neoplasia/Cervical Intraepithelial Neoplasia

Squamous cell carcinoma (SCC) is preceded by a substantial period of preinvasive disease. Tumor cells lose the cohesive properties of normal cells and can be easily scraped, making them very easily accessible for screening by cytological preparations. Epithelial tumors arise from the transformation zone of the cervix, and they are known to be associated with high-risk human papillomavirus (HPV) infection which begins at the basal cells of the cervical epithelium (Walbommers et al. 1999). Due to numerous years of research, mechanism of malignant transformation of the squamous epithelium by HPV is now well characterized. HPV gene product E6 attaches to the p53 tumor suppressor protein, and the E7 gene product binds the retinoblastoma gene product (pRB) causing deregulation of the host cell cycle. This leads to an increase in cellular proliferation and progressive involvement of the entire thickness of the cervical epithelium by HPV DNA (Burd 2003). HPV infection also causes disruption of cytokeratin framework in the cytoplasm of the host cell, leading to cytoplasmic clearing and perinuclear haloes (Lawson et al. 2009). Untreated infection by high-risk HPV can cause progression of cervical intraepithelial carcinoma to invasive carcinoma.

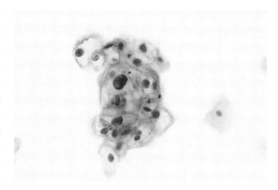

Fig. 2 LSIL: A cluster of large atypical cells is present with large irregular nuclei, clumped chromatin, perinuclear haloes, and a peripheral rim of dense cytoplasm

2.2.1 Cytology

On Pap smear, nuclear enlargement, hyperchromasia, irregular chromatin distribution, and clumping are the most common features of dysplastic cells. Based on the degree of these features, abnormal squamous cells can further be divided into low-grade squamous intraepithelial lesions (LSIL) and high-grade squamous intraepithelial lesions (HSIL). LSIL represents productive HPV infection and is self-limited in most patients. HSIL is a true neoplastic process with a capacity to progress to invasive disease if left untreated.

LSIL LSIL is characterized by at least a three-fold nuclear enlargement, hyperchromasia, and variation in nuclear shape as well as contour, in the superficial or intermediate cells of the squamous epithelium. Koilocytes are characteristic cells of LSIL and have well-defined perinuclear haloes surrounded by a rim of dense cytoplasm (Fig. 2). Binucleation and multinucleation are commonly seen.

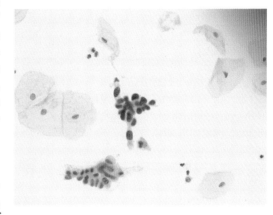

Fig. 3 HSIL: The center has an aggregate of atypical cells with high nuclear to cytoplasmic ratios, hyperchromatic nuclei, and absence of prominent nucleoli. Scattered benign squamous cells with small nuclei and abundant cytoplasm are present in the background for comparison

HSIL HSIL is characterized by cells that are less mature and have higher nuclear to cytoplasmic ratios than those seen in LSIL. The nuclear changes including hyperchromasia, chromatin clumping, and nuclear membrane irregularities are more severe in HSIL (Fig. 3).

HSIL can be further classified as small cell type, large cell non-keratinizing type, and large cell keratinizing type (Wright et al. 2011b). The small cell type consists of basal-type cells with very high nuclear to cytoplasmic ratios. The large cell non-keratinizing type has cells with large nuclei that form syncytial-like sheets where individual cell membranes cannot be discerned. The

large keratinizing cells consist of keratinized
orangeophilic atypical pleomorphic cells (Wright
et al. 2011b).

2.2.2 Histology

Definitive diagnosis of intraepithelial neoplasia is
made by histopathology usually on cervical
biopsy specimens. The hallmark of squamous
dysplasia is lack of polarity, the presence of
nuclear atypia, and frequent as well as atypical
mitosis. Once the diagnosis of dysplasia is made,
the next step is to classify it as low-grade cervical
intraepithelial neoplasia (CIN 1) or high-grade
dysplasia (CIN 2, 3) based on its severity.

Cervical Intraepithelial Neoplasia 1 (CIN1)
Low-grade dysplasia is defined as dysplastic
cells confined only to the lower third of the cervical squamous epithelium, signifying a mild delay
in epithelial cell maturation (Martin and O'Leary
2011). In addition, it is also defined by
koilocytosis which are superficial squamous epithelium cells with nuclear enlargement, atypia and
perinuclear haloes (Wright et al. 2011b). There is
generally a well-preserved polarity with uniform
transitions to mature epithelium (Crum et al.
2011). Marked atypia and abnormal mitotic
figures are not a feature of CIN1 (Fig. 4).

**Cervical Intraepithelial Neoplasia 2 and 3
(CIN2 and CIN3)** High-grade dysplasia is
defined by dysplastic cells occupying more than
half of the squamous epithelium thickness (CIN2)
or by involvement of the entire squamous epithelium thickness (CIN3). Because it is difficult to
differentiate between CIN2 and CIN3 and the
treatment is very similar for both, these are usually
referred as high-grade dysplasia (Fig. 5).

In few circumstances, differentiating between
low-grade and high-grade dysplasia can be very
challenging; immunohistochemistry using p16
and ki67 antibodies is used to overcome this issue.

p16 Cellular levels of p16 have been found to be
upregulated in high-risk HPV-infected cervical
cells. p16 is a cyclin-dependent kinase, whose
downstream effect is blocked by productive

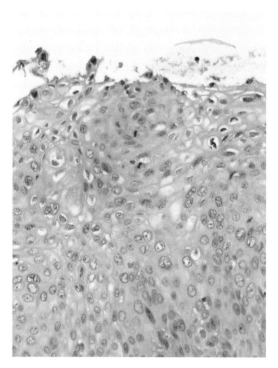

Fig. 4 CIN1: Superficial cells show koilotypic atypia with
nuclear enlargement, nuclear irregularities, chromatin
clumping, and sharp perinuclear haloes. Binucleation and
multinucleation of cells are identified

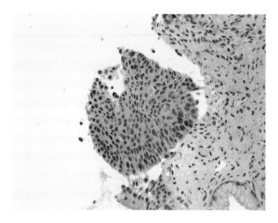

Fig. 5 CIN3: Large atypical cells that have lost their
polarity extend to the full thickness of the epidermis with
frequent Mitosis and absence of stromal invasion

HPV infection, causing accumulation and strong
overexpression of p16 in infected cells (Cuschieri
and Wentzensen 2008). Positive p16 immunostaining is expressed as a diffuse, strong,

parabasal nuclear staining pattern and is suggestive of a transforming infection by high-risk HPV and accompanied CIN2/3. The low-grade lesions which are associated with low-risk HPV infections tend to exhibit a focal and scattered weak blush of p16 rather than the diffuse strong granular staining pattern typical for HSIL (Martin and O'Leary 2011).

Ki67 Ki67 is an antigen that identifies proliferating cells. MIB-1 is a monoclonal antibody that detects this antigen in the cell's nuclei in paraffin tissue sections. Positive MIB-1 staining in parabasal cells of the squamous epithelium is found under normal conditions. Distinction of a CIN2/3 from nonneoplastic epithelium is based on the presence of MIB-1-positive cells in the middle and upper thirds of the epithelium. A high index of Ki67 nuclear staining and diffuse p16 nuclear and cytoplasmic expression involving most of the mucosal thickness are highly suggestive of high-grade dysplasia.

2.3 Invasive Squamous Cell Carcinoma

Histologically, the hallmark of invasive squamous cell carcinoma (SCC) is stromal invasion by malignant cells leading to a stromal loosening, desmoplasia, and/or increased epithelial cell cytoplasmic eosinophilia (Kurman et al. 2014). Squamous cells breach the basement membrane and invade the stroma. Malignant squamous cells are characterized by high nuclear/cytoplasmic ratio, hyperchromatic nuclei, pink cytoplasm, and frequent mitotic figures. On the other hand, desmoplastic reaction is defined by loose somewhat edematous stroma, associated with chronic and acute inflammation surrounding tumor cells (Kurman et al. 2014) (Fig. 6).

2.3.1 Microinvasive Squamous Cell Carcinomas (MicrSCCs)

Based on the International Federation of Gynecologic Oncologists (FIGO), they are defined as microscopic tumors that invade to less than 5 mm into the depth of the epithelium and have

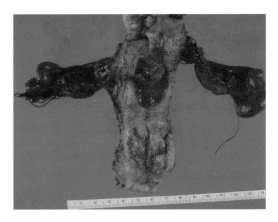

Fig. 6 Gross appearance of invasive squamous cell carcinoma: Irregular large tumor is seen to invade the endocervical mucosa. There is obliteration of the endocervical canal and invasion of the cervical stroma

a horizontal span of less than 7 mm. However, the Society of Gynecologic Oncologists definition uses a depth of invasion of less than 3 mm and an absence of lymphovascular invasion (Cebellos et al. 2006). MicrSCCs are associated with excellent long-term survival after surgical treatment.

2.3.2 Invasive Squamous Cell Carcinoma

Invasive SCCs can have multiple morphological variations and may present as sheetlike growth or single-cell invasion.

Conventional SCC Conventional SCCs are classified as keratinizing or non-keratinizing types. Keratinizing SCC shows the presence of keratin pearls, cytoplasmic keratinization, and/or keratohyaline granules (Kurman et al. 2014). The tumor cells have eosinophilic cytoplasm and prominent intracellular bridges (Fig. 7). Non-keratinizing tumors consist of polygonal squamous cells with intracellular bridges that lack the presence of keratin pearls. SCC are graded into three grades: well (G1), moderately (G2), and poorly (G3) carcinomas based on degree of atypia, mitotic figures, and presence of keratin pearls. Grading SCC seemed to have an impact on patient prognosis and outcome. Other variants of SCC include the following:

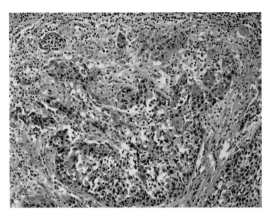

Fig. 7 Invasive SCC: Large irregularly arranged cells with keratin formation, large nuclei, and prominent nucleoli are seen invading the cervical stroma with a prominent desmoplastic response

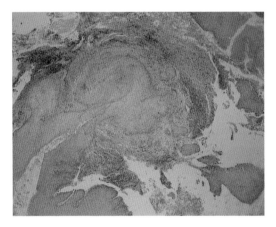

Fig. 8 Verrucous SCC: This is a well-differentiated SCC seen to be invading the cervical stroma with broad pushing borders

Verrucous Carcinoma Verrucous carcinoma is a rare variant of the cervical SCC that is frequently misdiagnosed as condyloma acuminatum on a superficial cervical biopsy. It is a well-differentiated exophytic SCC, and the epithelium lacks significant atypia or mitosis. The base of the tumor invades the underlying stroma with broad and expansile pushing borders (Fig. 8). These are differentiated from condyloma acuminatum by the absence of fibrovascular cores in the papillary cores of the verrucous carcinoma (Degefu et al. 1986; Jennings and Barclay 1972). They are very challenging and often missed on biopsy specimen. Verrucous

carcinomas are locally aggressive and only rarely metastasize.

Warty/Condylomatous Squamous Cell Carcinoma This is a variant of SCC with architectural similarities to condyloma acuminata. Microscopically koilocytic atypia is present in the tumor cells, and, however, the base of the tumors shows typical changes of SCC with stromal invasion (Wright et al. 2011b; Kurman et al. 2014).

Basaloid SCC Basaloid SCC is an aggressive variant of SCC formed of nests or cords of small, intermediate, or large basaloid cells which are hyperchromatic and have high nuclear to cytoplasmic ratios. The characteristic feature is the presence of peripheral palisading of the tumor cells (Grayson and Cooper 2002). High mitotic rate and geographical necrosis are frequently seen (Kurman et al. 2014). As these tumors are very aggressive, it is important to distinguish it from other solid tumors of the cervix, including adenoid cystic carcinoma, adenoid basal carcinoma, and small cell neuroendocrine carcinoma.

Lymphoepithelioma-Like Carcinoma This variant has distinct morphological appearance and is considered less aggressive than conventional SCC. The tumor is well circumscribed and consists of undifferentiated tumor cells present in sheets or nests. The tumor cells have large uniform vesicular nuclei with prominent nucleoli, scant cytoplasm, and poorly defined cell membranes. The mitotic rate is high. Tumor cells are surrounded by a dense inflammatory infiltrate consisting of lymphocytes and plasma cells (Martorell et al. 2002). A role of Epstein-Barr virus (EBV) infection is suggested in the pathogenesis of this variant.

Papillary SCC/Papillary Transitional Cell Carcinoma The tumor is architecturally composed of narrow or broad papillae that contain cores of edematous fibrous stroma with prominent capillaries and stromal inflammation. The papillae are covered with a layer of cytologically dysplastic cells resembling high-grade squamous intraepithelial neoplasia (Mirhashemi et al. 2003). The invasive part of the tumor resembles conventional SCC. These are aggressive lesions and may be difficult to differentiate from papillary squamous cell carcinoma in situ on biopsy sections.

2.4 Glandular Lesions of the Cervix

Adenocarcinomas are cervical epithelial tumors that show glandular differentiation. There has been a small increase in the incidence of endocervical adenocarcinoma over the past few decades. Most cervical adenocarcinomas are detected within the first three decades of life. Similar to squamous carcinoma, adenocarcinomas are linked to HPV infection; however increased prevalence of HPV type 18 and variants of HPV type 16 are found in adenocarcinomas compared to squamous cell carcinomas. Around 50% of endocervical tumors have a concurrent squamous lesion (Wilbur 2016). Intraepithelial neoplasia is a precursor lesion to invasive adenocarcinoma and is referred to as adenocarcinoma in situ (AIS). It may involve both the endocervical surface and endocervical glands.

2.4.1 Adenocarcinoma In Situ (AIS)

Preinvasive endocervical lesions are usually asymptomatic, and they are not easily visible by colposcopy as they lie high up in the endocervical canal. On Pap smears, adenocarcinoma in situ is identified as three-dimensional clusters or crowded group of cells with hyperchromatic nuclei and features of glandular differentiation which may include the presence of columnar cells, rosettes, or feathering of the nuclei at the edges (Cibas 2014). The neoplastic cells also demonstrate pseudostratification and inconspicuous nucleoli. Mitosis and apoptotic debris are frequently seen.

On histopathology, AIS is characterized by architecturally preserved endocervical glands lined by atypical columnar cells. The atypical cells have increased nuclear to cytoplasmic ratios, usually show mucin depletion, and some glands have abrupt transition between benign and malignant endocervical epithelium. The cytological features of pseudostratification, lack of prominent

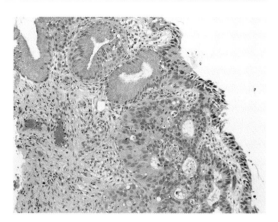

Fig. 9 AIS: There is sudden shift from benign endocervical glands with small basal nuclei and abundant cytoplasm to atypical glands with pseudostratification of epithelial cells with loss of polarity, nuclear hyperchromasia, and depletion of intracellular mucin. Atypical cells are limited to the ductal epithelium, and no invasion is identified

nucleoli, multiple mitoses, and apoptotic bodies should also be seen (Fig. 9).

The three most frequent subtypes are endocervical AIS, intestinal AIS, and endometrioid AIS. The endocervical type is the most common subtype and has atypical columnar cells with eosinophilic cytoplasm and depletion of mucin. Intestinal AIS is characterized by the presence of goblet cells. The endometrioid variant resembles proliferative endometrium and is characterized by cells with small nuclei and dense eosinophilic cytoplasm lacking mucin. The stratified mucin-producing intraepithelial lesion (SMILE) variant is a relatively rare subtype and has the following features: squamoid growth pattern along with intracellular mucin (Park et al. 2000). The mucin is present in the form of discrete vacuoles or as cytoplasmic clearing throughout all the layers (Kurman et al. 2014). In addition, cytological features of AIS with nuclear hyperchromasia, nuclear crowding, mitoses, and apoptotic bodies are present. AIS should be distinguished from benign lesions such as tubal and endometrioid metaplasia. This is extremely important due to their benign nature necessitating no further therapy for the latter and the need for conization and possible further therapy for the former. The major finding in tubal and endometrioid metaplasia is the presence of bland-looking columnar cells lacking hyperchromasia and nucleoli, ciliated brush in the glands lumen, and absence of significant mitosis.

Immunohistochemical studies using p16 and Ki67 are rarely used, and they act as markers of productive high-grade HPV infection and rapid cellular proliferation, respectively.

2.4.2 Invasive Adenocarcinoma

Invasive adenocarcinoma is characterized by the presence of cytologically and architecturally abnormal glands invading into the cervical stroma. On Pap smears, endocervical adenocarcinoma is usually seen as sheets of atypical cells with large round nuclei, prominent nucleoli, abundant cytoplasm, and tumor diathesis. Histopathologically, endocervical adenocarcinoma is further divided into multiple subtypes including conventional endocervical adenocarcinoma, endometrioid, adenocarcinoma, mucinous adenocarcinoma, clear cell adenocarcinoma, serous adenocarcinoma, and mesonephric adenocarcinoma (Loureiro and Oliva 2014).

Conventional Endocervical Adenocarcinoma (CEA) CEA exhibits a complex architectural glandular pattern including branching, cribriform, and papillary patterns. The lining epithelial cells are usually mucin poor and show pseudo-stratification with elongated hyperchromatic nuclei and prominent macronucleoli. These cells have an apical zone of eosinophilic cytoplasm. Apoptotic bodies are easily seen. Desmoplastic reaction is seen surrounding the invasive glands (Fig. 10). The stroma may show the presence of mucin pools (Kurman et al. 2014; Loureiro and Oliva 2014). Villoglandular papillary carcinoma is a well-differentiated variant of CEA that is characterized by the presence of tall and thin surface papillae lining spindled cells forming a fibrous core. The papillae are lined by endocervical-type cells. The invasive portion of the tumor is composed of elongated branching glands invading the stroma (Young and Clement 2002).

Endometrioid Endocervical Adenocarcinoma It is a rare subtype characterized by tubular glands lined by cells that lack mucin,

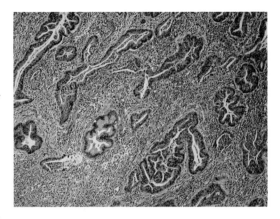

Fig. 10 Adenocarcinoma: Irregular large invasive glands lined by atypical cells showing pseudostratification and hyperchromatic nuclei surrounded by desmoplastic stroma

resembling endometrial cells, and has fewer mitosis and apoptotic bodies than the usual endocervical adenocarcinoma.

Mucinous Endocervical Adenocarcinoma These are characterized by the presence of mucin-rich cells, in contrast to mucin-depleted cells of the usual endocervical adenocarcinoma (Young and Clement 2002). These may resemble gastric epithelium, intestinal epithelium, or signet ring type. Gastric-type endocervical adenocarcinoma is rare and thought to be unrelated to HPV (Carleton et al. 2015). On morphology, the tumor cells have abundant eosinophilic cytoplasm, intracellular mucin, and distinct cell membranes. The neoplastic glands are present deeper than the expected level of benign endocervical glands and are architecturally more irregular, angulated, dilated, cribriform, or fused in appearance (Kurman et al. 2014). Desmoplasia may be noted in the cervical stroma surrounding the neoplastic glands. Adenoma malignum refers to the well-differentiated gastric-type adenocarcinoma. The intestinal-type mucinous adenocarcinoma has cells similar to the epithelial cells of the large intestine and may frequently have goblet cells. This type is frequently HPV and p16 negative (Wright et al. 2011b). Signet ring cells are formed when the intracellular mucin pushes the nucleus to the periphery and are usually seen in mixed adenosquamous carcinoma (Loureiro and Oliva 2014).

Clear Cell Endocervical Adenocarcinoma This subtype may have tubulocystic, solid, or papillary architecture. The malignant cells have clear cytoplasm and may show hobnailing. There is a historically an association between the presence of diethylstilbestrol exposure in utero and clear cell carcinoma of the ectocervix (Loureiro and Oliva 2014).

Serous Endocervical Adenocarcinoma It is very rare, and a diagnosis of primary serous cervical carcinoma should be made only after exclusion of origin in other organs of the female genital tract or the peritoneum (Loureiro and Oliva 2014). These have a distinct architecture, composed of papillae, with cellular budding and psammoma bodies (Kurman et al. 2014; Nofech-Mozes et al. 2006). The cells are markedly pleomorphic with high-grade atypia and frequent mitotic figures (Kurman et al. 2014).

Mesonephric Endocervical Adenocarcinoma It is an uncommon neoplasm that is not associated with HPV infection (Nofech-Mozes et al. 2006). These have a variety of architectural patterns including tubular, ductal, retiform, solid, or sex-cord like. The malignant cells are cuboidal, lack mucin, and may contain eosinophilic hyaline secretion in their lumen (Kurman et al. 2014).

Other rare epithelial tumors include adenosquamous carcinoma, glassy cell carcinoma, and adenoid cystic carcinoma (Fig. 11).

2.5 Neuroendocrine Tumors

Neuroendocrine tumors are very rare cervical epithelial tumors that range from well-differentiated (carcinoid tumors) to moderately differentiated (atypical carcinoid tumors) to poorly differentiated (small cell and large cell neuroendocrine carcinoma) neoplasms. They are also associated with HPV infection, and similar to cervical adenocarcinoma, HPV 18 has been more frequently observed in association with neuroendocrine neoplasms. Poorly differentiated neuroendocrine tumors are frequently associated with conventional neoplasms including CIN, SCC, AIS, and

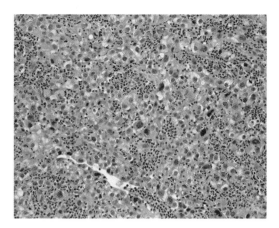

Fig. 11 Glassy cell variant: There are large polygonal atypical cells with ground-glass-like cytoplasm, large vesicular nuclei, and prominent nucleolus. The stroma shows marked infiltration by inflammatory cells

adenocarcinoma. It is postulated that HPV infection of the basal cell of the cervical epithelium may cause the pluripotent basal cell to differentiate along different cell lines, leading to coexistence of these epithelial tumors.

Poorly differentiated neuroendocrine tumors are aggressive and have a high propensity toward nodal metastasis.

Carcinoid Tumors Carcinoid tumors are well to moderately differentiated and have an organized architecture showing trabecular, solid, or cord-like pattern, with rosetting. The cells are monomorphic and lack atypia, frequent mitosis, and necrosis. The nuclei are small with finely granular chromatin, and the cytoplasm may contain neurosecretory granules. Atypical carcinoids resemble typical carcinoids architecturally; however they have more mitoses, nuclear atypia, and necrosis compared to the typical carcinoids (Rouzbahman and Clarke 2013).

Small Cell Neuroendocrine Tumors They are poorly differentiated and lose the organized architecture seen in carcinoids. On histology, these are highly cellular, formed of monomorphous small cells with high nuclear to cytoplasmic ratios, finely stippled chromatin, and inconspicuous nucleoli. Cells display prominent overlap or

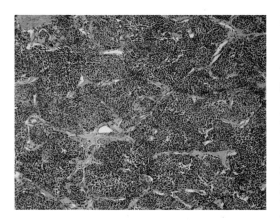

Fig. 12 Small cell carcinoma: Sheets of hyperchromatic small cell with high nuclear to cytoplasmic ratios, cell overlap, and molding are identified. The nuclear chromatin is finely stippled, and there is absence of prominent nucleolus

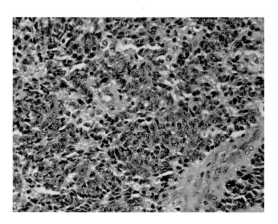

Fig. 13 Large cell carcinoma: Sheets of large cells with vesicular nuclei, prominent nuclei, and moderate cytoplasm are seen. Mitosis is frequently seen

nuclear molding, and geographic tumor necrosis is present. Mitotic rate is high, and lymphovascular space invasion is frequent (Rouzbahman and Clarke 2013) (Fig. 12).

Large Cell Neuroendocrine Carcinomas They have large cells with abundant cytoplasm, large nuclei, prominent nucleoli, and a high mitotic rate (Kurman et al. 2014) (Fig. 13).

Immunohistochemical studies using synaptophysin, chromogranin, CD56, and neuron-specific enolase may be needed for confirmation of diagnosis of neuroendocrine differentiation.

3 Mesenchymal Tumors

Sarcomas of the uterine cervix are uncommon tumors. A brief description of the common sarcomas of the cervix is provided below.

Leiomyosarcoma As primary cervical leiomyosarcomas (LMS) are rare, an attempt should be made to exclude the lower uterine segment as the site of origin (Fadare 2006). On morphology, these are spindle cell tumors with variable atypia, tumor necrosis, and atypical necrosis. They resemble similar tumors at the uterine corpus (Kurman 2014). Histological subtypes include epitheloid, myxoid, clear cell, and xanthomatous types (Crum et al. 2011). LMS should be distinguished from the most common benign mesenchymal tumors such as leiomyoma. The absence of tumor necrosis, atypia, and mitotic figures favors the latter. Immunohistochemistry is necessary to confirm the diagnosis of smooth muscle origin of LMS which usually express smooth muscle actin, desmin, and h-caldesmon.

Alveolar Soft Part Sarcoma These tumors have nested patterns that architecturally resemble alveoli of the lung (Feng et al. 2014). The malignant cells are large monomorphic, polygonal with eosinophilic cytoplasm, growing in a solid or dyscohesive pattern. The diagnosis is confirmed by cytogenetics as this tumor shows t(X;17) translocation resulting in *ASPL/TFE3* gene fusion..

Rhabdomyosarcoma Rhabdomyosarcomas are malignant tumors with skeletal muscle differentiation and are further classified as embryonal, alveolar, and pleomorphic subtypes. Alveolar rhabdomyosarcoma is most commonly seen and consists of malignant cells arranged in an alveolar pattern surrounded by fibrous tissue with vascular tissue. The tumor cells contain large hyperchromatic nuclei and can be large polygonal or small spindle shaped (Rivasi et al. 2008). Cytogenetic abnormalities t(2;13) (q35;q14), resulting in the fusion genes *PAX3-FKHR* and the less frequent t(1;13)(p36;q14), with fusion of *PAX7-FKHR*, are seen in majority of the cases.

Angiosarcoma Angiosarcomas are aggressive tumors consisting of interconnecting vascular channels lined by cuboidal cells with large atypical nuclei and high nuclear to cytoplasmic ratios. Tumor cells are positive for CD31, CD34, ERG, and factor VIII-related antigen by immunohistochemistry. Rarely, malignant peripheral nerve sheath tumor, primary malignant melanoma, germ cell tumors, lymphoid, and myeloid malignancies may arise in the cervix.

4 Mixed Epithelial and Mesenchymal Tumors

Mixed epithelial and mesenchymal tumors containing adenosarcoma and carcinosarcoma may be present. In adenosarcoma, a benign epithelial component is associated with a malignant mesenchymal part, while in carcinosarcoma, both the epithelial and mesenchymal components are malignant.

References

Burd EM. Human papillomavirus and cervical cancer. Clin Microbiol Rev. 2003;16:1–17.

Carleton C, Hoang L, Sah S, Kiyokawa T, Karamurzin YS, Talia KL, Park KJ, McCluggage WG. A detailed immunohistochemical analysis of a large series of cervical and vaginal gastric-type adenocarcinomas. Am J Surg Pathol. 2016;40:636-44.

Ceballos KM, Shaw D, Daya D. Microinvasive cervical adenocarcinoma (FIGO stage 1A tumors): results of surgical staging and outcome analysis. Am J Surg Pathol. 2006;30:370–4.

Cibas ES. Cervical and vaginal cytology. In: Cibas ES, Ducatman BS, editors. Cytology diagnostic principles and clinical correlates. Philadelphia: Saunders; 2014. p. 1–58.

Crum CP, Cibas ES, Rose PG, Peters WA. Cervical squamous neoplasia. In: Crum CP, Nucci MR, Lee KR, editors. Diagnostic gynecologic and obstetric pathology. 2nd ed. Philadelphia: Saunders; 2011.

Cuschieri K, Wentzensen N. HPV mRNA and p16 detection as biomarkers for the improved diagnosis of cervical neoplasia. Cancer Epidemiol, Biomark Prev: Publ Am Assoc Cancer Res, cosponsored by the American Society of Preventive Oncology 2008; 17:2536–45.

Degefu S, O'Quinn AG, Lacey CG, Merkel M, Barnard DE. Verrucous carcinoma of the cervix: a report of two cases and literature review. Gynecol Oncol. 1986;25:37–47.

Fadare O. Uncommon sarcomas of the uterine cervix: a review of selected entities. Diagn Pathol. 2006;1:30.

Feng M, Jiang W, He Y, Li L. Primary alveolar soft part sarcoma of the uterine cervix: a case report and literature review. Int J Clin Exp Pathol. 2014;7:8223–6.

Ferlay J, Soerjomataram I, Dikshit R, Eser S, Mathers C, Rebelo M, Parkin DM, Forman D, Bray F. Cancer incidence and mortality worldwide: sources, methods and major patterns in GLOBOCAN 2012. Int J Cancer. 2015;136(5):E359–86.

Grayson W, Cooper K. A reappraisal of "basaloid carcinoma" of the cervix, and the differential diagnosis of basaloid cervical neoplasms. Adv Anat Pathol. 2002; 9:290–300.

Jennings RH, Barclay DL. Verrucous carcinoma of the cervix. Cancer. 1972;30:430–4.

Kurman RJ, Carcangiu ML, Herrington S, Young RH. WHO classification of tumors of female reproductive organs. Lyon: IARC; 2014.

Lawson JS, Glenn WK, Heng B, Ye Y, Tran B, Lutze-Mann L, Whitaker NJ. Koilocytes indicate a role for human papilloma virus in breast cancer. Br J Cancer. 2009; 101:1351–6

Long ME, Dwarica DS, Kastner TM, Gallenberg MM, Chantigian PD, Marnach ML, Weaver AL, Casey PM. Comparison of dysplastic and benign endocervical polyps. J Low Genit Tract Dis. 2013;17:142–6.

Loureiro J, Oliva E. The spectrum of cervical glandular neoplasia and issues in differential diagnosis. Arch Pathol Lab Med. 2014;138:453–83.

Martin CM, O'Leary JJ. Histology of cervical intraepithelial neoplasia and the role of biomarkers. Best Pract Res Clin Obstet Gynaecol. 2011 Oct;25(5):605–15.

Martorell MA, Julian JM, Calabuig C, García-García JA, Pérez-Vallés A. Lymphoepithelioma-like carcinoma of the uterine cervix. Arch Pathol Lab Med. 2002; 126:1501–5.

Mirhashemi R, Ganjei-Azar P, Nadji M, Lambrou N, Atamdede F, Averette HE. Papillary squamous cell carcinoma of the uterine cervix: an immunophenotypic appraisal of 12 cases. Gynecol Oncol. 2003; 90:657–61.

Nofech-Mozes S, Rasty G, Ismiil N, Covens A, Khalifa MA. Immunohistochemical characterization of endocervical papillary serous carcinoma. Int J Gynecol Cancer. 2006 Jan-Feb;16(Suppl 1):286–92.

Park JJ, Sun D, Quade BJ, Flynn C, Sheets EE, Yang A, McKeon F, Crum CP. Stratified mucin-producing intraepithelial lesions of the cervix: adenosquamous or columnar cell neoplasia? Am J Surg Pathol. 2000;24:1414–9.

Rivasi F, Botticelli L, Bettelli SR, Masellis G. Alveolar rhabdomyosarcoma of the uterine cervix. A case report confirmed by FKHR break-apart rearrangement using a fluorescence in situ hybridization probe on paraffin-embedded tissues. Int J Gynecol Pathol. 2008; 27:442–6.

Rouzbahman M, Clarke B. Neuroendocrine tumors of the gynecologic tract: select topics. Semin Diagn Pathol. 2013;30:224–33.

Walboomers JM, Jacobs MV, Manos MM, et al. Human papillomavirus is a necessary cause of invasive cervical cancer worldwide. J Pathol. 1999;189:12–9.

Wilbur DC. Practical issues related to uterine pathology: in situ and invasive cervical glandular lesions and their benign mimics: emphasis on cytology-histology correlation and interpretive pitfalls. Mod Pathol. 2016; 29(Suppl 1):S1–S11.

Wright TC, Ronnett BM, Ferenczy A. Benign diseases of the cervix. In: Kurman RJ, Ellenson LH, Ronnett BM, editors. Blaustein's pathology of the female genital tract. 6th ed. New York: Springer; 2011a.

Wright TC, Ronnett BM, Kurman RJ, Ferenczy A. (Pre)cancerous lesions of the cervix. In: Kurman RJ, Ellenson HL, Ronnett BM, editors. Blaustein's pathology of the female genital tract. 6th ed. New York: Springer; 2011b.

Young RH, Clement PB. Endocervical adenocarcinoma and its variants: their morphology and differential diagnosis. Histopathology. 2002;41:185–207.

Pathology of the Uterine Corpus

Helena Hwang

Abstract

Endometrial cancer is the fourth most common cancer in women in the United States. Endometrial carcinomas can be divided into two types based primarily on association with excess estrogen. Endometrioid adenocarcinoma is the prototypical type 1 endometrial carcinoma, well known for its association with excess estrogen. It is the most common uterine malignancy and usually occurs in postmenopausal women. Endometrial hyperplasia is widely recognized as a non-obligate precursor to endometrioid adenocarcinoma. Type 2 endometrial carcinomas are not associated with excess estrogen and include serous and clear cell carcinomas. A wide variety of other neoplasms occur in the uterus. More common entities include biphasic tumors like malignant mixed Mullerian tumors (MMMT) and mesenchymal malignancies such as endometrial stromal sarcoma and leiomyosarcomas. More rare uterine tumors include perivascular epithelioid cell tumor (PEComa), primitive neuroectodermal tumor (PNET), lymphoma, and gestational trophoblastic disease.

Keywords

Endometrial hyperplasia • Endometrial intraepithelial neoplasia • Endometrioid adenocarcinoma • Clear cell carcinoma • Endometrial stromal sarcoma • Leiomyosarcoma • Malignant mixed Mullerian tumor • Gestational trophoblastic disease • Hydatidiform mole

Contents

H. Hwang (✉)
University of Texas Southwestern Medical Center, Dallas, TX, USA
e-mail: helena.hwang@utsouthwestern.edu

© Springer International Publishing AG 2017
D. Shoupe (ed.), *Handbook of Gynecology*,
DOI 10.1007/978-3-319-17798-4_63

1   Introduction

Endometrial carcinoma is the most common gynecologic malignancy in the United States, of which endometrioid adenocarcinoma is the most common type. Endometrial hyperplasia is a widely recognized non-obligate precursor to endometrioid adenocarcinoma. Other types of endometrial carcinomas include serous, clear cell, and malignant mixed Mullerian tumors (MMMT), among others. In addition to carcinomas, many different neoplasms can be found in the uterus. Leiomyoma is the most common tumor of the uterus; mesenchymal malignancies, such as endometrial stromal sarcoma and leiomyosarcomas, are less common. Other tumors that can be encountered in the uterine corpus include perivascular epithelioid cell tumor (PEComa), primitive neuroectodermal tumor (PNET), lymphoma, and gestational trophoblastic disease, all of which are rare. In this chapter, the histology of various tumors of the uterine corpus will be described with explanations of workup and differential diagnosis.

2   Histology of Normal Uterine Corpus

The uterine corpus consists of the endometrium, myometrium, and serosa. The endometrium is divided into stratum functionalis, the superficial portion that sheds into the uterine cavity, and stratum basalis, the deeper portion that abuts the myometrium. The appearance of the stratum functionalis varies depending on the time of the menstrual cycle while the basalis remains constant. Normal endometrium is composed of glands and stroma in an approximately 1:1 ratio. The stroma consists of a uniform population of small, round to spindled blue cells. In the proliferative phase, the glandular epithelium shows columnar cells with pseudostratification, and the stroma ranges from cellular to edematous. Both the glands and stroma show mitoses. The hallmark of secretory phase is vacuoles in glandular cells. Secretory phase shows features distinct enough to date day by day. In late secretory phase, a sawtooth pattern, the presence of neutrophils, and stromal predecidualization are seen. In predecidualization, the stromal cells become larger, plumper, and rounder, showing increased eosinophilic cytoplasm. During menstruation, glandular and stromal breakdown is seen with fibrin and necrosis. In postmenopause, the endometrium becomes atrophic, characterized by glands with a single layer of cuboidal or flat epithelial cells without stratification and without mitoses.

The myometrium is the thickest layer of the uterus and is composed of smooth muscle cells. The serosa is the outermost layer of the uterus and is composed of a single layer of mesothelial cells.

3   Endometrioid Adenocarcinoma Precursors

3.1   Endometrial Hyperplasia

Endometrial hyperplasia is a well-known non-obligate precursor to endometrioid adenocarcinoma. The most widely used classification system for endometrial hyperplasia is one that the World Health Organization (WHO) adopted in 1994, dividing endometrial hyperplasia into four categories: (1) simple hyperplasia, (2) complex hyperplasia, (3) simple hyperplasia with atypia, (4) and complex hyperplasia with atypia. In 2014, WHO revised this system, simplifying classification into two categories: hyperplasia without atypia and atypical hyperplasia/endometrial intraepithelial neoplasia (EIN) (Kurman et al. 2014). Both systems will be described below.

In endometrial hyperplasia, proliferative type endometrium is seen with an increased gland-to-stroma ratio with architectural complexity. Architectural complexity is defined as irregularity in gland size and shape. In simple hyperplasia, glandular crowding is present with mild to moderate architectural complexity, sometimes with cystic glands (Fig. 1). Complex hyperplasia shows increased glandular crowding and increased architectural complexity, including branching and outpouching of glands. Atypia refers to cytologic

Fig. 1 Simple hyperplasia without atypia. Glandular crowding with proliferative type endometrial glands showing irregular shapes

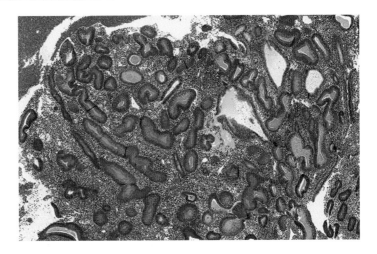

atypia defined by nuclear enlargement, loss of polarity with rounding of the nucleus rather than ovoid nuclei, irregular nuclear borders, pleomorphism, and prominent nucleoli. Among the four categories, simple hyperplasia without atypia and complex hyperplasia with atypia are most commonly seen while simple hyperplasia with atypia is very rare.

While widely used, this classification system is known to suffer from interobserver variability with suboptimal reproducibility. The binary system proposed in the most recent WHO aims to reduce interobserver reproducibility by simplifying classification. It is also based on the finding that cytologic atypia is the most significant factor in progression to endometrioid adenocarcinoma. The majority of hyperplasia without atypia regresses while 8% of simple hyperplasia with atypia and 29% of complex hyperplasia with atypia progress to endometrioid adenocarcinoma (Kurman et al. 1985).

3.2 Endometrial Intraepithelial Neoplasia

Endometrial intraepithelial neoplasia (EIN) is a monoclonal precursor lesion that was originally identified based on morphometric analysis and finding genetic alterations similar to that seen in grade 1 endometrioid adenocarcinomas (Mutter et al. 2000). The histologic criteria for EIN are (1) gland-to-stroma ratio greater than 1:1,

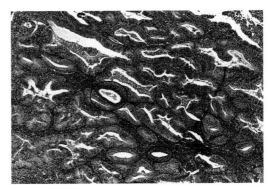

Fig. 2 Endometrial intraepithelial neoplasia (EIN). Marked glandular crowding with architectural complexity and enlargement and rounding of cells. Note that background glands (*circled*) are different from the neoplastic glands

(2) cytology of cells in lesional area is different from background glands or cytology is clearly abnormal, (3) greater than 1 mm focus, (4) and exclusion of benign mimics such as polyps, basalis, disordered proliferative endometrium, metaplastic change, and carcinoma (Fig. 2).

While most cases of atypical hyperplasia would fit the definition of EIN, these two categories are not interchangeable, as cases previously diagnosed as simple hyperplasia without atypia and complex hyperplasia without atypia have been reclassified as EIN.

The differential diagnosis of endometrial hyperplasia includes, but is not limited to, endometrial polyps, disordered proliferative endometrium, stratum basalis, metaplastic change, and endometrioid adenocarcinoma. Endometrial polyps may show disorganized glands resembling hyperplasia. Recognizing characteristic features of endometrial polyps such as thick-walled vessels and fibrotic stroma or polypoid architecture can help to distinguish between the two, although in an endometrial biopsy, distinction can be challenging at times. Disordered proliferative endometrium can also show irregular glands; however this change is more focal than in hyperplasia. The basalis may show glandular crowding; however the glands should be inactive, not proliferative type.

3.3 Metaplastic Change

The endometrium can demonstrate different types of metaplastic change, including eosinophilic, ciliated, squamous, mucinous, and clear cell change. Metaplasia can occur in benign endometrium, hyperplasia, and carcinoma, which can obfuscate the underlying process. Eosinophilic change, for example, shows rounding of cells that can be mistaken for cytologic atypia. Squamous differentiation is fairly common and has traditionally been thought to manifest in morular or non-morular forms. In morular metaplasia, round nests of bland oval or spindled cells are seen that resemble squamous epithelium, hence the name "squamous" morules. Morular metaplasia has been proposed as an alternative name as the squamous nature of these cells has been questioned recently due to different staining patterns than non-morular squamous differentiation. Morular metaplasia expresses CDX2 (a marker often associated with gastrointestinal differentiation) and does not express p63 (a marker of squamous differentiation) while non-morular squamous differentiation demonstrates the opposite staining pattern. Morular metaplasia is often seen with hyperplasia, and its presence should raise suspicion for possible hyperplasia or carcinoma. Distinguishing atypical hyperplasia from adenocarcinoma is discussed in the Sect. 4.1.1.

3.4 Progestin Effect

Progestin is commonly used to treat atypical hyperplasia as well as some cases of well-differentiated endometrioid adenocarcinoma. The characteristic histologic feature of progestin treatment is pseudodecidualized stroma where the stromal cells become large, round, and plump, with abundant pink cytoplasm. The glands may be inactive or show eosinophilic change that should be distinguished from residual atypia.

4 Uterine Tumors

4.1 Endometrial Carcinoma

Endometrial carcinomas occur more often in postmenopausal women and usually present with abnormal vaginal bleeding. They can be divided into two types: type 1 and type 2. Type 1 tumors are associated with unopposed estrogen and are usually low grade. Endometrioid adenocarcinoma is the prototypical type 1 tumor. Type 2 tumors are not associated with unopposed estrogen, tend to be high grade, and occur more frequently in an older age group than those who develop type 1 tumors. Serous carcinoma is an example of a type 2 carcinoma. Different types of endometrial carcinoma will be discussed below.

4.1.1 Endometrioid Adenocarcinoma

Endometrioid adenocarcinomas comprise 60–80% of endometrial carcinomas. Grossly, these tumors may be unifocal or multifocal and often present as an exophytic, friable mass (Fig. 3). However, in some cases, particularly in small, atrophic uteri, the tumor manifests primarily as thickened endometrium and myometrium and may be difficult to identify grossly. Identifying the tumor grossly is clinically significant since intraoperative consultation is often performed for staging purposes and the pathologist must identify the point of deepest invasion (whether tumor involves more than half of the myometrium) which may not always be evident on gross examination.

Fig. 3 Endometrioid adenocarcinoma. Gross photograph of a bivalved uterus showing a large, friable, tan-white mass filling the uterine cavity and invading into the myometrium

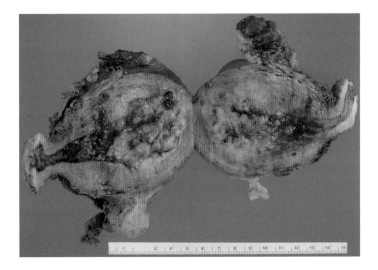

Microscopically, endometrioid adenocarcinoma consists of proliferative type endometrium with pseudostratified columnar cells showing crowded glands with complex architectural patterns and cytologic atypia. The extent of architectural and cytologic atypia should be greater than that seen in atypical hyperplasia/EIN. Differentiating between these two entities is further discussed below. The presence of invasive glands in the myometrium is pathognomonic for adenocarcinoma.

Endometrioid adenocarcinoma is graded using the International Federation of Gynecology and Obstetrics (FIGO) grading system. The tumor is divided into three grades based on both architecture and nuclear atypia. Architectural grade is based on the degree of gland formation: grade 1 = solid areas comprise less than 5% of the tumor, grade 2 = solid areas comprise 5–50% of the tumor, and grade 3 = solid areas comprise more than 50% of the tumor (Table 1) (Figs. 4 and 5). Nuclear grade is defined as follows: nuclear grade 1 = uniform round and oval nuclei, nuclear grade 2 = irregular nuclei with chromatin clumping, and nuclear grade 3 = large, pleomorphic nuclei that may show prominent nucleoli.

The nuclear grade of the tumor is usually consistent with the architectural features, e.g., endometrioid adenocarcinoma with low-grade architecture usually has low-grade nuclei. Under the FIGO grading system, if a tumor with grade

Table 1 Grading of endometrioid adenocarcinoma

	Architectural grade	Nuclear grade
Grade 1	Less than 5% solid areas	Uniform, round to oval nuclei; inconspicuous nucleoli
Grade 2	5–50% solid areas	Irregular nuclei with chromatin clumping
Grade 3	Greater than 50% solid areas	Large, pleomorphic nuclei with prominent nucleoli

Overall grade is based on both architecture and nuclear grade. Tumor grade is increased by one if nuclear grade is discordant with architectural grade, e.g., a tumor should be upgraded from grade 1 to 2 if it has grade 1 architecture and grade 2 nuclei

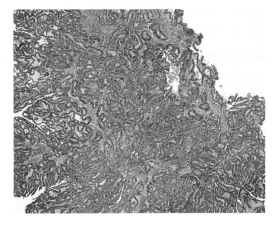

Fig. 4 Endometrioid adenocarcinoma, grade 1. The tumor is composed entirely of glands that are back to back and confluent with cytologic atypia

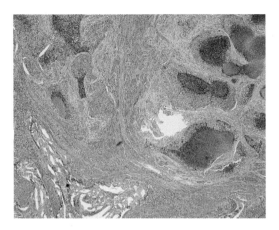

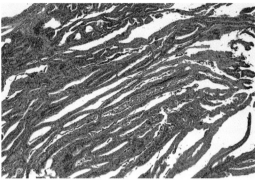

Fig. 6 Villoglandular carcinoma. The tumor shows long, villous papillae with low-grade nuclei

Fig. 5 Endometrioid adenocarcinoma, grade 3. The tumor shows predominantly solid nests of cells with central necrosis, invading the myometrium. In the lower left corner, gland formation is seen

1 architecture shows grade 2 nuclei, the tumor should be upgraded to an overall grade 2 tumor. Caution should be used in upgrading though as the presence of marked architectural/nuclear atypia dyssynchrony should raise suspicion that the tumor is actually serous carcinoma rather than endometrioid type as serous carcinomas show high-grade nuclei with gland formation. When evaluating tumor architecture, areas of squamous differentiation should not be included as solid areas.

4.1.2 Villoglandular and Secretory Carcinoma

Several variants of endometrioid adenocarcinoma exist. Two distinctive ones that can mimic serous and clear cell carcinomas are villoglandular and secretory carcinomas, respectively.

Villoglandular carcinomas are characterized by long, villous papillae with fibrovascular cores and bland, columnar cells (Fig. 6). The percentage of the tumor that should show villoglandular features in order to be classified as villoglandular carcinoma is not well-defined, but should be at least the majority of the tumor. Villoglandular carcinomas can resemble serous carcinomas due to papillary architecture; however marked nuclear atypia is not typical in villoglandular carcinomas as it is in serous carcinomas. The prognosis of villoglandular

carcinomas is based primarily on grade and stage as in other endometrioid adenocarcinomas and because these tumors are primarily low grade, they tend to have a good prognosis.

Secretory adenocarcinoma is rare and defined by the presence of cytoplasmic vacuoles as seen in secretory phase glands. It is a low-grade tumor with bland, uniform cells and is associated with a good prognosis. Secretory carcinoma is further discussed under clear cell carcinoma, a tumor it can mimic.

Other subtypes of endometrioid adenocarcinoma can show metaplastic change such as ciliated and clear cell change. The significance of recognizing variant features is to not misdiagnose endometrioid adenocarcinoma as a different tumor such as clear cell carcinoma. Mentioning such features also helps to identify the tumor on an excisional specimen or recurrence. Metaplastic change in endometrioid adenocarcinoma is not prognostically significant.

4.1.3 Commonly Encountered Problems in Pathologic Diagnosis and Staging of Endometrioid Adenocarcinoma

Several areas in diagnosis and staging of endometrioid adenocarcinoma can be problematic, with some issues more frequently encountered than others. The issues are enumerated below:

1. Endometrioid adenocarcinoma versus atypical hyperplasia/EIN

The line between atypical hyperplasia and adenocarcinoma can be blurry, and the diagnosis is subject to interobserver variability. Confluent glands, back-to-back glands with little to no intervening stroma, increased architectural complexity such as cribriforming or papillary architecture in more than a minute focus, greater nuclear atypia than that seen in atypical hyperplasia, and the presence of desmoplasia favor a diagnosis of adenocarcinoma. Desmoplasia however is rarely seen in endometrioid adenocarcinoma. In endometrial biopsy specimens, a diagnosis of "atypical hyperplasia bordering on low-grade endometrioid adenocarcinoma" may be appropriate in certain cases with the final diagnosis deferred to the excisional specimen.

2. Myometrial invasion

Myometrial invasion is measured from the endomyometrial junction to the deepest point of invasion. Several issues must be considered in determining both the presence of myometrial invasion and depth of invasion.

(a) The endomyometrial junction is irregular making it difficult to assess for invasion. Superficial myometrial invasion tends to be overdiagnosed. Clues to invasion are jagged, angular glands and desmoplasia. The diagnosis of superficial invasion can be highly subjective as borne out by data showing no difference in prognosis between those with tumors confined to the endometrium and those with tumors involving the upper half of the myometrium. Based on this evidence, in 2009, FIGO changed the staging system so tumors confined to the endometrium and involving the upper half of the myometrium are both now staged as Ia.

(b) Myometrial invasion can manifest as glands infiltrating the myometrium or as a pushing border. In cases of a pushing border, without the presence of normal endomyometrial junction for comparison, it can be difficult to diagnose invasion.

(c) Myometrial invasion should not be diagnosed when malignant glands involve adenomyosis. Adenomyosis is when benign endometrial tissue, both glands and stroma, are found in the myometrium. Adenocarcinoma involving adenomyosis is not true myometrial invasion. The rounded contour of adenomyosis versus the angulated glands of true invasion, the presence of benign glands adjacent to malignant glands, areas of uninvolved adenomyosis elsewhere, and the presence of endometrial stroma in adenomyosis favor a diagnosis of tumor involving adenomyosis. In some tumors, there can be both tumor involving adenomyosis and true myometrial invasion.

(d) An unusual type of invasion, microcystic, elongated, and fragmented (MELF) invasion, has been described. In this type of invasion, glands are surrounded by inflamed fibromyxoid stroma that can almost obscure the glands. The glands themselves may be flat and resemble lymphovascular spaces. The significance of MELF however is still controversial.

4.1.4 Serous Carcinoma

Serous carcinomas of the uterus are aggressive tumors that have a propensity to spread to peritoneal surfaces and commonly present at a late stage. They comprise 5–10% of endometrial cancers and are usually found in women over 65. Serous carcinomas of the uterus are by definition high grade. They can be found in pure form, admixed with other high-grade carcinomas such as high-grade endometrioid carcinoma or clear cell carcinoma, or found as a component of MMMT.

Grossly, serous carcinomas usually present as a friable, exophytic mass. Microscopically, serous carcinomas classically exhibit papillary or micropapillary architecture with fibrovascular cores; small glands and solid areas can also be seen. The cells often show tufting into the lumen and exfoliated cells are present. Cytologically, the cells are round to cuboidal, with large, pleomorphic, often vesicular nuclei and prominent nucleoli (Fig. 7). Brisk mitotic activity is common and hobnailing is not infrequent. Psammoma bodies

Fig. 7 Serous carcinoma.
Papillary architecture is
seen with markedly atypical
nuclei and detached cells

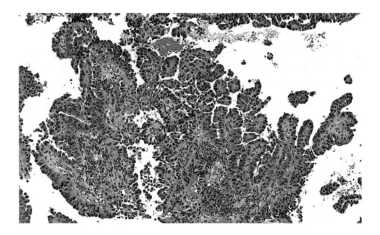

are another feature classically associated with
serous carcinomas.

The differential diagnosis of serous carcinoma
includes clear cell carcinoma, MMMT, villoglandular carcinoma, high-grade endometrioid
carcinomas, and eosinophilic syncytial change.
Distinguishing serous carcinoma from some of
these other lesions is discussed in the pertinent
sections of the aforementioned lesions. Serous
carcinomas tend to be either diffusely positive
or completely negative or "null" for p53 and
diffusely positive for p16 while endometrioid
carcinomas show heterogeneous staining with
p53 and p16. The combination of morphology
and pattern of immunostaining should help to
distinguish serous carcinoma from its mimics.
Eosinophilic syncytial change, also referred to
as eosinophilic syncytial metaplasia, is seen in
association with endometrial breakdown. The
epithelial cells are eosinophilic and can show
enlarged nuclei with pseudopapillary architecture
that can mimic serous carcinoma. The background of breakdown and minimal pleomorphism should help to distinguish this change
from malignancy.

Another problem that can be encountered with
serous carcinomas is determining the primary site.
When there is widespread tumor involving the
uterus, ovaries, and fallopian tubes, a fallopian
tube primary would be favored. Synchronous primaries should also be considered. The absence of
uterine serosal involvement would be more consistent with a uterine primary.

The precursor to serous carcinoma is serous
endometrial intraepithelial carcinoma (EIC).
Serous EIC involves only the surface epithelium,
showing markedly atypical cells lining the epithelium. An intraepithelial or in situ lesion should by
definition have no capacity to metastasize as it has
not yet invaded the stroma. In other tumors, such
is the case but serous EIC behaves differently than
other in situ lesions, demonstrating a propensity
to spread just like invasive serous carcinoma
(Sherman et al. 1992). Serous carcinoma confined
to endometrial polyps also demonstrates aggressive behavior (Silva and Jenkins 1990).

4.1.5   Clear Cell Carcinoma

Clear cell carcinomas are high-grade, aggressive
tumors that comprise less than approximately 5%
of uterine malignancies. They tend to occur in
women older than 65 and, like serous carcinoma,
are high-grade tumors by definition (Abeler and
Kjorstad 1991).

Grossly, clear cell carcinoma presents as a
uterine mass without any distinctive features.
Microscopically, the tumor shows papillary,
tubulocystic, and solid architecture, usually
exhibiting a mixture of patterns. Per its name,
cells with clear cytoplasm due to glycogen are
often seen (Fig. 8). Another characteristic feature
is hobnail cells. Hobnail refers to a cell with
bulbous nuclear protrusion and a narrow base;
hobnail is literally a short nail with a wide head.
The hobnail cells may have either clear or eosinophilic cytoplasm. The cells show high-grade

Fig. 8 Clear cell
carcinoma. Papillary
architecture is seen with
clear cells and stromal
hyalinization

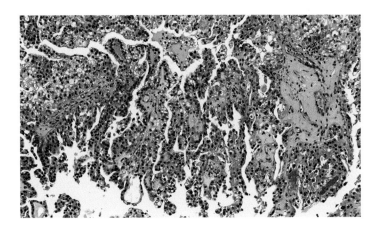

features such as pleomorphism and large nuclei with prominent nucleoli. Hyalinized stroma and hyaline bodies (homogeneous eosinophilic droplets) are also commonly seen.

Clear cells are not pathognomonic for clear cell carcinoma as clear cells can be encountered in a variety of lesions, both benign and malignant. Clear cell carcinomas should be distinguished from Arias-Stella reaction, secretory carcinoma, endometrioid carcinoma with clear cell change, and serous carcinoma.

Arias-Stella reaction is a benign change that usually occurs during pregnancy. It is characterized by atypical clear and hobnail cells mimicking malignancy. Features of Arias-Stella reaction that help to distinguish it from clear cell carcinoma include the following: it occurs in premenopausal women, does not show invasion, shows little to no mitotic activity, and is an incidental finding. Secretory carcinoma may show solid areas with clear cells that resemble clear cell carcinoma. The low-grade cytology of secretory carcinoma should help to distinguish it from the marked nuclear atypia seen in clear cell carcinoma. Serous carcinomas exhibit high-grade nuclei just as in clear cell carcinomas; however presence of extensive clearing or other features associated with clear cell carcinoma such as hyalinization would favor clear cell carcinoma. Endometrioid carcinoma with clear cell change is not likely to show marked nuclear atypia.

Immunostains have limited utility in the diagnosis of clear cell carcinomas, as these tumors do not show a specific pattern of immunostaining.

However, it can help in some instances. Clear cell carcinomas tend to be estrogen receptor/progesterone receptor (ER/PR) negative versus endometrioid adenocarcinomas that are clear cell carcinomas also tend to show heterogeneous expression of p53 which may help to differentiate them from serous carcinomas that tend to be diffusely positive or completely null for p53.

4.1.6 Undifferentiated Carcinoma

Undifferentiated carcinomas are rare tumors that, despite their name, have distinctive histologic features and should not be used as a wastebasket diagnosis for tumors that cannot be classified (Altrabulsi et al. 2005). Microscopically, these tumors are characterized by sheets of monotonous, epithelioid, medium-sized cells with cytokeratin expression in usually less than 10% of cells. Prominent nucleoli, vesicular nuclei, brisk mitoses, and necrosis are usually seen. A marked lymphoid infiltrate may also be present.

The differential diagnosis includes grade 3 endometrioid carcinoma, endometrial stromal sarcoma, high-grade sarcoma, neuroendocrine carcinoma, and lymphoma. Immunostains can help to differentiate between these entities: cytokeratin will show greater expression in pure endometrioid carcinomas, endometrial stromal sarcoma tends to be CD10 positive, high-grade sarcoma should show a pattern of immunostaining consistent with the differentiation seen, and lymphoma tends to be CD45 positive. Synaptophysin and chromogranin are markers of neuroendocrine differentiation that can be focally (usually less than 10%) expressed in undifferentiated carcinomas (Taraif et al. 2009) while neuroendocrine carcinomas should show greater expression of these two markers and also show neuroendocrine histology. Undifferentiated carcinomas are aggressive tumors with a poor prognosis.

4.1.7 Mixed-Type Carcinoma

Mixed carcinomas refer to tumors showing carcinomas of at least two different types. The most commonly encountered mixed carcinomas are endometrioid adenocarcinoma with serous carcinoma, endometrioid adenocarcinoma with clear cell carcinoma, and endometrioid adenocarcinoma with undifferentiated carcinoma. Endometrioid adenocarcinoma and its variants, such as secretory carcinoma, are not considered mixed carcinomas. When endometrioid adenocarcinoma is seen with variant features, it should be diagnosed as endometrioid adenocarcinoma with clear cell features, for example, rather than a mixed tumor. The percentage of each histologic type should be stated in mixed carcinomas as this can have prognostic value.

4.1.8 Lynch Syndrome

Lynch syndrome, or hereditary nonpolyposis colorectal cancer (HNPCC), is an autosomal dominant disorder with incomplete penetrance that increases the risk of various cancers, particularly colorectal and endometrial cancer. The lifetime risk for endometrial cancer has been found to be as high as 60% in Lynch syndrome. Endometrial cancers in Lynch syndrome demonstrate microsatellite instability (MSI) which is excessive repetition of short DNA sequences secondary to a defective DNA repair system. Twenty-five to 30% of sporadic endometrial tumors also exhibit MSI. Both endometrioid and non-endometrioid carcinomas can show MSI. Screening guidelines for Lynch syndrome are not standardized, but some groups recommend routine screening in women under the age of 50 who are diagnosed with endometrial carcinoma. Screening for MSI in Lynch-associated endometrial carcinomas can be performed with a panel of immunostains for the mismatch repair proteins, MLH1, MSH2, MSH6, and PMS2. Loss of expression in one or more of these stains suggests MSI and further genetic testing is then indicated.

4.2 Mesenchymal Lesions

4.2.1 Endometrial Stromal Tumors

Endometrial Stromal Nodule
Endometrial stromal nodules are the benign counterpart of endometrial stromal sarcomas. They are composed of small round to ovoid blue cells as seen in endometrial stromal sarcoma but are confined to the endometrium without myometrial involvement while endometrial stromal sarcoma involves the myometrium.

Endometrial Stromal Sarcoma
Endometrial stromal sarcomas were traditionally divided into low- and high-grade types. In 2003, WHO classified these tumors into two groups, endometrial stromal sarcoma, with no designation of low or high grade, and undifferentiated endometrial sarcoma. In the most recent WHO, these group of tumors are divided into low-grade and high-grade endometrial stromal sarcoma and undifferentiated endometrial sarcoma based on recent evidence showing a common translocation in the tumors now designated high-grade endometrial stromal sarcoma (Kurman et al. 2014).

Low-Grade Endometrial Stromal Sarcoma
Low-grade endometrial stromal sarcomas are low-grade malignant tumors that tend to occur in premenopausal women (median age 40). Women present with abnormal vaginal bleeding or abdominal pain.

Grossly, endometrial stromal sarcoma is classically described as showing a "wormlike" appearance that is primarily due to nodules of tumor in vascular spaces. It can also manifest as a solid mass with diffuse involvement of the myometrium.

Microscopically, the tumor consists of highly cellular, monotonous, small round to ovoid blue

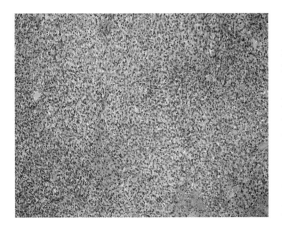

Fig. 9 Endometrial stromal sarcoma. Sheets of monotonous, small, round blue cells are seen

cells that forms large irregular nests and invades the myometrium as irregular tongues (Fig. 9); spindle cell forms can also be seen. Mitotic activity is usually low. A classic feature of endometrial stromal sarcoma is the presence of numerous small vessels resembling endometrial spiral arterioles. Vascular invasion is common. Endometrial stromal sarcoma can exhibit different elements, including smooth muscle differentiation, sex cord-like elements, and gland formation.

CD10 is the immunostain typically associated with endometrial stromal sarcoma; however it is not very specific. Endometrial stromal sarcomas also tend to express ER and PR. In the majority of typical endometrial stromal sarcomas, JAZF1-SUZ12 fusion is present secondary to t(7;17) (p15;q21) (Kurman et al. 2014).

The differential diagnosis of endometrial stromal sarcoma includes endometrial stromal nodule, smooth muscle lesions, adenomyosis, and adenosarcoma. As stated previously, the main difference between endometrial stromal sarcoma and endometrial stromal nodule is the presence of myoinvasion. In an endometrial biopsy, distinguishing between the two may be impossible, but endometrial stromal sarcoma would be more likely. In some cases, it can be difficult to distinguish endometrial stromal sarcoma from smooth muscle tumors, particularly cellular leiomyoma and intravenous leiomyomatosis. Since both endometrial stromal sarcomas and

smooth muscle tumors can express CD10 and smooth muscle markers, a panel of immunostains, rather than one or two immunostains, is recommended to differentiate between the two (see IHC chapter). Adenomyosis can be gland-poor such that only nests of endometrial stroma are seen in the myometrium that can raise suspicion for endometrial stromal sarcoma. Unlike endometrial stromal sarcoma, however, a mass should not be apparent, the stromal cells may appear atrophic, and adenomyosis with sparse glands is more likely to occur in postmenopausal women while endometrial stromal sarcoma is more common in premenopausal women. Adenosarcoma is discussed below.

High-Grade Endometrial Stromal Sarcoma

Recently, a specific genetic alteration was identified in a subset of tumors that are now designated as high-grade endometrial stromal sarcoma by WHO. High-grade endometrial stromal sarcoma exhibits a specific translocation, t(10;17)(q22; p13), which causes YWHAE-FAM22 fusion (Lee et al. 2012). Microscopically, the tumor consists of large, round cells with frequent mitoses and necrosis. Bland spindled cells may also be present. CD10 is negative in the high-grade round cells but tends to be expressed by the low-grade spindled cells. Cyclin D1 staining has also been found in these tumors.

Undifferentiated Endometrial Sarcoma

Undifferentiated endometrial sarcomas are aggressive, high-grade sarcomas. They are rare, occur primarily in postmenopausal women, and present with either abnormal vaginal bleeding or systemic symptoms related to late stage disease.

Microscopically, sheets of pleomorphic oval or spindled cells are seen, usually with necrosis and brisk mitoses. The tumor tends to replace the myometrium, rather than infiltrating it as endometrial stromal sarcoma does. The immunoprofile of undifferentiated endometrial sarcomas is not specific. Undifferentiated endometrial sarcoma may express CD10 and ER like endometrial stromal sarcoma but exhibits much weaker expression. Due to the fairly nonspecific histology of this tumor, the differential is broad, including other high-grade tumors such as high-grade leiomyosarcoma, sarcomatous component of MMMT, and undifferentiated endometrial carcinoma. Undifferentiated endometrial sarcoma is therefore a diagnosis of exclusion after ruling out other lesions.

4.2.2 Smooth Muscle Tumors

Leiomyoma

Leiomyomas are not only the most common tumor in the uterus; uterine leiomyomas are the most common neoplasm in humans. Grossly, classic features of uterine leiomyomas are circumscribed, tan-white solid masses with a whorled appearance on cut surface. Microscopically, leiomyomas show fascicles of uniform cigar-shaped spindle cells with little to no nuclear atypia, low to moderate cellularity, and little to no mitotic activity.

Leiomyosarcoma

Leiomyosarcomas are rare, aggressive tumors that are the most common pure mesenchymal malignancy of the uterus. It is most common in women in their 50s. Diagnosing a leiomyosarcoma requires recognition of two elements: (1) smooth muscle differentiation and (2) that it is malignant. Clinically, leiomyosarcoma may be suspected versus a leiomyoma when there is a single large mass versus multiple masses (leiomyomas) or a dominant large mass among multiple masses.

Grossly, leiomyosarcomas are usually large (10 cm or greater) and have a fleshy variegated appearance with infiltrative margins and necrosis. Microscopically, conventional leiomyosarcomas consist of fascicles of spindled cells with high cellularity, nuclear atypia, and brisk mitoses. Tumor cell necrosis may or may not be seen. The criteria for malignancy in smooth muscle tumors are moderate to marked nuclear atypia, mitotic rate ≥ 10 mitoses/10 HPF, and tumor cell necrosis. Leiomyosarcoma should be diagnosed when two of the three criteria are met.

Distinguishing between tumor cell necrosis and infarct-type necrosis is a well-known problematic issue in uterine smooth muscle neoplasms. Tumor cell necrosis is a criterion of

malignancy while infarct-type necrosis is not. Infarct-type necrosis can be seen in leiomyomas but tumor cell necrosis should not be present, while one or both types of necrosis may be present in leiomyosarcomas, but only tumor cell necrosis qualifies as a criterion of malignancy. Tumor cell necrosis shows abrupt transition from necrotic cells to viable tumor while infarct-type necrosis shows granulation tissue or fibrosis between necrosis and viable cells. Sometimes, the type of necrosis present is indeterminate and such cases, in combination with other features, may best be classified as smooth muscle tumors of unknown malignant potential (STUMP). Another confounding factor is that treated leiomyomas can be necrotic. Another criterion of malignancy, mitotic count, is also not always straightforward. Mitotic count can be overestimated if some cells showing nuclear condensation or smudging that can resemble mitotic figures are counted.

Two variants of leiomyosarcoma are epithelioid and myxoid types. The criteria for malignancy in these variants are somewhat different from conventional type, with both variants only requiring ≥ 5 mitoses/10 HPF rather than ≥ 10 mitoses/10 HPF. Epithelioid leiomyosarcomas have epithelioid or round cells, rather than spindled cells, that demonstrate smooth muscle differentiation by immunohistochemistry. Myxoid leiomyosarcomas, as their name states, show diffuse myxoid change and can have a deceptively bland appearance with low cellularity that may be construed as a benign lesion.

Smooth muscle differentiation can be confirmed with various smooth muscle markers if necessary. The most commonly used immunostains are smooth muscle actin (SMA), desmin, and h-caldesmon. In addition, ER/PR expression may be seen.

Several variants of leiomyomas are recognized that can be mistaken for leiomyosarcomas. They include cellular leiomyoma, leiomyoma with bizarre cells, mitotically active leiomyoma, among others. Cellular leiomyomas, per their name, show high cellularity. Mitotically active leiomyomas can have greater than 10 mitoses/10 HPF but should not show atypical mitoses. Leiomyomas with bizarre cells have also been referred to as symplastic leiomyomas or atypical leiomyomas and show scattered markedly atypical or bizarre cells that can show multinucleation. The aforementioned variants demonstrate a feature that is suspicious for malignancy or a criterion for malignancy; however, they do not have other criteria for malignancy.

The differential diagnosis of leiomyosarcoma depends on its type. Spindled or conventional leiomyosarcomas should be differentiated from cellular leiomyomas, MMMT, endometrial stromal sarcoma, spindle cell rhabdomyosarcoma, undifferentiated sarcoma, and other sarcomas. The differential diagnosis of epithelioid leiomyosarcoma is broad and includes carcinomas, PEComa, malignant melanoma, and other sarcomas. The differential diagnosis of myxoid leiomyosarcoma includes myxoid leiomyoma, myxoid variant of endometrial stromal sarcoma, and myxoid change within the myometrium. Careful attention to histologic features, immunostaining, and clinical information can help in differentiating between the different entities.

Smooth Muscle Tumor of Unknown Malignant Potential

Smooth muscle tumors with equivocal features between leiomyoma and leiomyosarcoma are best classified as smooth muscle tumor of unknown malignant potential or STUMP. Some have also referred to these lesions as atypical smooth muscle tumors, a designation that can be confusing as the term atypical leiomyoma has also been applied to a different lesion, leiomyoma with bizarre cells. STUMP shows some criterion for malignancy that is insufficient to render an unequivocal diagnosis of malignancy. An example would be a lesion with moderate nuclear atypia but no tumor cell necrosis and less than 10 mitoses/10 HPF.

4.3   Mixed Epithelial-Mesenchymal Tumors

4.3.1   Adenosarcoma

Adenosarcoma is a malignant biphasic tumor with a malignant mesenchymal component (sarcoma) and benign epithelial component. It can occur in all ages and usually presents with abnormal vaginal bleeding. Grossly, a polypoid mass is usually seen. Microscopically, adenosarcoma is morphologically similar to phyllodes tumor of the breast and classically shows broad polypoid fronds. The tumor consists of malignant spindled cells and dilated glands of varying shape lined by proliferative type endometrium. The sarcomatous component most often resembles endometrial stromal sarcoma but can exhibit heterologous differentiation. The mesenchymal component should show nuclear atypia, ≥ 2 mitoses/10 HPF, and periglandular cuffing. Periglandular cuffing refers to increased cellularity or condensation of cells around glands and is a distinctive feature of adenosarcomas. The epithelium can show metaplasia such as squamous and ciliated change and may exhibit some cytologic atypia but is not frankly malignant.

The differential diagnosis includes adenofibroma, adenomyoma, MMMT, and sarcomas. Adenofibroma is the benign counterpart of adenosarcoma. Adenomyoma is another polypoid lesion consisting of benign glands with benign stroma with a predominant smooth muscle component. Lack of malignant features of the mesenchymal component should help to identify both adenofibromas and adenomyomas. MMMT will show malignant epithelium, unlike adenosarcomas. A biopsy of an adenosarcoma may mimic pure sarcoma if the epithelial component is not evident; in some cases, diagnosis is best made on the excisional specimen. Immunostains are usually not necessary for diagnosis; if performed, the sarcomatous component will usually stain like endometrial stromal sarcomas, expressing CD10, ER, PR, and WT1.

Adenosarcomas may recur in 25% of cases. Cases with sarcomatous overgrowth ($\geq 25\%$ high-grade sarcomatous component) tend to be more aggressive (Clement 1989).

4.3.2   Malignant Mixed Mullerian Tumor

Malignant mixed Mullerian tumor (MMMT) or carcinosarcoma is a biphasic tumor with both epithelial and mesenchymal elements. They

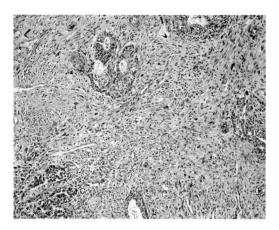

Fig. 10 Malignant mixed Mullerian tumor (MMMT). Biphasic pattern with glands and pleomorphic spindle cells is seen

comprise less than 5% of uterine malignancies and occur almost exclusively in postmenopausal women.

Grossly, MMMT may present as a polypoid mass and exhibit a fleshy appearance. Microscopically, the presence of malignant glands admixed with high-grade spindled cells is essentially diagnostic of MMMT (Fig. 10). These tumors however can exhibit varying histology. The epithelial component may show elements of endometrioid, serous, or other high-grade carcinomas, including unclassifiable carcinoma, while the mesenchymal component can be homologous and/or heterologous. Homologous elements refer to finding cells showing differentiation indigenous to the uterus, such as smooth muscle, while heterologous elements refer to the presence of tissue not usually found in the uterus, such as skeletal muscle. The homologous component in MMMT is often high-grade spindled or pleomorphic cells, while the heterologous component is often rhabdomyosarcoma (skeletal muscle differentiation) or chondrosarcoma (cartilaginous differentiation). The proportion of the epithelial to the mesenchymal component can vary. In some cases, the epithelial component may so predominate in an endometrial biopsy that MMMT can only be diagnosed on the excision. Lymphovascular invasion is common.

In MMMT, cytokeratin immunostains are not only expressed by the epithelial component but also tend to stain the mesenchymal component. The differentiation of the mesenchymal component can be demonstrated if necessary with stains such as desmin and myogenin for rhabdomyosarcoma but is usually not necessary.

The differential diagnosis of MMMT includes endometrioid carcinoma with spindle cells, endometrioid adenocarcinoma with heterologous elements, mixed endometrioid and undifferentiated carcinoma, and adenosarcoma. Endometrioid carcinoma with spindle cells should not show immunostaining for a mesenchymal component, heterologous elements in endometrioid adenocarcinoma should not be malignant as they are in MMMT, mixed endometrioid and undifferentiated carcinoma will usually show a low-grade epithelial component compared with the high-grade epithelial component seen in MMMT, and in adenosarcoma, the epithelial component is benign.

MMMT are aggressive tumors with a poor prognosis. Heterologous tumors had been thought to have a poorer prognosis at one time; however that is currently controversial. When MMMT metastasize, the epithelial component is more likely to be seen.

4.4 Other Uterine Tumors

4.4.1 Perivascular Epithelioid Cell Tumor

Perivascular epithelioid cell tumors (PEComas) are rare tumors of unclear origin that express both melanocytic (HMB-45, Melan-A) and smooth muscle markers (SMA, desmin). In some cases, PEComas are associated with tuberous sclerosis and lymphangioleiomyomatosis (LAM). Microscopically, fairly uniform, epithelioid or spindled cells with clear and eosinophilic cytoplasm are seen that classically show a nested growth pattern (Fig. 11). A prominent capillary pattern is usually present. Uterine PEComas may behave in a benign or malignant manner. One system proposed the following criteria for malignancy: size greater than 5 cm, high-grade nuclear atypia, necrosis, vascular invasion, ≥ 1 mitosis/

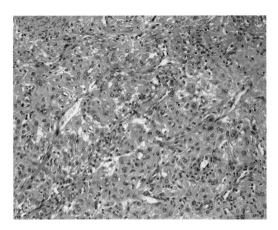

Fig. 11 Perivascular epithelioid cell tumor (PEComa). Nests of eosinophilic, epithelioid cells with mild pleomorphism are seen

50 HPF, and infiltrative growth pattern (Folpe et al. 2005). The differential diagnosis includes smooth muscle tumors, secondary involvement by gastrointestinal stromal tumors, malignant melanoma, and alveolar soft part sarcoma. Immunostains can help in diagnosis although smooth muscle neoplasms can also show expression of HMB-45 which can be a pitfall in diagnosis.

4.4.2 Primitive Neuroectodermal Tumor

Primitive neuroectodermal tumor (PNET) is an aggressive small round blue cell tumor thought to be of neuroectodermal origin that rarely occurs in the uterus. PNET is also referred to as Ewing sarcoma. Microscopically, sheets of monotonous, small, round cells are seen with brisk mitoses. A feature classically associated with PNET is rosettes; however they are not that commonly seen. Like PNET at other sites, uterine PNET tends to show membranous CD99 staining and FLI1 staining. They may also express neuroendocrine markers (synaptophysin, chromogranin). A characteristic translocation of these tumors is t(11;22) that leads to the fusion of EWS and FLI-1 genes. The differential diagnosis includes other round blue cell tumors such as small cell carcinoma, lymphoma, rhabdomyosarcoma, and endometrial stromal sarcoma.

4.4.3 Lymphoma

Non-Hodgkin lymphoma rarely involves the gynecologic tract. The female genital tract is the primary site of extranodal lymphomas in less than 2% of cases (Cohn et al. 2007). Secondary involvement is more common. Most cases are diffuse large B-cell lymphoma. Patients may be asymptomatic or present with abnormal vaginal bleeding or nonspecific complaints such as bloating. Lymphoma is a round blue cell tumor that shows a diffuse growth pattern. It tends to expand the endometrium and grows around the endometrial glands. The differential diagnosis includes other round blue cell tumors such as undifferentiated carcinoma, neuroendocrine carcinoma, particularly small cell carcinoma, PNET, and endometrial stromal sarcoma. Benign processes such as reactive lymphoid infiltrates and chronic endometritis should also be considered. Ancillary testing with immunohistochemical staining is necessary for a correct diagnosis; flow cytometry would also be helpful.

5 Gestational Trophoblastic Disease

Gestational trophoblastic diseases are diseases that occur related to pregnancy. Some understanding of normal placental histology is necessary to understand gestational trophoblastic diseases. The placenta is composed of amnion and chorionic villi. Chorionic villi consist of a core of stroma and capillaries lined circumferentially by cytotrophoblasts and syncytiotrophoblasts. Cytotrophoblasts are mononuclear, epithelioid cells with clear to eosinophilic cytoplasm. Syncytiotrophoblasts are multinucleated cells with hyperchromatic, smudgy nuclei. Intermediate or extravillous trophoblasts are another type of cell that helps anchor the placenta to the uterus and is usually found in the decidua. They can be epithelioid or spindled, have eosinophilic or amphophilic cytoplasm, and are usually mononuclear but can show multinucleation. Intermediate trophoblasts are thought to give rise to several gestational diseases, including exaggerated placental site, placental site nodule, placental site trophoblastic tumor (PSTT), and epithelioid trophoblastic tumor (ETT).

5.1 Hydatidiform Mole

Hydatidiform moles are products of abnormal fertilization and consist of partial and complete moles. Grossly, moles have a characteristic appearance often described as a "bunch of grapes" that consist of clear to opaque, small, delicate vesicles.

5.1.1 Complete Mole

Most complete moles develop when a single sperm or two sperm fertilize an egg that has lost its DNA, i.e., empty egg; hence all chromosomes in complete moles are usually paternally derived. Most complete moles have no fetal tissue and consist entirely of enlarged edematous villi or hydropic villi with circumferential trophoblastic proliferation. Cisterns or cavities are a characteristic feature. The stroma shows the absence of nucleated red blood cells that are seen in normal villi.

5.1.2 Partial Mole

Partial moles develop when a viable egg is fertilized by two sperm or by one sperm that duplicates itself leading to a triploid karyotype (69XXY or 69XXX). Partial moles have some fetal tissue and consist of a mixture of enlarged and normal-sized villi. Cisterns and nucleated red blood cells may be present. Fibrotic villi may be seen. Trophoblastic hyperplasia occurs but is less prominent than in complete moles.

Complete and partial moles need to be differentiated from hydropic villi of non-molar abortion or hydropic abortus as molar pregnancy has significant clinical implications. If histology is equivocal, ancillary studies can help to confirm the diagnosis. A fairly simple and cost-effective next step is p57 immunostaining. p57 is a biomarker expressed only in the maternal genome as it is paternally imprinted. In complete moles, p57 should be absent in cytotrophoblasts and villous stromal cells while in partial moles and hydropic villi, p57 is expressed. In some cases, p57

immunostaining may be equivocal and in these cases, further testing may be required.

DNA ploidy analysis can also be performed to determine whether a triploid (partial mole or hydropic abortus) or diploid (complete mole or hydropic abortus) population is present. Flow cytometry and fluorescent in situ hybridization (FISH) are two common methods of analysis; however one major limitation of these tests is that they will not distinguish hydropic abortus from partial moles. Currently, the best method for differentiating between the three entities is molecular genotyping with polymerase chain reaction (PCR) which requires maternal endometrial tissue.

Sequelae of molar pregnancy include persistent gestational disease (retained molar tissue and invasive moles), recurrence, and malignant gestational disease. Persistent and invasive moles occur in 15–20% of complete moles and less than 4% of partial moles (Conran et al. 1993). Beta-hCG is followed to monitor for persistent gestational disease, and methotrexate is used for treatment. As medical treatment is highly effective, histologic diagnosis of invasive moles is infrequent. However, if seen, invasive moles will show villi invading the myometrium. Distant metastasis can occur with invasive moles.

5.2 Malignant Gestational Disease

Choriocarcinoma, placental site trophoblastic tumor (PSTT), and epithelioid trophoblastic tumor (ETT) are all rare malignancies that are associated with previous gestation, particularly with molar pregnancy. Choriocarcinoma is more strongly associated with molar pregnancy than the other two tumors. Choriocarcinoma tends to occur months after pregnancy, while PSTT and ETT usually occur many years afterwards. Abnormal vaginal bleeding is commonly the presenting symptom. In cases of choriocarcinoma and PSTT, the tumor may have already metastasized at the time of presentation so the presenting symptoms will be related to metastasis. Beta-hCG is elevated in all three tumors; however it is much higher in choriocarcinoma than in PSTT and ETT.

5.2.1 Choriocarcinoma

Less than 3% of molar pregnancies lead to choriocarcinoma while half of choriocarcinomas are related to molar pregnancy. Twenty-five percent follow intrauterine gestation and 25% follow abortion or tubal pregnancy.

Grossly, choriocarcinoma presents as a markedly hemorrhagic mass with necrosis. Microscopically, a solid proliferation of cells consisting of three cell types, cytotrophoblasts, intermediate trophoblasts, and syncytiotrophoblasts, is seen. A "biphasic" pattern of cytotrophoblasts alternating with syncytiotrophoblasts is characteristic of this tumor. Both cytotrophoblasts and syncytiotrophoblasts show pleomorphism. In some cases, syncytiotrophoblasts may not be apparent and beta-hCG staining can be performed to identify their presence as syncytiotrophoblasts are necessary to render a diagnosis of choriocarcinoma. Hemorrhage is typical, necrosis is often seen, and villi are not present.

5.2.2 Placental Site Trophoblastic Tumor

Grossly, an ill-defined mass is seen deeply invading the myometrium. Microscopically, sheets of pleomorphic, mononuclear, epithelioid cells with clear, eosinophilic, or amphophilic cytoplasm are seen. The cells tend to split smooth muscle fibers of the myometrium. Nuclear grooves may be seen. Brisk mitoses are typical and necrosis and hemorrhage frequent. Sometimes, the neoplastic cells can show multinucleation that should not be mistaken for syncytiotrophoblasts.

5.2.3 Epithelioid Trophoblastic Tumor

Grossly, a well-circumscribed tumor that deeply invades the myometrium with hemorrhage and necrosis is seen. Microscopically, mononuclear epithelioid cells with abundant clear or eosinophilic cytoplasm are seen like in PSTT but are less pleomorphic than in PSTT. Multinucleated cells may be seen. Necrosis and lymphocytic infiltrate are often seen.

The differential diagnosis of both PSTT and ETT are placental site nodule, exaggerated placental site, choriocarcinoma, and squamous cell carcinoma. Placental site nodule is a benign lesion that can be found years after pregnancy as residue of gestation. It is most often an incidental finding. Small hyalinized nodules of intermediate trophoblasts with variable nuclear atypia and clear and eosinophilic cytoplasm are seen. Placental site nodule should not form a mass like PSTT and ETT, and it also should have low Ki67 (less than 10%) compared with Ki67 greater than 10% in PSTT and ETT. Exaggerated placental site can show similar morphology to these tumors but is usually found after recent gestation. It also should have Ki67 less than 1 (Kurman et al. 2011). Beta-hCG staining can be used to differentiate choriocarcinoma from these two entities. To distinguish squamous cell carcinoma from PSTT and ETT, immunostains can be used to identify squamous cells of squamous cell carcinoma versus the trophoblasts of PSTT and ETT. Both PSTT and ETT can show recurrence and metastasis, however do not appear to be as aggressive as choriocarcinoma.

6 Conclusion

Various lesions, both benign and malignant, occur in the uterus. The most common are benign leiomyomas and malignant endometrial carcinomas while more rare entities include gestational trophoblastic diseases. The mainstay of pathologic diagnosis is morphology; however, ancillary studies such as immunohistochemical staining can be instrumental in diagnosing a lesion. Advances in molecular pathology have led to the identification of certain mutations such as the recently identified translocation in tumors now designated high-grade endometrial stromal sarcomas; undoubtedly, more mutations will be discovered creating a larger role for molecular testing to better classify and possibly treat uterine tumors.

7   Cross-References

References

Abeler VM, Kjorstad KE. Clear cell carcinoma of the endometrium: a histopathological and clinical study of 97 cases. Gynecol Oncol. 1991;40(3):207–17.

Altrabulsi B, Malpica A, Deavers MT, Bodurka DC, Broaddus R, Silva EG. Undifferentiated carcinoma of the endometrium. Am J Surg Pathol. 2005;29(10): 1316–21.

Clement PB. Mullerian adenosarcomas of the uterus with sarcomatous overgrowth. A clinicopathological analysis of 10 cases. Am J Surg Pathol. 1989;13(1):28–38.

Cohn DE, Resnick KE, Eaton LA, deHart J, Zanagnolo V. Non-Hodgkin's lymphoma mimicking gynecological malignancies of the vagina and cervix: a report of four cases. Int J Gynecol Cancer. 2007;17(1):274–9.

Conran RM, Hitchcock CL, Popek EJ, Norris HJ, Griffin JL, Geissel A, et al. Diagnostic considerations in molar gestations. Hum Pathol. 1993;24(1):41–8.

Folpe AL, Mentzel T, Lehr HA, Fisher C, Balzer BL, Weiss SW. Perivascular epithelioid cell neoplasms of soft tissue and gynecologic origin: a clinicopathologic study of 26 cases and review of the literature. Am J Surg Pathol. 2005;29(12):1558–75.

Kurman RJ, Kaminski PF, Norris HJ. The behavior of endometrial hyperplasia. A long-term study of "untreated" hyperplasia in 170 patients. Cancer. 1985; 56(2):403–12.

Kurman RJ, Ellenson LH, Ronnett BM. Blaustein's pathology of the female genital tract. 2011. Springer, New York.

Kurman RJ, Carcangiu ML, Herrington CS, Young RH. WHO classification of tumours of female reproductive organs. Lyon: International Agency for Research on Cancer; 2014.

Lee CH, Marino-Enriquez A, Ou W, Zhu M, Ali RH, Chiang S, et al. The clinicopathologic features of YWHAE-FAM22 endometrial stromal sarcomas: a histologically high-grade and clinically aggressive tumor. Am J Surg Pathol. 2012;36(5):641–53.

Mutter GL, Baak JP, Crum CP, Richart RM, Ferenczy A, Faquin WC. Endometrial precancer diagnosis by histopathology, clonal analysis, and computerized morphometry. J Pathol. 2000;190(4):462–9.

Sherman ME, Bitterman P, Rosenshein NB, Delgado G, Kurman RJ. Uterine serous carcinoma. A morphologically diverse neoplasm with unifying clinicopathologic features. Am J Surg Pathol. 1992;16(6):600–10.

Silva EG, Jenkins R. Serous carcinoma in endometrial polyps. Mod Pathol. 1990;3(2):120–8.

Taraif SH, Deavers MT, Malpica A, Silva EG. The significance of neuroendocrine expression in undifferentiated carcinoma of the endometrium. Int J Gynecol Pathol. 2009;28(2):142–7.

Germ Cell Tumors of the Ovaries

Mohamed Mokhtar Desouki and Oluwole Fadare

Abstract

The basic classification of ovarian germ cell tumors has largely remained unchanged for several decades. Ovarian germ cell tumors develop from primordial germ and stem cells that differentiate into extraembryonal and somatic tissues. In most cases, benign and malignant ovarian germ cell tumors can be correctly diagnosed due to their characteristic morphologic profiles. Several immunohistochemical (IHC) markers are widely available and can significantly facilitate tumor typing of germ cell tumors, especially in high grade tumors or in atypical clinical scenarios. In this chapter, the clinicopathologic features of ovarian germ cell tumors will be reviewed, with emphasis on morphology and diagnostically useful IHC markers.

Keywords

Germ cell tumors • Mature teratoma • Immature teratoma • Struma ovarii • Dysgerminoma • Yolk sac tumor • Embryonal carcinoma • Choriocarcinoma

Contents

M.M. Desouki (✉)
Department of Pathology, Microbiology and Immunology, Vanderbilt University Medical Center, Nashville, TN, USA
e-mail: mokhtar.desouki@vanderbilt.edu

O. Fadare
Department of Pathology, University of California San Diego, San Diego, CA, USA
e-mail: ofadare@ucsd.edu

1   Introduction

Ovarian germ cell tumors (OGCTs) are derived from neoplastic transformation of the ovarian primordial germ and stem cells. These tumors are unique because they form imperfectly formed "normal" human body tissues (Nogales et al. 2014). Germ cell tumors (GCTs) can be classified into: (1) tumors with mature elements which include mature cystic teratoma (MCT), (2) tumors with immature elements exhibiting range of differentiation and include dysgerminoma, embryonal carcinoma (EC), choriocarcinoma (CC), yolk sac tumor (YST), and immature teratoma (IT), and (3) malignant transformations such as squamous cell carcinoma (SCC), carcinoid, malignant struma ovarii and other rare neoplasms arising in a preexisting mature teratoma (Table 1) (Prat et al. 2014). Most GCTs are benign with straightforward pathologic diagnosis. Only rarely these tumors present diagnostic issues especially when occur in unusual clinical scenarios. On the other hand, malignant ovarian germ cell tumors (MOGCTs) or malignant transformation in an existing MCT account for a small fraction of OGCTs (Nogales et al. 2014).

2   Epidemiology and Clinical Presentation

While OGCTs constitute 20–25% of all ovarian neoplasms, only <3% are malignant. The prevalence is significantly higher (15%) in Asian and

Table 1 World Health Organization (WHO) classification of ovarian germ cell tumors[a]

Mature teratoma
Immature teratoma
Monodermal teratoma
Struma ovarii
Carcinoid
Somatic tumors arising from dermoid cyst
Squamous cell carcinoma and others
Dysgerminoma
Yolk sac tumor
Embryonal carcinoma
Choriocarcinoma

[a]Only the most commonly encountered tumors in practice are included (Prat et al. 2014)

black populations as compared to Caucasian populations (5%) (Low et al. 2012). Clinical information including patient age, elevated serum markers, and presentation are important to report to the pathologic laboratory when specimens are being submitted, as they constitute a component of the pathologic evaluation and assessment. For example, benign MCTs predominate in reproductive-age women, immature teratomas and malignant GCTs predominate at young age (below 20), and somatic malignant transformation, e.g., SCC is more common in postmenopausal women (Nogales et al. 2014).

Patients are either asymptomatic with the tumor discovered incidentally on clinical or radiologic examinations or present with abdominal pain and/or a palpable abdominal mass. The mass may grow rapidly in a fraction of cases (~10%) resulting in acute abdominal pain due to capsular distention, ischemic necrosis, hemorrhage, rupture, or torsion (Nogales et al. 2014). MOGCT may present with metastases. Alpha-fetoprotein (AFP), lactate dehydrogenase (LDH), beta human chorionic gonadotropin (β-hCG), and cancer antigen 125 (CA-125) titers are some serum tumor markers used mainly for follow-up after treatment (Prat et al. 2014).

3   Mature Teratoma

Ovarian teratomas differentiate to mature tissues derived from the three germ layers. On the other hand, monodermal teratomas such as struma ovarii differentiate to one germ layer. Mature teratomas are the most common OGCTs accounting for ~20% of all ovarian tumors, more than 90% of OGCTs, and are the most common tumors seen in children (de Silva et al. 2004; Nogales et al. 2014).

3.1   Gross Pathology

Most lesions are mature cystic teratomas (MCTs). Approximately, 15% of MCTs are bilateral. MCTs usually measure from 5 to 10 cm and contain a mixture of hair, skin, and malodorous sebaceous or keratinaceous material

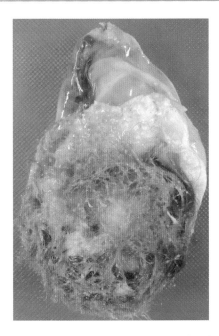

Fig. 1 Mature cystic teratoma containing hair tufts and sebaceous material

(Fig. 1). A raised protuberance (Rokitansky's tubercle) is often present and should be pathologically evaluated (Peterson et al. 1955). The cyst may be unilocular or multilocular, and the contents may appear hemorrhagic, similar to an endometriotic cyst. The more grossly complex the cyst is, the more likely the presence of other elements such as thyroid tissue (solid and brown mass).

3.2 Histopathology

Morphologically, MCTs are composed of various tissues derived from one or more germ layers. Ectodermal components, which are usually the most prominent, include skin with associated appendages (Fig. 2a) and mature neuroectodermal tissue (Fig. 2b), among others. Endodermal components include thyroid, salivary, and gastrointestinal tissues, among others (Fig. 2c, d). Mesodermal component includes muscle, cartilage (Fig. 2d), bone, and fat. MCTs may show minute neuroepithelial/ependymal areas which should not be reported as immature teratoma (Yanai-Inbar and Scully 1987). Gliomatosis

peritonei (GP) is a teratoma associated with peritoneal nodules composed of mature glial tissue. Despite its advanced clinical stage (stage III), its behavior is benign if immature elements are absent. The origin for GP may be related to capsular rupture from the ovarian teratoma, although this is still largely speculative (Perrone et al. 1986; Peterson et al. 1955).

Ovarian mucinous tumors may be associated with mature cystic teratomas. These mucinous tumors display an IHC profile that is similar to gastrointestinal tract adenocarcinomas, including expression of CK20, CDX2, and villin and lack thereof for CK7 (Vang et al. 2007). These features would point toward a germ cell origin for the mucinous component rather than metastasis from a gastrointestinal primary. Rarely, the teratoma component is overgrown by the mucinous tumor (Vang et al. 2007).

4 Immature Teratoma

Immature teratoma is the second (after dysgerminoma) most common MOGCT (Fig. 3). Grossly, the tumors are large, solid, and fleshy with hemorrhage, necrosis, and cyst formation. Immature element (mainly primitive neuroectoderm) is the diagnostic feature of the lesion. Primitive neuroectodermal units are composed of tubules and rosettes. The tubules are lined by atypical, hyperchromatic, stratified cells with frequent mitoses. Immature cartilage, fat, bone, and skeletal muscles are often present but by themselves are not enough to qualify a MCT as immature. Embryoid bodies are the most primitive element in immature teratomas and consist of yolk sac epithelium and germ disk with cells resembling embryonal carcinoma. In rare instances, the immature element consists of mitotically active cellular glia admixed with ectodermal and endodermal elements (Yanai-Inbar and Scully 1987). Assessment of the degree of immaturity (grading) is a highly reliable prognostic and therapeutic factor (Gershenson 2012). Grading is performed by assessing the relative amount of the immature neuroectodermal component as assessed microscopically. Two-tiered (low

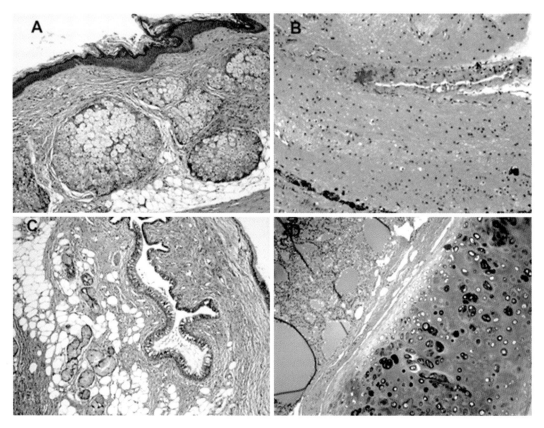

Fig. 2 Mature cystic teratoma containing tissues from all three germ lines. (**a**) Dermoid cyst lined by keratinized squamous epithelium with sebaceous glands in the dermis. (**b**) Mature glial (brain) tissue. (**c**) Glandular type epithelium. (**d**) Cartilage and variable sized colloid filled thyroid follicles (struma ovarii)

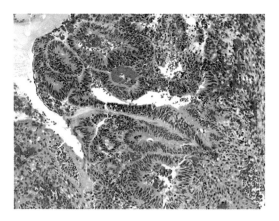

Fig. 3 Immature teratoma containing the diagnostic immature primitive neuroepithelium forming gland-like pseudo-rosettes with palisaded nuclei

and high grade) and three-tiered grading systems are in use (O'Connor and Norris 1994).

The three-tier grading system has been adopted by the most recent World Health Organization (WHO) classification of gynecologic tumors (Prat et al. 2014). Grade 1 tumors contain rare foci of immature elements occupying <1 low power field (x4) in any slide. The immature elements in grade 2 tumors occupy 1–3 low power field in any slide. On the other hand, the primitive neuroectodermal immature elements occupy >3 low power fields in grade 3 tumors (Norris et al. 1976). Any tumor with immature elements occupying more than one low-power field per any slide is a high-grade tumor in the two-tier grading system (i.e., all grade 2 tumors are high grade) (O'Connor and Norris 1994). The two-tier grade system may be more practical since most grade 2 tumors are more comparable in clinical behavior to grade 3 tumors than they are to grade 1 tumors in a three-tiered system. Additionally, unlike grade 1 tumors which are treated conservatively, grade 2 and 3 tumors are treated similarly with recommended chemotherapy (Patterson and Rustin 2006). A point of caution is the occasional presence of normal neuroepithelium in mature teratomas which should not be confused with immature neuroectodermal elements.

4.1 Serum Markers and Immunophenotype

One third of immature teratomas produce AFP. Positive markers include SOX2, SALL4, Glypican-3 (focal), and OCT3/4 (focal) (Liu et al. 2010).

5 Monodermal Teratomas

5.1 Struma Ovarii

Struma ovarii is a monodermal teratoma composed predominantly of thyroid tissue. The tumor occurs most frequently in the fifth decade of life. Clinical hyperthyroidism occurs in <5% of cases. Grossly, the tumor characteristically appears as greenish brown, firm to slightly gelatinous. Microscopically, struma ovarii varies from a classic macro- and microfollicles with abundant colloid to a cyst with small tubules (Fig. 2d). Solid patterns with hurthle or clear cells may be present and occasionally form trabecular configurations that may mimic carcinoid (Loughrey et al. 2003). The presence of morphologically benign thyroid tissue in the peritoneum (peritoneal strumosis) is now being recognized as a metastatic low-grade follicular neoplasm (Roth and Karseladze 2008).

5.2 Carcinoid Tumor

Carcinoid tumor is a well-differentiated neuroendocrine tumor that arises in MCTs. Grossly, these tumors are brown to tan masses. Microscopically, primary ovarian carcinoids exhibit insular, trabecular, strumal (see below), and goblet cell variants. Insular carcinoids are characterized by tubular glands arranged in garland-like patterns separated by fibrous stroma and sharply defined central lumina with uniform rounded nuclei with fine chromatin stippling (salt and pepper) (Figs. 4 and 5). Trabecular carcinoids display discrete linear cords and trabeculae. The rare

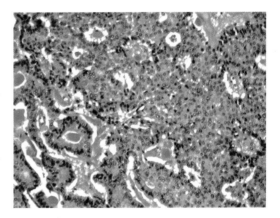

Fig. 4 Insular carcinoid forming broad interconnected sheets of cells

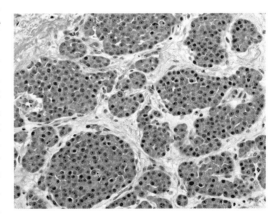

Fig. 5 Insular carcinoid forming sheets of cells with the characteristic granular (salt and pepper) chromatin

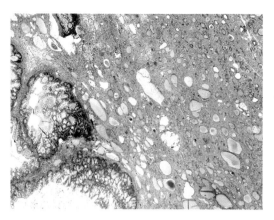

Fig. 6 Mucinous tumor (*left*) and goblet carcinoid (*right*). Notice the admixture of colloid-filled follicles of the thyroid stuma ovarii and the nests and cords of carcinoid component

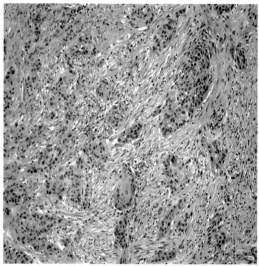

Fig. 7 Invasive squamous cell carcinoma arising in a mature cystic teratoma

goblet cell carcinoids exhibit range of differentiation, including well-differentiated tumors with glands lined by goblet cells in a mucinous background, confluent glands with cribriform or microcystic patterns, and frank carcinomas associated with the carcinoid (Baker et al. 2001).

5.3   Strumal Carcinoid

Strumal carcinoid is a mixed tumor composed of struma ovarii and carcinoid in a background of MCT elements. Grossly, strumal carcinoid exhibits both solid white-to-yellow appearance of carcinoid and fleshy brown areas of thyroid component. Histologically, the carcinoid merges abruptly with the thyroid follicles with variable colloid or both components may be morphologically indistinguishable (Fig. 6). TTF-1, PAX8, and thyroglobulin IHC stains will highlight the thyroid component (Prat et al. 2014).

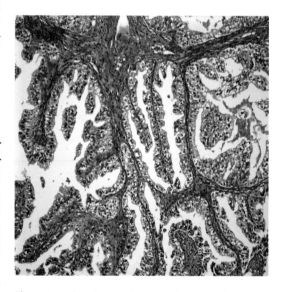

Fig. 8 Invasive adenocarcinoma arising in a mature cystic teratoma

6   Malignant Transformation in Teratomas

The reported incidence for an associated malignant tumor within an MCT is 1.2–14.2 cases per 100,000 more than 75–90% of which are squamous cell carcinoma (SCCs) (Fig. 7), especially in postmenopausal patients (Hackethal et al. 2008). Wide varieties of other malignancies have been reported including adenocarcinomas (Fig. 8), lymphomas, melanomas, thyroid carcinoma (mainly papillary thyroid carcinoma), and YSTs. Advanced age and larger tumor size are some factors that have been significantly associated with malignant transformation (Desouki et al. 2015).

7 Dysgerminoma

The morphology of dysgerminoma is identical to the testicular counterpart, seminoma and the midline germinoma (Low et al. 2012).

7.1 Epidemiology and Clinical Features

Dysgerminoma comprises 1–2% of malignant ovarian tumors and is the most common malignant primitive GCT. The tumor occurs almost exclusively in children and young adults, with an average age of 22 years. Patients with gonadal dysgenesis with partial or complete Y chromosome are more commonly susceptible to dysgerminomas arising in a gonadoblastoma (Fig. 9). The overall survival for treated cases is >90%. Clinical stage and tumor size are the most important prognostic factors (de Silva et al. 2004; Prat et al. 2014).

7.2 Gross and Histopathology

The tumors are large with an average diameter of 10 cm. They exhibit solid, tan, or fleshy-white cut surfaces, occasional hemorrhage, necrosis, and cyst formation. Histologically, the neoplastic germ cells are usually arranged in sheets and sometimes grow in individual cords with rare microcysts or pseudoglandular spaces. The tumor is composed of large, clear, primitive germ cells showing no specific pattern of differentiation. The cells are polygonal with abundant eosinophilic cytoplasm and distinct cell borders. The nuclei are uniform with vesicular chromatin, prominent nucleoli, and numerous mitotic figures. The nests of neoplastic cells are surrounded by fibrous stroma with characteristic infiltrating lymphocytes (mostly T cells) (Hadrup et al. 2006; Fig. 9). A minority of cases show a prominent population of syncytiotrophoblasts. Cases with minimal lymphocytic infiltration or an epithelioid eosinophilic cytoplasm should be differentiated from EC and YSTs (Kao et al. 2012). Cases with granulomatous pattern composed of isolated cells embedded in an extensive fibrosis or chronic inflammatory matrix can also represent a diagnostic challenge. Additionally, clear cell carcinomas with solid growth pattern may display morphologic similarity to dysgerminomas (Nogales et al. 2014).

7.3 Serum Markers and Immunophenotype

A small fraction of dysgerminomas (3–5%) have elevated LDH or low levels of β-hCG. Tumor cells are positive for PLAP, CD117 (c-KIT) (Lau et al. 2007; Fig. 9), D2-40 which is a relatively specific marker (Lau et al. 2007), OCT3/4 (POU5F1), SOX2, and SALL4 by IHC (Liu et al. 2010; Table 2).

7.4 Genetic Abnormalities

Most cases show isochromosome 12p. *C-KIT* mutation has been reported in up to 50% of cases (Prat et al. 2014).

8 Yolk Sac Tumor

YST is a primitive GCT with multiple patterns ranging from primitive gut and mesenchyme to somatic tissue as intestine and liver. These tumors generally have a favorable response to contemporary chemotherapy regimens (de Silva et al. 2004; Nogales-Fernandez et al. 1977).

8.1 Gross and Histopathology

YST is usually a large, soft, encapsulated tumor with gray yellow cut surfaces. Areas of necrosis, hemorrhage, and cyst formation are common. These tumors show complex histologic characteristics comprising early endodermal differentiation into secondary yolk sac elements. Multiple

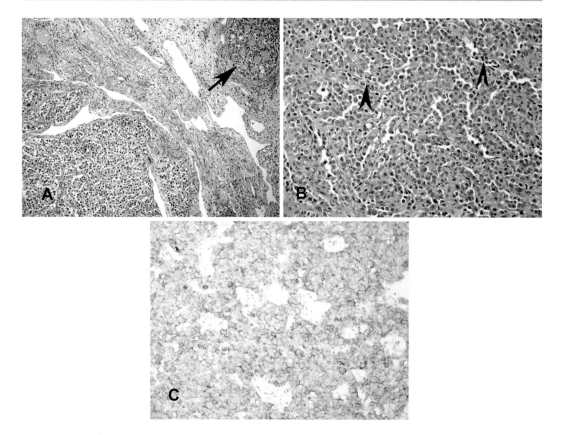

Fig. 9 Dysgerminoma. A germ cell tumor commonly arises in patients with gonadal dysgenesis in a gonadoblastoma (*arrow*) (**a**). The tumor cells grow in sheets of uniform neoplastic cells with centrally placed nuclei and well-defined cell membranes separated by a delicate stroma studied with lymphocytes (*arrow heads*) (**b**). The tumor cells are often positive for CD117 immunohistochemical stain (**c**)

terms have historically been used for these tumors, including endodermal sinus tumors and primitive endodermal tumors. The classic histologic features include reticular microcystic spaces with hyaline globules and amorphous acellular basement membrane like material (Nogales-Fernandez et al. 1977). The cells lining the cystic spaces are clear and flattened that form papillary fibrovascular structures with central blood vessels surrounded by tumor cells and projecting into the space lined by the tumor cells in a characteristic Schiller-Duval bodies (Fig. 10). The stroma is usually myxoid, loose, and hypocellular. Other patterns include polyvesicular type, hepatoid, and intestinal,

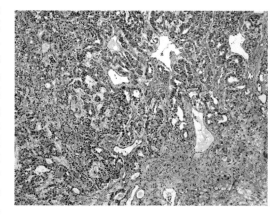

Fig. 10 Yolk sac tumor. The tumor cells grew in microcystic and glandular patterns

Table 2 Selected immunohistochemistry markers used in the diagnosis and/or differentiation of rare ovarian germ cell tumors

	Dysgerminoma	Yolk sac tumor	Choriocarcinoma	Embryonal carcinoma
HCG-Beta	7%	0	100%	23%
OCT 3/4	70%	0	0	100%
Glypican 3	16%	89%	78%	7%
CD117	92%	37%	0	11%
Alpha- fetoprotein	N/A	69%	0	31%
SALL4	53%	99%	50%	99%
PLAP	96%	46%	49%	100%
SOX2	67%	0	0	100%

The percentage represents the reported positive cases. See text for references
N/A not reported

which are rare and may mimic other neoplasms (Cohen et al. 1987; Kao et al. 2012).

8.2 Serum Markers and Immunophenotype

YSTs produce AFP which is considered the gold standard for the diagnosis and follow-up of YSTs. YSTs are positive for AFP, Glypican 3 (Kandil and Cooper 2009), SALL4, HepPar-1 in hepatoid areas, CDX2 and villin in intestinal areas, TTF 1, and CD117 by IHC (Liu et al. 2010; Table 2).

9 Embryonal Carcinoma

EC is an extremely rare malignant ovarian germ cell tumor. Due to its rarity, any diagnosis of EC in a female patient should prompt a chromosomal study. Differential diagnosis includes dysgerminoma and YST (Kao et al. 2012; Prat et al. 2014).

9.1 Clinical Features

ECs are aggressive but chemosensitive tumors that occur in children and young adults with an average age of 15 years. Precocious pseudopuberty and isochromosome 12p may be associated with EC (Gershenson 2012).

9.2 Gross and Histopathology

ECs are usually large tumors with an average diameter of 15 cm. The tumors are solid with soft, fleshy cut surfaces with cyst formation, hemorrhage, and necrosis. Histologically, the tumor grows in solid sheets with glandular differentiation. The cells are polygonal with vesicular nuclei, coarse chromatin, and prominent nucleoli. Mitotic figures are numerous. Areas of necrosis and hemorrhage are extensive. Syncytiotrophoblasts are common (Fig. 11; Pallesen and Hamilton-Dutoit 1988).

9.3 Serum Markers and Immunophenotype

EC may produce β-hCG and AFP with the former being more common. ECs are positive for cytokeratin, CD30 (Pallesen and Hamilton-Dutoit 1988), SOX2, PLAP, OCT3/4, and SALL4 (Liu et al. 2010; Table 2).

10 Choriocarcinoma

Pure nongestational CC is exceptionally rare in the ovaries. These tumors occur mostly in children and young adults (Prat et al. 2014). Grossly, these tumors are large with solid and cystic components, extensive hemorrhage, and necrosis. The tumors show mononuclear trophoblasts and sheets of multinucleated syncytiotrophoblasts arranged in plexiform pattern. Areas

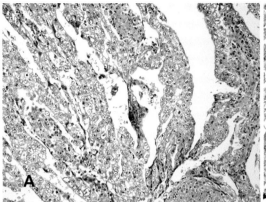

Fig. 11 Embryonal carcinoma. Tumor cells are polygonal and grow in solid sheets (**a**). The cells have vesicular nuclei, coarse chromatin, prominent nucleoli, and frequent mitotic figures (**b**). Notice areas of necrosis and hemorrhage. Syncytiotrophoblasts are common (*arrows*)

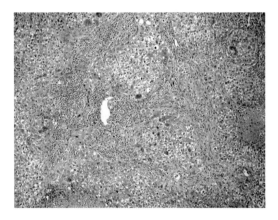

Fig. 12 Choriocarcinoma. The tumor composed of mononuclear trophoblasts and sheets of syncytiotrophoblasts arranged with areas of hemorrhage and necrosis

of hemorrhage and/or necrosis may be so extensive as to obscure the malignant cells (Fig. 12). β-hCG is a well-known serum marker that is frequently elevated in patients with choriocarcinoma, CC is positive for cytokeratin, β-hCG, α-inhibin (McCluggage 2001), SALL4, CD10, and glypican-3 (Liu et al. 2010; Table 2).

11   Conclusion

Ovarian germ cell tumors develop from primordial totipotential germ and stem cells that can differentiate into extraembryonal and somatic tissues. The most common OGCT is mature cystic teratoma. Dysgerminoma is the most common immature malignant OGCT followed by YST. Clinical information, morphology, and immunohistochemical profile are crucial to assign an ovarian mass to the right category of ovarian tumors.

References

Baker PM, Oliva E, Young RH, Talerman A, Scully RE. Ovarian mucinous carcinoids including some with a carcinomatous component: a report of 17 cases. Am J Surg Pathol. 2001;25(5):557–68.

Cohen MB, Friend DS, Molnar JJ, Talerman A. Gonadal endodermal sinus (yolk sac) tumor with pure intestinal differentiation: a new histologic type. Pathol Res Pract. 1987;182(5):609–16.

de Silva KS, Kanumakala S, Grover SR, Chow CW, Warne GL. Ovarian lesions in children and adolescents – an 11-year review. J Pediatr Endocrinol Metab. 2004;17(7):951–7.

Desouki MM, Fadare O, Chamberlain BK, Shakir N, Kanbour-Shakir A. Malignancy associated with ovarian teratomas: frequency, histotypes, and diagnostic accuracy of intraoperative consultation. Ann Diagn Pathol. 2015;19(3):103–6.

Gershenson DM. Current advances in the management of malignant germ cell and sex cord-stromal tumors of the ovary. Gynecol Oncol. 2012;125(3):515–7.

Hackethal A, Brueggmann D, Bohlmann MK, Franke FE, Tinneberg HR, Munstedt K. Squamous-cell carcinoma in mature cystic teratoma of the ovary: systematic review and analysis of published data. Lancet Oncol. 2008;9(12):1173–80.

Hadrup SR, Braendstrup O, Jacobsen GK, Mortensen S, Pedersen LO, Seremet T, Andersen MH, Becker JC, Straten PT. Tumor infiltrating lymphocytes in seminoma lesions comprise clonally expanded cytotoxic T cells. Int J Cancer. 2006;119(4):831–8.

Kandil DH, Cooper K. Glypican-3: a novel diagnostic marker for hepatocellular carcinoma and more. Adv Anat Pathol. 2009;16(2):125–9.

Kao CS, Idrees MT, Young RH, Ulbright TM. Solid pattern yolk sac tumor: a morphologic and immunohistochemical study of 52 cases. Am J Surg Pathol. 2012; 36(3):360–7.

Lau SK, Weiss LM, Chu PG. D2-40 immunohistochemistry in the differential diagnosis of seminoma and embryonal carcinoma: a comparative immunohistochemical study with KIT (CD117) and CD30. Mod Pathol. 2007; 20(3):320–5.

Liu A, Cheng L, Du J, Peng Y, Allan RW, Wei L, Li J, Cao D. Diagnostic utility of novel stem cell markers SALL4, OCT4, NANOG, SOX2, UTF1, and TCL1 in primary mediastinal germ cell tumors. Am J Surg Pathol. 2010;34(5):697–706.

Loughrey MB, McCusker G, Heasley RN, Alkalbani M, McCluggage WG. Clear cell struma ovarii. Histopathology. 2003;43(5):495–7.

Low JJ, Ilancheran A, Ng JS. Malignant ovarian germ-cell tumours. Best Pract Res Clin Obstet Gynaecol. 2012; 26(3):347–55.

McCluggage WG. Value of inhibin staining in gynecological pathology. Int J Gynecol Pathol. 2001;20(1):79–85.

Nogales-Fernandez F, Silverberg SG, Bloustein PA, Martinez-Hernandez A, Pierce GB. Yolk sac carcinoma (endodermal sinus tumor): ultrastructure and histogenesis of gonadal and extragonadal tumors in comparison with normal human yolk sac. Cancer. 1977;39(4): 1462–74.

Nogales FF, Dulcey I, Preda O. Germ cell tumors of the ovary: an update. Arch Pathol Lab Med. 2014;138(3): 351–62.

Norris HJ, Zirkin HJ, Benson WL. Immature (malignant) teratoma of the ovary: a clinical and pathologic study of 58 cases. Cancer. 1976;37(5):2359–72.

O'Connor DM, Norris HJ. The influence of grade on the outcome of stage I ovarian immature (malignant) teratomas and the reproducibility of grading. Int J Gynecol Pathol. 1994;13(4):283–9.

Pallesen G, Hamilton-Dutoit SJ. Ki-1 (CD30) antigen is regularly expressed by tumor cells of embryonal carcinoma. Am J Pathol. 1988;133(3):446–50.

Patterson DM, Rustin GJ. Controversies in the management of germ cell tumours of the ovary. Curr Opin Oncol. 2006;18(5):500–6.

Perrone T, Steiner M, Dehner LP. Nodal gliomatosis and alpha-fetoprotein production. Two unusual facets of grade I ovarian teratoma. Arch Pathol Lab Med. 1986;110(10):975–7.

Peterson WF, Prevost EC, Edmunds FT, Hundley Jr JM, Morris FK. Benign cystic teratomas of the ovary; a clinico-statistical study of 1,007 cases with a review of the literature. Am J Obstet Gynecol. 1955;70(2): 368–82.

Prat J, Cao D, Carinelli SG, Nogales FF, Vang R, Zaloudek CJ. Germ cell tumors. In: Kurman RJ, Carcangiu ML, Herrington CS, Young RH, editors. WHO classification of tumours of female reproductive organs. Lyon: World Health Organization; 2014. p. 57–68.

Roth LM, Karseladze AI. Highly differentiated follicular carcinoma arising from struma ovarii: a report of 3 cases, a review of the literature, and a reassessment of so-called peritoneal strumosis. Int J Gynecol Pathol. 2008;27(2):213–22.

Vang R, Gown AM, Zhao C, Barry TS, Isacson C, Richardson MS, Ronnett BM. Ovarian mucinous tumors associated with mature cystic teratomas: morphologic and immunohistochemical analysis identifies a subset of potential teratomatous origin that shares features of lower gastrointestinal tract mucinous tumors more commonly encountered as secondary tumors in the ovary. Am J Surg Pathol. 2007;31(6):854–69.

Yanai-Inbar I, Scully RE. Relation of ovarian dermoid cysts and immature teratomas: an analysis of 350 cases of immature teratoma and 10 cases of dermoid cyst with microscopic foci of immature tissue. Int J Gynecol Pathol. 1987;6(3):203–12.

Immunohistochemistry of Gynecologic Malignancies

Yan Wang and Paulette Mhawech-Fauceglia

Abstract

Since its first discovery in 1930, immunohisto-chemistry (IHC) became a staple in all pathology departments. Its usage gained popularity in early 1970 when "immunoperoxidase" method to formalin paraffin-embedded tissues was developed. In recent days, this ancillary technology becomes a routine and essential tool in diagnostic and research laboratories. Application of IHC in medical practice is commonly used in helping to identify the origin of malignancy, predicting prognosis, and helping select targeted therapy. Gynecologic pathology is not an exception. Example and just to name a few, pair box gene 8 (PAX8) has been used to identify the Müllerian origin of a carcinoma, alpha-inhibin and calretinin for sex cord tumor. In this chapter, we will describe the principle and the interpretation of IHC, and we will discuss various immunomarkers that are commonly used in gynecologic pathology.

Keywords

Immunohistochemistry • Principles • Gynecologic malignancies • Differential diagnosis • Prognostic diagnosis

Contents

Y. Wang (✉)
Department of Pathology, Kaiser Roseville Medical Center, Roseville, CA, USA
e-mail: yanw98@gmail.com

P. Mhawech-Fauceglia
Division of Gynecologic Oncologic Pathology, Department of Pathology, Keck School of Medicine, University of Southern California, Los Angeles, CA, USA
e-mail: pfauceglia@hotmail.com; mhawechf@usc.edu

© Springer International Publishing AG 2017
D. Shoupe (ed.), *Handbook of Gynecology*,
DOI 10.1007/978-3-319-17798-4_65

1   Introduction

Immunohistochemistry (IHC) refers to the process of detecting antigens (e.g., proteins) in cells of a tissue section by exploiting the principle of antibodies binding specifically to antigens in biological tissues. These antibodies can be cytoplasmic or nuclear or they can shuttle between the cytoplasm and the nucleus. In recent days IHC has become a routine and essential tool in diagnostic and research laboratories. In this chapter we will discuss the principle, interpretation, pitfalls, and role of the most common immunomarkers in gynecologic pathology.

2   Basic Principle of Immunohistochemistry

Modern immunohistochemistry (IHC) uses an indirect method, so-called "sandwich" method. It consists of three parts, (1) specific antibodies, (2) bridging compound, and (3) detection system that are described below:

1. Specific antibodies, also called primary antibodies, are commonly IgG and less frequently IgM. Specific antibodies react with antigens of interest, and they can be polyclonal or monoclonal antibodies. Polyclonal antibodies are collected from the antisera of immunized animals by antigen(s) of interest. The antisera is then purified and become commercially available for clinical use. They react with multiple epitopes of the same antigen, making them highly sensitive but less specific.

    Monoclonal antibodies are a population of homogeneous immunoglobulin reacting specifically with a single epitope. A monoclonal antibody is manufactured from a so-called hybridoma, a fused and immortalized cell line; a myeloma cell line/fusion partner fused with immunized B-lymphocytes isolated from animal spleen. B-lymphocytes confer the capability to produce specific immunoglobulin, while the fused partner cell line enables immortality and indefinite growth in culture. The advantage of monoclonal antibody comparing to polyclonal antibody is that it is very specific and very consistent.

2. Bridging compound, commonly called "secondary antibody," is a biotinylated nonspecific anti-antibody reacting with primary antibodies. It functions as a link between the primary antibody and detecting systems.

3. The detecting system witnessed significant changes since immunohistochemistry was first introduced. The immunoperoxidase bridging method and the peroxidase antiperoxidase (PAP) complex method were used earlier; however, the avidin-biotin is now the dominant method. It consists mainly of the avidin-biotin complex (ABC or BAC). Avidin or streptavidin has strong affinity for biotin with four biotin-binding sites. The biotin molecule is easily conjugated to second antibody and enzyme (peroxidase) then forming the avidin-biotin-peroxidase complex which catalyzes chemical reaction of substrate and chromogens.

2.1   Interpretation of Immunohistochemistry

Immunoreactivity of cells of interest can be nuclear, cytoplasmic, cell membranous, or a mixture of any of these patterns. Positivity of immunostains is defined by specific pattern of immunoreactivity of cells of interest. For example, S100 and TTF1 can be cytoplasmic, but they are considered positive when they exhibit only nuclear immunoreactivity. In general, immunostains can be interpreted for intensity and percentage as well as diffuse, focal, or rare expression. As for intensity, the result of an immunostain is reported as negative or as positive with weak, moderate, or strong intensity. On the other hand, the percentage of positive cells is arbitrary and somewhat subjective.

Immunostains can have false positive and false negative. Causes of false positive can be positive cells that are not the cells of interest, wrong staining pattern (e.g., cytoplasmic instead nuclear), intrinsic peroxidase (commonly seen in inflammatory cells), background staining, and edge effect. Causes of false negative can be loss of cells of interest on deeper cut, bad fixation, loss of antigen during tissue process, and technical problem. To get correct interpretation, it is essential that the pathologist is familiar with tumor morphology and staining interpretation and has good external and internal control. Therefore, experience in surgical pathology and deep knowledge of IHC can avoid these pitfalls.

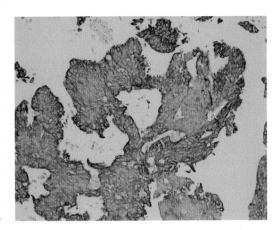

Fig. 1 Total cytokeratin (AE1/3) is positive in a cytoplasmic pattern, indicating that this malignancy is a carcinoma

3 Common IHC Markers Used in Gynecologic Malignancies

3.1 Epithelial Markers

3.1.1 Cytokeratin

Cytokeratin (CK) or simply called keratin is a group of intracytoplasmic proteins of keratin-containing intermediate filaments found in all type of epithelial tissue. It is a common epithelial marker and generally functioning as cytoskeleton. There are 20 common subtypes of keratins. All epithelial cells will express one or more subtypes of keratins. There are two types of keratins: type 1 (acidic) comprising CK 9, 10, 12, and 14–20 and type 2 (basic) comprising CK 1–8. Type 1 and type 2 cytokeratins are in pairs. Cytokeratins can also be divided into low and high molecular weight (LMW and HMW) based solely on their molecular weight. In general, type 1 keratins are low molecular weight keratins, and type 2 keratins are high molecular weight keratins. AE1/AE3 is a cocktail of anti-keratin antibodies. AE1 mainly includes CK10, 11, 13, 14, 15, 16, and 19 and AE3 contains CK1, 2, 3, 4, 5, 6, 7, and 8. It can be slightly variable from manufacture to another. In gynecologic pathology, AE1/AE3 has a cytoplasmic pattern, and it is used to identify cells of epithelial origin, like carcinomas (Fig. 1). However, it also can be positive in some non-epithelial

cells like epithelioid leiomyosarcoma and perivascular epithelioid cell neoplasm (PECOMA). The unique CK7 and CK20 expression by carcinomas has been proven to be useful to recognize the origin of these epithelial tumors, and they are regularly used in the IHC workup of malignancies of unknown origin. Tumors of the gynecologic tract are usually CK7+/CK20−, but exception occurs as ovarian mucinous adenocarcinomas can be CK7+/CK20+ (Chu et al. 2000).

3.1.2 Epithelial Membrane Antigen (EMA)

EMA is another epithelial marker. It is a membrane bound, glycosylated phosphoprotein, the product of the MUC-1 gene (1). It is often expressed in the cytoplasm of nearly all epithelial cells. Therefore it can be used as an alternative or subsidiary to other epithelial marker. However it can also be positive in some non-epithelial tumors, such as sarcoma, namely, synovial sarcoma.

3.1.3 Pair Box Gene 8 (PAX8)

It is a member of paired-box (PAX) family of transcription factors. It is involved in embryogenesis of the thyroid, Müllerian, and renal/upper urinary tracts as a nephric-lineage transcription factor. PAX8 is a nuclear stain that is highly sensitive and site-specific marker for thyroid, Müllerian, renal, and thymic neoplasms (Ozcan et al. 2011). In gynecologic pathology, it has been

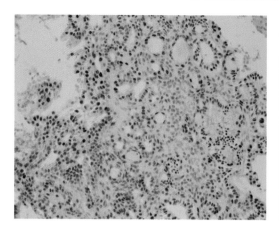

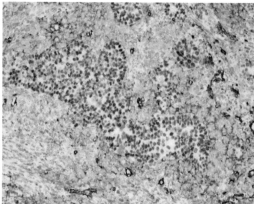

Fig. 2 PAX8 is positive in a nuclear pattern. PAX8 positivity in a tumor of unknown origin indicates that the tumor is of probable gynecologic tract origin

Fig. 3 WT1 is positive in nuclear pattern in a metastatic serous ovarian carcinoma to the vulva

widely used in identifying tumor of Müllerian origin, including most of ovarian epithelial neoplasms, endometrial carcinomas, and cervical adenocarcinoma (Fig. 2). It is usually negative in cervical squamous cell carcinoma and mesenchymal tumors of the female genital tract.

3.1.4   Wilm's Tumor 1 (WT1)

It is a marker traditionally used to diagnose Wilms' tumor. Wilms tumor protein is a transcription factor encoded by the WT1 gene on human chromosome 11p and serves an essential role in the normal development of the urogenital system. This gene is mutated in a subset of patients with Wilms' tumor. WT1 immunostain gains its popularity in gynecology-pathology due to its nuclear positivity in the vast majority of serous carcinoma of ovary (Fig. 3). Another use of WT1 is to help differentiating endometrial serous carcinoma versus ovarian serous carcinoma, as it is negative in the former and positive in the latter. Because WT1 is frequently positive in mesothelial cells, caution is needed when evaluating malignant cells in peritoneal cytology (Moritani et al. 2008).

3.2   Mesenchymal Markers

3.2.1   Vimentin

It is a type 3 intermediate filament protein that is expressed in mesenchymal cells and the major

cytoskeletal component of mesenchymal cells. Therefore, vimentin is often used as a marker of mesenchymally derived cells or cells undergoing an epithelial-to-mesenchymal transition (EMT) during both normal development and metastatic progression. It has a cytoplasmic pattern of expression. In gynecologic pathology it can be positive in endometrial glandular cells and its tumor derivatives. This characteristic feature is very helpful in distinguish adenocarcinoma originating from the endometrium versus the endocervix.

3.2.2   Actin

Actins are microfilaments existing essentially in all eukaryotic cells. They are expressed in many cellular processes, including muscle contraction, cell motility, cell division and cytokinesis, vesicle and organelle movement, cell signaling, and the establishment and maintenance of cell junctions and cell shape. Actins include both alpha-smooth muscle actin (SMA) and muscle-specific actin (MSA) that are equally expressed in skeletal muscle, smooth muscle, myofibroblasts, myoepithelial cells, and pericytes in a cytoplasmic pattern.

3.2.3   Desmin

Desmin is an intermediate filament in skeletal, cardiac, and smooth muscle. Desmin immunostain has a cytoplasmic pattern of expression, and it is useful to identify neoplasms of skeletal, cardiac, and smooth muscle origin, but not for myoepithelial cells, and less than actin for myofibroblasts.

3.2.4 Myoglobulin, MyoD1, and Myogenin

These are skeletal muscle-specific markers often used in identifying rhabdomyosarcoma and rhabdomyosarcomatous component in carcinosarcoma. Myoglobulin is present in well-differentiated skeletal muscle cells.

3.2.5 Transgelin

Transgelin is an actin-binding protein of the calponin family that correlates with smooth muscle differentiation. It is a good marker for smooth muscle differentiation, and recently it proved to be a good marker to differentiate leiomyosarcoma from endometrial stromal sarcoma, where it is positive in the former and negative in the latter.

3.3 Sex Cord Markers

3.3.1 Alpha-Inhibin

Alpha-inhibin is a subunit of an inhibitor of pituitary FSH secretion, encoded by the INHA human gene. Inhibin also participates in the negative regulation of gonadal stromal cell proliferation and has tumor suppressor activity. Alpha-inhibin has a cytoplasmic pattern, and it is widely accepted as a marker for sex cord tumor as it is positive in the vast majority of sex cord stromal tumors such as granulosa cell tumor, Sertoli cell tumor, or a Sertoli cell in Sertoli-Leydig cell tumor. When alpha-inhibin is combined with calretinin (another marker for sex cord stroma tumor), the sensitivity as well as the specificity is highly increased (Deavers et al. 2003; Jones et al. 2010).

3.3.2 CD30

CD30 is also known as ki-1. It is a member of the tumor necrosis family of cell surface receptors and is a lymphocytic activation antigen. It is mostly expressed in classic Hodgkin's lymphoma, large cell anaplastic lymphoma, and embryonal carcinoma of the testis and the ovary.

3.4 Trophoblastic Markers

3.4.1 Human Chorionic Gonadotropin (hCG)

hCG is a polypeptide hormone with two subunits: α- and β-subunits. Naturally, it is produced in the human placenta by the syncytiotrophoblast. β-subunit (β-hCG)-specific immunostain will highlight normal syncytiotrophoblasts, choriocarcinoma, hydatidiform mole, and syncytial trophoblastic cells in tumors containing syncytial trophoblastic cells.

3.4.2 Human Placental Lactogen (hPL)

hPL is another polypeptide hormone produced by syncytial and intermediate trophoblasts. The intensity of immunostain is stronger on intermediate trophoblastic cells than on syncytial trophoblastic cells. Intermediate trophoblastic cells can be positive, but they are most likely negative for hCG. hPL staining is very useful for the diagnosis of placental site trophoblastic tumor due to the predominance of proliferation of intermediate trophoblastic cells in this tumor.

3.5 Other Immunomarkers

3.5.1 Ki67/MIB 1

This marker was originally described in Kiel, Germany, where the name was originated. It is a cellular marker for cell proliferation, and it is encoded by MKI67 gene in human. Ki67 protein is a nuclear protein, and it is present in all cells during the proliferative phases (G1, S, G2, M) and is not present in cells in the resting phase. It has a nuclear staining pattern and provides a proliferation index (Ki67 index). Each given tumor has its own meaningful Ki67 index. In general, the higher Ki67 index associates with more aggressive tumor behavior and worse prognosis. In gynecologic pathology, Ki67 has been commonly used to distinguish between benign and dysplastic lesions of the cervix. It is very useful in differentiating endocervical adenocarcinoma from reactive endocervical glands and in distinguishing squamous cell atrophy from squamous dysplasia of the exocervix.

3.5.2   P53

P53 is an oncoprotein is encoded by TP53 gene that is located on chromosome 17. TP53 is called the "guardian of the genome." It is a tumor suppressor gene and is the most frequently mutated gene in human tumors. In gynecologic pathology, TP53 mutation has been associated with high-grade serous carcinoma. Positive p53 expression in approximately 60% of tumor cells or greater, or completely negative p53 expression (p53 null) are both indicative for TP53 mutation and, therefore, are considered helpful in confirming high-grade serous carcinoma. P53 immunostain has a nuclear pattern. It can be positive, such as clear cell type and high-grade endometrioid type, and mucinous type.

3.5.3   P16

P16 is a tumor suppressor protein and a surrogate marker for high-risk HPV-related neoplasia and carcinoma. A positive result is defined as diffuse, strong nuclear, and cytoplasmic expression by the cells of interest. It is very specific in differentiating squamous intraepithelial neoplasia/carcinoma of cervix from reactive changes. Because of overlapping immunoreactivity with adenocarcinoma of other origin, the use of p16 by itself to identify tumor origin is not of great use.

3.5.4   ER and PR

ER and PR are hormonal receptors seen in the entire female genital tract (Fig. 4). They are used

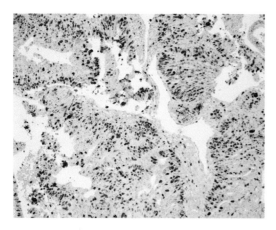

Fig. 4 ER is strongly positive in nuclear pattern in an endometrial adenocarcinoma endometrioid type, FIGO 1

to distinguish endocervical from endometrial cancer where they are negative in the former and positive in the latter. In addition, they are used for therapeutic options in patients with endometrioid adenocarcinoma and endometrial stromal sarcoma.

3.5.5   Insulin-like Growth Factor II mRNA Binding Protein 3 (IMP3)

IMP3 plays an important role in RNA trafficking, stabilization, cell growth, and cell migration during early stages of embryogenesis. IMP3 has a cytoplasmic and an apical pattern. It is useful to differentiate endometrioid adenocarcinoma from serous carcinoma of the endometrium where it is negative in the former and positive in the latter (Zheng et al. 2008; Mhawech-Fauceglia et al. 2010, 2013).

3.5.6   CD10

CD10 also known as CALLA (common acute lymphocytic leukemia antigen). It is a hematologic marker encoded by the MME gene and is expressed by many hematopoietic malignancies. In the gynecologic tract, it is expressed by the cytoplasm of endometrial stromal cells making it very useful in the diagnosis of endometrial stromal sarcoma (ESS) and for distinguishing ESS from smooth muscle tumor. Other tumors positive for CD10 include many renal cell carcinomas such as clear cell type, solid pseudopapillary type, as well as some urothelial tumors.

4   Application of IHC to Female Genital Tract

4.1   Vulvar Lesions

The most frequent lesion of the vulva is extramammary Paget disease of the vulva and Bowen's disease. Even though melanoma does not commonly occur in the vulva, it is still included in the differential diagnosis (Table 1). It is essential to distinguish among these lesions due to their different treatments and outcomes.

Table 1 Immunohistochemistry markers helpful in differentiating among different types of vulvar lesions

| | Primary Paget disease | Second Paget disease | | Bowen | Melanoma |
		Anorectal	Urothelial		
CK7	+ (100%)	−	+	−	−
CK20	−	+	+ (variable)	−	−
GCDFP-15	+ (88%)	− (100%)	− (100%)	−	−
CEA	+	+	−	−	−
Specific markers	**CAM 5.2**		Thrombomodulin		S100, HMB45 Melanan A
	Androgen		**Uroplakin III**		

4.2 High-Risk HPV-Related Cervical Neoplasms Versus Benign Reactive Cervical Lesions

High-risk HPV-related cervical neoplasms, squamous and adenocarcinoma, and their precursors are positive for both p16 (strong and diffuse) and Ki67. On the other hand, benign reactive lesions are negative or positive for only one marker but not for both p16 and Ki67.

4.3 Endometrial Endometrioid Adenocarcinoma Versus Endocervical Adenocarcinoma

The panel of immunohistochemistries (IHCs) such as CEA monoclonal, ER/PR, vimentin, and p16 are used to differentiate endometrial adenocarcinoma from endocervical adenocarcinoma. Endometrial adenocarcinomas are positive for vimentin, and ER/PR and endocervical adenocarcinomas are positive for CEAm and Muc1. P16 is unable to differentiate between the two as it is positive in both (Mhawech-Fauceglia et al. 2008; Reid-Nicholson et al. 2006).

4.4 Serous Carcinoma, Endometrial Versus Ovarian Origin

WT1 is very useful to differentiate ovarian serous adenocarcinoma (90% positive) from endometrial serous carcinoma (90% negative). WT1 is also useful to distinguish among histologic ovarian subtypes as we will be discussing in the next paragraph (Acs et al. 2004).

4.5 Ovarian Carcinomas Histologic Subtypes

There is no single reliable immunomarker that can distinguish among various ovarian carcinomas histologic subtypes (Baker and Oliva 2004; Kobel et al. 2008). However, a panel of antibodies including p53, WT1, and ER might be helpful (Table 2).

4.6 Clear Cell Carcinoma of Ovary

Clear cell carcinoma (CCC) can be very difficult to diagnose, and other tumors with similar morphology should be excluded:

1. **Metastatic Renal Cell Carcinoma**: ovarian CCC is negative for vimentin and CD10; renal cell carcinoma is positive for vimentin and CD10.
2. **Dysgerminoma:** CCC is positive for AE1/AE3 and EMA; dysgerminoma is negative for AE1/AE3 and EMA.
3. **Yolk Sac Tumor:** AFP and glypican-3 are positive in yolk sac tumor and negative in CCC (McCluggage and Young 2005).

4.7 Mucinous Carcinoma of Ovary Versus Lower Gastrointestinal (GI) Tract

Ovarian mucinous carcinomas are positive for CK7 and either positive or negative for CK20 and CDX2. Mucinous carcinomas of lower GI tract are negative for CK7 and positive for CK20 and CDX2.

Table 2 Immunohistochemistry markers expressions in ovarian surface epithelial malignancies

Carcinomas	WT1 (%)	TP53 (%)	ER (%)
LGSC	100	0	96
HGSC	92	93	80
Mucinous	0	50	6
Endometrioid	4	11	86
Clear cell	0	12	13

Table 3 Immunohistochemical markers useful in discriminating among different subtypes of germ cell tumors of the ovary

	Dysgerminoma	Yolk sac tumor	Embryonal carcinoma	Choriocarcinoma
AE1/AE3	− or +weak	+	+	+
EMA	−	+	−	+
CD30	−	−	+	−
CD117	+	+	−	−
OCT-4	+	−	+	−
Glypican-3	−	+	+	+
AFP	−	+	+ in rare cells	
HCG	+ rare cells		+ in rare cells	+

4.8 Endometrioid Adenocarcinoma Versus Metastastic Adenocarcinoma from the GI Tract

Endometrioid adenocarcinomas are positive for CK7, ER/PR, and vimentin and negative for CK20 and CDX2. However, metastatic carcinomas from the GI tract are negative for CK7 (except upper GI carcinomas which they are positive for CK7), positive for CK20 and CDX2, and negative for ER/PR and vimentin.

4.9 Endometrial Stromal Sarcoma (ESS) Versus Leiomyosarcoma

ESSs are positive for CD10 and negative or sometime weakly positive for SMA, transgelin, and desmin; leiomyosarcomas are strongly positive for SMA, transgelin, and desmin, and they are negative or occasionally weakly positive for

CD10. ER and PR are usually positive in ESS. These immunostains are not usually useful in high-grade ESS and leiomyosarcoma (Hwang et al. 2015).

4.10 Germ Cell Tumors

IHC is very useful and often done to differentiate among germ cell tumors including dysgerminoma, yolk sac tumor, embryonal carcinoma, and choriocarcinoma (Table 3). Making the right diagnosis is essential for patient management and outcome.

5 Conclusion

IHC is used regularly in medical practices and is commonly used in helping to identify the origin of malignancy, predicting prognosis, and helping select targeted therapy.

References

Acs G, Pasha T, Zhang PJ. WT1 is differentially expressed in serous, endometrioid, clear and mucinous carcinomas of the peritoneum, fallopian tube, ovary and endometrium. Int J Gynecol Pathol. 2004;23:110–8.

Baker PM, Oliva E. Immunohistochemistry as a tool in the differential diagnosis of ovarian tumors: an update. Int J Gynecol Pathol. 2004;24:39–55.

Chu P, Wu E, Weiss LM. Cytokeratin 7 and cytokeratin 20 expression in epithelial neoplasms; a survey of 435 cases. Mod Pathol. 2000;13:962–72.

Deavers MT, Malpica A, Liu J, Broaddus R, Silva EG. Ovarian sex cord-stromal tumors: an immunohistochemical study including a comparison of calretinin and inhibin. Mod Pathol. 2003;16:584–90.

Jones MW, Harri R, Dabbs DJ, Carter GJ. Immunohistochemical profile of steroid cell tumor of the ovary; a study of 14 cases and a review of the literature. Int J Gynecol Pathol. 2010;29:315–20.

Hwang H, Matsuo K, Duncan K, Pakzamir E, Pham HQ, Correa A, Fedenko A, Mhawech-Fauceglia P. Immunohistochemical panel to differentiate endometrial stromal sarcoma, uterine leiomyosarcoma and leiomyoma: something old and something new. J Clin Pathol. 2015;9:710–7.

Kobel M, Kalloger SE, Boyd N, McKinney S, Mehi E, Palmer C, Leung S, Bowen NJ, Ionescu DN, Rajput A, Prentice LM, Miller D, Santos J, Swenerton K, Gilks CB, Huntsman D. Ovarian carcinoma subtypes are different diseases: implications for biomarker studies. PLoS One. 2008;5:e232.

McCluggage WG, Young RH. Immunohistochemistry as a diagnostic aid in the evaluation of ovarian tumors. Semin Diagn Pathol. 2005;22:3–32.

Mhawech-Fauceglia P, Herrmann F, Bshara W, Zhang S, Penetrante R, Lele S, Odunsi K, Rodabaugh K. Intraobserver and interobserver variability in distinguishing between endocervical and endometrial adenocarcinoma on problematic cases of cervical curettings. Int J Gynecol Pathol. 2008;27:431–6.

Mhawech-Fauceglia P, Herrmann FR, Rai H, Tchabo N, Lele S, Izevbaye I, Odunsi K, Cheney RT. IMP3 distinguishes uterine serous carcinoma from endometrial endometrioid adenocarcinoma. Am J Clin Pathol. 2010;133:899–908.

Mhawech-Fauceglia P, Yan L, Liu S, Pejovic T. ER+/PR+/TTF3+/IMP3- immunoprofile distinguishes endometrioid from serous and clear cell carcinomas of the endometrium: a study of 401 cases. Histopathology. 2013;62(7):976–85.

Moritani S, Ichihara S, Hasegawa M, Endo T, Oiwa M, Yoshikawa K, Sato Y, Aoyama H, Hayashi T, Kushima R. Serous papillary adenocarcinoma of the female genital organs and invasive micropapillary carcinoma of the breast. Are WT1, CA125, and GCDFP-15 useful in differential diagnosis? Hum Pathol. 2008;39:666–71.

Ozcan A, Shen SS, Hamilton C, Anjana K, Coffey D, Krishnan B, Truong LD. PAX8 expression in non-neoplastic tissues, primary tumors, and metastatic tumors: a comprehensive immunohistochemical study. Mod Pathol. 2011;24:751–64.

Reid-Nicholson M, Iyengar P, Hummer AJ, Linkov I, Asher M, Soslow RA. Immunophenotypic diversity of endometrial adenocarcinomas: implications for differential diagnosis. Mod Pathol. 2006;19:1091–100.

Zheng W, Yi X, Fadare O, Liang SX, Martel M, Schwartz PE, Jiang Z. The oncofetal protein IMP3. A novel biomarker for endometrial serous carcinoma. Am J Surg Pathol. 2008;32:304–15.

Surface Epithelial Neoplasms of the Ovary

Paulette Mhawech-Fauceglia

Abstract

Surface epithelial tumors are the most frequent neoplasms of the ovary, occurring in both reproductive and menopausal aged women. They are classified as benign, borderline (low potential malignancy/LMP), and malignant. They are classified in different histologic subtypes, such as serous, endometrioid, mucinous, clear cell, and transitional cell. However, 2014 was a year that brought significant changes to the classification of ovarian tumors. This chapter reviews the latest histologic subtyping of surface epithelial tumors based on the new World Health Organization (WHO) classification and revised grading systems as well as the new International Federation of Gynecology and Obstetrics (FIGO) staging system.

Keywords

Immunohistochemistry • Principles • Gynecologic malignancies • Differential diagnosis • Prognostic diagnosis

Contents

1 Introduction

The Surveillance, Epidemiology and End Results (SEER) cancer statistics estimated 21.290 new ovarian cases in 2015 claiming almost 14.180 lives (SEER 2015). Surface epithelial tumors accounts for almost two-third of all ovarian tumors, and they are by far the most frequent ovarian cancer types in the western world. Their origin is likely the epithelium lining of the ovarian surface, invaginations of this lining into the superficial cortex of the ovary, and/or fallopian tube tissue. Surface epithelial tumor rates are highest in women aged 55–64 years with a median age of 6.3 years. Numerous changes concerning tumor staging and histologic subtypes were introduced

P. Mhawech-Fauceglia (✉)
Division of Gynecologic Oncologic Pathology,
Department of Pathology, Keck School of Medicine,
University of Southern California, Los Angeles, CA, USA
e-mail: mhawechf@usc.edu; pfauceglia@hotmail.com

© Springer International Publishing AG 2017
D. Shoupe (ed.), *Handbook of Gynecology*,
DOI 10.1007/978-3-319-17798-4_66

in 2014. Based on the new data regarding molecular alterations in ovarian carcinogenesis, the revised WHO classification eliminated transitional cell carcinoma subtype and reclassified them into high-grade serous and high-grade endometrioid carcinoma (Kurman et al. 2014). Second, a seromucinous category was newly introduced. There were also changes made in the 2014 FIGO staging (FIGO Committee on Gynecologic Oncology 2014) that are discussed below.

2   Benign Ovarian Cysts

The most common benign ovarian lesions are the corpus luteal cyst and solitary follicular cyst.

2.1   Corpus Luteal Cyst

Corpus luteal cysts usually occur in women in the reproductive age. They are unilocular cysts. Grossly, the cyst is lined by a convoluted golden brown rim. These cysts can become cystic, and large, filled with chocolate brown fluid (Fig. 1). Histologically, the cysts are lined by large

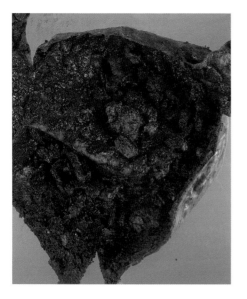

Fig. 1 The ovary is cystically dilated. The cyst is filled with *brown* chocolate fluid with blood clot

luteinized granulosa cells and an outer layer of smaller luteinized theca interna cells.

2.2   Solitary Follicular Cyst

Solitary follicular cysts occur in women of reproductive age [although they can occur even in postmenopausal women]. They are unilocular cyst with a size ranging from 3 to 8 cm. The cyst lining is composed of an inner layer of granulosa cells and an outer layer of theca interna cells. The evidence of the two layers are seen on reticulin stain where it is negative in former and positive in the later (Fig. 2).

3   WHO Classification of Epithelial Tumors

Serous Tumors
Benign
- Serous cystadenoma
- Serous adenofibroma
- Serous surface papilloma

Borderline
- Serous borderline tumor/low malignant potential/atypical proliferative serous tumor
- Serous borderline tumor micropapillary variant/noninvasive low-grade serous carcinoma

Malignant
- Low-grade serous carcinoma
- High-grade serous carcinoma

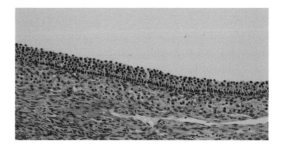

Fig. 2 Solitary follicular cyst where the cyst is lined by inner layer of granulosa cells and an outer layer of theca cells

Mucinous Tumors

Benign
- Mucinous cystadenoma
- Mucinous adenofibroma

Borderline
- Mucinous borderline tumor/low malignant potential/atypical proliferative mucinous tumor

Malignant
- Mucinous carcinoma

Endometrioid Tumors

Benign
- Endometriotic cyst
- Endometrioid cystadenoma
- Endometrioid adenofibroma

Borderline
- Endometrioid borderline tumor/low malignant potential/atypical proliferative endometrioid tumor

Malignant
- Endometrioid carcinoma

Clear Cell Tumors

Benign
- Clear cell cystadenoma
- Clear cell adenofibroma

Borderline
- Clear cell borderline tumor/low malignant potential/atypical proliferative clear cell tumor

Malignant
- Clear cell carcinoma

Brenner Tumors

Benign
- Brenner tumor

Borderline
- Borderline Brenner tumor/low malignant potential/atypical proliferative Brenner tumor

Malignant
- Malignant Brenner tumor

Seromucinous Tumors

Benign
- Seromucinous cystadenoma
- Seromucinous adenofibroma

Borderline
- Borderline seromucinous tumor/low malignant potential/atypical proliferative seromucinous tumor

Malignant
- Seromucinous carcinoma

Undifferentiated Carcinoma

3.1 Serous Tumors

3.1.1 Serous Cystadenoma and Adenofibroma

Serous cystadenoma and adenofibroma are common tumors accounting for 25% of all benign ovarian neoplasms. It occurs at any age with peak incidence during the fourth and fifth decades [highest at age 40.]. Bilaterality rate is variable and is around 20–30% of cases. Grossly, the cyst is filled with clear serous fluid. The inner layer of the cystadenoma is smooth, while the adenofibroma has focal excrescences. These excrescences are very different than those seen in borderline tumor as they are soft in the later and chalky white and very hard on touch in the former. Microscopically, serous cystadenomas are cysts lined by single cell layer which can be cuboidal or flattened due to the fluid pressure in the cyst content. The stroma may appear as normal ovarian parenchyma or it can be fibrotic. In adenofibroma, the excrescences seen grossly are large broad clefts of fibrous tissue lined by simple single layer of epithelial cells. Some cases have a focal area of pseudostratified epithelium with mild atypia. The tumor is classified as borderline if the pseudostratified epithelium with atypia is present in 10% or more of the tumor. Since this is a very arbitrary cutoff, it has been suggested to classify this finding as a serous cystadenoma with focal epithelial proliferation with a comment explaining the presence of focal areas of borderline tumor which constitute ≥10% of overall histological material" (Longacre et al. 2005).

3.1.2 Serous Borderline Tumor/Low Malignant Potential/Atypical Proliferative Serous Tumor

Serous borderline tumors (SBTs) represent 25–30% of nonbenign serous tumors and occur in women 30–50 years of age. In the majority of cases, they are unilateral and usually present at an early stage (stage I). Grossly, the ovarian mass is typically unilocular although it can present as a multilocular cyst, usually measuring >5 cm. The outer surface of the cyst may appear smooth, but it is important to do a close gross examination to note any surface projections/involvement as it changes the tumor FIGO staging as discussed below. The cyst is usually filled with serous fluid and the cyst lining usually exhibits very soft, friable white projections (Fig. 3). Microscopically, the cyst lining shows papillary projections lined by stratified cuboidal cells. In places, these cells are marked by hobnail features reflected by eosinophilic cytoplasm, mild to moderate atypia, and high nuclear/cytoplasmic ratio. The critical finding of a borderline tumor is the lack of invasion of the ovarian stroma (Fig. 4).

Serous borderline tumor may be associated with omental implants. Peritoneal implants are classified as noninvasive epithelial implants, invasive epithelial implants, or desmoplastic implants. Since implants are a heterogeneous group and various types may coexist, it is important that multiple biopsies of numerous foci of suspicious lesions are done at the time of surgery and that extensive tumor sampling by the pathologist is done to accurately exclude an invasive implant.

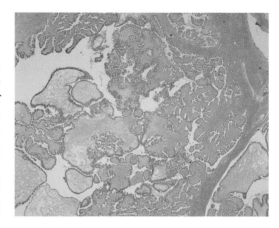

Fig. 4 The cut surface of these projections show papillary structure lined by stratified cuboidal cells. These cells exhibit mild to moderate atypia and few mitotic figures are also present. There is no stromal invasion

The diagnosis of peritoneal implants is very challenging and very difficult. It is therefore recommended of the opinion that the final diagnosis is cleared by an expert gynecologic pathologist, especially in cases where the diagnosis may change a patient's treatment options and management.

3.1.3 Serous Borderline Tumor (SBT) Micropapillary Variant (MSBT)

Serous borderline tumors account for 5–10% of all SBTs. Microscopically, MSBT shows highly complex micropapillary growth in a filigree pattern, growing in a nonhierarchical fashion from stalk. It has been described as "Medusa head" like appearance. Micropapillae are at least five times as long as they are wide (Fig. 5). The significance of this subtype has generated a lot of debate in pathology. Some authors have found a close association between MSBT and invasive implants and have urged that this lesion be labeled as a "micropapillary serous carcinoma." Others prefer the terminology of MSBT, avoiding the use of the term of "carcinoma," to minimize the possibility of overtreating patients (Chang et al. 2008). The general agreement on the significance of micropapillary architecture in SBTs is that they are related to significant increases in the incidence of invasive peritoneal implants. Molecular studies show that MSBTs

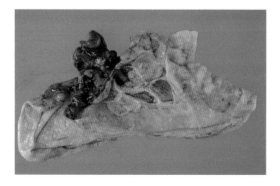

Fig. 3 The ovarian cyst is multilocular. The inner surface is smooth, but some areas of very soft friable vegetations

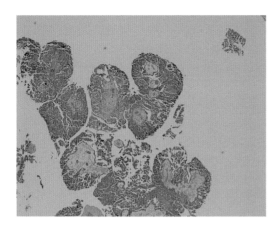

Fig. 5 Serous borderline, micropapillary variant where there is highly complex micropapillary growth in a filigree pattern looking like "medusa head." These micropapillae are long and wide

have a similar gene expression profile to low-grade serous carcinomas (LG-serous carcinoma) that are distinct from typical SBT (May et al. 2002). The underlying genes involved in the pathogenesis of LG-serous carcinoma and in MBST include mutations in a number of different genes including *KRAS* and *BRAF*. MSBT is the only surface epithelial-stromal tumor with a well-defined adenoma-carcinoma sequence, whereas LG-serous tumors are thought to arise in a stepwise fashion from a benign cystadenoma (through BST to an invasive LG-serous carcinoma) (Shih and Kurman 2005). Since micropapillary foci of less than 5 mm have no bearing on clinical outcome, these tumors with low levels of micropapillary foci and atypia can be classified as SBT with focal micropapillary features (Slomovitz et al. 2002).

3.1.4 Low-Grade and High-Grade Serous Carcinoma

The majority of epithelial ovarian carcinomas are of serous histology. The new WHO classification of ovarian serous carcinomas places them into two distinct categories: high grade and low grade. The two types are distinct in terms of site of origin, molecular pathways, and treatment response. Low-grade serous carcinomas (LG-SC) are type I tumors that are relatively rare. They are genetically very stable, and they frequently harbor

alterations in the mitogen-activated protein kinase (MAPK) signaling pathway. Recent pathologic evidence showed that there are three possible origins for LG-SC: ovarian surface epithelium, fallopian tube origin, and endometrial cells ectopically located in the ovary by retrograde menstruation. They are cytologically very low grade with mild atypia and low mitotic rate. LG-SC are usually cisplatin resistant leading to new clinical trials with tyrosine kinase inhibitors in several cancer centers (Kurman et al. 2014).

High-grade serous carcinomas (HG-SC) are the most common histotype (70%) of the epithelial ovarian cancer. They are considered type II ovarian cancers. They occur in women a bit older than women with SBT, with an average age of 56 years. Patients with serous adenocarcinoma often present with advanced stage disease (stages III and IV) at first presentation. They are characterized by multiple gene abnormalities such as *TP 53* mutation in almost 97%, and BRCA1/BRCA2 loss is frequent (30–45%, including germline and somatic alterations). Many of these tumors are thought to originate from the fallopian tube (serous tubal intraepithelial carcinoma/STIC). Grossly, the tumor varies considerably in size from a few cm to 30 cm (Fig. 6). They can be multicystic or solid. When these tumors are diagnosed at advanced stage frequently, the omentum is replaced by tumor creating what is called "omental caking." Cytologically the tumor exhibits moderate to severe atypia

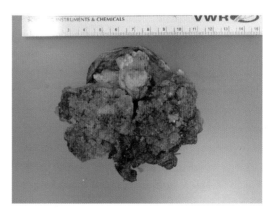

Fig. 6 Ovarian mass with serous carcinoma. The cut surface is partially cystic and partially solid, soft, and friable

with a high mitotic rate (Mhawech-Fauceglia and Pejovic 2015).

3.2 Mucinous Tumors

3.2.1 Mucinous Cystadenoma

Mucinous cystadenomas are the most common type (75%) of mucinous tumors. They can be very large (up to 20 cm) and can be unilocular or multilocular. They are filled with mucoid fluid and in 95% of cases they are unilateral. The cyst is lined by one layer of cells that have small bland looking nuclei with ample mucin-filled cytoplasm creating what is called "picket fence" appearance.

3.2.2 Mucinous Borderline Tumor/ Mucinous Tumor of Low Malignant Potential

Mucinous borderline tumors (MBT) (mucinous tumors of low malignant potential), as defined by the WHO, are tumors exhibiting an epithelial proliferation of mucinous-type cells greater than those seen in their benign counterparts but without evidence of stromal invasion. MBT can be of intestinal type or endocervical-like type. Mucinous borderline tumors account for 10% of mucinous tumors. They can be multilocular and are bilateral in 40% of the cases. MBT are cystic tumors with a visible solid vegetating mass protruding from the cystic wall. Careful gross examination of the cyst wall to identify these lesions is crucial. Histologically, the lining of the cyst is composed of stratified epithelial cells having high N/C ratio and prominent nucleoli. Goblet cells and Paneth cells are present in the intestinal type. No stromal invasion is seen. Borderline tumors remain a controversial issue concerning their pathogenesis, progression, and treatment (Fischerova et al. 2012).

3.2.3 Mucinous Adenocarcinoma

Mucinous adenocarcinoma (MAC) accounts for 15% of mucinous tumors and 2–4% of all ovarian surface epithelial tumors. They are rare and unilateral in 95% of cases. Therefore, when they are bilateral, metastatic tumors especially from the

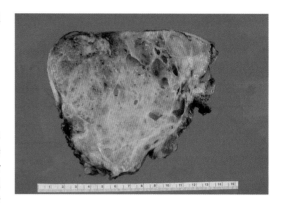

Fig. 7 Cut surface of mucinous adenocarcinoma where it is spongy with numerous tiny cystic spaces. These cysts were filled with mucin

gastrointestinal tract, namely, the colon, should be in question. They can be very large masses reaching more than 10 cm in the vast majority of the cases. They can be multicyctic/partially cystic and partially solid or solid tumors (Fig. 7). They have two patterns of invasion, the first and most common, pushing or expansile pattern where there are complex glands with back to back architecture and no intervening stroma. The glands are evidently malignant exhibiting mild to moderate cytologic atypia, high nuclear/cytoplasmic ratio, and lack of mucin. The second pattern is infiltrative pattern where single or groups of malignant cells are seen to invade the ovarian stroma with desmoplastic reaction. The origin of MAC is very elusive but some cases have been associated with endometriosis. They harbor Ras pathway alterations, and like LG-SC they may contain a spectrum of mucinous cystadenoma to borderline tumor to MAC in the same tumor (Brown and Frumovitz 2014).

3.2.4 Pseudomyxoma Peritonei

Pseudomyxoma peritonei (PP) is a clinical term used to describe the finding of mucoid, gelatinous material in the abdominal cavity, often accompanied by an ovarian or gastrointestinal tumor. In 1995, Ronnett et al. classified PP as either a low-grade variety "diffuse peritoneal adenomucinosis" (DPAM) or a high-grade variety "peritoneal mucinous carcinomatosis" (PMCA). The classification of the tumor is prognostically significant with 5-year survival rates of 84% for DPAM and 6.7% for PMCA (Ronnett et al. 2001). PP may originate from an ovarian primary or from an appendiceal primary. Cytoreductive surgery involves removal of the peritoneum and it is common to remove the ovaries, fallopian tubes, uterus, and parts of the large intestine, including the appendix. Whether the primary origin of this tumor is from an ovarian mucinous tumor or from an appendiceal primary or has synchronous origins is still a subject of great debate.

3.2.5 Mucinous Tumors with Mural Nodule

Mucinous tumors of the ovary, whether benign, borderline, or malignant, may contain one or more mural nodules. These nodules are more frequent in borderline and malignant tumors. Grossly, mural nodules are different than the overlying mucinous neoplasm. Grossly, nodules are yellow and pink with areas of hemorrhage and necrosis. Morphologically, they are classified as benign (sarcoma-like) or malignant anaplastic carcinoma and sarcoma. It is important to distinguish between benign and malignant mural nodules, because benign mural nodules are of no prognostic significance (Mhawech-Fauceglia et al. 2015). Whether malignant mural nodules represent a form of dedifferentiation or a collision of two divergent tumor types is still unsolved mystery.

3.3 Clear Cell Tumor

3.3.1 Borderline Clear Cell Tumor

Borderline clear cell tumors are extremely rare. The gross appearance is nonspecific as it can range from solid to spongy. Microscopic findings include a proliferation of small glands with or without cystic dilatation that are lined by flat and hobnail atypical cells. No stromal invasion is present.

3.3.2 Clear Cell Carcinoma

Clear cell carcinomas (CCC) represent 6–10% of surface epithelial tumors. They occur in postmenopausal women, with a mean age of

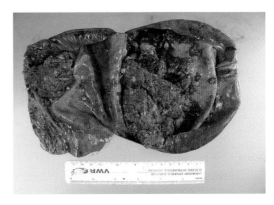

Fig. 8 Cut surface of a clear cell carcinoma. It is unusually cystic. The surface is hemorrhagic and friable

57 years. CCC of the ovary have a few notable characteristics. (1) They are almost always unilateral (Fig. 8), and when they are bilateral, a metastatic renal cell carcinoma should be excluded. (2) They are admixed with endometrioid-type adenocarcinoma in 20–25% of cases. (3) They are often accompanied by endometriosis of the same ovary. (4) They may be associated with paraneoplastic hypercalcemia. And (5) they have frequent mutations of ARID1A and PIK3CA genes and express HNF1B. CCC are generally chemoresistant. They have numerous histological patterns including tubulocystic, papillary, solid, or a mixture of any of those patterns. Typically, the cysts are lined by atypical hobnail cells with clear cytoplasm and numerous intracytoplasmic hyaline globules (Fig. 9) (Okamoto et al. 2014).

3.4 Endometrioid Tumors

3.4.1 Endometriotic Cyst

Endometriotic cyst or endometriomas are simply endometriosis cells that have undergone a cystic dilation. They are among the most common ovarian cystic lesions in the fourth and fifth decade. Grossly, they consist of a large simple cyst. The content is characteristic of chocolate brown fluid. Microscopically, they are a simple cyst lined by cuboidal endometrial cells with hemorrhage, hemosiderin deposits, and macrophages present in the cyst wall.

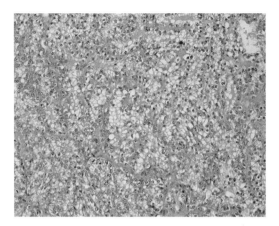

Fig. 9 Microscopic section shows diffuse sheets of tumor cells. These cells have clear cytoplasm. The nuclei are round with prominent nucleoli

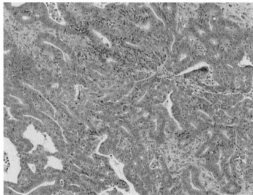

Fig. 10 Endometrioid adenocarcinoma characterized by glands back to back with no intervening stroma

3.4.2 Borderline Endometriotic Tumor

Borderline endometriotic tumors are such rare tumors that some gynecologic pathologists doubt their existence. Morphologically, they are very similar to endometrial hyperplasia occurring in the endometrium. There are composed of crowded glands that are embedded in very fibrotic stroma. The glands exhibit mild atypia and focal squamous morules.

3.4.3 Endometrioid Adenocarcinoma

Endometrioid adenocarcinoma (EAC) accounts for 10–20% of ovarian carcinomas. They occur in postmenopausal women in the fifth and sixth decade, with an average age of 56 years. They are associated with endometriosis in the same ovary or pelvis, and they can coexist with endometrioid adenocarcinoma of the endometrium in 15–20% of cases. PTEN, CTNNB1, PIK3CA, and ARID1A are commonly mutated in EAC and tumors frequently express estrogen/progesterone receptors and TFF3 by immunohistochemistry (Kobel et al. 2013). They are bilateral in 20% of cases. About half of EAC cases present as low-grade/well-differentiated tumors and with early stage disease (stages I and II). Grossly, the ovary may be cystic or solid with friable cut surface. EAC is microscopically very similar to those occurring in the endometrium, where there is back to back glandular architecture, with no intervening stroma and squamous differentiation in the form of squamous morules and keratin pearls (Fig. 10). However, EAC is the most chameleon ovarian cancer in existence as it can have numerous histologic variants such as tubular/tubulovillous, spindle shape, mucin-rich, eosinophilic, secretory, ciliated, and resembling sex-cord stromal tumors. In these cases, immunohistochemistry is necessary for accurate diagnosis.

3.5 Brenner Tumors

3.5.1 Benign Brenner Tumor

Benign Brenner tumors account for 5% of benign ovarian epithelial tumors. They occur at a wide range group age, between 30- and 60-year-old women. They are usually asymptomatic and can be totally accidental finding. In 20–30% of cases, Brenner tumors develop synchronously with other neoplasms including mucinous neoplasm, dermoid cyst, or mature cystic teratoma. They are small generally less than 2 cm in size. They are unilateral in 95% of cases. Grossly, they are a sharply delineated mass seen in a normal ovary with a whitish firm cut surface. Microscopically, benign Brenner tumors appear as islands of transitional cells with nuclear grooving embedded in a fibrotic stroma. Sometimes, cystic dilation lined by transitional or mucinous epithelium can be seen. No atypia, mitotic figures, and necrosis are seen.

3.5.2 Malignant Brenner Tumor

Malignant Brenner tumors are the least common of the surface epithelial tumors of the ovary. They occur in women over 50 years of age. They are usually large and they might be cystic or solid. Histologically, they resemble urothelial/ transitional carcinoma of the urinary tract. They are composed of sheets of transitional-like epithelium exhibiting moderate atypia and fair numbers of mitotic figures. Cystic areas can be present. With extensive sampling, islands of benign Brenner tumor are seen in the background. However, if no benign Brenner tumor cells are seen after extensive sampling, a high-grade serous or endometrioid adenocarcinoma should be suspected.

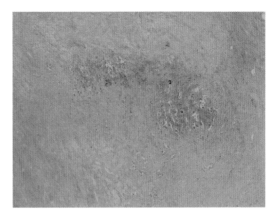

Fig. 11 Residual serous adenocarcinoma post neo-adjuvant chemotherapy. Tumor cells are in single files or clusters with abundant fibrous stroma

3.6 Seromucinous Tumors

Seromucinous tumors is a new entity that was introduced in the 2014 WHO classification. It has three categories: benign, borderline, and malignant (carcinoma). They are rare neoplasms. They are composed of a variable admixture of serous and mucinous (endocervical) epithelial lining. They are likely derived from endometriosis cells but this is still subject to speculation.

3.7 Undifferentiated Carcinoma

By the WHO definition "undifferentiated tumor is a malignant tumor showing no differentiation of any specific Mullerian cell type." Undifferentiated carcinomas usually present at the late stage. They are characterized by proliferation of high-grade tumor cells with high mitotic rate in a diffuse pattern with areas of necrosis.

3.8 Ovarian Carcinoma After Neoadjuvant Therapy

Traditionally, advanced stage ovarian carcinoma is treated by debulking surgery followed by chemotherapy. In some circumstances, neoadjuvant chemotherapy followed by debulking surgery may be done. Neoadjuvant chemotherapy is increasingly being used in the management of patients with advanced ovarian cancer, and pathologists should be aware of the morphologic changes in ovarian cancer after neoadjuvant chemotherapy. Treated tumors may be mistaken for metastatic carcinoma from breast primary or other sites. The morphologic changes seen in response to neoadjuvant chemotherapy include small groups or single tumor cells in a densely fibrotic stroma (Fig. 11). The tumor cells are characterized by nuclear and cytoplasmic alteration making the grading and sometimes the tumor typing impossible and inaccurate. Nuclear changes include nuclear enlargement, hyperchromasia, irregular nuclear outlines, and chromatin smudging. Cytoplasmic alterations include eosinophilic cytoplasm, vacuolation, and foamy cell changes (Fig. 8). The stroma may have pronounced fibrosis, inflammation, foamy histiocytic infiltrates, hemosiderin deposits, necrosis, calcification, and numerous free psammoma bodies (McCluggage et al. 2002; Miller et al. 2008). Fortunately, tumor cells seem to keep their antigens and therefore express antibodies similar to those seen in pretreatment including CK7+, WT1+, and p53+ (Chew et al. 2009).

3.9   Ovarian Grading Systems

Ovarian cancer is a very challenging task and it is still performed haphazardly with several systems and nonsystems used in different institutes and in different research studies. The lack of uniformity in grading has resulted in little consensus as to whether ovarian tumor grade has any significance in predicting disease outcome. The grading systems used most commonly worldwide are the International Federation of Gynecology and Obstetrics (FIGO) system and the World Health Organization (WHO) system. The FIGO grading system for the ovary is similar to the grading system used in the uterus. It is based on architectural features. The grade depends on the ratio of glandular or papillary structures versus solid tumor growth. Grade 1 is equivalent to <5% solid growth, grade 2 to 5–50% solid growth, and grade 3 to =>50% solid growth. In the **WHO** system, the grade is assessed by both the architectural and cytologic features, without any quantitative evaluation. The Gynecologic Oncology (GOG) system is the most commonly used system in the United States (Bendaj and Zaino 1994). It employs a method based on the histologic type. For example, ovarian carcinoma of endometrioid type is graded similarly to the endometrial adenocarcinoma of endometrioid type. Ovarian carcinoma of transitional type is graded similar to transitional cell carcinoma (TCC) of the bladder. Clear cell carcinomas are not graded at all. Silverberg et al. proposed a new grading system similar to that used in breast carcinoma, and it depends on architectural features (glandular 1, papillary 2, and solid 3), cytologic atypia (mild 1, moderate 2, severe 3), and mitotic rate (1 0–9 mitosis/10HPF, 2 10–24, 3 >25). A score is given by adding the parameters, a score of 3–5 is grade 1, a score of 6–7 is grade 2, and a score of 8–9 is grade 3 (Silverberg 2000). Figure 12 and 13 is an example of grade 1 and grade 3 serous carcinomas. This grading system was confirmed to be reproducible in subsequent studies (Ishioka et al. 2003).

Another study from MD Anderson Cancer Center group suggested adopting a two-tier system that is based primarily on the assessment of

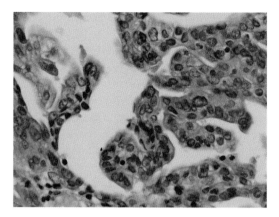

Fig. 12 Low-grade serous carcinoma defined by mild atypia and few mitotic figures

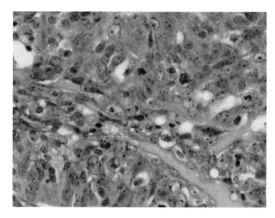

Fig. 13 High-grade serous carcinoma defined by moderate to severe atypia and high mitotic figures

nuclear atypia (uniformity vs. pleomorphism) in the worst area of the tumor (Malpica et al. 2004). The tumor is graded into low grade (Fig. 12) and high grade (Fig. 13). A few years after its introduction, the authors confirmed its reproducibility and urged its use to facilitate the clinical trials and protocols (Malpica et al. 2007). This grading system has gained huge popularity and even it was adopted by the 2014 WHO classification. However, this grading could be applied to only serous carcinomas.

3.10   Ovarian Staging FIGO 2014

The International Federation of Gynecology and Obstetrics (FIGO) staging has revised the staging for ovarian cancer, and the approved and new ovarian cancer staging went into effect on 1 January 2014. There were some major differences between the old FIGO and new FIGO staging system.

Stage I: IC (ovaries with any of the following: capsule rupture, tumor on surface, positive washings/ascites) was subdivided in IC1 (surgical spill), IC2 (capsule rupture before surgery or tumor on surface ovarian surface), and IC3 (malignant cells in the ascites or peritoneal washings).

Stage II: IIC in the old system (IIA or IIB with positive washings/ascites) was canceled. So in the new system is only stage IIA and IIB.

Stage III: IIIA was modified and subclassified into IIIA1 (positive retroperitoneal lymph nodes only) and IIIA2 (microscopic, extrapelvic peritoneal involvement ± positive retroperitoneal lymph nodes).

4 Conclusion

Epithelial ovarian tumors are very interesting and fascinating tumors. They still are a subject of debate regarding their pathogenesis, molecular pathways, diagnosis, and treatment. However, the discovery of new genetic mutations and pathways had revolutionized our understanding of ovarian cancer and has provided us with a fresh outlook based on their molecular fingerprints. In the past, histologic classification of surface epithelial tumor had poor interobserver agreement (60%), but because of the advancement of the molecular testing, the immunohistochemistry agreement has risen to 80–90% (Kobel et al. 2010). Due to these advancements in reclassification, it will not be a surprise if 10 years from now, ovarian tumors will be reclassified using not just morphology alone but will heavily incorporate the molecular findings. All the gynecologic oncologic communities are excited about these developments. Targeted therapy and personalized medicine are very promising venues for patients' care.

References

Bendaj A, Zaino R. GOG pathology manual. Buffalo: Gynecologic Oncologic Group; 1994.

Brown J, Frumovitz M. Mucinous tumors of the ovary: current thoughts on diagnosis and management. Curr Oncol Rep. 2014;16(6):389.

Chang SJ, Ryu HS, Chang KH, Yoo SC, Yoon JH. Prognostic significance of the micropapillary pattern in patients with serous borderline ovarian tumors. Acta Obstet Gynecol Scand. 2008;87:476–81.

Chew I, Soslow RA, Park KJ. Morphologic changes in ovarian carcinoma after neoadjuvant chemotherapy: report of a case showing extensive clear cell changes mimicking clear cell carcinoma. Int J Gynecol Pathol. 2009;28(5):442–6.

Fischerova D, Zikan M, Cibula D. Diagnosis, treatment and follow-up of borderline ovarian tumors. Oncologists. 2012;17(12):1515–33.

Ishioka S-I, Sagae S, Terasawa K, Sugimura M, Nishioka Y, Tsukada K, Kudo R. Comparison of the usefulness between a new universal grading system for epithelial ovarian cancer and the FIGO grading system. Gynecol Oncol. 2003;89:447–52.

Köbel M, Kalloger SE, Baker PM, Ewanowich CA, Arseneau J, Zherebitskiy V, Abdulkarim S, Leung S, Duggan MA, Fontaine D, Parker R, Huntsman DG, Gilks CB. Diagnosis of ovarian carcinoma cell type is highly reproducible: a transcanadian study. Am J Surg Pathol. 2010;34(7):984–93.

Köbel M, Kalloger SE, Lee S, Duggan MA, Kelemen LE, Prentice L, Kalli KR, Fridley BL, Visscher DW, Keeney GL, Vierkant RA, Cunningham JM, Chow C, Ness RB, Moysich K, Edwards R, Modugno F, Bunker C, Wozniak EL, Benjamin E, Gayther SA, Gentry-Maharaj A, Menon U, Gilks CB, Huntsman DG, Ramus SJ, Goode EL; Ovarian tumor tissue analysis consortium. Biomarker-based ovarian carcinoma typing: a histologic investigation in the ovarian tumor tissue analysis consortium. Cancer Epidemiol Biomark Prev. 2013;22(10):1677–86. doi: 10.1158/1055-9965.EPI-13-0391. Epub 2013 Jul 23.

Kurman RJ, Carcangiu ML, Herrington CS, Young RH. WHO classification of tumors of female reproductive organs. 124th ed. Lyon: International Agency of Research on Cancer (IARC); 2014.

Longacre TA, McKenney JK, Tazelaar HD, Kempson RL, Hendrickson MR. Ovarian serous tumors of low malignant potential (borderline tumors), outcome-based study of 276 patients with long term (> or = 5 year) follow-up. Am J Surg Pathol. 2005;29:707–23.

Malpica A, Deavers MT, Lu K, Bodurka DC, Atkinson EN, Gershenson DM, Silva EG. Grading ovarian serous carcinoma using two-tier system. Am J Surg Pathol. 2004;28:496–504.

Malpica A, Deavers MT, Tornos C, Kurman RJ, Soslow R, Seidman JD, Munsell MF, Gaertner E, Frishberg D, Silva EG. Interobserver and intraobserver variability of a two-tier system for grading serous carcinoma. Am J Surg Pathol. 2007;31:1168–74.

May T, Virtanen C, Sharma M, Milea A, Begley H, Rosen B, Murphy KJ, Brown TJ, Shaw PA. Low malignant potential tumors with micropapillary features are molecularly similar to low-grade serous carcinoma of the ovary. Gynecol Oncol. 2002;117:9–17.

McCluggage WG, Lyness RW, Atkinson RJ, Dobbs SP, Harley I, McClelland HR, Price JH. Morphological effects of chemotherapy on ovarian carcinoma. J Clin Pathol. 2002;55:27–31.

Mhawech-Fauceglia, Pejovic T. Hypothesis on the origin and risk genes of high grade serous ovarian carcinoma. IJGORMR. 2015;1(2):1–5.

Mhawech-Fauceglia P, Ramzan A Walia S, Pham HQ, Yessaian A. Microfocus of anaplastic carcinoma arising in mural nodule of ovarian mucinous borderline tumor with very rapid and fatal outcome. Int Gynecol Pathol. 2015 [epud ahead of print} PMID 26598983.

Miller K, Price JH, Dobbs SP, McClelland RH, Kennedy K, McCluggage WG. An immunohistochemical and morphological analysis of past-chemotherapy ovarian carcinoma. J Clin Pathol. 2008;61:652–7.

National Cancer institute, Surveillance, Epidemiology, and End Results Program (SEER) Ovarian Cancer Statistics, [internet] 2015; available from http://www.seer.cancer.gov/statfacts/ovary.

Okamoto A, Glasspool RM, Mabuchi S, Matsumura N, Nomura H, Itamochi H, Takano M, Takano T, Susumu N, Aoki D, Konishi I, Covens A, Ledermann J, Mezzanzanica D, Steer C, Millan D, McNeish IA, Pfisterer J, Kang S, Gladieff L, Bryce J, Oza A. Gynecologic Cancer InterGroup (GCIG) consensus review for clear cell carcinoma of the ovary. Int J Gynecol Cancer. 2014;24(9 Suppl 3):S20–5. doi:10.1097/IGC.0000000000000289.

Prat J, FIGO Committee on Gynecologic Oncology. Staging classification of cancer of the ovary, fallopian tube and peritoneum. Int J Gynaecol Obstet. 2014;124:1–5.

Ronnett BM, Yan H, Kurman RJ, Shmookler BM, Wu L, Sugarbaker PH. Patients with pseudomyxoma peritonei associated with disseminated peritoneal adenomucinosis have a significantly more favorable prognosis than patients with peritoneal mucinous carcinomatosis. Cancer. 2001;92:85–91.

Shih I-M, Kurman RJ. Molecular pathogenesis of ovarian borderline tumors: new insights and old challenges. Clin Cancer Res. 2005;11(20):7273–9.

Silverberg SG. Histopathologic grading of ovarian carcinomas: a review and proposal. Int J Gynecol Pathol. 2000;19:7–15.

Slomovitz BM, Caputo TA, Gretz HF 3rd, Economos K, Tortoriello DV, Schlosshauer PW, Baergen RN, Isacson C, Soslow RA. A comparative analysis of 57 serous borderline tumors with and without a noninvasive micropapillary component. Am J Surg Pathol. 2002;26(5):592–600.

Sex Cord–Stromal Tumors of the Ovaries

Mohamed Mokhtar Desouki and Oluwole Fadare

Abstract

Ovarian sex cord–stromal tumors (SCSTs) are uncommon neoplasms that are known to have a wide morphologic spectrum and which accordingly may be diagnostically challenging. The keys to accurately diagnosing the tumors in this group is to recognize the full pathologic spectrum of every constituent entity and to consider the possibility for each ovarian neoplasm encountered that is plausibly in the differential diagnosis.

Keywords

Ovary • Sex cord–stromal tumors • Fibroma • Fibrothecoma • Fibrosarcoma • Sertoli–Leydig cell tumor • Sertoli cell tumor • Granulosa cell tumor • Leydig cell tumor • Steroid cell tumor

Contents

M.M. Desouki (✉)
Department of Pathology, Microbiology and Immunology, Vanderbilt University Medical Center, Nashville, TN, USA
e-mail: mokhtar.desouki@vanderbilt.edu; mohamed.desouki@vanderbilt.edu

O. Fadare
Department of Pathology, University of California San Diego, San Diego, CA, USA
e-mail: ofadare@ucsd.edu

1 Introduction

Patient age, clinical manifestations (e.g., hormone production), morphologic features, and occasionally ancillary diagnostic studies (e.g., immunohistochemistry (IHC)) are important tools in assigning an ovarian neoplasm to one of the tumors among the diverse sex cord–stromal tumors (SCSTs) (Kurman et al. 2014). SCSTs are derived from or display differentiation towards ovarian cortical stroma, hilar, and other steroidal cells and granulosa-theca cells of the ovarian follicles. Apart from fibroma, all other SCSTs are uncommon. The differential diagnosis for a given case typically includes many other SCST. Similarly, SCST is frequently in the differential diagnosis for a wide variety of non-SCST. Accordingly, familiarity with the morphologic spectrum of SCST is crucial to their accurate pathologic categorization (Kurman et al. 2014).

2   Epidemiology and Clinical Presentation

SCSTs constitute <10% of all ovarian tumors. Benign tumors, e.g., fibromas and thecomas account for approximately 85% of all SCSTs. Adult granulosa cell tumors (AGCTs), Sertoli–Leydig cell tumors (SLCTs), and sclerosing stromal tumors account for approximately 15% of SCSTs. The remaining tumors collectively are very rare constituting <1% of the SCSTs (Kurman et al. 2014). Diagnostic issues are mainly due to the rarity of most entities. Clinical information including endocrine manifestations and patient age are important parameters to clinically investigate and communicate to the pathologist. The patient age is especially significant since there are clear age-related differences in the incidence of several tumors in this category: (a) juvenile granulosa cell tumors (JGCTs) occur primarily in the <20 age group (Young et al. 1984a); (b) JGCTs and SLCTs predominate between menarche and 25 years (Young et al. 1982, 1984a); (c) fibrothecomas and AGCTs most commonly occur between 25- and 50-year age group (Burandt and Young 2014; Schumer and Cannistra 2003); and (d) and fibrosarcomas commonly emerge after menopause (Irving et al. 2006; Seidman et al. 1995; Young and Scully 1988). Patients are either asymptomatic with the tumor discovered incidentally on clinical or radiologic examination or present with abdominal pain and/or abdominal mass. Endocrine related symptoms due to hyperestrinism and hyperandrogenism may be the presenting symptoms (Kurman et al. 2014). A small subset of SCSTs have known associations with specific syndromes, including Gorlin's (fibroma), Meigs' (fibroma), Ollier's disease (JGCT), *DICER1* (SLCT, JGCT, gynandroblastoma), Maffucci's (JGCT), and Peutz–Jeghers (sex cord tumor with annular tubules (SCTATs)) (Gorlin 1987; Samanth and Black 1970; Seidman 1996; Young

Table 1 World Health Organization classification of ovarian sex cordstromal tumors[a]

Pure stromal tumors
Fibroma
Fibrosarcoma
Thecoma
Steroid cell tumor
Pure sex cord tumors
Granulosa cell tumor
Sertoli cell tumor
Mixed sex cord–stromal tumors
Sertoli–Leydig cell tumors
Sex cord–stromal tumors, unclassified

[a]A non-exhaustive listing of commonly encountered tumors in practice (Kurman et al. 2014)

et al. 1982) and may accordingly present with extraovarian manifestations reflecting these syndromes.

Patient outcomes for SCSTs are largely histotype dependent, although histotypes such as SLCTs and steroid cell tumors may display a wide spectrum of outcomes even within a single diagnostic group. This chapter highlights the most common tumors encountered in clinical practice (Table 1) with an emphasis on the clinicpathologic profile of each entity.

2.1   Fibromas and Cellular Fibromas

2.1.1   Epidemiology and Clinical Features

Fibromas are benign tumors composed of variably cellular neoplasm and collagen deposition. Fibromas with tumors showing thecomatous differentiation (fibrothecomas) constitute the largest group of SCSTs (~85%). Fibromas commonly affect women in the fifth decade, with a mean age of 48 years. Meigs' syndrome is a constellation of ovarian fibroma, ascites, and pleural effusion (Samanth and Black 1970). Gorlin's (nevoid basal cell) syndrome is another autosomal dominant syndrome described with ovarian fibroma and cutaneous basal cell carcinomas (Gorlin 1987). Cellular fibromas are much less common than conventional fibromas (10%) and commonly present with rupture and surface adhesions (Prat and Scully 1981).

2.1.2   Gross Pathology

Fibromas are typically unilateral (9% bilateral) and range in size from less than 1 to 16 cm (average of 3.8 cm). They typically have a smooth outer surface, solid to rubbery consistency, and white to tan cut surfaces. Edema and calcification are common. Infarction and hemorrhage occasionally present. Fibromas associated with Gorlin syndrome are usually bilateral (~75%) and more commonly multinodular rather than smooth (Gorlin 1987). Cellular fibromas may have a softer consistency and a tan to yellow color (Young and Scully 1988).

2.1.3   Histopathology

Fibromas are composed of uniformly distributed, bland spindle-shaped cells which usually arrange in a swirling (storiform) pattern. The nuclei are elongated with tapered ends and have inconspicuous nucleoli. No cytological atypia is present, and mitotic figures are usually infrequent (Fig. 1). Calcification, intercellular edema, sex cord–like elements, and hyaline fibrosis may be focally present. The cellularity is typically mild to moderate (Young and Scully 1988).

Cellular fibromas tend to have increased cellularity with haphazard rather than uniform growth pattern with focal areas of conventional fibroma. Usually, no hyaline bands in the hypercellular areas and edema is not as frequent as that of conventional fibromas (Fig. 2). The mitotic index may be >4 per 10 HPF in a subset of cases (Prat and Scully 1981), and these tumors should be categorized as mitotically active fibromas, as long as cytologic atypia is absent.

2.1.4   Differential Diagnosis

Fibromas are easily diagnosed lesions. However, small tumors may be confused with cellular cortex or stromal hyperplasia. These distinctions are based on the presence of a distinct mass lesion separate from the background stroma in fibromas. Pure thecoma is another challenging differential.

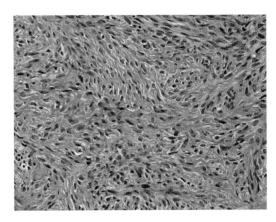

Fig. 1 Ovarian fibroma. The tumor is morphologically characterized by spindled stromal fibroblasts and intervening collagen. No mitotic figures are appreciated

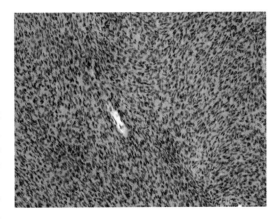

Fig. 2 Ovarian cellular fibroma. Compared to fibroma in Fig. 1, this tumor is hypercellular with vague storiform pattern. No atypia, mitotic figures, or necrosis is seen

In contrast to fibromas, thecoma (see below) typically display scattered collagenous plaques and the constituent cells have abundant pale to vacuolated cytoplasm (Young and Scully 1988).

2.2   Fibrosarcoma

2.2.1   Epidemiology

Ovarian fibrosarcoma is a rare malignant fibroblastic tumor which occur predominantly in the fifth decade (Prat and Scully 1981).

Fig. 3 Ovarian fibrosarcoma. Gross photograph of soft mass with foci of hemorrhage and gross necrosis

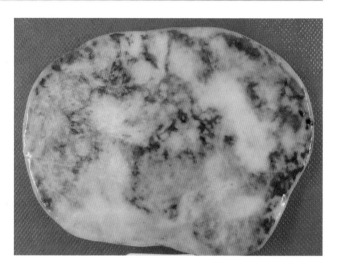

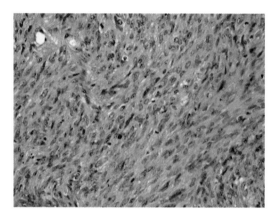

Fig. 4 Ovarian fibrosarcoma. High power (40×) showing increased, cellularity, moderate to severe atypia, and mitotic figures

2.2.2 Gross Pathology

Fibrosarcomas are unilateral tumors which usually reach large size compared to fibromas. Solid to cystic heterogeneous consistency and associated hemorrhage and necrosis are common gross findings (Prat and Scully 1981) (Fig. 3).

2.2.3 Histopathology

Fibrosarcoma, like those of other organs, is composed of spindle cell proliferation with a storiform or herringbone growth pattern with moderate to severe nuclear atypia (Fig. 4). Despite the fact that high mitotic activity is a feature of fibrosarcoma and can be easily found, high mitotic count also encountered in cellular fibromas and by itself is not an indicative of malignancy (Irving et al. 2006; Prat and Scully 1981).

2.2.4 Differential Diagnosis

Fibrosarcomas should be distinguished from other malignant spindle cell neoplasms that may involve the ovary, most notably primary or metastatic leiomyosarcomas or other sarcomas, poorly differentiated SLCTs, or sarcoma-dominant carcinosarcomas.

2.3 Thecoma and Luteinized Thecoma

2.3.1 Epidemiology and Clinical Features

Thecomas are benign tumors that occur typically in postmenopausal women with an average age of 49.6 years. Approximately half of cases will present with manifestations of hyperestrinism. Some cases (~20%) may be associated with endometrial adenocarcinoma. Another 10% of thecomas are associated with androgenic symptoms (Burandt and Young 2014). Compared with typical thecomas, luteinized thecomas are more likely to be associated with androgenic manifestations and less likely to be associated with estrogenic manifestations

2.3.2 Gross Pathology

Thecomas are mostly (95%) unilateral tumors with firm, smooth surfaces and homogeneous yellow and lobulated cut surfaces. The tumor may reach up to 22.5 cm with an average dimension of 4.9 cm (Burandt and Young 2014).

2.3.3 Histopathology

Thecomas are a group of stromal tumors resembling thecal cells of the ovarian follicles. Pure forms composed of theca cells only with no admixture of fibroblasts (fibrothecomas) or granulosa cells (granulosa-theca cell tumors) are extremely rare. The fusiform tumor cells usually grow in a diffuse pattern with alternating hyaline plaques or rarely in a nodular pattern. The cells have ill-defined membranes and pale gray cytoplasm. Calcifications and keloid-like sclerosis are common in these tumors. Vesicular nuclei with delicate membranes are usually appreciated (Burandt and Young 2014) (Fig. 5).

Luteinized thecomas exhibit single or clusters of lutein cells which are ovoid cells containing abundant cytoplasm interspersed between the neoplastic spindle cells (Fig. 6). Luteinized thecomas in rare occasions are associated with sclerosing peritonitis which typically occurs in women less than 30 years. Patients with this rare association typically present with ascites and bowel symptoms and bilateral ovarian tumors. Morphologically, the peritoneal surface exhibits a fascicular growth pattern with mitotically active but cytologically bland fibroblasts admixed with inflammatory cells (Burandt and Young 2014; Clement et al. 1994). The term "thecomatosis" has been proposed for this phenomenon (Staats et al. 2008).

2.3.4 Differential Diagnosis

The differential diagnosis with fibromas has been previously discussed. The cells of GCT, an important differential diagnostic consideration, do not display the pale, eosinophilic cytoplasm of thecomas unless they are luteinized. In comparison to GCTs, reticulin stain will delineate individual cells in thecoma/fibroma (Fig. 7) versus

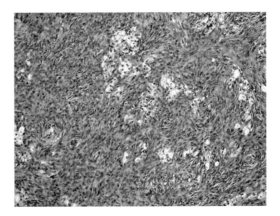

Fig. 6 Ovarian luteinized thecoma. The tumor is composed of fascicles of spindled cells with abundant eosinophilic cytoplasm. Clusters of luteinized cells containing vacuolated cytoplasm are interspersed between the tumor cells

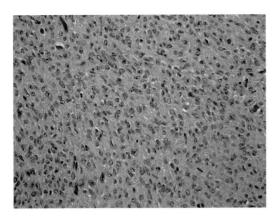

Fig. 5 Ovarian thecoma. The tumor is composed of plump to spindle cells with abundant pale cytoplasm and central nuclei

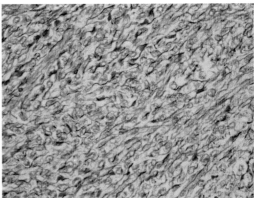

Fig. 7 Reticulin special stain. A reticulin stain surround individual cells in fibrothecoma

surrounding clusters of cells in GCTs (Burandt and Young 2014) (Fig. 15). Other potential considerations (relative to luteinized thecoma) include stromal hyperthecosis (bilateral, minimal collagen), pregnancy luteoma (commonly multiple, no fibromatous background, minimal lipid), and steroid cell tumor, not otherwise specified (NOS) (a designation that would be used if the spindle cell to steroid cell ratio of the tumor is less than 1:10)

2.4 Steroid Cell Tumors

This group of tumors are very rare constituting less than 1.0% of all SCSTs. The group includes hilus cell tumor, stromal luteoma, Leydig cell tumor, pregnancy luteoma, and lipid cell tumor. The term "lipid cell tumor" is not recommended because it is nonspecific since most of these tumors contain lipid in the cytoplasm (Seidman et al. 1995). The pregnancy luteoma is considered by some as an exaggerated hyperplasia of theca-lutein during pregnancy rather than a neoplasm (Norris and Taylor 1967). The most recent World Health Organization (WHO) classification of tumors of the female reproductive organs included Leydig cell tumors and steroid cell tumors under this category (McCluggage et al. 2014).

2.4.1 Clinical Manifestations

Leydig cell tumors occur in the sixth and seventh decades with symptoms related to hormone production mainly testosterone in most cases in the form of hirsutism (Zhang et al. 1982). The tumors are typically unilateral and relatively small in size. The biology of most of these tumors is favorable with benign behavior (Zhang et al. 1982). On the other hand, the age range of patients with steroid cell tumors, NOS is very wide with a mean age of 43 years. Steroid cell tumors, NOS are typically unilateral with a mean diameter of 8 cm. The behavior of steroid cell tumors NOS have a guarded prognosis with a reported rate of 34% with malignant behavior (Hayes and Scully 1987).

2.4.2 Steroid Cell Tumor Types

Leydig Cell Tumor

Leydig cell tumor occurs mostly in the hilus of the ovary or rarely in the ovarian parenchyma. Crystalloids of Reinke should be present to qualify for this classification otherwise the tumor will be classified as steroid cell tumor. The crystalloids of Reinke are rod or spherical eosinophilic structures in the cytoplasm. Histologically, Leydig cell tumors exhibit lobular aggregates of eosinophilic to vacuolated cells with centrally located nuclei and abundant cytoplasm (Fig. 8). Additionally, anuclear eosinophilic material intervening the cells is a clue to the diagnosis. Nuclear atypia in the form of enlarged, bizarre nuclei is not uncommon and does not imply malignant behavior (Zhang et al. 1982).

Steroid Cell Tumors, Not Otherwise Specified

Absence of crystalloid of Reinke is the main morphologic feature which qualifies for this nomenclature (Hayes and Scully 1987). Worrisome (malignant) features include large size (>7 cm), high mitotic index (> two per 10 HPFs), necrosis, and severe nuclear atypia (Hayes and Scully 1987). The gross morphology is yellow to dark brown (Fig. 9). The cells form diffuse aggregates in linear or circular pattern separated by thin fibrous septae. The nuclei are centrally placed

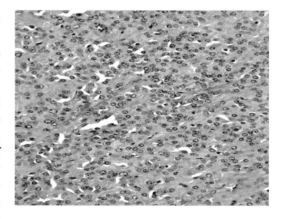

Fig. 8 Ovarian Leydig cell tumor. Aggregates of eosinophilic cells with centrally located nuclei and abundant cytoplasm

Fig. 9 Ovarian steroid cell tumor. Gross photograph showing well circumscribed yellow mass

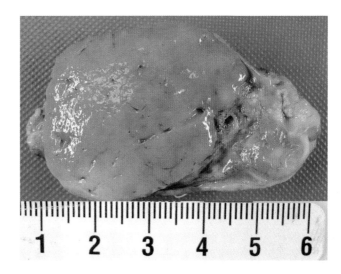

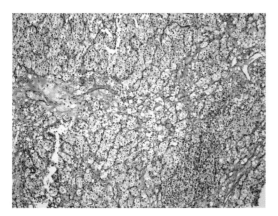

Fig. 10 Ovarian steroid cell tumor, not otherwise specified. The cells form diffuse aggregates separated by thin fibrous stroma. The cytoplasm is vacuolated and lipid rich. The nuclei are centrally placed with prominent nucleoli

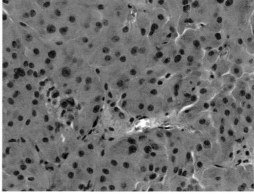

Fig. 11 Ovarian stromal luteoma. The tumor composed of a uniform cell population with centrally placed nuclei and prominent nucleoli. The cytoplasm is finely granular with demarcated cellular outlines

with prominent nucleoli and minimal atypia. The cytoplasm is frequently vacuolated and lipid rich (Hayes and Scully 1987) (Fig. 10).

Stromal Luteoma

This tumor presents with estrogenic symptoms mainly vaginal bleeding and a few cases present with androgenic symptoms. The lesion is characterized by centrally located neoplasm within the ovarian parenchyma. A uniform cell population with centrally placed nuclei and prominent nucleoli are evident. The cytoplasm is pale, finely granular, pink to vacuolated with demarcated cellular

outlines (Fig. 11). Hyperthecosis with vacuolated cells in the surrounding ovarian stroma is common (Vilain et al. 1992).

2.5 Granulosa Cell Tumors

Granulosa cell tumors (GCTs) are rare tumors constituting 1–2% of all ovarian tumors. The tumors contain at least 10% of follicular granulosa cells. Despite the fact that GCTs are rare, they are the second most common SCSTs after fibromas (Schumer and Cannistra 2003).

2.5.1 Clinical Features

Traditionally GCTs are classified into adult and juvenile types. As the name implies with exceptions both ways, adult type predominates in postmenopausal women and juvenile type in younger age (average age of 13 years) (Schumer and Cannistra 2003; Young et al. 1984a). The tumor may produce estrogenic or androgenic effects, including abnormal uterine bleeding with cystic hyperplasia due to anovulation. Associated endometrial carcinoma have been reported in ~5% of cases with GCTs. Juvenile GCTs are rarer (less than 5% of GCTs) and commonly associated with hyperestrinism resulting in isosexual pseudoprecocity in prepubertal girls (Young et al. 1984a).

2.5.2 Gross Pathology

GCTs are unilateral in ~91% of cases, and stage I is the most common stage at diagnosis. Grossly, GCTs are typically solid with variable cystic spaces and hemorrhagic. Tumors with prominent theca component are often yellow and firm. Rupture at the time of surgery is not uncommon and do occur in up to 15% of cases (Schumer and Cannistra 2003; Young et al. 1984a).

2.5.3 Histopathology

Adult GCTs exhibit a range of epithelioid to spindle cell pattern with organoid or diffuse architecture. Combination of patterns is usually seen in a single tumor. Morphologic patterns include trabecular, insular, gland-like, microfollicular and macrofollicular, diffuse, "watered silk," pseudopapillary, and cystic. The nuclei are uniform, with evenly dispersed chromatin and nuclear grooves (Figs. 12 and 13). Call–Exner bodies are characteristic of GCTs and defined as granulosa cells which arrange haphazardly around a space filled with eosinophilic material. Focal marked atypia is more common in juvenile GCT and is not independently correlated with malignant behavior. Luteinization of cells with plump pale cytoplasm is a common finding (Schumer and Cannistra 2003).

The morphology of juvenile GCT is characterized by a nodular or diffuse proliferation of neoplastic cells in a myxoid and edematous

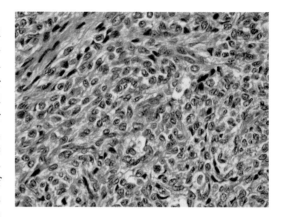

Fig. 12 Adult granulosa cell tumor of the ovary. The tumor composed of monotonous cells with scant cytoplasm, uniform nuclei with evenly dispersed chromatin and nuclear grooves

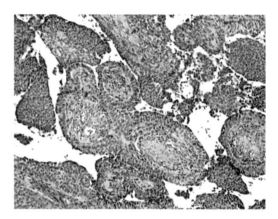

Fig. 13 Adult granulosa cell tumor of the ovary. The characteristic tumor cells grow in a pseudopapillary pattern

background. Follicle-like spaces of different sizes and shapes containing proteinaceous material are characteristic with rare Call–Exner bodies (Fig. 14). In contrast to adult GCTs, the nuclei are larger and hyperchromatic with no to scarce grooves (Young et al. 1984a). JGCTs are known to display a notably higher mitotic index than AGCTs, whose mitotic index is generally <5 MF/10 HPF. GCTs stain positive for inhibin, and FOXL2 by IHC. Reticulin stain usually surrounds nests and groups of cells (Fig. 15).

2.5.4 Differential Diagnosis of GCTs

- High grade endometrioid adenocarcinoma. Carcinomas usually exhibit a higher nuclear

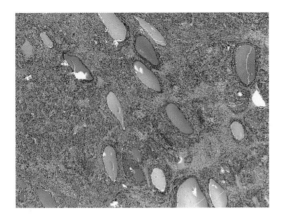

Fig. 14 Juvenile granulosa cell tumor of the ovary. Diffuse proliferation of tumor cells among follicle-like spaces of different sizes and shapes

grade, are more mitotically active than the typical AGCT, and by IHC are negative for sex cord–stromal markers and are positive for epithelial membrane antigen (EMA).

- Metastatic lobular carcinoma of the breast. Lobular carcinoma grows in cord-like and single file patterns, typically involves both ovaries and is EMA and GATA3-positive and is negative for inhibin and FOXL2.
- Carcinoid tumor. Insular pattern carcinoid is usually associated with teratoma, the nuclear chromatin is granular "salt and pepper," and the cells are positive for neuroendocrine markers, e.g., synaptophysin and chromogranin.
- Luteinized thecoma/fibrothecoma. A reticulin stain will surround individual cells in fibrothecoma and nests of cells in GCT (Figs. 7 and 15).
- Small cell carcinoma, hypercalcemic type (SCCH). Hypercalcemia and lack of estrogenic manifestations may help in differentiating this tumor from the juvenile GCT. Morphologically, SCCH lacks the nodular growth pattern of JGCTs, shows a lesser tendency for follicle-like spaces, mucinous cells in a subset, lacks inhibin and FOXL2 positivity, and shows loss of SMARCA4 (BRG1) expression.
- Undifferentiated carcinoma. More mitotically active than most AGCTs and are negative for inhibin and calretinin.

- Other entities. Endometrioid carcinoma with sex cord elements, endometrioid stromal sarcoma, SCTATs, gonadoblastoma, melanoma, steroid cell tumor, and yolk sac tumor.

2.6 Sertoli–Leydig Cell Tumor

SLCTs differentiate towards testicular counterparts. These tumors are rare, usually unilateral and classified according to the tumor grade and associated morphologic changes (Young and Scully 1985).

2.6.1 Epidemiology and Clinical Features

SLCTs predominate in the third decade with an average age of 25 years (Young and Scully 1984). Androgenic symptoms, e.g., virilism, amenorrhea, deepening of voice, and clitoromegaly are the main symptoms in approximately half of patients (Young and Scully 1985).

2.6.2 Gross Pathology

SLCTs tend to be partially cystic mass and some may be either completely cystic or completely solid. Solid tumors are yellow with lobulated outer surfaces. Higher grade lesions show gross hemorrhage and necrosis. As the case with GCTs, SLCTs present at an early stage at initial diagnosis (Young and Scully 1985).

2.6.3 Histopathology

SLCTs are classified according to tumor differentiation and clinical behavior into well-differentiated (11% of cases, clinically benign), intermediately differentiated (54% of cases, 11% malignancy rate), and poorly differentiated (11% of cases, 59% malignancy rare) (Young and Scully 1985).

Well-Differentiated

The neoplastic cells form tubules forming either compact lobules of round tubules, or tubules which are infiltrative between the intervening collagen bundles. The tubules usually have open lumina and rarely are compact with inconspicuous lumens. The Leydig cells are present throughout

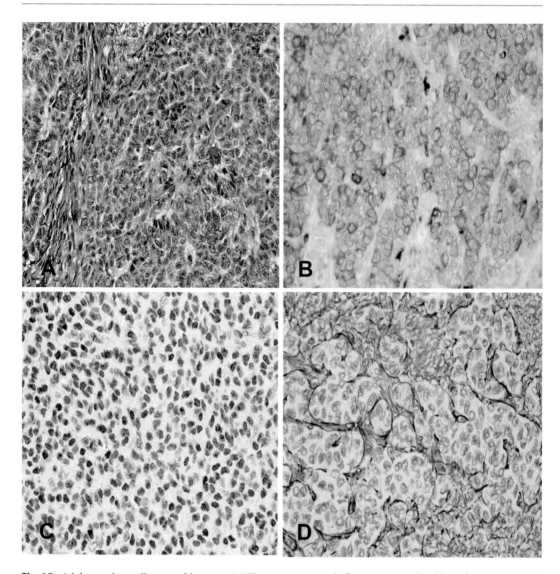

Fig. 15 Adult granulosa cell tumor of the ovary. (**a**) The tumor composed of monotonous cells with uniform nuclei which stain positive for inhibin (**b**) and FOXL2 (**c**) by immunohistochemistry. (**d**) Reticulin stain surrounds nests of cells

the tumor with variable density in a single or cluster pattern (Young and Scully 1984). The tubules are lined by cells with elongated nuclei arranged perpendicular to the surrounding basement membranes. The cytoplasm is uniform and may be lipid rich or oxyphilic (Ferry et al. 1994) (Fig. 16).

Intermediately Differentiated

The characteristic morphology is the presence of alternating cellular areas separated by

hypocellular edematous stroma in lobulated pattern. The neoplastic cells grow as sheets, tubules, nests, cords, or microcysts. The cells have small, round nuclei and scant cytoplasm. Leydig cells are usually rimming the nodules at the periphery and populating the hypocellular stroma (Young and Scully 1985) (Fig. 17).

Poorly Differentiated

These tumors are characterized by sarcomatoid growth pattern. They are formed of spindle cells

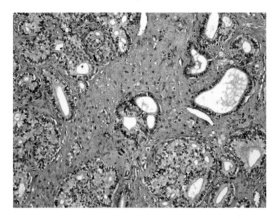

Fig. 16 Well-differentiated Sertoli–Leydig cell tumor. The neoplastic cells form tubules with elongated nuclei which arrange perpendicular to the basement membranes. The cytoplasm is uniform and contains lipid. The Leydig cells are present throughout the tumor

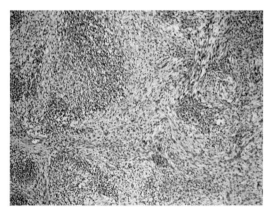

Fig. 17 Intermediately differentiated Sertoli–Leydig cell tumor. The characteristic morphology is shown in this photomicrograph with alternating cellular areas separated by hypocellular edematous stroma in lobulated pattern. The cells have small, round nuclei and scant cytoplasm. Leydig cells are scattered in the hypocellular areas

mimicking sarcoma with high nuclear grade and absent tubule formation. Leydig cells are rare. Inhibin stain by IHC (see below) is positive (Young and Scully 1985) (Fig. 18).

SLCT with Retiform Pattern

These tumors as the name implies are characterized by growth pattern simulating the rete testis. Morphologically they include poorly formed tubules, gland-like structures, and intraglandular

micropapillary pattern. The papillae are short and blunt with hyalinized cores.

SLCT with Heterologous Elements

Twenty-two percent of SLCTs display heterologous elements, in the form of gastrointestinal-type mucinous epithelium, skeletal muscles, bone, cartilage, and other mesenchymal structures (Young and Scully 1985). Mucinous epithelium is the most common, constituting ~90% of the heterologous differentiation (Fig. 19a). The average age is 24 years and androgenic symptoms are the main presentation. Apart from the associated heterologous elements, these tumors are morphologically similar to intermediately or poorly differentiated ones. Tumors with mucinous elements have a favorable outcome (Young et al. 1982). On the other hand, tumors with cartilage (Fig. 19b) and skeletal muscle elements have less favorable prognosis (Prat et al. 1982).

2.6.4 Differential Diagnosis

- Endometrioid and clear cell carcinomas. Clinical presentation in older age group, at least focal recognized areas of conventional carcinoma, positive EMA, and negative inhibin IHC stains favor carcinoma.
- Metastases. Bilaterality, signet rings and severe atypia favor a metastatic lesion.
- A wide variety of other possibilities, including other SCSTs, sarcomas, carcinosarcomas, teratomas (versus heterologous tumors), female adnexal tumor of probable Wolffian origin (FATWO), struma ovarii are worthy of consideration.

2.7 Sertoli Cell Tumors

2.7.1 Clinical Features

Less than 5% of tumors with Sertoli component are pure Sertoli cell tumors (SCTs). The mean age of patients is 30 years. In contrast to SLCTs (see above), the pure ones are typically (~70%) hormonally inert and minority of cases produce estrogen instead of androgen. Abdominal mass/ swelling, pain, or menstrual irregularities are common presentations (Oliva et al. 2005).

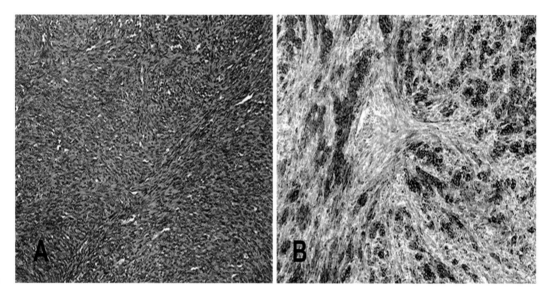

Fig. 18 Poorly differentiated Sertoli–Leydig cell tumor. (**a**) The tumor cells exhibit sarcomatoid growth pattern. They are formed of spindle cells mimicking sarcoma with high nuclear grade and absent tubule formation. (**b**) Inhibin stain by IHC is positive in tumor cells

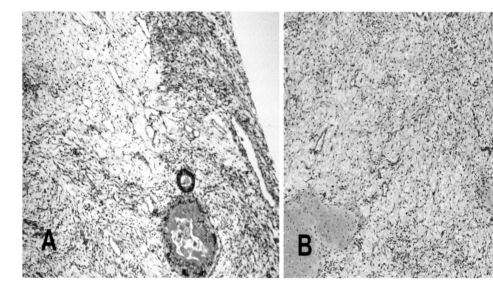

Fig. 19 Sertoli–Leydig cell tumor with heterologous elements. The tumor exhibits the morphology of intermediately differentiated tumor with alternating cellular and hypocellular stroma in lobulated pattern. Notice the presence of gastrointestinal mucinous elements in (**a**) and cartilaginous elements in (**b**)

2.7.2 Gross Pathology

As that with SLCT, SCTs are typically unilateral, solid, yellow tumors. Unlike SLCTs, cystic change is uncommon in SCTs. The average size is 9 cm (Oliva et al. 2005).

2.7.3 Histopathology

SCTs composed of well-formed tubules in most cases. Other patterns, e.g., cord-like, trabecular, and diffuse could also be encountered. The glands are lined with cells with basally located round nuclei with grooves and moderate amounts of eosinophilic or lutenized cytoplasm. Mild cytologic atypia and few mitoses are the characteristic features in most cases. In cases with abundant lipid-rich cytoplasm, the term "lipid-rich" SCT is used. The background stroma is variable and occasionally sclerotic. As the case with SLCTs, these tumors are typically EMA and CK-7 negative and inhibin positive (Oliva et al. 2005).

2.7.4 Differential Diagnosis
- Sertoli cell tumor is differentiated from SLCT by the absence of Leydig cells in the former.
- Endometrioid carcinoma sometimes composed of closely packed tubules simulating Sertoli cell tumor. The older age, squamous differentiation, positive EMA, and negative inhibin support the diagnosis of carcinoma.
- Carcinoid tumors have characteristic morphology with "salt and pepper" chromatin, cytoplasmic granules, positive neuroendocrine markers, and negative inhibin.

2.8 Sex Cord–Stromal Tumors, Unclassified

A fraction (10–20%) of SCSTs fall into this category. Clinical situation as pregnancy may cause difficulty in classifying SCSTs due to prominent edema, increased luteinization in GCTs, and prominent Leydig cells in SLCTs (Young et al. 1984b). Mixed patterns seen in different tumors as fibrothecomas, GCTs, and SLCTs may also qualify for the term unclassified (Seidman 1996).

2.9 Immunohistochemistry

The typical ovarian sex cord–stromal tumor is negative for EMA and is positive for calretinin, inhibin (Figs. 15 and 18), and to various extents, MART-1/melan-A, CD99, steroidogenic factor 1 (SF-1, adrenal 4-binding protein), WT1, and FOXL2 (Rabban and Zaloudek 2013) (Fig. 15). These markers have varying performances and some are more useful than the others for particular entities. However, a judiciously selected panel of markers can provide ample diagnostic information.

3 Conclusion

In summary, ovarian SCSTs have a wide pathologic spectrum. Clinical information and morphologic and immunophenotypic profiles are important tools employed by the pathologist to accurately classify these tumors and to exclude differential diagnostic considerations that may be managed differently.

References

Burandt E, Young RH. Thecoma of the ovary: a report of 70 cases emphasizing aspects of its histopathology different from those often portrayed and its differential diagnosis. Am J Surg Pathol. 2014;38(8):1023–32.

Clement PB, Young RH, Hanna W, Scully RE. Sclerosing peritonitis associated with luteinized thecomas of the ovary. A clinicopathological analysis of six cases. Am J Surg Pathol. 1994;18(1):1–13.

Ferry JA, Young RH, Engel G, Scully RE. Oxyphilic Sertoli cell tumor of the ovary: a report of three cases, two in patients with the Peutz-Jeghers syndrome. Int J Gynecol Pathol. 1994;13(3):259–66.

Gorlin RJ. Nevoid basal-cell carcinoma syndrome. Medicine (Baltimore). 1987;66(2):98–113.

Hayes MC, Scully RE. Ovarian steroid cell tumors (not otherwise specified). A clinicopathological analysis of 63 cases. Am J Surg Pathol. 1987;11(11):835–45.

Irving JA, Alkushi A, Young RH, Clement PB. Cellular fibromas of the ovary: a study of 75 cases including 40 mitotically active tumors emphasizing their distinction from fibrosarcoma. Am J Surg Pathol. 2006;30(8):929–38.

Kurman RJ, Carcangiu ML, Herrington CS, Young RH. WHO classification of tumours of the female reproductive organs, IARC WHO classification of tumours. Lyon: International Agency for Research on Cancer (IARC); 2014.

McCluggage W, Staats RN, Kiyokawa T, Young RH. Sex cord-stromal tumors. In: Kurman RJ, Carcangiu ML, Herrington CS, Young RH, editors. WHO classification of tumours of the female reproductive organs, series editors: Bosman FT, Jaffe ES, Lakhani SR, Ohgaki H. IARC WHO classification of tumours. Lyon: International Agency for Research on Cancer (IARC); 2014.

Norris HJ, Taylor HB. Nodular theca-lutein hyperplasia of pregnancy (so-called "pregnancy luteoma"). A clinical and pathologic study of 15 cases. Am J Clin Pathol. 1967;47(5):557–66.

Oliva E, Alvarez T, Young RH. Sertoli cell tumors of the ovary: a clinicopathologic and immunohistochemical study of 54 cases. Am J Surg Pathol. 2005;29(2): 143–56.

Prat J, Scully RE. Cellular fibromas and fibrosarcomas of the ovary: a comparative clinicopathologic analysis of seventeen cases. Cancer. 1981;47(11):2663–70.

Prat J, Young RH, Scully RE. Ovarian Sertoli-Leydig cell tumors with heterologous elements. II. Cartilage and skeletal muscle: a clinicopathologic analysis of twelve cases. Cancer. 1982;50(11):2465–75.

Rabban JT, Zaloudek CJ. A practical approach to immunohistochemical diagnosis of ovarian germ cell tumours and sex cord-stromal tumours. Histopathology. 2013;62(1):71–88.

Samanth KK, Black 3rd WC. Benign ovarian stromal tumors associated with free peritoneal fluid. Am J Obstet Gynecol. 1970;107(4):538–45.

Schumer ST, Cannistra SA. Granulosa cell tumor of the ovary. J Clin Oncol. 2003;21(6):1180–9.

Seidman JD. Unclassified ovarian gonadal stromal tumors. A clinicopathologic study of 32 cases. Am J Surg Pathol. 1996;20(6):699–706.

Seidman JD, Abbondanzo SL, Bratthauer GL. Lipid cell (steroid cell) tumor of the ovary: immunophenotype with analysis of potential pitfall due to endogenous biotin-like activity. Int J Gynecol Pathol. 1995;14(4): 331–8.

Staats PN, McCluggage WG, Clement PB, Young RH. Luteinized thecomas (thecomatosis) of the type typically associated with sclerosing peritonitis: a clinical, histopathologic, and immunohistochemical analysis of 27 cases. Am J Surg Pathol. 2008;32(9): 1273–90.

Vilain MO, Cabaret V, Delobelle-Deroide A, Duminy F, Laurent JC. Stromal luteoma of the ovary. Differential diagnosis of steroid cell tumors. Ann Pathol. 1992; 12(3):193–7.

Young RH, Scully RE. Well-differentiated ovarian Sertoli-Leydig cell tumors: a clinicopathological analysis of 23 cases. Int J Gynecol Pathol. 1984;3(3):277–90.

Young RH, Scully RE. Ovarian Sertoli-Leydig cell tumors. A clinico-pathological analysis of 207 cases. Am J Surg Pathol. 1985;9:543–69.

Young RH, Scully RE. Ovarian sex cord-stromal tumors. Problems in differential diagnosis. Pathol Annu. 1988;23(Pt 1):237–96.

Young RH, Prat J, Scully RE. Ovarian Sertoli-Leydig cell tumors with heterologous elements. I. Gastrointestinal epithelium and carcinoid: a clinicopathologic analysis of thirty-six cases. Cancer. 1982;50(11):2448–56.

Young RH, Dickersin GR, Scully RE. Juvenile granulosa cell tumor of the ovary. A clinicopathological analysis of 125 cases. Am J Surg Pathol. 1984a;8(8):575–96.

Young RH, Dudley AG, Scully RE. Granulosa cell, Sertoli-Leydig cell, and unclassified sex cord-stromal tumors associated with pregnancy: a clinicopathological analysis of thirty-six cases. Gynecol Oncol. 1984b;18(2): 181–205.

Zhang J, Young RH, Arseneau J, Scully RE. Ovarian stromal tumors containing lutein or Leydig cells (luteinized thecomas and stromal Leydig cell tumors) – a clinicopathological analysis of fifty cases. Int J Gynecol Pathol. 1982;1(3):270–85.

Index

A

ABCDE scheme, 979
Abdominal aortic aneurysm (AAA), 527
Abdominal radical trachelectomy, 838
Abdominal uterosacral ligament suspension, 733
Abnormal bleeding, 14–15
Abnormal discharge, 222
Abnormal genital bleeding, 588
Abnormal menstruation, 103–107
Abnormal uterine bleeding (AUB), 14–15, 103, 188, 421–423, 642, 643, 883
  causes of, 588
  endometrial destruction, 611–613
  equipment, 613
  heavy menstrual bleeding, 195–201
  infrequent menses, 192
  intermenstrual bleeding, 194
  post-coital bleeding, 194
  secondary amenorrhea, 189
  second generation endometrial ablation technique, 613–614
  TCRE (transcervical resection of the endometrium), 613
Abnormal vaginal bleeding, 316
Aborting fibroid, 136
Abortion, 96
  medical, 32
  surgical, 33
Abscess, 399, 759
Abuse, 116–117, 284, 581
  sexual, 561–562, 589
  substance abuse, 44, 96, 99, 117, 257
Acanthosis, 1010
Acetylcholine, 751
Acini, 1014
Acne, 445
  and hirsutism (*see* Hirsutism)
  treatment of, 456
ACOG (American College of Obstetricians and Gynecologists), 199
Acquired platelet aggregation, 198
Acquired uterine abnormalities
  hysteroscopic treatment of, 614
  intrauterine adhesions, 614–615
  retained products of conception, 615–616

Acrochordon, 595
Acromegaly, 161, 462
ACTH stimulation, 161
Actin, 1074
Actinomycin D, 777
Acute heavy bleeding, 196–198
Acute pelvic pain, 136
  ectopic pregnancy, 318
  ovarian torsion, 315
  ruptured ovarian cysts, 322
  tuboovarian abscesses, 320–322
Adenocarcinoma, 847
Adenocarcinoma in situ (ACIS), 61, 869–870, 873, 1035–1036
Adenocarcinoma of cervix, 55
Adenofibroma, 1053
Adenomas, 460, 461, 465
Adenomyoma, 1053
Adenomyosis, 143, 188, 417, 562, 563, 644, 1047, 1051
Adenosarcoma, 965, 1053, 1054
Adenosquamous carcinoma, 847
Adequate vaginal access, 699
Adhesion, cervical stenosis, and a loss of cervical function, 842
Adhesions, 560, 672
Adjuvant chemotherapy, 841, 860, 929
Adjuvant hysterectomy, 779
Adjuvant radiotherapy, 841
Adnexal mass, 316, 550–554, 630
Adolescence, 81–90, 96
Adolescent, 122, 124, 126, 128, 131
  CAH (*see* Congenital adrenal hyperplasia (CAH))
  sexual development, 100
Adrenal insufficiency, 80, 84
Adrenal rest tumors, 81, 85–86
Adrenarche, 446
Adult type granulosa cell tumor, 935
Adverse obstetric outcomes, 642
Afibrinogenemia, 126
Agenesis, 172
Aggressive angiomyxoma, 1024
AGO score, 916–917
Alcohol, 49
Alcohol consumption, 522–524

© Springer International Publishing AG 2017
D. Shoupe (ed.), *Handbook of Gynecology*,
DOI 10.1007/978-3-319-17798-4

Printed by Printforce, the Netherlands